PEARLS of WISDOM

Urology

BOARD REVIEW

Fourth Edition

Stephen W. Leslie, MD, FACS

Associate Professor of Surgery and Chief, Division of Urology
Department of Surgery
Creighton University School of Medicine
Omaha, Nebraska

Mc Graw Hill Education | Medical

New York   Chicago   San Francisco   Lisbon   London   Madrid   Mexico City
Milan   New Delhi   San Juan   Seoul   Singapore   Sydney   Toronto

Urology Board Review: Pearls of Wisdom, Fourth Edition

Copyright © 2013, 2009, 2006 by McGraw-Hill Education LLC. All rights reserved. Printed in the United States of America. Except as permitted under the United States Copyright Act of 1976, no part of this publication may be reproduced or distributed in any form or by any means, or stored in a database or retrieval system, without the prior written permission of the publisher.

1 2 3 4 5 6 7 8 9 0 WCK/QVR 18 17 16 15 14 13

ISBN 978-0-07-179926-3
MHID 0-07-179926-5

Notice

Medicine is an ever-changing science. As new research and clinical experience broaden our knowledge, changes in treatment and drug therapy are required. The authors and the publisher of this work have checked with sources believed to be reliable in their efforts to provide information that is complete and generally in accord with the standards accepted at the time of publication. However, in view of the possibility of human error or changes in medical sciences, neither the authors nor the publisher nor any other party who has been involved in the preparation or publication of this work warrants that the information contained herein is in every respect accurate or complete, and they disclaim all responsibility for any errors or omissions or for the results obtained from use of the information contained in this work. Readers are encouraged to confirm the information contained herein with other sources. For example and in particular, readers are advised to check the product information sheet included in the package of each drug they plan to administer to be certain that the information contained in this work is accurate and that changes have not been made in the recommended dose or in the contraindications for administration. This recommendation is of particular importance in connection with new or infrequently used drugs.

This book was set in Adobe Garamond by Thomson Digital.
The editors were Catherine A. Johnson and Peter J. Boyle.
The production supervisors were Sherri Souffrance and Richard Ruzycka.
Project management was provided by Garima Sharma, Thomson Digital.
The cover designer was Handel Low.
Quad Graphics Versailles was printer and binder.

This book is printed on acid-free paper.

Library of Congress Cataloging-in-Publication Data

Urology board review / [edited by] Stephen W. Leslie. — 4th ed.
     p. ; cm. — (Pearls of wisdom)
  Includes bibliographical references and index.
  ISBN-13: 978-0-07-179926-3 (pbk. : alk. paper)
  ISBN-10: 0-07-179926-5
  I. Leslie, Stephen W. II. Series: Pearls of wisdom.
  [DNLM: 1. Urologic Diseases—Examination Questions. WJ 18.2]
  RC873
  616.60076—dc23
                                                    2013010626

McGraw-Hill Education books are available at special quantity discounts to use as premiums and sales promotions, or for use in corporate training programs. To contact a representative, please e-mail us at bulksales@mcgraw-hill.com.

DEDICATION

To Scott Plantz, MD, who decided at the last minute to give me this unique editorial opportunity; to all of my urological colleagues who worked hard as contributing authors to review, update, and expand their chapters and who spared me from having to do all that work myself; to Neil Baum, MD, who was happy to provide a useful and interesting article as an extra added "bonus"; and to my administrative assistant, Amanda Biehle, who discovered on her first day on the job that, in addition to all of her other responsibilities, she also had to organize and coordinate all the chapters and contributing authors for this book.

Stephen

CONTENTS

CONTRIBUTORS

Himanshu Aggarwal, MD, MSc
Resident of Urology
Division of Urology
Albany Medical College
Albany, New York

Treatment of Locally Advanced or Recurrent Prostate Cancer

Madhu Alagiri, MD
Associate Professor of Surgery
University of California, San Diego
Vice Chair
Department of Pediatric Urology
Rady Children's Hospital
San Diego, California

Megaureter, Ectopic Ureter, and Ureterocele

David M. Albala, MD
Chief of Urology
Crouse Hospital
Medical Director
Associated Medical Professionals
Syracuse, New York

Radionuclide Studies
Upper Urinary Tract Obstruction
Adult Urinary Tract Infections

Anthony Atala, MD
Professor and Chair
Department of Urology
Wake Forest Baptist Medical Center
Winston-Salem, North Carolina

Congenital Disorders of the Lower Urinary Tract

Marcus W. Balters, MD
Assistant Professor of Surgery
Department of Surgery
Creighton University School of Medicine
Division of Cardiovascular and Thoracic Surgery
Creighton University Medical Center
Omaha, Nebraska

Renovascular Hypertension

Daniel A. Barocas, MD, MPH
Assistant Professor
Department of Urologic Surgery
Vanderbilt University Medical Center
Nashville, Tennessee

Adrenal Physiology

Neil Baum, MD
Clinical Associate Professor
Department of Urology
University of Tulane Medical School
New Orleans, Louisiana

Getting to the Top of Google in 5 Steps

Mark F. Bellinger, MD
Emeritus Clinician
Children's Hospital of Pittsburgh
University of Pittsburgh
Pittsburgh, Pennsylvania

Embryology of the Genitourinary Tract

Jay Laurence Bloch, MD*
Chief
Department of Urology
Urological Specialists of Southern New Jersey
Voorhees, New Jersey

Renovascular Hypertension

Emily Blum, MD
Resident Physician
Department of Urology
Beaumont Health System
Royal Oakland, Michigan

Bladder Cancer

William O. Brant, MD, FACS
Assistant Professor
Division of Urology
University of Utah
Salt Lake City, Utah

Urethral Strictures

---

*Dr. Bloch was contributing author from the previous edition of the work.

Benjamin N. Breyer, MD, MAS
Assistant Professor
Department of Urology
University of California, San Francisco
San Francisco, California

Urethral Lesions

Thomas Chi, MD
Clinical Instructor
Department of Urology
University of California, San Francisco
San Francisco, California

Genitourinary Tuberculosis

Bilal Chughtai, MD
Assistant Professor
Department of Urology
Weill Cornell Medical Center
New York, New York

Surgical Anatomy of the Pelvis

Christopher L. Coogan, MD, FACS
Professor of Urology
Department of Urology
Rush University Medical Center
Chicago, Illinois

Urinary Diversion and Undiversion

Paul L. Crispen, MD
Assistant Professor
Department of Urology
University of Florida
Gainesville, Florida

Adrenal Tumors
Renal Tumors, Adults

James M. Cummings, MD
Professor
Department of Surgery
University of Missouri School of Medicine
Columbia, Missouri

Genitourinary Trauma

John W. Davis, MD
Assistant Professor of Urology
The M.D. Anderson Cancer Center
The University of Texas
Houston, Texas

Penile Cancer

David A. Diamond, MD
Professor of Surgery (Urology)
Harvard Medical School
Urologist-in-Chief
Boston Children's Hospital
Boston, Massachusetts

Disorders of Sexual Development

Kevin M. Feber, MD, FAAP
Associate Professor of Urology
Department of Urology
Oakland University
William Beaumont School of Medicine
Beaumont Health System
Royal Oakland, Michigan

Congenital Disorders of the Upper Tracts

Fernando A. Ferrer, MD, FAAP, FACS
Vice Chairman
Department of Surgery
Associate Professor
Surgery (Urology) and Pediatrics (Oncology)
University of Connecticut School of Medicine
Farmington, Connecticut
Executive Vice President, Medical Affairs
Surgeon-in-Chief
Director Division Pediatric Urology
Connecticut Children's Medical Center
Hartford, Connecticut

Urological Emergencies in the Newborn
Pediatric Oncology

Andrew I. Fishman, MD
Attending
Department of Urology
New York Medical College
Valhalla, New York

Renal/Ureteral Stone Surgery

Matthew T. Gettman, MD
Professor of Urology
Department of Urology
Mayo Clinic
Rochester, Minnesota

Adrenal Tumors
Renal Tumors, Adults

Cameron Ghaffary, BS
Medical Student, Class of 2014
Division of Urology
Creighton University School of Medicine
Omaha, Nebraska
Surgical Anatomy of the Pelvis

Reza Ghavamian, MD
Professor and Chairman
Department of Urology
Montefiore Medical Center
Albert Einstein College of Medicine
Bronx, New York
*Squamous Cell Carcinoma and Adenocarcinoma
    of the Bladder*

Gamal M. Ghoniem, MD, FACS
Professor and Vice Chairman
Department of Urology
University of California
Orange, California
Urodynamics

Leonard Glickman, MD
House Staff Physician
Department of Urology
Lenox Hill Hospital
New York, New York
Neurogenic Voiding Dysfunction

Marc Goldstein, MD, DSc (Hon), FACS
Matthew P. Hardy Distinguished Professor of
    Reproductive Medicine and Urology
Surgeon-in-Chief
Male Reproductive Medicine and Microsurgery
New York Presbyterian Hospital–Weill Cornell
    Medical College
New York, New York
Male Infertility

Michael Grasso III, MD
Professor and Vice Chairman
Department of Urology
New York Medical College
Valhalla, New York
Renal/Ureteral Stone Surgery

Graham F. Greene, MD, FACS
Chief Medical Officer
Director Urologic Oncology
Lakeland Regional Health System
Lakeland, Florida
Retroperitoneal Anatomy

A. Ari Hakimi, MD
Urologic Oncology Fellow
Department of Surgery, Urology Service
Memorial Sloan-Kettering Cancer Center
New York, New York
*Squamous Cell Carcinoma and Adenocarcinoma
    of the Bladder*

J. Nathaniel Hamilton, MD
Affiliate Instructor
Department of Surgery
Brody School of Medicine
East Carolina University
Greenville, North Carolina
*Interstitial Cystitis and Other Inflammatory Conditions
    of the Lower Urinary Tract*

Brian J. Hamm, MD
Chief Radiology Resident
Department of Radiology
Creighton University Medical Center
Omaha, Nebraska
*Uroradiology
Radiology: CT/Ultrasound/MRI*

Sang Won Han, MD, PhD
Professor and Chairman
Department of Urology and Pediatric Urology
Yonsei University College of Medicine/Severance Hospital
Seoul, Korea
Enuresis

Miriam Harel, MD
Pediatric Urology Fellow
Division of Urology
Connecticut Children's Medical Center
University of Connecticut School of Medicine
Hartford, Connecticut
*Urological Emergencies in the Newborn
Pediatric Oncology*

George P. Hemstreet III, MD, PhD
Chief of Urology
Veterans Administration Hospital
Consult in Urology
Creighton University
University of Nebraska Medical Center
Children's Hospital
Omaha, Nebraska

Diagnosis and Staging of Prostate Cancer
Surgical Therapy for Prostate Cancer

Michael P. Hoeh, MD
Resident Physician
Department of Urology
Rush University Hospital
Chicago, Illinois

Urinary Diversion and Undiversion

Johann P. Ingimarsson, MD
Urology Resident
Department of Surgery, Section of Urology
Dartmouth Hitchcock Medical Center
Lebanon, New Hampshire

Testicular and Paratesticular Tumors

Sudhir Isharwal, MD
Department of Urology
University of Nebraska Medical Center
Omaha, Nebraska

Diagnosis and Staging of Prostate Cancer
Surgical Therapy for Prostate Cancer

Jonathan I. Izawa, MD, FRCSC
Associate Professor
Departments of Surgery, Oncology and Pathology
Divisions of Urology and Surgical Oncology
Schulich School of Medicine and Dentistry
Western University
Victoria, London

Surgical Anatomy of the Pelvis

Thomas W. Jarrett, MD
Professor and Chairman
Department of Urology
George Washington University
School of Medicine
Washington, District of Columbia

TCC of the Upper Urinary Tracts

Forrest Jellison, MD
Clinical Instructor Fellow
Department of Urology
David Geffen School of Medicine
University of California, Los Angeles
Los Angeles, California

Female Incontinence and Vesicovaginal Fistula

Justin D. Johnson, MD
Resident Physician
Department of Surgery
Section of Urology
University of Nebraska Medical Center
Omaha, Nebraska

Laparoscopic and Robotic Urologic Surgery

Kelly C. Johnson, MD
Clinical Instructor
Department of Urology
Medical University of South Carolina
Charleston, South Carolina

Interstitial Cystitis and Other Inflammatory Conditions
of the Lower Urinary Tract

Evan J. Kass, MD, FACS, FAAP
Professor of Urology
Oakland University
William Beaumont School of Medicine
Beaumont Health System
Chief, Division of Pediatric Urology
Beaumont Children's Hospital
Royal Oakland, Michigan

Congenital Disorders of the Upper Tracts

Howard H. Kim, MD
Director, Male Reproductive Medicine and Microsurgery
Cedars-Sinai Medical Center
Los Angeles, California

Male Infertility

Ja-Hong Kim, MD
Assistant Professor
Department of Urology
David Geffen School of Medicine
University of California, Los Angeles
Los Angeles, California

Female Incontinence and Vesicovaginal Fistula

Neil A. King, MD
Resident Physician
Department of Surgery
University of Medicine and Dentistry of New Jersey
New Jersey Medical School
Newark, New Jersey

Cryptorchidism: Diagnosis and Management

Zachary Klaassen, MD
Resident
Department of Surgery, Section of Urology
Georgia Health Sciences University
Augusta, Georgia

Prostatic Hyperplasia

Laurence Klotz, MD
Professor of Surgery
University of Toronto
Sunnybrook Health Sciences Centre
Toronto, Ontario

Intestinal Segments in Urology

Michael O. Koch, MD
Chairman and John P. Donohue Professor
Department of Urology
Indiana University School of Medicine
Indianapolis, Indiana

Urothelial Carcinoma of the Bladder

Badrinath R. Konety, MD, MBA
Chair at University of Minnesota
Department of Urology
University of Minnesota Medical School
Minneapolis, Minnesota

Urethral Lesions

Harry P. Koo, MD, FAAP, FACS
Chief, Pediatric Urology
Hackensack University Medical Center
Hackensack, New Jersey

Cryptorchidism: Diagnosis and Management

Howard J. Korman, MD, FACS
Attending Physician
Department of Urology
William Beaumont Hospital
Royal Oakland, Michigan

Bladder Cancer

Gregory J. Kubicek, MD
Assistant Professor
Department of Radiation Oncology
Cooper University Hospital
Camden, New Jersey

Radiation Therapy for Prostate Cancer

Udaya Kumar, MD, FRCS Urol, Dip Urol (Lon)
Advanced Urology Specialist
Homosassa, Florida
Attending Urologist
Seven Rivers Regional Medical Center
Crystal River, Florida
Attending Urologist
Citrus Memorial Hospital
Inverness, Florida

Radionuclide Studies
Upper Urinary Tract Obstruction
Adult Urinary Tract Infections

Chad A. LaGrange, MD, FACS
Associate Professor and Chief
Division of Urology
University of Nebraska Medical Center
Omaha, Nebraska

Laparoscopic and Robotic Urologic Surgery

Hyeyoung Lee, MD, MS
Clinical Assistant Professor
Department of Urology and Pediatric Urology
Yonsei University College of Medicine
Severance Hospital
Seoul, Korea

Enuresis

Stephen W. Leslie, MD, FACS
Associate Professor of Surgery
Chief, Division of Urology
Department of Surgery
Creighton University School of Medicine
Omaha, Nebraska

Prostatic Hyperplasia
Peyronie Disease and Penile Fractures
Urological Grab Bag Challenge
Just for Fun: Urology Trivia

Mary Ann C. Lim, MD
Athens, Georgia
Renal Physiology

Jessica C. Lloyd, MD
Resident
Division of Urology
Duke University Medical Center
Durham, North Carolina
Renal Tumors, Children

Tom F. Lue, MD, ScD (Hon), FACS
Professor
Department of Urology
University of California, San Francisco
San Francisco, California
Urethral Strictures
Male Sexual Function and Dysfunction

John H. Makari, MD, MHA, MA
Assistant Professor of Surgery (Urology)
University of Connecticut
School of Medicine
Farmington, Connecticut
Attending, Pediatric Urologist
Connecticut Children's Medical Center
Hartford, Connecticut
Urological Emergencies in the Newborn

Elizabeth Malm-Buatsi, MD
Fellow
Pediatric Urology
University of Oklahoma
Oklahoma City, Oklahoma
Prune-Belly Syndrome

David Margel, MD
Urologic Oncology Fellow
Division of Urology
Department of Surgical Oncology
University of Toronto
Toronto, Ontario
Intestinal Segments in Urology

Patrick H. McKenna, MD, FACS, FAAP
Professor and Chief
Division of Pediatric Urology
Department of Urology
University of Wisconsin
School of Medicine and Public Health
Madison, Wisconsin
Urological Emergencies in the Newborn

Akanksha Mehta, MD
Fellow in Male Reproductive
    Medicine and Microsurgery
Department of Urology
Weill Cornell Medical College
New York, New York
Male Infertility

Badar M. Mian, MD, FACS
Associate Professor of Surgery
Division of Urology
Albany Medical College
Albany, New York
Treatment of Locally Advanced or Recurrent
    Prostate Cancer

Michael C. Morris, MD, FACS
Associate Professor of Surgery
Surgical Director, Kidney/Pancreas Program
Transplant Surgeon
University of Nebraska Medical Center
Omaha, Nebraska
Renal Transplantation

Jeremy B. Myers, MD, FACS
Assistant Professor
Division of Urology
University of Utah
Salt Lake City, Utah
Urethral Strictures

Durwood E. Neal, Jr, MD, FACS
Professor and Chair of Urology
Department of Surgery
School of Community Medicine
University of Oklahoma
Medical Director
Urology Center at Hillcrest
Hillcrest Medical Center
Tulsa, Oklahoma
Prostatitis

Elizabeth A. Phillips, MD
Urology Resident
Department of Urology
Boston Medical Center
Boston, Massachusetts
Medical Aspects of Urolithiasis

Derek Prabharasuth, MD
Urology Resident
Department of Urology
New York Medical College
Valhalla, New York
Renal/Ureteral Stone Surgery

Pramod P. Reddy, MD
Professor of Clinical Surgery
University of Cincinnati
Division Director of Pediatric Urology
Cincinati Children's Hospital Medical Center
Cincinnati, Ohio
Radionuclide Studies

Matthew J. Resnick, MD
Instructor
Department of Urologic Surgery
Vanderbilt University Medical Center
Nashville, Tennessee
Adrenal Physiology

Kevin R. Rice, MD
Urologic Oncology Fellow
Department of Urology
Indiana University School of Medicine
Indianapolis, Indiana
Urothelial Carcinoma of the Bladder

Julie M. Riley, MD
Assistant Professor
Division of Urology
University of New Mexico
Albuquerque, New Mexico
Prune-Belly Syndrome

Ron Romano
President, Instant Marketing Systems
Carlisle, Ontario
Getting to the Top of Google in 5 Steps

Jonathan C. Routh, MD, MPH
Assistant Professor
Division of Urology
University Medical Center
Durham, North Carolina
Renal Tumors, Children

Eric S. Rovner, MD
Professor of Urology
Department of Urology
Medical University of South Carolina
Charleston, South Carolina
*Interstitial Cystitis and Other Inflammatory Conditions
of the Lower Urinary Tract*

Megan S. Schober, MD, PhD
Chief Resident
Department of Urology
Beaumont Health System
Royal Oakland, Michigan
Congenital Disorders of the Upper Tracts

John D. Seigne, MB, FACS
Associate Professor of Surgery (Urology)
Geisel School of Medicine
Dartmouth-Hitchcock Medical Center
Lebanon, New Hampshire
Testicular and Paratesticular Tumors

Alan W. Shindel, MD
Assistant Professor in Residence
Department of Urology
University of California, Davis
Sacramento, California
Male Sexual Function and Dysfunction

W. Bruce Shingleton, MD
Professor of Urology
Division of Urology
Georgia Health Science University
Augusta, Georgia
Prostatic Hyperplasia

Gopi Kiran Reddy Sirineni, MBBS, MD
Assistant Professor
Department of Radiology
Creighton University Medical Center
Omaha, Nebraska
*Uroradiology
Radiology: CT/Ultrasound/MRI*

Emil Tanagho, MD
Professor
Chairman Emeritus
Department of Urology
University of California, San Francisco
San Francisco, California

Genitourinary Tuberculosis

Alexis E. Te, MD
Professor of Urology
Weill Medical College of Cornell University
New York, New York

Surgical Anatomy of the Pelvis

Mark R. Wakefield, MD, FACS
Associate Professor and Chief
Division of Urology
University of Missouri School of Medicine
Columbia, Missouri

Prune-Belly Syndrome

David S. Wang, MD
Associate Professor
Department of Urology
Boston University School of Medicine
Boston, Massachusetts

Medical Aspects of Urolithiasis

John Chandler Williams, MD, MS
Chairman
Department of Surgery
Baptist Medical Center–Beaches
Attending Urologist
Beaches Urology
Jacksonville Beach, Florida

Benign Renal Cystic Disease

Michael B. Williams, MD, MS
Assistant Professor
Department of Urology
Leroy T. Canoles, Jr. Cancer Research Center
Eastern Virginia Medical School
Norfolk, Virginia

Penile Cancer

Jeffrey P. Wolters, MD, MPH
Resident Physician
Division of Urology
Virginia Commonwealth University
    School of Medicine
Richmond, Virginia

Cryptorchidism: Diagnosis and Management

George P. H. Young, MD, FACS
Attending Urologist
Department of Urology
Lenox Hill Hospital
New York, New York

Neurogenic Voiding Dysfunction

Ashraf Youssef, MD, MBA
Assistant Professor
Department of Radiation Oncology
Cooper University Hospital
Camden, New Jersey

Radiation Therapy for Prostate Cancer

Richard N. Yu, MD, PhD
Instructor in Surgery (Urology)
Department of Urology
Boston Children's Hospital and
    Harvard Medical School
Boston, Massachusetts

Disorders of Sexual Development

Vladimir Yutkin, MD
Urologic Oncology Fellowship Program
Departments of Surgery and Oncology
University of Western Ontario
London, Ontario

Surgical Anatomy of the Pelvis

INTRODUCTION

Congratulations! *Urology Board Review: Pearls of Wisdom* will help you pass urology and improve your board scores. *Urology Board Review's* unique format differs from all other review and test preparation texts. Let us begin, then, with a few words on purpose, format, and use.

The primary intent of *Urology Board Review* is to serve as a rapid review of urology principles and serve as a study aid to improve performance on urology written and practical examinations. With this goal in mind, the text is written in rapid-fire, question/answer format. The reader receives immediate gratification with a correct answer. Questions themselves often contain a "pearl" reinforced in association with the question/answer.

Additional hooks are often attached to the answer in various forms, including mnemonics, evoked visual imagery, repetition and humor. Additional information not requested in the question may be included in the answer. The same information is often sought in several different questions. Emphasis has been placed on evoking both trivia and key facts that are easily overlooked, are quickly forgotten, and yet somehow always seem to appear on urology exams.

Many questions have answers without explanations. This is done to enhance ease of reading and rate of learning. Explanations often occur in a later question/answer. It may happen that upon reading an answer the reader may think—"Hmm, why is that?" or, "Are you sure?" If this happens to you, GO CHECK! Truly assimilating these disparate facts into a framework of knowledge absolutely requires further reading in the surrounding concepts. Information learned, as a response to seeking an answer to a particular question is much better retained than that passively read. Take advantage of this. Use this book with your urology text handy and open, or, if you are reviewing on train, plane, or camelback, mark questions for further investigation.

Urology Board Review risks accuracy by aggressively pruning complex concepts down to the simplest kernel. The dynamic knowledge base and clinical practice of medicine is not like that! This text is designed to maximize your score on a test. Refer to your mentors for direction on current practice.

Urology Board Review is designed to be used, not just read. It is an interactive text. Use a 3×5 card and cover the answers; attempt all questions. A study method we strongly recommend is oral, group study, preferably over an extended meal or pitchers. The mechanics of this method are simple and no one ever appears stupid. One person holds the book, with answers covered, and reads the question. Each person, including the reader, says "Check!" when he or she has an answer in mind. After everyone has "checked" in, someone states his or her answer. If this answer is correct, on to the next one. If not, another person states his or her answer, or the answer can be read. Usually, the person who "checks" in first gets the first shot at stating the answer. If this person is being a smarty-pants answer-hog, then others can take turns. Try it—it's almost fun!

Urology Board Review is also designed to be re-used several times to allow, dare we use the word, memorization. I suggest putting a check mark every time a question is missed. A hollow bullet has been arbitrarily provided. Another suggestion is to place a check mark when the question is answered correctly once; skip all questions with check marks thereafter. Utilize whatever scheme of using the check boxes you prefer.

We welcome your comments, suggestions, and criticism. Great effort has been made to verify these questions and answers. There will be answers we have provided that are at variance with the answer you would prefer. Most often this is attributable to the variance between original source. Please make us aware of any errata you find. We hope to make continuous improvements in a subsequent edition and would greatly appreciate any input with regard to format, organization, content, presentation, or about specific questions. Please write to Stephen W. Leslie, M.D. at StephenLeslie@creighton.edu. We look forward to hearing from you.

Study hard and good luck!

S. W. L.

TEST-TAKING TIPS

BEFORE THE TEST

Review old tests to become familiar with the format and type of questions. Prepare all the materials you're allowed to bring and make sure they work. Bring extra pens, pencils, and erasers. Bring a watch so that you can pace yourself.

Make a quick study sheet or flash cards of all the material, from *Urology Board Review*, that you have trouble remembering or keep getting wrong. Go over the flash cards or study sheet repeatedly until the material becomes familiar. Review the study sheet/flash card material just before bed and first thing in the morning. This will help reinforce the information.

THE DAY BEFORE

Trying to cram the night before won't help, so get a good night's sleep. Set your alarm and have a backup. Avoid any sleeping pills that can have side effects the next morning.

Make sure you know exactly where the test is being given and how to get there. Have a backup plan for transportation just in case.

Bring or wear a sweater. If the room is too warm, you can always take it off. A slightly cool room is ideal. Have a good meal before the test. Having food in your stomach will help, but avoid having too many heavy foods that can make you groggy. Carry a protein bar in case you get hungry. Use the bathroom before the test. You don't need any bodily distractions.

TAKING THE TEST

Try to pick a comfortable spot in the room with plenty of space. Scan the entire test before actually starting. Read the directions and rules carefully and make sure you understand them. It's amazing how often mistakes are made because the rules and directions weren't followed exactly.

Read the entire question carefully, even if you think you know the question type and the answer right away. Be certain you've answered all parts of the question and didn't leave anything out.

Answer the easiest questions first. Mark the questions you're passing in the test booklet, if allowed, so you can quickly find them later. When you reach the end of the test, go back and finish the skipped questions. With multiple-choice questions, try to determine the correct answer before you read the possible solutions. Don't get worried or anxious if others finish before you do. It's not a race.

DEALING WITH TOUGH QUESTIONS

When dealing with a tough question, start by eliminating the answers that are clearly wrong, are probably wrong, or just don't seem to fit. Go back and read the entire question again. Test preparers don't usually add unnecessary words and details to their questions; every word is important. Look for a keyword or phrase that might be the key to the solution and circle it.

If two answers are virtually identical, chances are both are incorrect. Work on a problem question until you get stuck. Think about it for a minute or two, but if nothing else comes, go on to the next question. If allowed, place a mark by that question so that you can find it easily later. Sometimes there will be clues in later questions—these can help you with an earlier problem.

Look for grammatical clues. For example, the word "an" before a blank indicates that the answer starts with a vowel. Go with your first impulse as it's usually right. If you try to overthink the question, you'll probably get it wrong. If you really can't decide between two or more answers, the longer and more detailed answer is usually correct more often. If all else fails and there's no penalty for guessing, go for it!

Don't panic. You are probably not going to get every question right, but getting anxious over it won't help. If you feel yourself hyperventilating, getting anxious, or sweating, just do the following: Put down the pencil, close your eyes, take a few deep breaths, and consciously relax any muscle groups that you're clenching (jaw, neck, stomach). When you've calmed down, go back to the examination.

THE BIG FINISH

Use all of your time. Even if you finish early, check for silly mistakes and make sure all your marks are clear, legible, and in the correct space. Don't go back and change an answer unless you misread or misinterpreted the question. Make sure there are no stray marks on the answer sheet and that each answer completely fills in the little bubble.

Every few pages, make sure the test numbers and the answer numbers match. It's very easy to put an answer in the wrong place, especially if you skipped a question but forgot to skip marking the answer sheet, and then all the subsequent answers will be mismatched and incorrect. Make absolutely sure that your name and identification numbers are correct.

Good luck!

CHAPTER 1 Uroradiology

Gopi Kiran Reddy Sirineni, MBBS, MD and Brian J. Hamm, MD

○ **What are the specific radiological findings depicted below and what diagnosis do they suggest?**

Diffuse bladder wall and distal ureteral calcifications suggest schistosomiasis of the bladder and ureters. Nodular bladder wall thickening occurs in the acute phase, which is followed by bladder wall fibrosis and calcification. Calcification of the ureter and seminal vesicle may also occur. This diagnosis should be suspected when a patient gives a history of travel to an endemic region (the Middle East, India, Africa, and Central and South America) and presents with frequency, urgency, hematuria, and dysuria. Abnormal appearance of the bladder is secondary to deposition of eggs, which subsequently calcify, into the bladder wall from the pelvic venous plexus. Squamous cell carcinoma can be a long-term complication. The computed tomography (CT) axial image on the left demonstrates circumferential bladder wall thickening and calcification extending into the left ureter in a patient with schistosomiasis. Abdominal x-ray in a similar patient, a 27-year-old refugee from Africa, also demonstrates diffuse bladder wall and bilateral ureteral calcifications. Diagnosis is confirmed by a blood test for parasitic antigens or by finding eggs in the urine or stool. Treatment is with a single dose of praziquantel. A total of 240 million people worldwide are affected by this parasite, which uses a snail as an intermediate host.

○ **A 23-year-old man has a history of microscopic hematuria and an intravenous urogram (IVU) is planned for evaluation. The patient reports a history of an allergy to shellfish. He has not previously received IV contrast. The next step should be?**

Patients with a history of asthma, drug allergy, or allergy to shellfish have approximately a 2-fold greater risk of a contrast reaction. Minor reactions include hot flushes, nausea, vomiting, or urticaria while major reactions include bronchospasm, hypotension, laryngeal edema, and cardiac arrest. The overall incidence of contrast reactions is estimated to be 13% with high-osmolality agents and only 3% with low-osmolality agents. The alternatives to consider in this patient include substitution of a different study (particularly had there been a severe prior reaction), the use of lower osmolality contrast agents, and pretreatment with steroids and antihistamines. A reasonable pretreatment regimen for adults consists of 50-mg prednisone at 13, 7, and 1 hour prior to the study, and 50 mg of diphenhydramine 1 hour before the examination. H1 and H2 blockers can also be used.

Another option would be to use either ultrasound and/or noncontrasted CT scan to examine the kidneys in a case of microscopic hematuria, particularly when the patient is only 23 years old.

Contraindications to IVP include previous anaphylactic reactions to IV contrast and positive azotemia (creatinine >2.0). Relative contraindications include dehydration, diabetes, multiple myeloma, and pregnancy.

○ **A 30-year-old female is undergoing a workup for microhematuria. Her serum pregnancy test is negative. The 15-minute film from the IVU is shown. The next step should be?**

The patient should have a cystoscopy to complete the workup. The IVU is normal. (It is not uncommon to have a normal study appear on a board examination.) While the film as shown is normal, it is important to point out that the top of the left kidney is "cropped." The entire kidney should be visible on an IVU. If not, additional films should be taken.

○ **Describe the proper technique for performing and reviewing an IVU.**

In a normal IVU, a kidneys, ureters, bladder (KUB) or scout film is obtained following which approximately 1 cm^3/kg of IV contrast is administered. On the KUB, careful attention should be paid to any and all unusual calcifications, organs outside the urinary tract, and bony abnormalities as well as any technical flaws. A 30-second film shows the nephrogram phase of the IVU and is regarded as the best film to assess renal masses and renal contour. During the excretion phase, 5-, 10-, and 15-minute films are generally taken. There should be symmetric excretion. The left kidney should be no more than 2-cm longer than the right kidney. Kidneys should be approximately 3 to 5 vertebral bodies in length. Forniceal angles should be sharp. Blunting of the forniceal angles is said to be the earliest radiographic sign of hydronephrosis on IVU. Three major infundibula should be visualized along with roughly 13 to 14 calyces for each kidney. The angle, orientation, outlines, shape, and position of the kidneys should be reviewed and tomograms should be taken if there is any doubt about the integrity of the kidneys. The ureter should not show a standing column (columnization) of contrast and the bladder contour, best seen on the 15-minute film, should be smooth. A postvoid film should also be done. Posterior oblique films can be performed to better visualize the distal ureters.

○ **A 70-year-old man presents with microhematuria and a portion of the initial KUB done for the IVU is shown. Prior to cystoscopy, what should be the next step?**

Four things to look for on the scout film are "masses, gasses, bones, and stones." Each time you look at a scout film review those 4 things and comment about whether they are normal or abnormal. Symmetry is also important. In this case, there is asymmetry on either side of the pubic symphysis with sclerosis evident on the left. There is a somewhat moth-eaten appearance to the periosteum on the left superior and inferior pubic rami as well. Sclerotic bone lesions are found in patients with breast and prostate cancer. On plain films, a 50% change in cortical density is required to visualize metastatic disease. In this elderly man, the next step should be a prostate-specific antigen and a prostate examination.

○   **A child with multiple birth defects had a renal ultrasound suggestive of duplication and hydronephrosis. An IVU was performed to further evaluate the finding. The KUB obtained prior to the study is shown. What is the radiographic finding demonstrated?**

The radiograph is a classic picture of complete sacral agenesis. The sacrum is absent causing the pelvic ring to look like an inverted teardrop. Incomplete agenesis may be more difficult to diagnose. The diagnosis may be delayed until failed attempts at toilet training prompt urological evaluation for neurogenic bladder. Sacral agenesis may be one component of the VACTERL syndrome (V = **V**ertebral anomalies, A = imperforate **A**nus, C = **C**ardiac anomalies, TE = **T**rach**e**oesophageal fistula, R = **R**enal anomalies, and L = **L**imb anomalies).

○   **This KUB accompanied the IVU done for evaluation of congenital urological problems in a child. What is the radiographic finding demonstrated?**

The 3 conditions that are associated with widening of the symphysis pubis include pregnancy, trauma, and the congenital condition of exstrophy/epispadias, of which this is an example. The femurs are rotated laterally. There is no separation of the sacroiliac (SI) joint to suggest trauma. This abnormality is thought to occur as a result of failed mesodermal ingrowth and consequent failure of descent of the cloacal membrane that produces eventration of the bladder onto the abdominal wall. The spectrum ranges from pure epispadias with a dorsal penile meatus and urethra to cloacal exstrophy with eventration of both bowel and bladder.

○ **A 35-year-old female presents many years after a sterility procedure in which silicone was injected into the fallopian tubes. She has had significant microscopic hematuria. The likely diagnosis is?**

The diagnosis is a bladder stone secondary to foreign body, which in this case was the silicone that eroded through the bladder wall producing a nidus for stone formation. It is important to consider the possibility of outlet obstruction or foreign body when treating a patient with a bladder stone.

○ **This plain film was obtained in a patient undergoing a workup for microhematuria and pyuria. A routine urine specimen submitted for culture was negative. What is the likely diagnosis?**

This film shows the classic "paste" stones of genitourinary tuberculosis. The stones are faint on plain film and represent dystrophic calcification of the caseating granulomas that infiltrate the parenchyma of the kidney. The tissue sloughs into the collecting system giving rise to these stones.

○   **A 20-year-old diabetic female presents to the emergency department with fever to 104°C and a white count of 33,000 associated with a left shift. The scout film from an IVU is shown. What is the most likely diagnosis?**

There is gas essentially replacing the left renal outline in a classic case of emphysematous pyelonephritis. The treatment is broad-spectrum antibiotics and nephrectomy. A CT scan, if the patient is stable enough to tolerate the procedure, may help to distinguish a perinephric abscess caused by a gas-forming organism. Gas may outline the kidney in cases of duodenal or colon (retroperitoneal) trauma as well.

○ **An elderly man presents with obstructive voiding symptoms, microhematuria, and a palpable abdominal mass. A KUB was obtained prior to the IVU. The next step should be?**

The plain film while overpenetrated shows a midline abdominal mass extending from the pelvis to well above the presumed umbilicus. The next step should be to place a Foley catheter, which in this case resulted in resolution of the mass. This is a bad case of urinary retention.

○ **A patient undergoing a workup for microhematuria has the following KUB obtained prior to the IVU. What is the radiologic finding and what are the top 3 possible diagnoses associated with this radiographic finding?**

The film shows medullary nephrocalcinosis. This finding is seen most commonly with medullary sponge kidney, type 1 renal tubular acidosis, and hyperparathyroidism. Cortical nephrocalcinosis is rarely seen in the present era. In the past, it typically was seen as a consequence of postpartum hypotension and renal infarction that produced atrophic kidneys with calcified cortices.

○   **This scout film was obtained to evaluate left flank pain and fever. The urinalysis shows a pH of >7.2 and many gram-negative rods. What are the significant findings on the film? What is the most likely organism cultured from the urine? In addition to antibiotics, what immediate procedure is probably necessary?**

This film shows a large staghorn calculus on the right and multiple stones in both the kidneys. To be classified as a staghorn calculus, the stone should fill and outline at least one calyx and infundibulum. In addition, there appears to be a large calcification medial to the left kidney, which could represent ureterolithiasis. These are likely magnesium ammonium phosphate (struvite or triple phosphate) stones associated with urea splitting organisms such as a *proteus* species accounting for the alkaline urinary pH. Subsequent films confirmed obstruction on the left and a left nephrostomy was placed. *In a septic patient with obstruction, a percutaneous nephrostomy is safer than a double J stent.*

○   **A 50-year-old homeless woman presents with gross hematuria and severe dysuria. This KUB was obtained as part of the initial workup. What is the significant radiographic finding?**

This KUB shows a retained ureteral stent with a large bladder calculus incorporated into the distal coil. Further questioning this patient revealed a history of ureterolithiasis and ureteral stent placement at an outside facility 18 months ago. *It is imperative to secure follow-up in all patients with ureteral stents.* The management should be based on functional findings on the right kidney with a study such as a diuretic renogram.

○   **A 30-year-old female involved in a motor vehicle accident presents with gross hematuria and underwent an IVU. What is the significant finding on the IVU?**

The IVU shows a pelvic fracture with obvious displacement of the SI joint on the right. *It is important on any film presented to look at surrounding structures.* Be especially careful if you are given only one film from a series to review. In this case, the Foley catheter has already been successfully placed. A cystogram and drainage film did not show any evidence of bladder rupture.

○ **A 75-year-old female is evaluated for an episode of gross painless hematuria. The IVU obtained is significant for 2 abnormalities. Identify these problems.**

In elderly patients, it is especially important to look for associated findings. In this film, the left ureter deviates laterally in the upper third. There is a fine rim of calcification and a suggestion of a midline mass. On the left side, these findings are suspicious for an aortic aneurysm, which this proved to be. In addition, there is a large calcified pelvic mass displacing the bladder, which ultimately proved to be a Brenner tumor of the ovary. Not well seen is the invasive transitional cell carcinoma of the bladder, which was diagnosed by cystoscopy. *Always remember that finding renal pathology does not exclude bladder and lower urinary tract pathology.*

○ **A 40-year-old man undergoes an IVU to evaluate microhematuria. The 15-minute film is shown. What is the abnormality shown?**

Close inspection of the IVU shows a portion of a calyceal system just below the right pelvic brim and overlying the sacrum. This is an example of an ectopic kidney. The plain film in this case demonstrated a stone in the pelvic kidney. Up to 50% of pelvic kidneys will have hydronephrosis or reflux.

○ **A 42-year-old man who presented with a history of a febrile UTI was evaluated with an IVU. What is the likely diagnosis?**

This is an IVU that we do not often see in adults. There is duplication of the collecting system on the left. **Duplication of one collecting system should immediately raise suspicion about duplication in the other kidney.** The right collecting system is notable for only 2 major infundibula and tilts to the right, a finding labeled as the "drooping lily" sign. The collecting system is missing the upper pole calyx, which often bears close resemblance to a "ball peen hammer." Additionally, there is a large lucent smooth filling defect in the bladder, which could be confused with a tumor or benign prostatic hypertrophy (BPH). However, putting the whole picture together, it is likely that this is an ectopic ureterocele with obstruction of an upper pole ureter in a complete duplication on the right. Ectopic refers to the location of the ureteral orifice, which is likely to be outside the trigone. The Meyer–Weigert rule governing the configuration of duplicate orifices is "the upper pole drains lower and lower pole drains lateral." The lower pole orifice is located more laterally on the trigone and is therefore more prone to reflux, while the upper pole orifice enters more medially and is more often obstructed, ectopic, or associated with a ureterocele.

○   **A 27-year-old man presents with right flank pain. His urinalysis shows 0 RBCs/hpf, 2 to 4 WBCs/hpf, and no bacteria. An IVU is ordered. A delayed film of the IVU is shown. The left kidney was normal on the earlier films. Also a film from a later retrograde ureteropyelography is shown. What radiographic diagnosis is most likely?**

The IVU shows massive hydronephrosis on the right side with no hydroureter, an appearance consistent with an ureteropelvic junction obstruction. A Lasix renogram may give a better estimate of relative function and degree of obstruction but, more importantly, may give a more sensitive test to use to assess outcome after repair. Retrograde ureteropyelography confirms the diagnosis. Many times the formal repair is done in the same setting as the cystoscopy with retrogrades.

○ **A retrograde pyelogram was attempted in a 10-year-old male with intermittent flank pain and hydronephrosis on ultrasound. The ureter is incompletely filled. What is the diagnosis?**

This film shows the classic appearance for a distal adynamic segment associated with a primary obstructed megaureter. The pathology is believed to be due to disordered smooth muscle in the distal segment of the ureter associated with increased collagen deposition. This segment fails to conduct the peristaltic wave and creates a functional obstruction. A similar mechanism is postulated for the majority of ureteropelvic junction (UPJ) obstructions.

○ **A 30-year-old man presented with right-sided flank pain. His urinalysis showed 0 RBC/hpf. An IVU was obtained. A 10-minute film is shown. What are the 2 likely diagnoses?**

The lower pole of the left kidney has a medially based calyx, which is suggestive of a horseshoe kidney. In addition, the renal axis is shifted laterally. Approximately one-third of horseshoe kidneys may have a contralateral ureteropelvic junction obstruction. The renal pelves are oriented anteriorly, so the pyeloplasty is performed transabdominally. Ureterolithiasis with hydronephrosis is a possibility, but no stone is seen and the patient had no significant hematuria making this diagnosis less likely. A retrograde pyelogram at the time of surgery would confirm the diagnosis and rule out a stone or distal adynamic segment.

○   **An IVU was obtained to evaluate microhematuria in a young man. The radiographic diagnosis is?**

While a medially based calyx is suggestive of a horseshoe kidney, here is the exception. The left kidney has medial calyces, but the right does not. This is a malrotated left kidney. The renal pelvis is oriented anteriorly during renal ascent and the kidney then rotates medially. Most malrotated kidneys rotate laterally instead so the vessels cross anteriorly.

○   **A retrograde pyelogram was obtained to evaluate an abnormality seen on IVU for microhematuria. A representative film is shown. What is the abnormality?**

The abnormality is a blind-ending ureter on the left associated with an aborted partial duplication. Blind-ending ureters commonly have a 2:1 length-to-width ratio. They are histologically identical to normal ureters. Ureteral diverticula fail to meet these criteria. The management is individualized but may include excision where either symptoms or infection supervene.

○ **A 19-year-old male had an IVU performed for intermittent right flank pain. He has had a prior left nephrectomy. The IVU suggested obstruction of the upper one-third of the ureter. A representative film from a retrograde pyelogram is shown. What is the diagnosis?**

The film is classic for retrocaval ureter with medial deviation of the upper third of the right ureter. The embryologic derivation of the condition is best remembered by referring to the condition as persistent subcardinal vein. The first description of a dismembered pyeloplasty performed for this condition was by Andersen and Hynes.

○ **A 45-year-old man presented with left flank pain and gross hematuria. A representative film from the IVU is shown. What is the likely diagnosis?**

This film shows a different kind of "drooping lily" on the left. There appear to be 3 major infundibula suggesting normal collecting system architecture and arguing against a duplication. However, the "ball peen hammer" appearance has been modified by what appears to be compression due to a large mass. There are several densities seen in the middle of the mass and while those could represent pooling of contrast, a more likely explanation would be the presence of parenchymal calcification, which of course implies cancer. The differential would include renal cell carcinoma versus adrenal tumor, but statistics favor the former. One must consider the possibility of adrenal disease when the kidney is displaced in this fashion.

○   **An IVU is obtained on a 50-year-old man who presents with gross hematuria. What is the most likely diagnosis?**

This film illustrates the principle that masses frequently stretch and distort portions of the urinary tract. The left kidney is displaced cephalad and the ureter is stretched and bowed medially. These findings suggest a lower pole renal mass, which is suspicious for renal cell carcinoma. An ultrasound or CT scan would confirm that it is solid and not a simple cyst.

○   **A 28-year-old man presents with a history of gross hematuria. A retrograde pyelogram is undertaken because of the findings on an IVU showing delayed function and hydronephrosis of the right kidney. What is the radiographic sign demonstrated? What is the likely diagnosis?**

This is Bergman sign or the "goblet sign." There is dilation of the ureter distal to a ureteral mass. The cause of this phenomenon is not well known but it may be caused by "to and fro" peristalsis of the mass. This leads to a radiographic appearance resembling a chalice or goblet on retrograde pyelogram. The likely diagnosis is transitional cell carcinoma of the ureter.

○ **A 70-year-old man who has a long smoking history presents with painless gross hematuria. A retrograde pyelogram has been done to evaluate the right ureter for hydronephrosis seen on the IVU. The most likely explanation for the findings is?**

We like to apply the "rat bite" guideline of film interpretation in this case. **If the film looks like a rat has been at work, it is cancer until proven otherwise.** The retrograde pyelogram demonstrates a filling defect in the upper third of the ureter. The initial decision is to determine whether the defect is an intraluminal or extraluminal process. Extraluminal processes tend to displace and compress the ureter. In this case, a portion of the ureter appears to be "eaten" away and the diagnosis is most likely transitional cell carcinoma of the ureter. Other causes of lucent filling defects would be a lucent stone, sloughed papilla, polyp, blood clot, fungus ball, or malakoplakia/ cystitis cystica. However, the classic "rat bite" appearance points to malignancy as the likely cause in this case. Ureteroscopy will confirm the diagnosis.

○   **A 70-year-old man with a long smoking history presents with painless gross hematuria. An IVU is performed as part of the diagnostic evaluation. What is the likely diagnosis?**

This IVU is notable for nonvisualization of the left kidney. There is a filling defect in the bladder, which could be mistaken for BPH except that it is somewhat irregular. In addition, the right kidney has a standing column of contrast to the middle third of the ureter and early hydronephrosis evidenced by blunting of the forniceal angles. Given the history, the likely diagnosis is muscle invasive transitional cell carcinoma of the bladder, with obstruction of the left ureter causing nonfunction of the left kidney. In addition, the findings on the right are suspicious for transitional cell cancer of the ureter, which proved to be the case as the retrograde showed. This film makes the point that **transitional cell carcinoma can be a bilateral process and the contralateral kidney must be evaluated carefully.** Ureteral obstruction signals invasive cancer up to 90% of the time.

○   **Shown is a representative film from the IVU of a patient who presented with painless gross hematuria. The patient has a long smoking history. What are the 2 significant findings on this study?**

The IVU shows a bladder diverticulum with a filling defect present in the diverticulum. The filling defect is slightly irregular and given the history, the mass most likely represents a transitional cell cancer in a diverticulum. This usually carries a more ominous prognosis.

○ **An IVU is performed for gross hematuria and the collecting system is not well visualized. A retrograde pyelogram is performed. What is the likely diagnosis?**

There is a nice goblet sign in the upper ureter, and the collecting system architecture has been destroyed. A "rat" has been at work here and the diagnosis is most likely transitional cell carcinoma. However, the differential should also include xanthogranulomatous pyelonephritis and tuberculosis.

○ **This IVU was performed on a 65-year-old male presenting with gross hematuria and a serum creatinine of 1.8. What are the radiographic findings?**

The IVU shows no right nephrogram and a large filling defect in the bladder, which appears to originate from the right bladder wall. This likely represents a bladder tumor and the right kidney is completely obstructed. Upper tract obstruction is worrisome for ureteral involvement of the tumor. A CT scan of the abdomen would be helpful in this setting in addition to transurethral resection of the bladder tumor for therapy and staging.

○   **A 15-year-old nonsmoker presents with an episode of gross hematuria. An IVU shows delayed function of the left kidney. The CT scan findings suggest a soft tissue mass in the ureter. A retrograde pyelogram was performed. What are the significant findings on the study? What are the 2 most likely diagnoses?**

The retrograde pyelogram shows a somewhat lobulated filling defect in the upper ureter. Transitional cell carcinoma is always a possibility, but in a younger patient, the differential would include a fibroepithelial polyp, which, in fact, this turned out to be. The CT scan is useful to rule out a radiolucent stone. Ureteroscopy will confirm the diagnosis.

○   **A middle-aged man referred for microhematuria has 10 RBCs/hpf and 20 WBCs/hpf. A urine culture is negative. Urine cytology is negative. A representative film from the IVU is shown for the right kidney. What is the most likely diagnosis?**

The diagnosis is tuberculosis. Most of the features of tuberculosis are illustrated in this film. Tuberculous strictures occur classically in the infundibula, ureteropelvic junction, and ureterovesical junction. In this film, there are strictures of the upper pole infundibulum and UPJ with some degree of "beading" of the upper ureter. There is evidence of papillary necrosis and actual tissue slough in the film. Damage to parenchyma may progress to calyceal amputation or frank autonephrectomy. Faint amorphous calcifications were evident on the plain film.

○ **This patient has a history of pyuria and vague right flank pain. Routine urine cultures have been negative. This film is the 15-minute film from an IVU. What is the most likely diagnosis?**

The diagnosis is again tuberculosis. The film illustrates something that both tuberculosis and transitional cell carcinoma do and that is to amputate calyces. The upper pole calyx of the right kidney is seen as just a whisp of irregular contrast (arrow). There is a distal ureteral stricture, which is not well demonstrated on the film. The bladder is contracted and the left kidney is not working and has undergone a functional autonephrectomy.

○   **This film shows bilateral retrograde pyelograms obtained in a patient who had a chronic indwelling stent on the right, which had recently been removed. What diagnosis is suggested by the radiographic finding shown?**

The retrograde pyelogram on the right shows extensive notching of the ureter with smooth, small round filling defects. The history and radiographic findings are most consistent with ureteritis cystica. Other possibilities in the differential would be tuberculosis, malakoplakia, persistent fetal ureter, or transitional cell carcinoma.

○   **This patient underwent an evaluation for microhematuria and pyuria. Past history was remarkable for an extensive travel history including trips to Africa and China. An IVU was obtained and shown are a portion of the scout and 5-minute films. What is the most likely diagnosis?**

There are few things that will calcify the bladder wall and the first one that should come to mind in this clinical scenario is *Schistosoma.* Schistosomiasis is found in rivers in Africa and other parts of the world. Once in the host, the *Schistosoma hematobium* reside in the perivesical venous plexus and lay their eggs in the bladder wall and venous tributaries of the bladder. The eggs are then shed in the urine completing its life cycle. The result of this process is an intense inflammatory reaction in the bladder. Schistosomiasis can acutely present with hematuria and inflammatory changes in the bladder wall on IVU. Late findings include calcification of the bladder and ureteral walls. Similar to tuberculosis, there may be extensive ureteral strictures. Nonfunction, stones, polypoid masses, and hydronephrosis are also seen. The risk of bladder cancer is high in these patients. Consistent with the intense inflammatory reaction, there is a higher risk of squamous cell cancer and adenocarcinoma. **When there is a suspicion of an inflammatory condition involving the urinary tract, ask about the travel history.**

○   **A 45-year-old female presented with a history of recurrent urinary tract infection. A catheterized urine specimen grew multiple gram-negative organisms. An IVU was obtained. The significant findings on the film are? The most likely diagnosis to explain the film is?**

The IVU shows a large amount of gas in the bladder and outlining of the left upper pole calyx. Gas can occur in the urinary tract in association with infection caused by a gas-forming organism. Gas in the amounts seen on this film should raise suspicion for a vesicoenteric fistula, particularly given the history of a polymicrobial infection. Sometimes gas will appear in the wall of the bladder in association with a urinary tract infection known as emphysematous cystitis. Gas outlining the collecting system with no parenchymal gas occurring in the presence of a urinary tract infection is because of emphysematous pyelitis, which responds to antibiotics more favorably than emphysematous pyelonephritis. Renal pelvic gas can also be caused by reflux of air associated with instrumentation. The most likely diagnosis in this case is colovesical fistula caused by diverticulitis. Crohn disease, colon cancer, and other pelvic malignancies can also cause fistulas.

○   **A 50-year-old female presented with a history of malaise, left-sided flank pain, and a low-grade fever. On physical examination, a hard mass was palpable in the left upper quadrant. A urine culture grew *Proteus*. The IVU suggested a left renal mass associated with several calcifications, which appeared to be stones, and the kidney was essentially nonfunctional. A representative film from the retrograde pyelogram is shown. What is the likely diagnosis?**

The constellation of renal mass and stones raises the differential of xanthogranulomatous pyelonephritis versus squamous cell carcinoma of the kidney. The presence of the proteus infection makes the former more likely. Renal calculi are seen in one-third of cases and a mass is found in two-thirds. *Proteus* is the most common organism, but *E. coli* is also common. The retrograde pyelogram shows destruction of parenchyma and collecting system with multiple abscess cavities. There is a suggestion of a filling defect in the renal pelvis corresponding to the stone seen on plain film.

○   **A middle-aged female presented with a history of recurrent urinary tract infection. The infections have all been characterized by dysuria and frequency but without fever. A postvoid film from the IVU is seen. The likely diagnosis is?**

The film shows a relatively smooth double-contrast density at or just distal to the bladder neck. In a female, the likely diagnosis is a urethral diverticulum. Urethral diverticula may be a cause of recurrent UTI. They may be difficult to diagnose. The diagnosis should begin with a good physical examination that includes palpation of the urethra. An IVU and particularly the postvoid bladder film may identify the diverticulum. A voiding cystogram, "double bubble" urethrogram using a special double balloon urethral catheter, and cystoscopy may also be useful.

○ A 25-year-old female presented with a history of intermittent right flank pain and hematuria. A faint stone was seen overlying the right bladder shadow on plain film. Hexagonal crystals were present in the urine. What is the significant radiographic sign demonstrated in this IVU and what is the most likely diagnosis?

The IVU shows a "cobra head" deformity of the distal right ureter consistent with a simple orthotopic ureterocele. The orifice is likely to be on the trigone. The faint lucency seen in the middle of the ureterocele is likely to be a "relatively" radiolucent stone composed of cystine. The crystalluria confirms this and a sodium nitroprusside test on the urine would be positive. Unlike uric acid stones, which are not seen on a plain film, cystine stones are faintly seen on the plain film but appear lucent versus contrast on the IVU. Cystine and uric acid stones are both visible on noncontrast CT scans. Only medication stones (indinavir) are invisible on both noncontrast CT scans and plain films. IVU should be used for diagnosis of possible stones in patients on indinavir and similar medications.

○ This patient had an IVU performed for hematuria. A urinalysis showed numerous RBCs, no WBCs or bacteria, and a pH of 5.0. The plain film did not show a stone. What are the significant findings and what is the most likely diagnosis? What test should be performed next to confirm the diagnosis?

This film shows a smooth lucent filling defect in the lower pole system of a partial duplication. The surface of the defect is smooth. While the usual differential of tumor, stone, clot, papilla, and fungus ball applies, the findings are most consistent with a radiolucent uric acid stone. This could be confirmed with a noncontrast (renal colic) spiral CT scan since uric acid stones appear bright white, while the other possibilities would show only soft tissue. An ultrasound would show a solid stone if the calculus is large enough.

○   **This man presented with gross hematuria. The scout film from the IVU and a set of retrograde pyelograms are shown. A urine culture is sterile. What is the diagnosis and what is the stone composition likely to be?**

This patient has bilateral staghorn calculi. The stones are relatively radiolucent. Staghorn calculi are most often composed of struvite or magnesium ammonium phosphate and are accompanied by infection with urea-splitting organisms such as *Proteus*. Struvite has a relative density of 0.20, while cystine is slightly lower at 0.15 compared to bone that has a relative radiographic density of 1. These stones are relatively radiolucent and the diagnosis in this patient was staghorn calculi composed of cystine.

○   **A 35-year-old man presented with a history of hypertension, gross hematuria, and abdominal masses. A representative film from the IVU and a retrograde pyelogram are shown. The diagnosis is most likely?**

This is a set of films we do not see too often in the era of CT scanning. A normal kidney should be roughly 3 vertebral bodies in length. The IVU shows large kidneys bilaterally with diffuse splaying of both collecting systems due in this case to multiple cysts. The retrograde pyelogram confirms the IVU findings but also shows some degree of ureteral displacement because of the large kidneys. The diagnosis is autosomal dominant polycystic kidney disease. The patient may have a strong family history. Because of the risk of infecting cysts, the decision to perform retrograde pyelograms in these patients is a serious one and prophylactic antibiotics should be given. The differential diagnosis for large kidneys is long and includes bilateral hydronephrosis, bilateral duplication, bilateral renal tumors, acute bilateral renal vein thrombosis, renal lymphoma, leukemic infiltrates, acute tubular necrosis, diuretic or contrast administration, preeclampsia, lupus, Wegener, Goodpasture syndrome, and myeloma with amyloidosis.

○ **This patient with an ileal conduit and a history of transitional cell carcinoma of the bladder had an IVU performed as part of a routine follow-up evaluation. The serum creatinine was elevated to 1.7 mg/dL. The likely diagnosis is?**

This is a classic film demonstrating stomal stenosis. The presence of bilateral hydronephrosis and a large dilated ileal loop is the conduit equivalent of bladder outlet obstruction confirming the diagnosis of stomal stenosis. A gentle digital examination of the stoma would confirm this.

○   **This young man sustained a gunshot wound to the abdomen and underwent a laparotomy with closure of several small bowel perforations. Two weeks later, he presented with a history of fever to 104°C and flank pain. An ultrasound revealed left hydronephrosis. A representative film of the IVU is shown. What is the likely diagnosis and how should it be managed?**

The IVU shows marked extravasation of contrast into a large urinoma. The likely diagnosis is a missed ureteral injury with an infected urinoma. Management in this case consisted of percutaneous drainage of the kidney and urinoma, antibiotics, and delayed repair. **As a general radiologic principle of trauma, whether blunt or penetrating, medial extravasation of contrast should raise suspicion for a ureteral injury.**

○   **This 20-year-old male was involved in a motor vehicle accident. He had multiple long bone fractures. His blood pressure in the field was 70 mm Hg, but he responded quickly to fluids. He had no hematuria. A trauma IVU was performed in the trauma suite. What is the likely diagnosis?**

The film shows the left kidney to be functioning normally, but there is absence of a nephrogram and function of the right kidney. In addition, there is a fracture of the right L1 transverse process. **Fractures of transverse processes in the region of the renal hilum raise concern for a right renovascular injury.** An expeditious angiogram or contrasted CT scan would confirm the diagnosis. The presence of shock, hematuria, or high suspicion as with major decelerating trauma in the absence of hematuria should prompt urological evaluation. The advent of high-speed CT scanning has largely supplanted the use of IVU in the evaluation of the trauma patient. The 2-shot trauma IVU consists of a scout film followed by an injection of 1 mL/kg of IV contrast. A second film is taken at 10 minutes postcontrast injection.

○ **This 50-year-old man presented with poorly localized abdominal pain and was found by ultrasound to have bilateral hydronephrosis and a serum creatinine of 6.0 mg/dL. Past history is significant for migraine headaches. The prostate examination is normal and a trial of catheter drainage does not improve things. Bilateral retrograde pyelograms were obtained and the film for the right side is shown and the film on the left was nearly identical. A stent was passed easily on both sides and the creatinine responded and decreased to 2.0 mg/dL. What is the most likely diagnosis?**

The retrograde pyelograms show medial deviation of the ureter over the spine. The fact that a stent passed easily makes the diagnosis of a stricture less likely and with medial deviation, the diagnosis is most likely retroperitoneal fibrosis. Migraine headaches provide an additional clue to the possible use of methysergide, which has been used to treat migraines and has been associated with retroperitoneal fibrosis. A CT scan may be useful to confirm the presence of a fibrous mass encircling the aorta and vena cava and encasing the ureters as well. **Remember that on examinations, the examiners usually don't usually give you any information that isn't relevant to the case in some way, such as travel, medications, allergies, or surgical history.**

○   **The prenatal ultrasound of a newborn male showed bilateral hydronephrosis. A follow-up study confirmed the presence of bilateral hydronephrosis. A serum creatinine was 1.7 mg/dL 3 days postpartum. A representative film of the voiding cystourethrogram is shown. What is the likely diagnosis?**

Any history of bilateral hydronephrosis should prompt a look at the bladder outlet. A normal bladder outlet should be funneled and nondilated. This film shows the three-key radiographic characteristics of posterior urethral valves, which are dilation and elongation of the posterior urethra and indentation of the bladder neck. The voiding film also shows high-grade vesicoureteral reflux, which is frequently seen with posterior urethral valves. The differential would include membranous urethral stricture or external sphincter dyssynergia, neither of which fit the history.

○   **This KUB and voiding cystourethrogram were obtained in a male infant with undescended testes and bilateral hydronephrosis on ultrasound. What is the likely diagnosis?**

This classic film which needs little history is a case of the Eagle-Barrett or "prune-belly" syndrome. The classic triad consists of a male with absent abdominal wall musculature, bilateral undescended testes, and urological anomalies. The rib cage is flared and the flanks are bulging. There is massive reflux bilaterally into tortuous and dilated ureters. In this patient, the posterior urethra is nondilated making the diagnosis of posterior urethral valves unlikely. However, the prostate may be hypoplastic in these patients causing the posterior urethra to appear dilated. The bladder is usually large, but smooth walled as obstruction is not generally present.

○ **Here is another voiding cystourethrogram performed in a male infant with hydronephrosis on antenatal ultrasound confirmed in the postnatal period by repeat ultrasound. What is the diagnosis?**

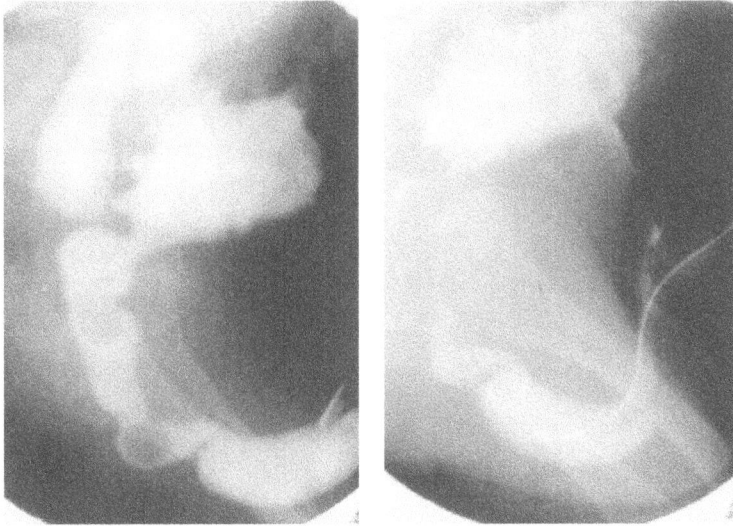

In this case, both the posterior and anterior urethra are dilated and the catheter identifies a "flap" of tissue at the distal end of a diverticulum. There is a heavily trabeculated bladder and at least unilateral massive reflux. The film demonstrates an anterior urethral diverticulum or anterior urethral valves. This is a very rare cause of outlet obstruction in newborn males.

○ **This cystogram was obtained in a young male with recurrent febrile urinary tract infections. His physical examination is normal. What is unusual about the film and what is the diagnosis?**

The diagnosis is bilateral vesicoureteral reflux. The cystogram shows high-grade vesicoureteral reflux into duplicate collecting systems on either side. The unusual finding on the film is the presence of reflux into both collecting systems. In association with the Meyer–Weigert rule, the upper-pole ectopic orifice more commonly obstructs and is located more inferomedially while the lower-pole system refluxes. However, reflux can occur into both segments. An alternative explanation for this film might be a low-lying, incomplete duplication with reflux into the solitary orifice on each side.

○   **This cystogram was obtained in a child who had a febrile urinary tract infection. What is the most likely diagnosis?**

The right ureter is opacified due to reflux, and it inserts into the urinary tract at a site distal to the bladder neck. The diagnosis is a refluxing ectopic ureter. In females, ectopic ureters are more often associated with the upper pole segment of duplication, while in males, the ureter more commonly drains a nonduplicated system. In females, the ureter may insert into the uterus, vagina, cervix, bladder neck, vestibule, or urethra, while in males, insertion is most commonly in the bladder neck, prostatic urethra, seminal vesicles, vas deferens, or ejaculatory duct.

○   **This child presented with umbilical discharge. A voiding cystogram was obtained. What is the diagnosis?**

The cystogram shows a patent urachus. While persistence of the urachus has been attributed to intrauterine bladder outlet obstruction, the majority of patients with a patent urachus do not have obstruction.

○ **This is a voiding cystourethrogram obtained in a child who presented with a history of voiding with 2 streams. What is the diagnosis?**

The cystogram shows a sagittal or epispadiac complete urethral duplication. Collateral or side-by-side duplications also exist and are more often associated with other pelvic anomalies such as imperforate anus or penile duplication.

○ **In the previous case, which urethra is the normal one?**

In the overwhelming majority of cases, the ventral urethra is the normal variant.

○ **This cystogram lateral view was obtained in a young male who had obstructive urinary symptoms. What is the likely diagnosis?**

The study shows bilateral congenital bladder diverticula. While bladder diverticula may be associated with posterior urethral valves or neurogenic bladder, they may occur as an isolated entity. In this case, the posterior urethra is nondilated and the bladder is relatively smooth making these 2 diagnoses less likely. Diverticula may be associated with infection, but also may cause outlet obstructive symptoms. In this case, simple resection of only diverticula relieved the symptoms.

○   **This 3-year-old female had an episode of gross hematuria. A cystogram was obtained. What is the likely diagnosis?**

The classic cystographic appearance of a botryoid rhabdomyosarcoma of the bladder is that of a **"cluster of grapes,"** which the filling defect in this cystogram certainly resembles. Sarcoma botryoides is a variant of embryonal type rhabdomyosarcoma, which forms polypoid tumor masses.

○   **This patient was involved in a motor vehicle trauma and had gross hematuria. The patient initially had abdominal CT scanning, which was unremarkable. A cystogram was then obtained. What is the likely diagnosis?**

This film illustrates the importance of obtaining a scout film prior to the introduction of bladder contrast. In this case, the diagnosis is suspicious for an intraperitoneal bladder rupture. However, the contour of the bladder is smooth and appears to be intact. In fact, it was subsequently proven that the contrast seen was actually oral contrast, which had been given to the patient at the time of CT scanning. **Drainage films are also important since extravasation can hide behind the opacified bladder.** Oblique views should also be obtained.

○ **This older male had just undergone a transurethral resection of the prostate. A cystogram was obtained at the conclusion of the procedure because of a concern about a possible bladder perforation. What is the most likely diagnosis and how should it be treated?**

This film shows a classic extraperitoneal bladder rupture. The pattern of contrast extravasation is **"flame shaped"** and "whispy" in appearance and extends from the base of the bladder cephalad. Treatment is with catheter drainage. A repeat cystogram should be done in 7 to 10 days. Eighty-five percent of patients will be healed by that time. Virtually, all will be healed by 3 weeks after the injury.

○ **This patient was involved in a motor vehicle accident and sustained a pelvic fracture. A retrograde urethrogram was normal and a cystogram was performed. What is the likely diagnosis and how should it be treated?**

The cystogram shows a classic **"teardrop"** shape caused by compression by the pelvic hematoma. There is "flame-shaped" extravasation extending in a whispy fashion from the base of the bladder. The picture is typical for an extraperitoneal bladder rupture. Some concern for intraperitoneal rupture might be raised because of contrast-located cephalad to the bladder, but there is no obvious contrast outlining loops of bowel. While only 10% of pelvic fractures manifest bladder rupture, virtually 100% of traumatic extraperitoneal bladder ruptures are associated with pelvic fracture. Roughly 10% are combined intra- and extraperitoneal injuries. **In adults, at least 300 mL of a water-soluble iodinated contrast should be instilled into the bladder by gravity pressure for a cystogram in order to exclude bladder rupture. A retrograde urethrogram should always be done first.**

○   **What is the formula used to calculate the estimated bladder capacity in children?**

Bladder capacity equals 60 mL + (30 mL × age in years).

○   **This patient presented following a motor vehicle accident. The patient had been drinking at the local bar prior to the accident. On presentation, he had suprapubic tenderness and a urinalysis showed gross hematuria. He did not have a pelvic fracture by plain film. An abdominal CT scan with a passive "CT cystogram" was normal. In spite of this, a standard trauma cystogram was performed. What does the study show and what is the diagnosis?**

The study shows a classic intraperitoneal bladder rupture. As opposed to extraperitoneal ruptures, the contrast outlines loops of bowel and the direction of extravasation is cephalad. **Bladder ruptures in which there is significant contrast-located cephalad to the bladder should raise suspicion for intraperitoneal rupture.** A diagnostic maneuver that may help in equivocal cases is placing the patient in Trendelenburg position and repeating the film. Contrast may be seen over the liver or spleen. An active CT cystogram is usually a very sensitive test, but it should be done with the standard 300 mL contrast instillation into the bladder rather than using just the passive filling by the IV contrast used with CT. **Cystograms are best done before any oral, rectal, or IV contrast.**

○   **This 20-year-old male presents to the emergency room after a motor vehicle accident with blood at the urethral meatus. The patient is hemodynamically stable and undergoes a retrograde urethrogram after a failed single passage of a Foley catheter. What are the significant radiographic findings?**

This retrograde urethrogram film shows significant pubic diastasis and urethral extravasation of contrast material consistent with urethral disruption. With this mechanism of injury, the most common place for a urethral injury is at the membranous urethra; however, this particular patient has sustained a bulbar urethral injury. No contrast material can be seen within the bladder. The patient will likely require a suprapubic cystostomy. Careful flexible urethroscopy and subsequent Foley catheter placement over a guidewire could be considered as a primary therapy.

○   **This retrograde urethrogram was obtained on a 35-year-old male presenting with a history of perineal trauma 2 years ago. What is the significant radiographic finding and how should it be treated?**

This urethral stricture extends from the distal bulbar urethra to the proximal pendulous urethra. Its length is estimated at 3.5 cm. **Remember that length of a urethral stricture must be measured from the point where tapering begins.** Options for repair include excision and primary anastomosis, augmented anastomotic repair, graft repair, and flap repair. Primary anastomosis can be attempted, but is usually reserved for strictures 2.5 cm or less. Augmented anastomotic repair would be a good choice for this length of stricture and the buccal mucosa would be an ideal graft material.

○   **This 40-year-old male with diabetes presented with fever, chills, and severe scrotal pain. What is the significant finding on KUB and what is the next step?**

This film shows a likely left scrotal abscess. Air is seen but appears to be confined to the tunica vaginalis. Air on KUB in a diabetic, febrile patient should be considered a surgical emergency because of the possibility of Fournier gangrene. Physical examination findings of subcutaneous crepitus and a rapidly expanding erythema would be worrisome. Wide excision and debridement is mandatory and potentially lifesaving along with antibiotics.

○ **Which common medication is specifically contraindicated and must be stopped prior to IV contrast administration; how long should it be held and why?**

Metformin (Glucophage) needs to be stopped before IV contrast studies and not resumed for at least 48 hours. A renal function test should be done to verify normal renal function before resuming the medication. Lactic acidosis is associated with the concomitant use of metformin and IV contrast. If it develops, severe lactic acidosis is associated with a 50% mortality rate.

○ **What prophylactic treatments can be used to prevent IV contrast-induced nephropathy?**

The most effective appears to be acetylcysteine and sodium chloride hydration. Sodium bicarbonate may be more effective than plain saline hydration, but reports are conflicting. Other possible preventive therapies include theophylline and fenoldopam (a selective dopamine-receptor agonist), but their roles are still unclear with conflicting reports on their efficacy. Lasix, steroids, and mannitol have not shown any benefit.

○ **Gadolinium can cause what potentially serious complication when used in patients with renal failure?**

Nephrogenic systemic fibrosis.

CHAPTER 2 Radionuclide Studies

David M. Albala, MD,
Udaya Kumar, MD, FRCS Urol, Dip Urol (Lon),
and Pramod P. Reddy, MD

○ **What are the half-lives of ^{99m}Tc, ^{123}I, and ^{131}I?**

The half-lives are 6 hours, 13.2 hours, and 8 days, respectively.

○ **What exactly is a rad?**

The amount of radiation energy absorbed by a patient's tissue is expressed in rad. The rad is defined as 100 erg absorbed per gram of tissue.

○ **What is the difference between a roentgen and rad?**

A roentgen is a measure of ionization of the air by x-rays or gamma rays. Although the terms roentgen and rad are often used interchangeably, it should be remembered that roentgen is a measure of exposure, whereas the rad is a measure of energy absorbed by tissue.

○ **What are the most common instruments used to clinically detect ionizing radiation?**

Although gas detectors such as Geiger–Müller counters are used in nuclear medicine laboratories, solid crystal detectors are most commonly employed to detect ionizing radiation. The Anger camera used in most departments uses a sodium iodide crystal.

○ **What isotopes are used to measure the glomerular filtration rate (GFR)?**

Although ^{14}C-inulin would give an accurate measurement of GFR, it is impractical to use. ^{51}Cr-EDTA and ^{99m}Tc-DTPA are alternatives. In practice, ^{99m}Tc-DTPA is usually used, as it also provides excellent renal images.

○ **Which isotopes are useful in measuring renal blood flow (RBF)?**

^{131}I-hippuran, ^{123}I-hippuran, and ^{99m}Tc-MAG3 are useful. ^{99m}Tc-MAG3 is most commonly used in the United States for these purposes.

○ **How is ^{99m}Tc-DTPA processed in the kidney?**

^{99m}Tc-DTPA is filtered and concentrated in the tubules and is then excreted through the collecting system. In a normal kidney, activity in the renal pelvis and ureter decreases after 5 to 10 minutes making it a useful test to detect obstruction.

○ **What does a DMSA scan demonstrate?**

^{99m}Tc-DMSA accumulates progressively in the kidneys over several hours and images the renal cortex well. It is useful to detect renal scarring and early stages of renal damage from infection, and to differentiate functioning from nonfunctioning renal masses.

○ **What are the common uses of radionuclide studies after renal transplantation?**

They are useful in evaluating complications such as complete renal artery occlusion, urinary obstruction, or leakage. Acute tubular necrosis and rejection cause reduced perfusion and prolonged parenchymal transit times.

○ **What isotopes are useful in investigating occult suppuration in the abdomen or pelvis?**

Gallium-67 citrate–labeled or indium-111-labeled leukocytes are used.

○ **What is the advantage of scanning with indium-111-labeled leukocyte over gallium-67 citrate in localizing infection?**

Studies with indium-111-labeled leukocytes often can be completed in 24 hours, whereas those using gallium-67 may take 48 to 72 hours to complete. In addition, the latter may be taken up by certain tumors such as lymphomas and hepatomas and is taken up by kidneys, which may confuse the diagnosis.

○ **How is mercaptoacetyltriglycine (MAG3) cleared by the kidneys?**

MAG3 is cleared by the kidneys primarily by tubular secretion and to a lesser extent by glomerular filtration. Therefore, it is an excellent agent for estimating the effective renal plasma flow. It is used to define ureteropelvic junction (UPJ) obstruction and differential renal function.

○ **What is nuclear cystography and what is its value in ureteral reflux?**

It is the scintigraphic equivalent of conventional cystography. It is an accurate method for detecting and following reflux, although it does not provide the anatomic detail of fluoroscopic studies.

○ **True/False: In screening siblings for reflux, the nuclear scan is preferable to a standard voiding cystography.**

True. The radiation exposure in a nuclear scan is lower than that in a cystogram and when anatomic detail of VCUG is not essential, the nuclear scan is preferable.

○ **What are the nuclear scan findings in testicular torsion?**

The testicle appears avascular. In cases of epididymitis hypervascularity is noted. However, in cases of intermittent torsion and late torsion, hypervascularity may result from an inflammatory response. Occasional false-positive and false-negative results and limited availability of the nuclear scan 24 hours a day limit its usefulness in the diagnosis of torsion.

○ **What is the "doughnut sign" on the nuclear scan in testicular torsion?**

In a missed torsion (ie, one that is several days old), there is often an area of hyperemia surrounding the central ischemic region of the testis. The central area appears photopenic surrounded by a rim of increased activity (doughnut).

○ **What factors affect the drainage curve of the nuclear scan in patients with UPJ obstruction?**

In addition to the severity of obstruction, the size and compliance of the collecting system, and the hydration of the patient, the timing of diuretic and bladder drainage influences the drainage curve. A poorly functioning kidney may not respond adequately to the diuretic.

○ **True/False: The advantages of the ^{99m}Tc-DMSA scan over IVU in the evaluation of renal damage from pyelonephritis include (a) lack of study impairment by bowel gas, (b) earlier detection of renal damage, (c) clear visualization of kidneys despite overlying bony structures, (d) improved ability to image the kidneys in various positions to delineate specific lesions, and (e) more clear visualization of the collecting system.**

False. All are true except that the visualization of the collecting system in the DMSA scan is not nearly as good as with an IVU.

○ **True/False: Captopril is used to improve the accuracy of nuclear scan findings of renovascular hypertension.**

True. Captopril exaggerates the differences between the perfused and nonperfused areas of the kidney in patients with renovascular hypertension.

○ **What is the rationale behind the performance of a captopril renogram in the diagnosis of obstructive uropathy?**

Renin is secreted by the juxtaglomerular apparatus in renovascular hypertension and/or obstructive uropathy as a result of poor tissue perfusion. The local vascular regulatory mechanisms of the kidney are:

• Release of thromboxane, causing vasoconstriction of the afferent arteriole, resulting in a further decrease of RBF
• Activation of the renin–angiotensin system (RAS) that results in the formation of angiotensin II, which in turn increases the efferent arteriolar tone and is primarily responsible for restoring and maintaining glomerular filtration pressure

Use of an angiotensin-converting enzyme inhibitor (ACEI) such as captopril can block this mechanism by preventing the formation of angiotensin II that reduces the vasoconstriction of the efferent arteriole, thereby causing a drop in GFR and relative renal function. This decrease is demonstrable with captopril renography.

○ **What is the correct dose of captopril administered for a captopril renogram?**

0.3 mg/kg is administered orally 1 hour prior to the radioisotope injection. A change of at least 5% (baseline scan vs captopril scan) is considered significant when interpreting the results.

○ **What is an MIBG scan and what is it used for?**

Metaiodobenzylguanidine (MIBG) is taken up by adrenal neurons. It is labeled with iodine and used to image the adrenal medulla and other active adrenergic tissues such as pheochromocytomas and neuroblastomas.

○ **How are nuclear scans helpful in carcinoma of the prostate?**

Bone scans with ^{99m}Tc-methylene diphosphonate (MDP) are most useful in the staging of prostate cancer. They are more than 95% sensitive in detecting bony metastases from carcinoma of the prostate.

○ **What is a "superscan" in a patient with prostate cancer?**

When there is extensive involvement of the bony skeleton with metastases in a patient with prostate cancer, the isotope is extensively taken up by the bone and the kidneys are not visualized.

○ **Bone scans typically are almost always negative and therefore not particularly useful until the PSA level reaches what point?**

A PSA level of 20 or more is usually necessary before a bone scan will be positive.

○ **Can nuclear scans be used in renal failure?**

Yes. ^{123}I and ^{131}I-hippurate and MAG3 can be concentrated even in kidneys with minimal renal function. They are of immense value in patients with renal failure or renal transplantation.

○ **What are the features of renal obstruction in a patient with hydronephrosis on a nuclear scan?**

During the excretory phase of the scan, the renogram demonstrates increasing activity over time, even after administration of furosemide, but the test may be unreliable in patients with poorly functioning kidneys or massively dilated collecting systems.

○ **How accurate is the MIBG scan in localizing pheochromocytomas and neuroblastomas?**

^{123}I-MIBG scan is 85% to 90% sensitive and nearly 100% specific for localizing pheochromocytomas. It is almost 100% specific and 100% sensitive for neuroblastomas.

○ **What constitutes a "well-tempered renogram" and how is it done?**

The Society for Fetal Urology and the Pediatric Nuclear Medicine Council of the Society of Nuclear Medicine published guidelines for the "well-tempered diuresis renogram" in 1992:

- Small field of view gamma camera is used for pediatric studies.
- If the child is younger than 4 months, MAG3 should be the radioisotope used for the study.
- In children older than 4 months, MAG3 is still the preferred radioisotope. However, DTPA may be substituted instead.
- The patient is well hydrated. A normal saline IV (15 mL/kg) bolus given over 30 minutes is begun 15 minutes prior to the administration of the radioisotope. For the remainder of the study, a maintenance IV at 200 mL/kg/24 h is administered. The child's bladder should be catheterized to prevent any lower urinary tract dysfunction from influencing the results of the study.

○ **What is the recommended dose of diuretic (furosemide) for a "well-tempered diuresis renogram?"**

The dose of diuretic (Lasix) used should be 1 to 2 mg/kg IV.

○ **What is an indirect radionuclide cystogram (IRC)?**

The IRC is a diagnostic test to detect vesicoureteral reflux (VUR). It employs ^{99m}Tc-DTPA as the radionuclide tracer. It provides information about the emptying phase of the bladder and can demonstrate VUR. Since it does not provide any information about the filling phase, it will miss the 3% of VUR known to occur during this phase of the bladder cycle. The high sensitivity of the IRC combined with the advantages of lower radiation and avoidance of bladder catheterization makes it a valuable alternative to the VCUG.

○ **Match the following radionuclide tracers with method of action tracers:**

1. DTPA	A. Eighty percent tubular secretion
2. OIH	B. Both GFR-dependent and tubular secretion for clearance
3. MAG3	C. Localizes to the proximal convoluted tubules (PCT)
4. DMSA	D. Mostly tubular secretion
5. GH	E. GFR-dependent for clearance

1—E; 2—A; 3—D; 4—C; 5—B.

○ **What advantages does radionuclide cystography (RNC) have over a standard VCUG?**

The RNC is more sensitive and specific for the detection of VUR than a VCUG. It also has a significantly lower gonadal radiation dose (RNC = 0.001-0.005 rad vs VCUG = 0.208 rad).

○ **What are the disadvantages of RNC?**

- Limited ability to grade reflux and less anatomic detail.
- It does not provide additional radiographic data, that is, the presence of constipation or bony abnormalities, etc.

○ **In a child presenting with flank pain, high fever, and dysuria, which radionuclide study would be appropriate to order?**

The child has features suggesting an acute pyelonephritis. DMSA renal imaging has been shown to demonstrate areas of decreased perfusion (inflammation vs scar) in the kidneys. In order to differentiate between scar and inflammation, a renal ultrasound could be used or one could repeat the DMSA scan in 6 months. Persistent cortical defects represent parenchymal scars.

○ **What is the role of radionuclide imaging in the management of a duplex collecting system with an obstructed upper pole moiety?**

Radionuclide scanning (with a cortical agent) can provide information about the degree of function and amount of functioning renal tissue in each moiety of the duplex kidney. In the case of an obstructed upper pole moiety, it will also serve as a diagnostic test to determine efficacy of surgical intervention.

○ **Are there any potential complications to keep in mind or to counsel the parents about while ordering a radionuclide study?**

For the most part, nuclear medicine studies are quite safe and the radiation dose involved is minimal. There is a small risk of a nosocomial UTI from urethral catheterization in RNC. Some children may experience significant abdominal discomfort during a Lasix renogram, especially if they have intermittent obstruction and the study reproduces an obstructive episode.

○ **What are the contraindications to performing a radionuclide study on a patient?**

There are no absolute contraindications to the use of radionuclides for diagnostic purposes. A relative contraindication is pregnancy; therefore, nuclear medicine scanning should not be performed on patients in the reproductive age group without first performing a pregnancy test.

○ **Is there a role for radionuclide scanning in the acute evaluation of a trauma patient?**

The advent of ultrafast spiral CT scanners has changed the imaging algorithm for the evaluation of the trauma patient, so there is little need for radionuclide scanning in these cases. In certain select cases, radionuclide scanning with a renal cortical agent might be indicated to evaluate the degree of function and amount of functioning renal tissue.

○ **What is the best radionuclide agent to use in a 1-month-old infant with severe hydronephrosis, suggestive of bilateral UPJ obstruction?**

Normally, it is not recommended to perform a Lasix scan on children younger than 3 months because of the relative functional immaturity of the kidneys, which limits the reliability of the results. However, there are instances where the physician has to perform the test sooner, as in the above clinical case. In such instances, MAG3 is the agent of choice, as it has lower uptake in the liver and spleen and higher renal extraction providing a better target to background ratio.

○ **In what clinical setting is "static" radionuclide imaging utilized?**

Static radionuclide imaging is used to evaluate VUR, urinary tract infections, hypertension, and cystic diseases of the kidney. It can document renal scarring, acute pyelonephritis, and differential renal function.

○ **In what clinical settings is "dynamic" radionuclide imaging utilized?**

Dynamic renal functional imaging is useful for evaluating a suspected obstruction in cases of possible UPJ obstruction and megaureters (although the $t_{1/2}$ values are of limited clinical relevance in light of the compliance of the dilated ureter). It is also useful in evaluating renal function in cystic kidney diseases and hypertension, as well as after a renal transplant or pyeloplasty.

○ **What is "SPECT" radionuclide scanning?**

Single-photon emission computed tomography (SPECT) is an imaging technique associated with single gamma ray–emitting radiopharmaceuticals. The images are obtained using a scintillation camera that moves around the patient to capture images from multiple angles for tomographic image reconstruction. It results in better image quality and improves the sensitivity of the test.

○ **What agent is used for a positron emission tomographic (PET) scan?**

The PET scan uses a radioactive glucose molecule as the radiotracer to identify metabolically active tissues. The radiotracer is a glucose analog called FDG ([18F]-2-fluoro-2-deoxy-D-glucose).

○ **What is the mechanism/physiologic principle on which a PET scan is based?**

During a PET scan, the patient is injected with a radiotracer, a glucose analog called FDG. FDG is preferentially taken up by tumor cells and phosphorylated by the enzyme hexokinase to $FDG-6-PO_4$. Unlike glucose-6-PO_4, $FDG-6-PO_4$ cannot enter into the glycolytic pathway and be further broken down; it therefore remains trapped intracellularly. This allows the hypermetabolic tissue of a tumor to be distinguished from the surrounding normal tissue.

○ **What are 18F-Sodium Fluoride (NaF) PET/CT Bone Scan Indications?**

18F-NaF PET/CT is an important tool for detecting and evaluating metastatic bone cancer. These bone studies are particularly useful, since some of the most prevalent cancers are commonly associated with metastatic bone disease, such as breast and prostate cancer, as well as carcinoma of the thyroid, kidney, and lung. This expansion of coverage for 18F-NaF studies provides a superior clinical alternative for bone scanning, with significant advantages over "conventional" ^{99m}Tc-MDP bone scans, including higher sensitivity and specificity, shorter uptake and scan times, and radiation doses comparable to ^{99m}Tc-MDP studies.

○ **List some of the desirable characteristics of 18F-NaF as a bone-imaging agent.**

- Bone uptake is 2 times higher and blood clearance is much faster than that with ^{99m}Tc-MDP, offering superior bone to background ratios and high contrast images within 45 to 60 minutes after injection.
- Improved sensitivity compared with that of traditional nuclear medicine SPECT or planar bone imaging, due to ability of 18F-NaF to demonstrate variation in bone metabolism, combined with the PET/CT scanner's high-resolution/tomographic images. Bone metastases are seen indirectly, with uptake depending on skeletal reaction to tumor.
- Little residual retention in soft tissues and the renal parenchyma.
- Deposition favors sites of high bone turnover and remodeling.
- Radiation dose comparable to that of conventional ^{99m}Tc-MDP bone scan.

○ **What GU malignancy is best suited for imaging with a PET scan?**

PET scanning is best suited for radiographic staging in testis cancer. Testis cancer and its metastatic lesions have a high glycolytic rate, and therefore accumulate a high concentration of the radiotracer FDG.

○ **What is the role of PET scanning in the management of prostate cancer?**

PET scanning does not currently have a significant role in the diagnosis and imaging of prostate cancer as the cancerous prostatic tissue has a relatively low glycolytic rate, and therefore does not accumulate high concentrations of the radiotracer FDG.

○ **In testicular cancer, which modality has the higher diagnostic accuracy in detecting metastases: PET or CT scanning?**

PET scanning has a higher diagnostic accuracy than a CT scan for both initial staging of testis cancer and restaging after surgical and chemotherapeutic interventions.

○   **What is fanolesomab (FNB) and what is its utility in nuclear medicine imaging?**

FNB is a ^{99m}Tc–labeled murine anti-CD15 IGM monoclonal antibody that specifically targets neutrophils. It is a radiopharmaceutical agent that has been designed to specifically target and localize acute infections. It is much more sensitive than an indium-111- or gallium-tagged white blood cell scan that is the current gold standard.

○   **What factors can limit the utility of the Lasix renogram?**

The following are the factors that can significantly alter the results of a Lasix scan being performed to detect an obstructive lesion at the UPJ:

- The volume of the collecting system. (A very large pelvis is compliant and can hold a lot of tracer, falsely affecting the drainage time.)
- Renal insufficiency.
- The hydration status of the patient.
- Renal tubular disorders, that is, acute tubular necrosis and Fanconi syndrome.

○   **What are some of the pitfalls and limitations of the ACEI renogram?**

The rationale of the ACEI renogram is that the ACEI blocks the vasoconstriction of the efferent arteriole and causes a decrease in the glomerular filtration pressure and a demonstrable decrease in the GFR:

- Patient hydration—overhydration can cause a false-negative result and underhydration can cause a false-positive result.
- Selection of the radiotracer—DTPA is better than MAG3.
- Choice of the ACEI—captopril versus enalapril.
- Asymmetric small kidney with poor function often is unresponsive to the effects of ACEI.
- Renal insufficiency results in a nondiagnostic ACEI renogram.
- Bilateral disease limits the diagnostic ability of the test.

CHAPTER 3 Retroperitoneal Anatomy

Graham F. Greene, MD, FACS

○ **What forms the lateral boundaries used to take down the bladder during an anterior approach to a robotic-assisted laparoscopic prostatectomy?**

The obliterated umbilical arteries, which form the medial umbilical folds.

○ **Retractor compression on the psoas muscle during surgery can affect which nerve?**

The femoral branch of the genitofemoral nerve.

○ **It is necessary to take care in placing the stitch in the psoas muscle during a bladder hitch procedure, so that what nerve is not injured?**

The femoral nerve.

○ **When performing a transverse colon conduit what cavity is exposed?**

The lesser sac.

○ **When exposing the infrahepatic inferior vena cava (IVC) what critical structure anteromedially that is associated with the liver can be injured?**

The common bile duct.

○ **What ligamentous attachments of the liver to the diaphragm need to be divided in order to rotate (flip) the liver and gain access to the suprahepatic and transhepatic IVC?**

The gastrophrenic ligament, the falciform ligament, and the coronary ligament.

○ **When closing a flank incision, which muscle layer has an obvious free border?**

The external oblique muscle has a free border laterally that extends from the lower border of the 12th rib to its aponeurotic insertion along the iliac crest.

○ **Between which 2 muscle layers do the intercostal nerves and vessels course?**

They course between the transversus abdominis and the internal oblique muscles. This is important when closing incisions to avoid entrapment of these structures.

○ **What is another name for Gerota fascia?**

Perirenal fascia. It is a specialized condensation within the intermediate stratum of the retroperitoneal connective tissue. It forms a barrier to benign and malignant processes.

○ **Does Gerota fascia form a tight seal around each kidney?**

No. Gerota fascia is weakest at its caudal aspect along the course of the gonadal vessels and ureter.

○ **When resecting a large left upper pole renal mass from an anterior approach, what medial attachments need to be divided to allow reflection of the spleen, pancreas, and stomach?**

Division of the phrenicocolic, splenorenal, gastrosplenic, and gastrophrenic ligaments will allow reflection of the spleen, pancreas, and stomach from the craniolateral aspect of the retroperitoneum exposing the upper pole of the left kidney and adrenal gland.

○ **What surgical maneuver will allow access to the intra- and suprahepatic vena cava?**

Division of the right and left triangular ligaments and continuing the incision along the cranial and caudal coronary ligaments will allow reflection of the right lobe of the liver, providing dramatic exposure to the inferior vena cava as it receives the hepatic veins and perforates the diaphragm.

○ **What nerve is commonly seen coursing anterolaterally in the inguinal canal?**

The ilioinguinal nerve (L1) courses through the inguinal canal on the cord to exit the external ring and provide sensation to the pubic area.

○ **What other nerve besides the ilioinguinal nerve follows the cord through the inguinal canal?**

The genital branch of the genitofemoral nerve (L1, L2). It is less conspicuous than the ilioinguinal nerve and has a dual function supplying motor innervation to the cremasteric muscle and sensation to the anterior scrotum or labia majora.

○ **What nerve is clearly visualized coursing along the ventrum of the psoas muscle and proves useful in defining the lateral border for a complete pelvic lymph node dissection?**

The genitofemoral nerve (L1, L2) serves a dual purpose in supplying motor function to the cremasteric muscle and sensation to the perineum and anterior thigh.

○ **Define the arterial blood supply of the right adrenal gland.**

The right adrenal receives its blood supply from 3 main sources. The 2 obvious ones include branches from the inferior phrenic artery as well as branches from the right renal artery. A branch that is often forgotten that passes behind the inferior vena cava is the middle adrenal artery. This can lead to significant bleeding if unrecognized and cut during a right adrenalectomy.

○ **Into what structures do the gonadal vessels on either side drain?**

The right gonadal vein enters the inferior vena cava on its ventral lateral aspect at an oblique angle. The left gonadal vein empties into the left renal vein.

○ **What is the significance of a varicocele that does not diminish when examined in the supine position?**

Suspect a retroperitoneal mass or process that is impairing venous drainage such as lymphoma, testicular cancer, renal cell carcinoma, or retroperitoneal fibrosis.

○ **What are the primary sites of lymphatic drainage from the left testis?**

The most common site on the left side is the left para-aortic lymph nodes followed by the preaortic, interaortocaval, left common iliac, and left suprarenal lymph nodes in decreasing order. Left-to-right lymphatic drainage tends not to occur unless there is lymphatic obstruction.

○ **What are the primary sites of lymphatic drainage from the right testis?**

The most common site on the right side is the interaortocaval lymph nodes followed by precaval, preaortic, right paracaval, right common iliac, and left para-aortic lymph nodes in decreasing order. Lymphatic drainage proceeds from the right to left side of the retroperitoneum. Alternative routes can occur when there is lymphatic obstruction.

○ **Which division of the renal artery supplies the majority of the kidney?**

The anterior division supplies more than 75% of the kidney, including apical, upper, middle, and lower vascular segments of the kidney. The posterior renal artery supplies the majority of the dorsal aspect of the kidney.

○ **How often can a surgeon anticipate accessory renal arteries?**

In 25% to 40% of cases, there is more than one renal artery arising from the lateral aorta at the level of the second lumbar vertebra. Accessory renal arteries to the right lower pole will often cross anterior to the vena cava. It becomes important to recognize such branches so that they are not divided when exposing the right renal hilum.

○ **Where do the renal pelvis and the upper ureter receive their arterial blood supply?**

There are 3 anastomosing arteries providing the upper ureter and renal pelvis with blood supply. They include the renal artery, aorta, and gonadal artery.

○ **Which adrenal gland is more intimate with the cranial aspect of the kidney?**

The left adrenal gland is most intimate with the cranial aspect of the left kidney. It often will drape over the ventral aspect of the upper pole. The right adrenal gland is decidedly cranial to the right kidney, and care must be given when removing it because of its short adrenal vein entering dorsolaterally into the inferior vena cava.

○ **What is an alternate route for venous drainage of the left adrenal gland?**

The left inferior phrenic vein. The adrenal gland vein drains into the left renal vein. Close to where it enters, it is joined by the inferior phrenic vein that cranially also empties into the inferior vena cava above the level of the hepatic veins. This means that you can divide the adrenal vein at the level of the renal vein without compromising its venous drainage.

○ **Does ligation of the gonadal arteries at the level of the aorta compromise the gonads?**

No. The rich collateral circulation provided by the artery to the vas deferens and external spermatic artery in the male and the uterine artery in the female provide collateral blood supply to the gonad.

○ **What are the first branches of the intra-abdominal aorta?**

The paired inferior phrenic arteries are the first branches of the intra-abdominal aorta. They give origin to the superior supra-adrenal arteries.

○ **What are the 3 main arterial blood supplies to the small bowel and colon?**

They include the superior mesenteric artery, inferior mesenteric artery, and the inferior and middle hemorrhoidal arteries, which are branches from the internal iliac artery.

○ **When is it possible to completely resect the infrahepatic vena cava for renal cell carcinoma and an IVC thrombus?**

It is possible to resect the infrahepatic vena cava when removing a large right renal mass and associated renal vein thrombus. This is due to the rich collateral venous drainage of the left kidney through the lumbar (azygos) system. The right kidney is not afforded a similar venous drainage.

○ **Other than the gonadal vein, what other vein drains into the caudal aspect of the left renal vein?**

A left lumbar vein. This large lumbar vein provides collateral venous drainage as well as a potential source of bleeding when ligating the left renal vein.

○ **If the inferior mesenteric artery is ligated during a retroperitoneal lymph node dissection, what artery insures blood supply to the upper rectum, sigmoid colon, descending colon, and part of the left transverse colon?**

The marginal artery of Drummond. This artery provides collateral circulation between the superior mesenteric artery and the inferior and middle hemorrhoidal vessels.

○ **When assessing left para-aortic lymphadenopathy on CT scan, what clue helps you distinguish retroperitoneal structures from mesenteric structures?**

At the level of the L3 vertebra (or inferior pole of the kidneys), the inferior mesenteric artery and inferior mesenteric vein run in a craniocaudal direction. The ureter can be seen posterolateral to these distinct vessels. Any structures dorsomedial are in the retroperitoneal space as compared to ventrolateral structures that are in the mesentery or coelomic space.

○ **In what direction does most lateral lumbar lymphatic flow proceed?**

Right to left. The lymphatics coalesce posterior to the aorta to form a localized dilation of lymphatic chain known as the cisterna chyli. This structure lies in a retrocrural position, just anterior to the first or second lumbar vertebra, and empties into the thoracic duct through the aortic hiatus of the diaphragm.

○ **What is Kocher maneuver?**

The Kocher maneuver refers to the surgical reflection of the second and third part of the duodenum craniomedially, to provide access to the right renal vessels and inferior vena cava. When combined with mobilization of the small bowel mesentery, this maneuver exposes the great vessels in anticipation of retroperitoneal dissection. It is important to recognize that the Kocher maneuver also mobilizes the head or uncinate process of the pancreas. Carefully placed retraction in this area will help prevent pancreatic injury.

○ **What happens to the ipsilateral adrenal gland in cases of renal ectopia or agenesis?**

They will present in their normal anticipated location within the retroperitoneum. The adrenal glands are embryologically and functionally distinct from the kidneys. Physically they are separated from the kidneys by connective tissue septa that are in continuity with Gerota's fascia as well as varying amounts of perinephric fat.

○ **During embryologic development the adrenal medulla has received what specialized cells and from where?**

The adrenal medulla consists of chromaffin cells, which are derived from the neural crest and are intimately associated with the sympathetic nervous system. Chromaffin cells belong to the family of amine precursor uptake decarboxylase (APUD) cells and produce neuroactive catecholamines that are released directly into the blood stream.

○ **What zone of the adrenal cortex produces glucocorticoids?**

The zona fasciculata. The adrenal gland consists of 3 zones or strata. The outermost layer of cells makes up the zona glomerulosa that produces aldosterone (mineralocorticoids). The next layer is the zona fasciculata that produces glucocorticoids, and in the normal adrenal gland is usually the thickest of the 3 layers. The innermost zona reticularis is responsible for producing sex steroids.

○ **Which layer of the adrenal cortex is not regulated by pituitary release of adrenocorticotropic hormone (ACTH)?**

The zona glomerulosa is not under direct pituitary regulation by ACTH. The zona glomerulosa, which is the outermost layer of the adrenal cortex, produces aldosterone in response to stimulation by the renin–angiotensin system.

○ **On which kidney can you find a dromedary hump?**

Both. This normal variation of renal contour is found much more commonly on the left than the right side. It is seen as a focal bulge on the midlateral border of the kidney.

○ **Between which 2 layers is the pararenal (paranephric) fat located?**

Between the transversalis fascia and Gerota fascia. Within Gerota fascia, the kidney is suspended in the perirenal fat. Depending upon the body habitus of the patient, varying amounts of pararenal fat can be found external to Gerota fascia. When surgically approaching the kidney, the transversalis fascia can sometimes be mistaken for Gerota fascia due to the underlying pararenal fat. Failure to incise transversalis fascia impends access to the retroperitoneum.

○ **Which segmental branch of the main renal artery is most constant?**

The posterior segmental artery is most constant. Prior to entering the renal hilum, the main renal artery divides into an anterior and posterior division. The posterior segmental artery supplies the majority of the dorsum of the kidney, whereas the anterior division gives rise to 4 anterior segmental arteries (apical, upper, middle, and lower) supplying the rest of the kidney. During nephron sparing surgery, mistaking the often long posterior segmental artery for the main renal artery can lead to incomplete arterial occlusion and blood loss.

○ **Describe intrarenal arterial anatomy.**

The renal artery divides into 4 or 5 segmental branches including the posterior, apical, upper, middle, and lower segmental renal arteries. The segmental arteries travel through the renal sinus and branch to give rise to lobar arteries. These lobar arteries divide again and enter the renal parenchyma as interlobar arteries and traverse the renal parenchyma through the renal columns of Bertin. At the base of the renal pyramids, the interlobar arteries branch into the arcuate arteries. In turn, the arcuate arteries branch to give rise to multiple interlobular arteries. These interlobular arteries branch within the renal cortex giving rise to the afferent arterioles of the glomerular capsule and contributing small branches to the renal capsular plexus. Blood leaves the glomerulus via the efferent arteriole and meets the venous system at the vasa recta within the renal medulla or through a capillary network within the cortex.

○ **What is implied when renal arteries are referred to as end arteries?**

The renal artery and its successive branches do not have anastomosis or collateral circulation. Therefore, occlusion of any of these vessels will result in ischemia and infarction of the renal parenchyma that it supplies.

○ **Describe renal venous drainage.**

The capillary bed within the cortex and the vas recta drain into interlobular veins, and then into arcuate, interlobar, lobar, and segmental veins, respectively. There are usually 3 to 5 segmental veins that empty into a main renal vein. Unlike renal arteries, renal parenchymal veins anastomose freely, especially in the arcuate vessels.

○ **Within the kidney where would the stellate veins be located?**

The stellate veins form a subcapsular venous plexus that form a communication between the interlobular veins and veins within the perinephric fat.

○ **How can renal vasculature obstruct the urinary collecting system?**

Accessory lower pole arteries may cross anterior to the urinary collecting system. In that orientation, they can become an extrinsic cause of ureteral pelvic junction obstruction.

○ **What is the significance of the anatomic landmark along the convex border of the kidney called "Brodel white line?"**

It is often mistaken for the relative avascular plane of the kidney used to gain access to the renal collecting system during an anatrophic nephrolithotomy. The white line of Brodel is a longitudinal crease 1 to 2 cm ventral to the convex border of the kidney. The actual location of the avascular longitudinal plane lies 1 to 2 cm dorsal to the convex border of the kidney between the posterior segmental circulation and the anterior.

○ **Within the nephron of the kidney, describe the location and function of the juxtaglomerular apparatus.**

The juxtaglomerular apparatus is a specialized association between the proximal aspect of the distal convoluted tubule and the afferent renal arteriole. Specialized macula densa cells within the renal tubule detect changes with intratubular sodium concentration. They communicate with juxtaglomerular cells of the afferent arteriole that are responsible for secreting renin into the afferent arteriole and renal lymph. The juxtaglomerular cells will respond to changes in wall tension and receive input from renal nerves that can stimulate renin secretion.

○ **Within the renal collecting system, what is the significance of compound papillae?**

When 2 renal pyramids fuse during their development, they form a "compound" papillae. They usually occur at the renal poles. Their physiologic significance lies in the fact that the configuration of the collecting ducts (of Bellini) allows for reflux of urine and potentially bacteria into the kidney. Renal parenchymal scarring secondary to infection is typically most severe, overlying these compound papillae.

○ **Describe the anatomy of a major calyx.**

There are usually 2 to 3 major calyces within a kidney. Each major calyx receives 2 or more infundibula, each of which drains 2 or more minor calyces.

○ **Describe the muscle layers of the ureter.**

The smooth muscle layers of the ureter orient themselves in 2 layers: the inner longitudinal layer and an outer layer of circular and oblique muscle. The ureter's muscle wall is thickest in its pelvic portion. The circular and oblique fibers become integrated into the smooth muscle of the bladder and Waldeyer ring. The inner longitudinal muscle fibers traverse the intramural ureter toward the ureteral orifice and trigone.

○ **What are the 3 distinct narrowings normally present along the course of the ureter?**

The first of these is the ureteropelvic junction, the second is the crossing of the iliac vessels, and the third is the ureterovesical junction within the bladder.

○ **Which of these is the smallest?**

The ureterovesical junction is usually the most narrow.

○ **What is the nomenclature used to describe ureteral segments intraoperatively and for radiologic purposes?**

The ureter can be divided into an abdominal and pelvic portion. The abdominal ureter extends from the renal pelvis to the iliac vessels. The pelvic portion extends from the iliac vessels down to the bladder. For radiologic purposes, the ureter can be divided into proximal, middle, and distal segments. The proximal segment extends from the renal pelvis to the upper border of the sacrum. The mid-ureter lies between the upper and lower borders of the sacrum. The distal ureteral segment extends from the lower border of the sacrum to the bladder.

○ **Describe the innervation of the kidney.**

The kidney receives preganglionic sympathetic fibers from T8 (thoracic) through L1 (lumbar) spinal segments. Postganglionic fibers arise from celiac and periaortic ganglia. Parasympathetic innervation arises from the lesser and lower splanchnic nerves as well as the vagus nerve.

○   **Describe the innervation of the ureter.**

The ureter receives preganglionic sympathetic fibers from T10 through L2 spinal segments. Postganglionic fibers arise from ganglia in the aortorenal, superior, and inferior hypogastric plexus. Parasympathetic input arises from the second through fourth sacral spinal segments.

○   **Does the ureter require autonomic innervation to maintain peristalsis?**

Intrinsic pacemaker sites located in the minor calices of the collecting system initiate the contraction, which is then propagated down the ureter.

○   **What is necessary for any abdominal hernia (including inguinal hernias) to occur?**

A defect (weakness) in the transversalis fascia, which is the outer stratum of the retroperitoneal connective tissue, is essential for a hernia to occur.

○   **When performing laparoscopic port placement in the lower abdomen, what vessels of the anterior abdominal wall can be injured leading to significant, often unrecognized bleeding?**

Inferior epigastric vessels; these vessels originate from the external iliac arteries and traverse in a cranial direction posterior to the body of the rectus muscle and anterior to the posterior rectus sheath. Laparoscopic ports will often tamponade (mask) injury to these vessels only later to be recognized at the time of port removal or postoperatively as a posterior rectus hematoma. The surgical principle of checking all port sites prior to proceeding will identify this injury early, which is amenable to either open or laparoscopic suture ligation.

○   **What perforating vessels of the anterior abdominal wall help identify the midline of the fascia?**

The musculocutaneous perforators from the superior and inferior epigastric arteries that perforate the anterior rectus fascia providing circulation to the dermis and skin. They emerge at regular intervals, approximately 2 to 4 cm cranial caudally and 2 cm off midline. Encountering these vessels can help the surgeon correct their midline approach. Ligation or cautery of these vessels can lead to fat necrosis and devascularization of the skin.

○   **What is the lymphatic drainage of the left kidney and the right kidney?**

Left kidney drains into the left para-aortic nodes; right kidney drains into the right paracaval lymph nodes. In either case, the lymph nodes can lie anterior, lateral, or posterior to the aorta and vena cava, respectively. Infrequently, lymph nodes may be classified as hilar lymph nodes based on their association with renal hilum instead of regional lymph nodes. To insure adequate lymph node sampling during radical nephrectomy, a staging lymphadenectomy may be required.

○   **What is the Pringle maneuver?**

It is the compression of the portal triad in order to arrest hepatic blood flow during complicated inferior vena cava thrombectomy. Care is taken not to injure the structures of the portal triad, including the hepatic artery, portal vein, and common bile duct as well as minimizing the warm ischemia time during clamping.

○   **What vessel associated with the posterior lateral border of Gerota fascia can lead to persistent annoying bleeding during radical nephrectomy?**

The renal capsular vein that connects the renal capsular plexus with the venous drainage of the posterior abdominal wall exiting at the intersection of the transversus abdominis and quadratus lumborum muscles with the iliac crest. This vessel is one of many that can get quite large if parasitized by a renal tumor.

○ **What fascia layer is often mistaken for Gerota (perirenal fascia) during an open-flank approach to the kidney?**

Transversalis fascia, lying deep to the thoracolumbar fascia and covering the pararenal fat, together mimicking the perirenal fascia and perirenal fat that surrounds the kidney.

○ **What are the most ventral renal structures coursing over the isthmus of a Horseshoe kidney?**

The ureters.

○ **What is the cisterna chyli and where is it located?**

The cisterna chili is located posterior medial to the aorta. It drains into the thoracic duct that enters the chest medial to the right crus of the diaphragm. The cisterna chyli is the confluence of the left and right lymphatic trunks, each with anterior and posterior branches to the renal vessels. Injury to the lymphatics at this level can result in chylous ascites.

○ **Do the lumbar sympathetic nerves travel anterior or posterior to the vena cava?**

Posterior, often located cranial to the junction of the lumbar veins and the posterior vena cava.

○ **What structures lie anterior to the hilum of the left kidney?**

The tail of the pancreas, the splenic artery, and the splenic vein.

○ **What are the various orientations of the right ureter to the vena cava?**

Paracaval (normal) and retrocaval (circumcaval).

○ **Where do the gonadal arteries originate?**

From the ventral abdominal aorta, cranial to the inferior mesenteric artery and caudal to the renal arteries.

○ **What nerve is seen exciting behind the psoas major muscle at the L2 level, traveling on top of the quadratus lumborum muscle in a lateral direction over the iliacus muscle?**

The lateral femoral cutaneous nerve of the thigh. Other obvious nerves in this area include the genitofemoral nerve, which is more medial and runs on top of the psoas muscle, and the ilioinguinal and iliohypogastric nerves, which lie lateral and more cranial to the lateral femoral cutaneous nerve.

○ **Describe the association of the pleura to the 11th and 12th ribs.**

The majority of the 11th rib and the dorsal–lateral half of the 12th rib. The 11th and 12th ribs are free-floating ribs that help the surgeon plan percutaneous, laparoscopic, and open surgical approaches to the kidneys. The pleura lie on the inner surface of the rib, medial to the insertion of the intercostal muscles, and superior to the diaphragmatic insertion.

○ **The most important lumbar nerves for preserving antegrade ejaculation arise from which sympathetic ganglia?**

L3 and L4 sympathetic ganglia.

○ **Parasympathetic fibers reach the inferior mesenteric plexus via what nerves?**

Pelvic splanchnic nerves via the superior hypogastric plexus.

CHAPTER 4

Surgical Anatomy of the Pelvis

Bilal Chughtai, MD, Alexis E. Te, MD,
Vladimir Yutkin, MD,
Jonathan I. Izawa, MD, FRCSC, and
Cameron Ghaffary, BS

BONY ANATOMY AND PELVIC SPACES

○ **Which is the thinnest of the pelvic bones?**

The pubic bones, which are often fractured in blunt pelvic trauma. Their fragments may injure the bladder, urethra, and vagina.

○ **True/False: The sacroiliac (SI) joint is often fractured in pelvic trauma.**

False. The synovial SI joint gains additional strength from anterior and posterior ligaments and fractures rarely involve this joint.

○ **Where is Bogros space, what does it represent, and what are its anatomical limits?**

Bogros space is located at the pelvic opening of the spermatic cord. It is lateral and superior to Retzius space. It represents the retroinguinal preperitoneium. Its limits are:

- Medially: Epigastric vessels, spermatic cord, iliac vessels, and space of Retzius.
- Anteriorly: Transversalis muscle.
- Laterally: Psoas muscle and lateral cutaneous nerve.

○ **Where is the border between the true and false pelvis?**

The boundary between the 2 is the arcuate line that starts at the superior pubic ramus and extends to the sacral promontory.

○ **How many openings are there in the true bony pelvis? Name them.**

Eight. Paired—greater and lesser sciatic foramina, obturator foramina; nonpaired—pelvic inlet and pelvic outlet.

○ **What effect has congenital nonunion or resection of the pubic symphysis on the ambulation of the patient?**

It does not have any significant effect owing to the strength of the SI joint.

○ **What are the major osseous ligaments of the pelvis?**

Sacroiliac, pubic symphysis, sacrococcygeal, and sacrosciatic.

○ **What passes through the anourogenital hiatus?**

Urethra, vagina (females), and rectum.

○ **What are the boundaries of the greater sciatic foramen?**

Laterally and superiorly: Greater sciatic notch.
Medially: Sacrotuberous ligament.

○ **What structures are found in Alcock canal and what is another name for Alcock canal?**

The pudendal (Alcock) canal runs approximately 4 cm above the lower ridge of ischial tuberosity and contains the pudendal artery, pudendal veins, and the pudendal nerve; all are invested in connective tissue, binding these structures to the perineal surface of the obturator internus fascia.

VASCULAR ANATOMY

○ **True/False: As the dorsal vein of the penis passes within the pelvis under the pubic arch it forms a venous complex and part of this complex runs within the anterior and lateral walls of the striated urinary sphincter.**

True. One must be cautious during ligation and division of the dorsal venous complex, as damage to the striated sphincter can occur.

○ **What anatomic reason may account for the relatively higher incidence of axial skeletal and pelvic bone metastases in patients with metastatic prostate cancer, as opposed to lung metastases for example?**

There are numerous interconnections between the pelvic venous plexuses and the emissary veins of the pelvic bones and vertebral venous plexuses, which may be routes of dissemination of infection or tumor from the diseased prostate.

○ **What artery has its origin off the inferior epigastric artery and can be identified medial to the femoral vein during pelvic surgery?**

The accessory obturator artery arises from the inferior epigastric artery in 25% of patients and continues on through the obturator canal.

○ **Following a radical dissection of inguinal lymph nodes for penile carcinoma, the surgeon decided to cover the area with a rectus myocutaneous flap. Where does the blood supply come from for this flap?**

Ipsilateral inferior epigastric artery.

○ **What is the most common origin of the superior vesical artery?**

The proximal portion of the obliterated umbilical artery.

○ **What structures besides the rectum does the middle rectal artery supply?**

The middle rectal artery anastomoses with the superior and inferior rectal arteries to supply the rectum. It also gives small branches to provide additional arterial supply to the seminal vesicles and prostate.

○ **What accessory vein drains into the inferior surface of the external iliac vein in at least 50% of patients?**

The accessory obturator vein. Care must be taken to not tear this vein at the time of pelvic lymph node dissection.

○ **True/False: Intramural longitudinal vessels run the length of the ureter in 75% of patients.**

True. These vessels are formed by anastomoses of segmental ureteral vessels. In the other 25% of patients, the intramural ureteral vessels form a fine interconnecting mesh with less collateral flow and render the ureter more prone to ischemic insult. This intramural, interconnecting meshlike vascular pattern is often found in the pelvic ureter, and therefore, this portion of the ureter is less suited for ureteroureterostomy.

○ **What is one of the main reasons that the primary repair of the pelvic ureter is often prone to strictures?**

The blood supply of the pelvic ureter is based on longitudinal collaterals that run along it, which are often severed following both the primary injury to the ureter and subsequent mobilization during its repair, thus limiting its blood supply with a high risk for ischemic strictures.

○ **What arteries usually supply the ureter with its largest pelvic branches?**

The inferior vesical and uterine arteries.

○ **In a normal adult male, at what anatomic location are the ureters closest to each other?**

The ureters are closest and are located within 5 cm of each other as they cross the iliac vessels.

○ **What is the principal arterial supply to prostatic adenomas in benign prostatic hyperplasia and where are the origin and principal branches of the prostatic artery?**

The inferior vesical arteries have urethral artery branches that enter the prostate posterolaterally at its junction with the bladder and these branches are the principal arterial supply to the adenomas. There is also a capsular branch. The short segment at the end of the inferior vesical artery after all the branches to the bladder but before the bifurcation between the capsular and urethral branches is called the prostatic artery. It can be embolized in selected cases for treatment of benign prostatic hyperplasia (BPH) or intractable prostatic bleeding.

○ **What structures do the uterine arteries supply?**

The proximal vagina, uterus, and medial two-thirds of the fallopian tubes.

○ **When an accessory pudendal artery is present and is supplementing or replacing the penile arterial supply by the common penile artery, what is its origin?**

An accessory pudendal artery is present in approximately 4% of patients undergoing a radical retropubic prostatectomy and arises from the inferior vesical artery, superior vesical artery, and obturator artery.

○ **What are the anatomic relations of the internal pudendal artery in the male?**

The internal pudendal artery in the male lies anterior to the piriformis muscle, sacral plexus of nerves, and the inferior gluteal artery. As it crosses the ischial spine, it is covered by the gluteus maximus muscle and overlapped by the sacrotuberous ligament. The pudendal nerve is medial to the artery while the nerve to the obturator internus muscle is lateral to the internal pudendal artery.

○ **What is the anatomic course of the accessory pudendal artery in relation to the prostate gland?**

It runs anterolateral to or within the prostate to reach the penis.

○ **What is the relation of spermatic cord to the deep external pudendal artery?**

The spermatic cord is crossed posteriorly by it.

○ **If the right internal iliac artery was ligated, what principal vessels might contribute to collateral circulation?**

The following would possibly allow collateral circulation:
- The ovarian artery from the aorta with the uterine artery.
- The vesical arteries of the contralateral side with the same vessels on the ligated side.
- The middle rectal artery branches of the internal iliac artery with the superior rectal artery from the inferior mesenteric artery.
- The obturator artery with the inferior epigastric artery and the medial femoral circumflex artery, and by means of the pubic branch of the obturator artery, with the same vessels from the contralateral side.
- The circumflex artery with perforating branches of the deep femoral artery and the inferior gluteal artery.
- The superior gluteal artery with the posterior branches of the lateral sacral arteries.
- The iliolumbar artery with the last lumbar artery.
- The lateral sacral artery with the middle sacral artery.
- The iliac circumflex artery with the iliolumbar and the superior gluteal arteries.

○ **Where is the aortic bifurcation relatively to the spine?**

The aorta gives rise to 2 common iliac arteries at the level of 4th lumbar vertebra.

○ **What artery arises posteriorly at the level of the aortic bifurcation and what does it supply?**

It is the middle sacral artery and it supplies the sacral foramina and the rectum.

○ **Does the blood supply to the pelvic ureter enter laterally or medially?**

Laterally. The pelvic peritoneum should be incised only medial to the ureter.

○ **What are the branches of the internal iliac artery?**

The posterior trunk gives rise to 3 parietal branches: The superior gluteal, the ascending lumbar, and the lateral sacral branches. The anterior trunk gives rise to 7 branches: The superior vesical, the middle rectal, the inferior vesical, the uterine, the internal pudendal, the obturator, and the inferior gluteal branches.

○ **What are the sources of collateral blood supply to the pelvic organs in the case of bilateral ligation of the internal iliac arteries due to massive hemorrhage?**

Aortic branches (middle sacral and lumbar arteries) and inferior mesenteric branches (inferior mesenteric artery).

○ **What are the pelvic organs that do not receive blood supply from the internal iliac artery?**

Gonads (testicles and ovaries) and superior part of the rectum.

○ **True/False: In a nerve-sparing cystoprostatectomy, the unilateral internal iliac artery should be ligated and divided to improve hemostasis and facilitate the nerve-sparing procedure, thereby possibly maintaining erectile function.**

False. The internal iliac artery should be preserved and the superior vesical artery should be ligated and divided proximally in order to maintain the integrity of the internal pudendal artery and to prevent vasculogenic erectile dysfunction.

○ **Which blood vessels run in Camper fascia?**

The superficial circumflex iliac, external pudendal, and superficial inferior epigastric vessels. They are branches of the femoral vessels.

○ **What 2 branches of the external iliac artery are within the pelvis?**

The inferior epigastric and the deep circumflex iliac arteries.

○ **At what anatomic site does the internal iliac artery branch into its anterior and posterior trunks?**

The greater sciatic foramen.

○ **Where is the origin of the obturator artery?**

The obturator artery has a variable origin. It can arise from the anterior trunk of the internal iliac artery, the inferior epigastric artery, or the inferior gluteal artery.

○ **What are the branches of the obturator artery within the pelvis?**

The iliac, vesical, and pubic arterial branches. The iliac branches ascend in the iliac fossa and supply the iliacus muscle and ilium, while anastomosing with branches of the iliolumbar artery. The vesical branch courses medially and posteriorly to help supply the bladder. The pubic branch arises from the obturator artery just before it leaves the pelvis and ascends inside the pelvis to communicate with the same vessel on the contralateral side and with the inferior epigastric vessels.

○ **The middle sacral vein is usually a tributary of which vein?**

The left common iliac vein.

○ **What are the origins of the arteries that supply the seminal vesicles?**

These arteries are derived from the middle vesical, inferior vesical, and middle rectal arteries.

○ **What is the venous drainage of the vagina?**

The venous drainage occurs by means of the vaginal plexus of veins along the lateral aspect of the vagina. These are in continuity with the uterine, vesical, and rectal venous plexuses. The vaginal plexuses are drained by 1 or 2 vaginal veins on each side that flow into the internal iliac veins either directly or through the connections with the internal pudendal veins.

○ **During a radical cystectomy (anterior exenteration) and an ileal conduit in a 65-year-old female, the vagina is observed to have very good vascular supply when the anterior wall is resected en bloc with the specimen. What is the main arterial supply to the vagina?**

The vaginal arteries, which can be represented by 1, 2, or 3 arterial vessels. These include arterial branches that can arise from the uterine artery, inferior vesical artery, or separate arterial branches directly from the anterior trunk of the internal iliac artery.

○ **In what percentage of patients undergoing radical retropubic prostatectomy does the superficial dorsal vein of the penis appear to be absent?**

Approximately 10%.

○ **During a radical cystectomy and pelvic lymph node dissection, care should be taken to avoid dissection below the presacral fascia. Why?**

This dissection may disturb the presacral veins and cause unnecessary blood loss.

○ **What is the arterial supply to the rectum?**

- Inferior mesenteric artery to superior rectal
- Internal iliac artery to middle rectal
- Internal iliac to internal pudendal to inferior rectal

○ **What 2 tubular structures can be identified near the cervico-uterine junction upon opening the broad ligament between the round ligament and the infundibulopelvic ligament?**

Uterine artery and, beneath it, the ureter.

○ **What life-threatening complication can occur while dissecting posterior to the rectum?**

Damage to the presacral venous plexus can be massive and very difficult to control.

LYMPH NODES AND DRAINAGE

○ **To what nodal locations do the lymphatics of the vas deferens and seminal vesicles drain?**

The external and internal iliac lymph nodes.

○ **True/False: The external iliac lymph nodes can be further separated anatomically and functionally into 3 chains.**

True. The external, middle, and internal chains. For example, the external chain does not receive any lymphatic drainage from organs within the pelvis and these lymph nodes are located lateral to the external iliac vessels.

○ **What is the lymph node of Cloquet anatomic location?**

The lymph node of Cloquet lies within the femoral canal, medial to the external iliac vein, and beneath the inguinal ligament.

○ **Lymphatics from the pelvis and testes cross the midline at what level?**

At the level of the renal hilum.

○ **How many external iliac lymph nodes are usually present in the normal adult and what is their anatomic arrangement?**

There are usually 8 to 10 external iliac lymph nodes that lie along the external iliac vessels. They are arranged in 3 groups. One group is on the lateral aspect, another on the medial aspect, and a third group on the anterior aspect of the external iliac vessels. The third group of lymph nodes on the anterior aspect of the vessels is sometimes absent.

○ **What are the primary lymph nodes that drain the uterus?**

The external and internal iliac nodes, obturator nodes, para-aortic nodes (accompanying the drainage of ovary), and superficial inguinal nodes (through round ligament).

○ **How does a previous inguinal surgery (ie, orchiopexy) influence the possible distribution of metastatic disease in testicular cancer?**

It can alter the lymphatic drainage, hence allowing additional routes for lymphogenic spread, for example to inguinal, iliac, and obturator lymph nodes.

NERVES AND INNERVATION

○ **During a psoas hitch procedure (fixation of the urinary bladder to the psoas muscle with sutures), in which direction should the sutures be placed and why?**

The sutures should be placed in the direction of the muscle fibers and femoral nerve to avoid femoral nerve entrapment or damage due to the nerve passing within the substance of the psoas muscle. Caution must also be taken with retractor blades on the psoas muscle for prolonged periods, as this may also cause a femoral nerve palsy affecting ipsilateral knee extension.

○ **Which nerve is located lateral to the psoas muscle in the iliacus fascia?**

The lateral femoral cutaneous nerve.

○ **During a radical cystectomy in a 65-year-old male patient for clinical T3a transitional cell carcinoma of the bladder, you notice a nerve visible on the surface of the right psoas major muscle has been damaged by an electrosurgical injury. Which nerve is this and what sensory loss do you anticipate this patient may experience if the nerve function cannot be salvaged?**

The right genitofemoral nerve has been injured. Sensory loss to the anterior right thigh below the inguinal ligament and the anterior right hemiscrotum may occur.

○ **A 67-year-old male patient, 3 months postradical retropubic prostatectomy, but otherwise healthy, describes difficulty in moving his left leg into the car when he is on the driver's side. He has noticed this only in the postoperative period. What nerve injury likely occurred during his surgery?**

The patient likely sustained a left obturator nerve injury. The obturator nerve supplies the adductor muscles of the ipsilateral thigh.

○ **Where is the obturator nerve located in relation to the obturator artery and vein?**

The obturator nerve lies lateral and superior to the obturator vessels.

○ **During a sacrospinous colposuspension, which nerve or nerve plexus is at relatively high risk of injury?**

The risk of injury is to the sacral plexus, as it leaves the pelvis via the greater sciatic foramen and is immediately posterior to the sacrospinous ligament. If injured, there may be sensory and motor nerve supply compromise to the posterior thigh and lower leg.

○ **Where is the sacral plexus located?**

The sacral plexus is located on the surface of the piriformis muscle, deep to the endopelvic fascia, and posterior to the internal iliac vessels.

○ **Which nerve passes through the greater sciatic foramen and supplies sensory branches to the perineum and posterior aspect of the scrotum?**

The posterior femoral cutaneous nerve.

○ **Can a local anesthetic alone achieve a complete prostatic block?**

Yes. It must be instilled into the pelvic plexus to block all afferent neurons.

○ **During a radical retropubic prostatectomy, where are the cavernosal nerves most vulnerable?**

At the apex of the prostate, where they closely approach the prostatic capsule at the 5- and 7-o'clock positions.

○ **What are the anatomic relations of the communicating nerve fibers of the left and right components of the pelvic plexus?**

These fibers communicate posterior to the rectum, as well as anterior and posterior to the bladder neck.

○ **True/False: There is no pelvic parasympathetic efferent innervation to the descending and sigmoid colon.**

False. Some pelvic parasympathetic efferent fibers travel up the hypogastric nerves to the inferior mesenteric plexus, where they will subsequently provide innervation to the descending and sigmoid colon.

○ **True/False: The pelvic ureter has rich adrenergic and cholinergic autonomic nerve supply and will lose its peristaltic activity if it is denervated.**

False. The ureter will continue to have peristaltic activity despite its pelvic denervation. This is driven from pacemakers in the upper urinary tract.

○ **True/False: Bilateral pudendal nerve injury will cause loss of striated external sphincter function at the level of the membranous urethra.**

False. The striated sphincter has additional somatic nerve supply from a branch of the sacral plexus and it is located on the levator ani. Autonomic innervation from the cavernous nerves is also present, but this may not be sufficient for urinary continence.

○ **What course do the nerves from the pelvic plexus travel to reach the female pelvic viscera?**

The nerves from the pelvic plexus travel through the cardinal and uterosacral ligaments. During a hysterectomy, these ligaments are divided and therefore may result in a neurogenic bladder.

○ **Which nerve crosses the distal end of the external iliac artery?**

The genital branch of the genitofemoral nerve.

○ **True/False: Presacral neurectomies are reasonably effective in relieving bladder pain.**

False. Afferent innervation from the bladder travels with the parasympathetic nerves as well as the sympathetic nerves, which travel via the hypogastric nerves.

○ **What spinal nerve root or roots supply the cremasteric muscle?**

Spinal nerve root S-4.

○ **Describe the course of the cavernosal nerves in the pelvis.**

They originate from the most caudal portion of the pelvic plexus, then pass the tips of the seminal vesicles and lie within leaves of the lateral endopelvic fascia near its juncture with, but outside, Denonvilliers fascia. They travel at the posterolateral border of the prostate on the surface of the rectum and are lateral to the prostatic capsular vessels.

○ **Where is the location and anatomic orientation of the pelvic plexus?**

The pelvic plexus is rectangular, 4 to 5 cm in length, oriented in the sagittal plane and is located at its midpoint at the tip of the seminal vesicles.

○ **What structure is often described as the inferolateral limit of a pelvic lymph node dissection in a radical cystectomy?**

The genitofemoral nerves. The fibroareolar tissue is divided medial to this structure in a pelvic lymph node dissection during a radical cystectomy.

○ **What neural structure can be damaged while performing radical inguinal orchiectomy?**

The ilioinguinal nerve, which lies inferior to the spermatic cord as it traverses the inguinal canal.

○ **While extracting the seminal vesicles during a radical prostatectomy the surgeon encountered difficulty in dissection. What neural structures can be damaged while removing the seminal vesicles?**

Hypogastric (pelvic) neural plexus carries within it presynaptic parasympathetic nerve fibers which further on their course become the cavernosal nerves, injury to which can cause postoperative impotence.

○ **What sensory and motor deficits can follow Gibson and inguinal abdominal wall incisions?**

Iliohypogastric (L1) and ilioinguinal (L1) nerves emerge from the lumbosacral plexus and provide the muscle innervation to internal oblique and transversus muscles and sensory supply to the skin of the posterior gluteal and suprapubic regions (iliohypogastric) and the skin of the medial thigh and genital region (ilioinguinal).

○   **What is the location of the presynaptic sympathetic and parasympathetic cell bodies that project to the pelvic autonomic plexus?**

Sympathetic: Lateral column of gray matter in T10-12 and L1-2.

Parasympathetic: Intermediolateral cell column of the sacral cord.

○   **What effect will stimulation of parasympathetic nerve fibers from S2-4 segments have?**

Vasodilatation of the cavernosal artery of penis with resultant tumescence.

MUSCLES, LIGAMENTS, AND FASCIAL LAYERS

○   **What is the origin of the muscles of the pelvic diaphragm?**

The origin of the pubococcygeus and iliococcygeus muscles is the tendinous arch of the levator ani.

○   **What types of muscle fibers make up the pelvic diaphragm?**

Type 1 (slow-twitch), for tonic support to the pelvic structure, and type 2 (fast-twitch), for rapid increases in intra-abdominal pressure, muscle fibers.

○   **What are the walls of the pelvic cavity?**

Posterior: Sacrum, piriformis muscles.

Lateral: Hip bones, obturator internus muscles.

Anterior: Bodies of pubic bones, pubic symphysis.

Inferior wall: Muscular pelvic diaphragm.

○   **What are the muscles of the false pelvis?**

Rectus abdominis, psoas major, and iliacus.

○   **True/False: Longitudinal smooth muscle fibers from the rectum join Denonvilliers fascia.**

True. The fibers are located anteriorly at the inferior portion of the rectal ampulla.

○   **During a radical cystectomy/anterior exenteration in a 65-year-old female patient with clinical T3a transitional cell carcinoma of the bladder, what ligaments are part of the lateral and posterior bladder pedicles that will be divided?**

The cardinal and uterosacral ligaments.

○   **What is the muscle that connects the rectum, posterior Denonvilliers fascia, and the posterior striated urinary sphincter?**

The rectourethralis muscle.

○ **Is smooth muscle present within the puboprostatic ligaments?**

Yes. There are smooth muscle fibers within the puboprostatic ligaments derived from the outer layer of detrusor musculature. Once the puboprostatic ligaments are divided during a radical retropubic prostatectomy, the ligaments contract due to their smooth muscle components and are no longer apparent.

○ **What 3 muscles combine to make up the pubococcygeus muscle in the female?**

The pubococcygeus muscle is a thick "V-shaped" muscle band comprising 3 sections—the pubovaginalis muscle anteriorly, the puborectalis muscle, and the puboanalis muscle. These muscles pull the rectum, vagina, and urethra anteriorly against the pubic bone to compress the lumen of each.

○ **What is the primary muscular component of urethral support in the female?**

The pubovaginalis muscle, which is the most anterior part of the levator ani.

○ **While performing the incision for a radical retropubic prostatectomy, the pyramidalis muscle is observed to be present. What is the innervation of this muscle and what happens when it contracts?**

The 12th thoracic nerve. Contraction of this muscle tenses the linea alba.

○ **Is the configuration of the pelvic diaphragm flat, bowl-shaped, or near vertical?**

At the urogenital and anal hiatus, the muscles lie in a near-vertical configuration.

○ **Name the muscles of the true pelvis.**

Piriformis, coccygeus, obturator internus, and the Levator ani.

○ **What are the parts of levator ani muscle?**

Ischiococcygeus, iliococcygeus, and pubococcygeus. Pubococcygeus is further subdivided into puboperinealis, puboprostaticus or pubovaginalis, puboanalis, and puborectalis.

○ **What are the insertion points of levator ani muscle?**

Ischiococcygeus: From pelvic surface and tip of ischial spine to lateral margin of coccyx and lower sacral segments. Iliococcygeus: From inner surface of ischial spine and tendinous arch of levator ani to the tip of the sacrum and the coccyx and anococcygeal ligament. Pubococcygeus: From inferior part of the pubic bone and to urethra (including external sphincter complex), prostate/vagina, perineal body, anal canal, and anococcygeal ligament.

○ **What is the origin and insertion of the pyramidalis muscle?**

It arises from the pubic crest and inserts into the linea alba.

○ **What abdominal muscle layer is in continuity with the cremasteric muscle?**

The internal oblique muscle.

○ **The endopelvic fascia is continuous with which layer of the abdominal wall?**

The transversalis fascia.

○ **What structures can be injured if the incision in the endopelvic fascia made during a radical retropubic prostatectomy is too deep?**

The pudendal artery and nerve, which are located just deep to iliococcygeus muscle and run along the inferior pubic ramus.

○ **What organs does the inner stratum cover in the pelvis and what is its clinical importance?**

The inner stratum covers the rectum and the dome of the bladder. It also forms Denonvilliers fascia, which acts as a barrier between the rectum and prostate, which contributes to the low rate of local extension of prostate cancer into the rectum.

○ **What forms the arcus tendineus fascia pelvis?**

Fusion of the visceral and parietal components of the pelvic fascia forms the arcus tendineus fascia pelvis. It appears as a white line of condensation within the pelvis that runs in a sulcus lateral to the prostate from the puboprostatic ligaments to the ischial spine.

○ **What fascial structure extends medially from the arcus tendineus fascia in the female pelvis and what is its clinical significance?**

This structure is referred to as the periurethral, pubovesical, or urethropelvic ligament, and it provides support to the urethra and anterior vaginal wall. Compromise to this fascia may contribute to stress urinary incontinence, bladder neck hypermobility, cystocele, or urethrocele formation.

○ **During a radical retropubic prostatectomy, the endopelvic fascia is divided lateral to the arcus tendineus fascia pelvis and is mobilized off the levator ani medially with the prostate. Is this endopelvic fascia visceral or parietal?**

It is the parietal endopelvic fascia.

○ **What is unique about the Cherney incision?**

This incision involves access to the pelvic cavity and detaches the rectus muscles from the symphysis.

○ **Describe the medial and inferior limits of Scarpa fascia.**

Inferiorly, it fuses with the deep fascia of the thigh 1 cm below the inguinal ligament along a line from the anterior superior iliac spine to the pubic tubercle. Medially, it is continuous with Colles fascia of the perineum.

○ **What is the anatomical basis for a butterfly hematoma in the perineum?**

Colles fascia attaches to the ischiopubic rami laterally and to the posterior edge of the perineal membrane, hence limiting the spread of blood and urine following injury.

○ **Colles fascia is continuous with what other fascia of the penis and scrotum?**

Colles fascia is continuous with the dartos fascia of the penis and scrotum.

○ **Where is the arcuate line and what is its significance?**

The arcuate line is located two-thirds of the distance from the pubis to the umbilicus, and is the point at which all aponeurotic layers abruptly pass anterior to the rectus abdominis leaving this muscle clothed only by transversalis fascia and peritoneum posteriorly.

○ **What is the difference in the posterior lining of rectus abdominis muscle above and below the arcuate line?**

The aponeurosis of internal oblique muscle passes anterior to the rectus abdominis below the arcuate line.

○ **What are the boundaries of the inguinal canal?**

Floor—Inguinal ligament and lower border of external oblique aponeurosis.

Posterior wall—Transversalis fascia and conjoint tendon in medial third.

Roof—Fibers of conjoint tendon.

External oblique aponeurosis and internal oblique muscle in lateral third.

○ **What is the origin of the external spermatic fascia?**

The aponeurosis of external oblique muscle.

○ **What hernia has its internal opening between the inguinal ligament from above and the superior pubic ramus from below?**

A femoral hernia.

○ **What structures can be injured by a paramedian incision lateral to the rectus and what problems ensue?**

The last 6 thoracic segmental nerves enter the rectus abdominis laterally to supply it; division of these nerves can cause atrophy of the rectus and may predispose to ventral hernia. The inferior epigastric vessels may also be injured.

○ **At the start of a robotic transperitoneal radical prostatectomy, what folds are visible on the internal surface of the anterior abdominal wall and what do they contain?**

Approached laparoscopically, 3 elevations of the peritoneum, referred to as the median, medial, and lateral folds, are visible below the umbilicus. The median fold overlies the urachus; the medial fold covers the obliterated umbilical artery; and the lateral fold is over the inferior epigastric vessels.

○ **Why is the medial umbilical fold an important landmark for the surgeon?**

It contains the obliterated umbilical artery, which may be traced to its origin from the internal iliac artery to locate the ureter, which lies on its medial side.

○ **What are the narrowest sites of the pelvic ureter?**

Where the ureter crosses the iliac vessels and at ureterovesical junction.

○ **What layers of the abdominal wall are encountered during a Gibson incision?**
- The aponeurosis of the external oblique.
- The internal oblique muscle.
- The transversus abdominis muscle.

○ **What are the components of the broad ligament of the uterus?**
Mesosalpinx, mesovarium, and mesometrium.

○ **What structures will be found upon opening the infundibulopelvic ligament near its attachment to the lateral pelvic wall?**
External iliac vessels, ureter, and genitofemoral nerve.

○ **During radical cystectomy and anterior pelvic exenteration in a young female patient the decision was made to preserve the ovaries—which uterine support structures should be preserved and which ligated?**
The infundibulopelvic ligament (with blood supply to the ovary) should be preserved, while the utero-ovarian and round ligaments are divided.

○ **What stratum of pelvic fascia gives the origin to the suspensory ligaments of inner pelvic organs?**
Suspensory ligaments (eg, cardinal, posterior vesical, and uterosacral) arise from the intermediate stratum of pelvic fascia.

○ **Which of the pelvic floor muscles do not insert into the perineal body?**
All the pelvic muscles and fascia insert into the perineal body.

○ **What structure forms the superior, lateral, and inferior borders of the saphenous opening?**
The superficial stratum of the fascia lata.

○ **What are the compartments of the femoral sheath?**
Femoral artery (lateral), femoral vein (intermediate), and the femoral canal that contains lymph vessels and the occasional lymph node (medial).

○ **What muscles are attached to the pubic tubercle?**
Cremaster muscle and partially the rectus abdominis and pyramidalis muscles.

○ **How would you define the border between the sigmoid colon and the rectum?**
At the level of third sacral vertebra, the sigmoid mesocolon disappears, thus the rectum is technically situated in the retroperitoneum.

○ **What structure will be found upon incision of the anterior wall of the rectovesical pouch in the male?**
The seminal vesicles.

○　**Describe the course of the right ureter in the female pelvis.**

Passing medially at the level of the ischial spine, it lies behind the ovary in close association with the suspensory ligament of the ovary and forms the posterior limit of the ovarian fossa. The ovarian vessels make an oblique crossing over the ureter. Entering the parametrium of the broad ligament, it runs successively through the uterosacral ligament, the cardinal ligament, and the vesicouterine ligament. In its course, the ureter runs for a short distance with the uterine artery, which originates from the internal iliac artery and lies lateral and anterior to it.

BLADDER AND URETHRA

○　**What areas of a normal bladder may be more prone to diverticular formation?**

The dome of the bladder, where the urachus anchors the apex of the bladder to the anterior abdominal wall due to a paucity of detrusor muscle at this site. The hiatus in the detrusor, where the intramural ureter passes, is also more prone to diverticular formation.

○　**During cystoscopic examination of a normal bladder, the urothelium over the trigone appears relatively smooth compared to the surrounding urothelium. How is this explained?**

The urothelium over the trigone is usually 3 cells thick and the lamina propria is dense here with strongly adherent epithelial cells. Therefore, during changes in bladder volume, the trigonal epithelium remains smooth in appearance endoscopically.

○　**When completely filled, what is the approximate maximum capacity of the normal bladder?**

450 to 500 mL.

○　**What are the layers of the bladder?**

- Transitional epithelium
- Lamina propria
- Detrusor
- Inner longitudinal
- Middle circular
- Outer longitudinal

○　**What is the thickest part of the bladder?**

The bladder base.

○　**What are the distinct muscle layers of the trigone of the bladder?**

There are 3 layers:

1. A superficial layer, derived from the longitudinal muscle of the ureter.
2. A deep layer, which continues from Waldeyer sheath.
3. A detrusor layer, formed by the longitudinal and middle circular smooth muscle layers of the bladder wall.

○ **Where does the ureteral smooth muscle terminate distally?**

The verumontanum. The muscle of the trigone is made up of 3 distinct layers; the superficial layer, derived from the longitudinal smooth muscle of the ureter, extends down to the verumontanum.

○ **Is the bladder more richly supplied with sympathetic or parasympathetic nerves?**

Parasympathetic cholinergic nerve endings (mostly M2 and some M3) predominate.

○ **True/False: The bladder wall has many postganglionic cell bodies.**

True. The vast majority of these synapse with parasympathetic cholinergic nerve endings.

○ **What will be the effect of adrenergic sympathetic stimulation of the region of bladder neck and prostate?**

Contraction of smooth muscle of the area resulting in bladder neck closure and seminal emission.

○ **In what part of the spinal cord do you find the nerve fibers that mediate awareness of the bladder distention?**

In the posterior column (fasciculus gracilis).

○ **True/False: Presacral neurectomies are reasonably effective in relieving bladder pain.**

False. Afferent innervation from the bladder travels with the parasympathetic nerves as well as the sympathetic nerves, which travel via the hypogastric nerves.

○ **What arteries, besides the superior and inferior vesical, carry blood supply to the urinary bladder?**

Obturator and inferior gluteal arteries; in females, there are also branches from uterine and vaginal arteries.

○ **How is the venous drainage of the bladder different from normal venous drainage?**

Instead of following the arteries, the veins of the bladder drain into the lateral plexuses about the ureters and into the prostatovesical plexuses along with the deep dorsal vein of the penis and the cavernous vein. From the plexus, the veins run in the lateral prostatic ligaments to empty into the internal iliac veins.

○ **Where does the bulk of the lymphatic fluid from the bladder drain?**

The external iliac lymph nodes. Some drainage may go to the obturator, internal iliac, and common iliac lymph nodes.

○ **What are the 3 distinct sets of lymphatic vessels draining the bladder?**

1. Channels from the trigone area exit on the exterior of the bladder to run superolaterally.
2. Channels from dome join to the posterolateral angle and pass superolaterally.
3. Channels from the inferolateral surface go up to join those from the dome or run to the lymph nodes in the obturator fossa.

Most of these vessels end up in the obturator, hypogastric, and external iliac nodes, and can also reach common iliac, presacral, and even aortocaval regions.

○ **Does the urachus reach the umbilicus?**

The urachus does not usually reach the umbilicus in the adult; rather, it may terminate adjacent to one of the obliterated hypogastric arteries, or it may join both arteries, or it may be short and partially degenerate into the subumbilical fibrous plexus of Luschka.

○ **What is the type of epithelium that lines the urachus?**

In majority of cases it is transitional cell epithelium, sometimes colonic and small intestinal epithelium can be found.

○ **During emergency cesarean section the gynecologic surgeon noticed urine leaking into the field. What is the most common site of bladder injury during hysterectomy or cesarean section?**

At the posterior bladder wall just superior to the intraureteric ridge.

○ **What are the posterior relations of the urinary bladder in males and in females?**

Male: Rectum, sigmoid colon, and ileum.

Female: Proximal vagina, cervix and uterus, sigmoid colon, and ileum.

○ **What is the arterial blood supply of bulbar and penile urethra?**

Bulbourethral artery, which runs from bulbous urethra of the penis distally and the dorsal penile artery.

○ **What is the arterial blood supply of penile skin?**

Right and left superficial external pudendal arteries, which arise from the first portion of the femoral artery.

○ **What is the arterial blood supply of female urethra?**

Mainly from the vaginal artery and the inferior vesical artery.

○ **What are the parts of male urethra?**

Proximal (posterior) urethra: preprostatic, prostatic, membranous; distal (anterior): bulbar or bulbous, penile or pendulous, and the fossa navicularis.

○ **What does the verumontanum contain?**

It contains the prostatic utricle and the ejaculatory ducts.

○ **What anatomical structures are responsible for urinary continence at the level of membranous urethra?**

Folds of urethral mucosa, submucosal connective tissue, intrinsic urethral smooth muscle fibers, striated muscle fibers, and the pubourethral component of levator ani muscle.

○   **What will be the area of urine extravasation in the case of isolated bulbar urethral transection or the limits of extent of necrotizing fasciitis of the scrotum (Fournier gangrene)?**

Anteriorly and superiorly—toward the anterior and lateral abdominal wall deep to Scarpa fascia up to the clavicles. In the perineum, it is limited by the fusion of Colles fascia to the perineal membrane posteriorly and the ischiopubic rami laterally, thus the resulting collection will resemble a butterfly.

○   **What is the lining of the female urethra?**

Its lining changes gradually from transitional to nonkeratinized stratified squamous epithelium.

THE TESTIS

○   **What are the contents of the spermatic cord?**

Vas deferens, testicular artery and veins (pampiniform plexus), cremasteric artery, artery of vas deferens, the genital branch of the genitofemoral nerve, cremasteric nerve, and the sympathetic components of the testicular plexus.

○   **What are the origins of the collateral blood supply to the testis?**

Testicular artery—branch of aorta, cremasteric artery—branch of inferior epigastric artery, artery of vas deferens—branch of the superior vesical artery.

○   **Is there subcutaneous adipose tissue in the scrotum?**

No, the scrotal skin lacks this layer. The dartos muscle lays immediately beneath the skin.

○   **Where does the lymphatic drainage from the scrotal skin go?**

To the superficial inguinal nodes.

○   **What are the relations of the right testicular artery to other organs on its course from the aorta to the testis?**

Anterior to the inferior vena cava and posterior to the horizontal part of the duodenum, the right colic and ileocolic arteries, the root of the mesentery and terminal ileum.

○   **Where does the lymphatic drainage from the testes go?**

To the retroperitoneal lymph nodes.

○   **What is the type of germinal epithelium that lies outside the blood–testis barrier?**

Type A spermatogonia.

○   **True/false: The seminal vesicles and rectum are invested in the common fascial layer.**

False. The seminal vesicles are divided from the rectum by Denonvilliers fascia.

○   **Do the seminal vesicles have contact with parietal peritoneum?**

Yes, at their tips.

○ **True/false: The final stage of spermatozoa maturation occurs in the seminal vesicles.**

False. The spermatozoa are not stored in the seminal vesicles, but rather in the epididymis.

○ **What is the usual location of the appendix testis and what embryologic remnant does it represent?**

Located in the upper pole of the testis, it is a remnant of the Müllerian (paramesonephric) duct.

○ **What part of the epididymis gives rise to the vas deferens?**

The tail of the epididymis.

THE PENIS

○ **What are the 3 commonly recognized patterns of blood supply to the human penis?**

  1. Exclusively from internal pudendal arteries
  2. Both from accessory and internal pudendal arteries
  3. Exclusively from accessory pudendal arteries

○ **True/false: The 2 corpora cavernosa of the human penis freely communicate with each other through a deficient septum.**

True.

○ **What is the thinnest part of the tunica albuginea of the penis?**

The ventro-lateral part, where it can tear following abnormal bend (penile "fracture").

○ **What structures are enclosed between Buck fascia and the tunica albuginea of the penis?**

The deep dorsal vein, the dorsal penile arteries, and the dorsal nerves of the penis.

THE PROSTATE

○ **True/False: Normal prostatic glands may be within the striated urethral sphincter.**

True. There is no fibromuscular stroma or prostate capsule with these glands.

○ **True/False: The entire prostate is enclosed by a capsule composed of collagen, elastin, and abundant smooth muscle.**

False. The prostate is devoid of a capsule at the apex and base; therefore, no true capsule separates the prostate from the striated urethral sphincter or the bladder. The capsule is composed of collagen, elastin, and abundant smooth muscle and is continuous with the prostatic stroma.

○ **What is the zonal anatomy of the human prostate?**

Transition zone, peripheral zone, central zone, anterior fibromuscular stroma.

○ **What are the layers of prostate capsule left in a patient after open prostatectomy for benign disease?**

In these patients the capsule is comprised of true (prostatic fascia) and false (compressed transition zone) capsular layers.

○ **In what areas of the prostate is the capsule deficient and why is this important?**

At the apex and at the base. Normal prostatic glands can be found to extend into the striated urethral sphincter with no intervening "capsule." At the base of the prostate, outer longitudinal fibers of the detrusor fuse and blend with the fibromuscular tissue of the capsule. As with the apex, no true capsule separates the prostate from the bladder. This makes assessment of margins somewhat difficult in radical prostatectomy specimens.

○ **True/false: Part of the arterial blood supply of the prostate comes through the puboprostatic ligaments.**

False. The puboprostatic ligaments are virtually avascular structures.

○ **What is the arterial blood supply to the prostate?**

Branches from inferior vesical, middle rectal, and internal pudendal arteries.

○ **Which nerves carry sympathetic and parasympathetic innervation to the prostate?**

The cavernosal nerves.

CHAPTER 5

Embryology of the Genitourinary Tract

Mark F. Bellinger, MD

○ **For a normal kidney to form, the ureteric bud must unite with what embryonic tissue?**

It must join with the metanephric mesenchyme.

○ **Although one theory proposes that the renal vasculature develops in situ during development of the embryonic kidney, the classical teaching is that the renal vessels develop by what mechanism?**

They develop as branching vessels from the aorta.

○ **Remnants of the mesonephric duct in females may be seen in the ovarian mesentery. What are these structures called?**

The epoophoron and the paroophoron.

○ **What is the name given to the cystic remnants of the mesonephric duct in the anterolateral wall of the vagina?**

Gartner duct cysts.

○ **The urorectal septum divides the cloaca into the posterior anorectal canal and what anterior structure?**

The urogenital sinus.

○ **To initiate gonadal development, specialized undifferentiated cells must migrate to the location of the future genital ridge. What are these cells called and where do they migrate from?**

They are primordial germ cells and migrate from the yolk sac.

○ **What embryological process initiates the development of the prostate?**

The outgrowth of solid epithelial cords from urogenital sinus epithelium into the surrounding mesenchyme.

○ **Name the müllerian duct remnants that may persist in males.**

The appendix testis and the prostatic utricle.

○ **What is the mesonephric duct remnant that may persist near the inferior pole of the testis?**

The paradidymis.

○ **What is the potential significance of finding an upper pole renal cyst on fetal sonography? What else should the sonographer look for?**

The upper pole renal cyst may represent a complete ureteral duplication with a ureterocele or upper pole ectopic ureter. The sonographer should look for hydroureter and a ureterocele in the bladder.

○ **Describe the appearance of Type 1 and Type 3 posterior urethral valves.**

Type 1 valves are a pair of sail-like leaflets, and Type 3 valves look like an iris diaphragm in configuration.

○ **Name 2 pressure pop-off mechanisms in fetuses with posterior urethral valves that vent pressure from the bladder and may help prevent the development of renal dysplasia.**

Two mechanisms are contralateral vesicoureteral reflux and a patent urachus.

○ **What may be one consequence of oligohydramnios?**

Pulmonary hypoplasia may be a consequence of oligohydramnios.

○ **Explain the embryological basis for the finding of a bifid scrotum.**

Failure of fusion of the labioscrotal folds may produce a bifid scrotum.

○ **Explain the clinical significance of an atypical median presacral dimple.**

An atypical presacral dimple may be a cutaneous manifestation of occult spinal dysraphism.

○ **Describe the genetics and transmission of "infantile" polycystic kidney disease (ARPKD). Also describe the pulmonary and liver diseases that may be associated with it.**

ARPKD is transmitted as an auto recessive trait. This is a bilateral disease with a variable spectrum of severity. Congenital hepatic fibrosis is associated with the renal disease. Pulmonary hypoplasia may be a consequence of oligohydramnios in severe cases.

○ **Explain why an ectopic ureter in females may be associated with incontinence, whereas in males, normal continence is the rule.**

In females, the ectopic ureter may insert into the lower urinary tract or the lower genital tract below the external sphincter (distal to the bladder neck, in the urethra or vagina). In males, the ectopic ureter always inserts above the external sphincter.

○ **Describe the 3 main physical characteristics of the prune belly syndrome. What is the most important pathological aspect of this syndrome in terms of prognosis?**

The prune belly (triad) syndrome consists of 3 major physical findings: deficiency of the abdominal musculature, anomalous urinary tract with dilated and tortuous ureters, and bilateral intra-abdominal testes. The degree of renal dysplasia is the most important prognostic factor.

○ **A female infant is found to have unilateral renal agenesis. Ultrasound examination of the contralateral kidney and bladder and pelvis are normal. What concern should lead the urologist to recommend long-term monitoring of this child?**

Females with unilateral renal agenesis have a significant incidence of ipsilateral müllerian anomalies, and may present in early adolescence with a pelvic mass indicative of hydrometrocolpos due to any of a spectrum of uterine or vaginal anomalies, commonly uterus didelphys with an obstructed uterine horn.

○ **Ectopic and fused kidneys often have anomalous collecting systems. What is the orientation of the renal pelvis in most anomalous kidneys?**

The renal pelvis begins development in an anterior position and the kidneys rotate during ascent so that the pelves come to lie in a medial position. Most kidneys that are anomalous in location display incomplete rotation. The pelves are likely to be located in an anterior position.

○ **A 1-month-old female has a duplex left kidney with hydroureteronephrosis of the lower pole segment, which has a thin cortex. What is the most likely explanation for the hydronephrosis?**

In a completely duplicated collecting system, the upper pole is most likely to be hydronephrotic because of ureteral obstruction (ectopic ureter, ureterocele), while hydronephrosis of the lower pole system is most likely caused by vesicoureteric reflux.

○ **A 2-month-old male is found to have a right ureteral duplication with upper pole hydroureteronephrosis and a cystic mass in the bladder. What is the first logical therapeutic intervention to consider?**

The child's most likely diagnosis is ureteral duplication with a ureterocele subtending the upper pole ureter. In most cases, transurethral incision of the ureterocele is an appropriate first therapeutic intervention.

○ **A 7-year-old boy is found to have a complete right ureteral duplication with hydroureteronephrosis of the upper pole system during evaluation for nocturnal enuresis. Is this anomaly likely to be a cause of his incontinence?**

No. Ectopic ureters in males insert into the lower genitourinary tract above the external sphincter, including insertion into the Wolffian duct system (vas, seminal vesicle).

○ **An infant is found to have a right multicystic dysplastic kidney. What studies should be done to evaluate the left kidney?**

An ultrasound should be done to rule out hydronephrosis, and a voiding cystourethrogram should be performed since there is greater than 30% incidence of contralateral vesicoureteric reflux.

○ **An infant has drainage of clear fluid from the umbilicus. A small catheter is placed into the umbilical sinus and contrast injected is seen to pass into the gastrointestinal tract. What is the diagnosis?**

The child has persistence of the omphalomesenteric (vitelline) duct that connects with the terminal ileum at the site at which a Meckel diverticulum would be found.

○ **Early rupture of the cloacal membrane may result in a spectrum of urological anomalies. List them.**

Cloacal exstrophy, exstrophy of the bladder, and epispadias.

○ **Horseshoe kidneys have an incidence of hydronephrosis that in some cases is caused by anomalous renal vasculature. Why is the incidence of this type of ureteral obstruction so high?**

Horseshoe kidneys take their vascular supply from a ladder of vessels that alternately appear and involute as the kidneys ascend toward the flank. Persistence of such "anomalous" vessels may result in ureteral obstruction, most commonly at the ureteropelvic junction (UPJ) obstruction.

○ **In cases of unilateral renal agenesis, is ipsilateral adrenal agenesis likely to occur?**

No. Ipsilateral adrenal agenesis occurs in less than 10% of cases.

○ **In crossed renal ectopia, are the kidneys more likely to be fused or nonfused?**

Fused renal ectopia is more common.

○ **In cross-fused renal ectopia, where does the ureter of the crossed kidney usually enter the bladder?**

The ureter draining the ectopic kidney usually crosses the midline to enter the contralateral trigone.

○ **Explain the Meyer–Weigert law in relation to ureteral duplication.**

The law states that in complete ureteral duplication, the orifice to the lower pole ureter inserts into the bladder in a more lateral and cranial position, while the ureter to the upper pole inserts in a more caudal and medial position.

○ **A 14-year-old male is found to have right ureteral obstruction secondary to retrocaval ureter. What is the embryologic explanation for this anomaly?**

Retrocaval ureter is a result of persistence of (failure of involution of) the right subcardinal vein.

○ **The fetal testis produces 2 hormones that are essential for the development of the internal genitalia. Name these hormones and indicate what effect they have on the developing genital structures.**

Testosterone supports the development of the Wolffian duct structures (seminal vesicles, vas, etc). Müllerian-inhibiting substance acts ipsilaterally to suppress the development of the müllerian structures (fallopian tube, uterus, and upper vagina).

○ **A 1-month-old male is found to have a left flank mass. What are the 2 most likely diagnoses and what would be your first imaging study in this case.**

The most likely diagnoses are hydronephrosis and multicystic renal dysplasia. The primary imaging technique for infants with abdominal masses should be ultrasound.

○ **A female neonate has a midline pelvic abdominal mass and a bulging interlabial mass. What is the most likely diagnosis?**

The most likely diagnosis is hydrometrocolpos secondary to imperforate hymen.

○ **A 12-year-old male presents with terminal hematuria and is found to have a polyp in his posterior urethra arising from the verumontanum. What is the cause of this polyp and the most likely pathologic diagnosis? Where else in the urinary tract are similar lesions occasionally found?**

The polyp is most likely a benign fibroepitheliomatous polyp of congenital origin. Similar polyps may be found in the ureter and renal pelvis.

○ **A 15-year-old male with dysuria is found to have a cystic lesion in the bulbous urethra. What is its most likely embryologic origin?**

This is most likely a Cowper duct cyst.

○ **A 12-year-old boy with dysuria and bloody urethral spotting is found to have a small diverticulum on the roof of the distal urethra in the fossa navicularis. What is the correct term for this diverticulum?**

This lesion is known as a lacuna magna.

○ **A 1-month-old female is found to have a cystic mass prolapsing through the urethral meatus, and ultrasound of the abdomen shows hydronephrosis of the upper pole of the left kidney. What is the most likely diagnosis?**

The mass is a prolapsed ureterocele, which subtends the upper ureter of a completely duplicated left collecting system.

○ **A 3-year-old girl is found to have grade 3 left vesicoureteric reflux. What is the most likely anatomic location of the left ureteral orifice as seen at cystoscopy, and what is the embryologic explanation for its position?**

The ureter will likely be positioned in the bladder in a position lateral to the normal trigonal position. This is thought to be the result of a ureteral bud arising from the mesonephric duct in a position more caudal than usual. As a result, as the caudal mesonephric duct becomes absorbed into the trigonal structure, the ureteral orifice will migrate into a dorsolateral position in the bladder base.

○ **A 3-year-old boy is found to have a small, hydronephrotic left kidney and ureter. At cystoscopy, no left ureteral orifice can be identified. Where does the ureter most likely insert?**

The ureter most likely is inserted into the Wolffian system (seminal vesicle, vas). This anomaly represents failure of the ureteral bud to separate from its Wolffian duct origin.

○ **An infant being evaluated after urinary tract infection has an intravenous urogram performed. The study shows small folds in the upper portion of the left ureter without significant hydronephrosis. What is the nature and significance of these ureteral findings?**

The IVP has demonstrated "fetal folds" in the upper ureter. These persistent fetal infoldings generally are insignificant and disappear with time.

○ **What is the embryologic explanation for bifid ureters?**

Bifid ureters are thought to be the result of bifurcation of the ureteral bud during its ascent toward the renal mesenchyme.

○ **What is the most proximal extent of the ureteral bud in the renal collecting system?**

The ureteral bud ascends to join the metanephric blastema and unite with the glomerular structures. The collecting ducts of the kidney are the most proximal extent of the ureteral bud.

○ **Explain the differences in embryogenesis between multicystic renal dysplasia and autosomal dominant polycystic disease.**

The cysts in multicystic renal dysplasia are a reflection of failure of normal organogenesis; immature renal parenchyma and cystic dysplasia are found. In polycystic disease, the normal architecture of the nephron is destroyed by the obstruction of the nephron and resulting cystic deformation.

○   **At what stage of fetal development does the kidney begin to produce urine?**

At approximately 9 to 12 weeks.

○   **Congenital spinal anomalies may be associated with what urinary tract anomaly?**

Congenital spinal anomalies may be found in association with renal anomalies, in particular unilateral renal agenesis.

○   **Describe the syndrome in which urethral valves may be associated with unilateral renal dysplasia.**

In the VURD syndrome (vesicoureteric reflux, renal dysplasia), a dysplastic kidney may be found to be associated with massive unilateral vesicoureteric reflux.

○   **What ureteral anomaly is found in conjunction with multicystic renal dysplasia?**

Ureteral atresia.

○   **Explain the anomalies found in the triad syndrome.**

The triad, or prune belly syndrome is a constellation of abnormal abdominal musculature, intra-abdominal undescended testes, and an abnormal (dysmorphic) urinary tract.

○   **What embryologic explanations have been proposed to explain the prune belly syndrome?**

The explanations offered have been primarily those of anomalous development of the mesenchyme and a transient infravesical obstruction during early embryogenesis.

○   **What is the state of the prostate in boys with prune belly syndrome?**

The prostate is hypoplastic.

○   **It is very difficult to pass a urethral catheter into the bladder of a boy with hypospadias. What is the likely explanation for this?**

The child most likely has an enlarged prostatic utricle.

○   **A 1-year-old male has a nonpalpable right testis. At the time of exploration, the inguinal canal is empty. Where should the surgeon look to be sure that the testis is absent?**

The testis descends from a position above the internal inguinal ring. Testes above the ring are located in the abdominal cavity if they are not congenitally absent. In most cases, a testis or blind-ending vas and vessels can be found in the abdomen by laparoscopy or open exploration. Retroperitoneal dissection, as practiced in the past, may allow the surgeon to miss an abdominal testis.

○   **At the time of exploration, an undescended testis is found outside of the external inguinal ring. The cord structures are long enough to reach the scrotum easily. Should the tunica vaginalis overlying the testis be opened?**

Yes. Since most undescended testes have a persistently patent processus vaginalis that does not close after the testis descends into the inguinal canal. This processus should be ligated at the internal inguinal ring.

○ **At exploration for an undescended testis, a blind-ending vascular structure is noted in the inguinal canal. Is exploration complete?**

No. To be sure that a testis is not present, the vas deferens should be identified. The vas and vessels may, in a small number of cases, be separate.

○ **At the time of inguinal herniorrhaphy in a 2-year-old boy, a bright yellow circular nodule approximately 3 mm in diameter is noted in the inguinal canal attached to the cord structures. What does this represent?**

This is an adrenal rest. No therapy is necessary. It represents the common precursor of the genitourinary ridge in early development.

○ **A 30-week-gestation neonate is noted to have bilateral canalicular testes. Is there any chance that descent will occur after birth?**

Yes. The incidence of cryptorchidism in premature infants is approximately 30%, while it is approximately 3% in full-term neonates and less than 1% at 1 year of age.

○ **In the classical literature of urology, what is the embryologic importance of epididymitis in a prepubescent male?**

The worry is that the boy may have an ectopic ureter draining into the vas deferens or seminal vesicle. Renal ultrasound examination is warranted in these cases.

○ **Describe the anatomy of the exstrophic tissue seen in cloacal exstrophy.**

The exstrophic tissue classically consists of a midline segment of hindgut, frequently with a prolapsed ileum and one or more openings to at least one appendix. The bladder is split into 2 hemibladders by the hindgut. Widely separated genital tubercles are seen as a hemiscrotum and hemipenis on each side, or a hemiclitoris on each side. The anus is imperforate. Most children also have a myelomeningocele and an omphalocele.

○ **Primary obstructive megaureter is most commonly caused by what anatomic entity?**

Obstructive megaureter is thought in most cases to be due to an adynamic distal ureteral segment.

○ **Vaginal atresia may be associated with anomalies of the urinary tract. What is the most commonly recognized urinary tract anomaly seen?**

Unilateral renal agenesis.

○ **What is the embryologic origin of the vagina?**

The upper portion of the vagina originates from the müllerian duct. The lower portion (distal to the hymen) originates from the urogenital sinus.

○ **The appendix testis is an embryologic remnant of what structure?**

The müllerian duct.

○ **A neonate with imperforate anus is seen to pass meconium per urethra. What is the most likely site of the connection between the urinary and gastrointestinal tracts?**

Embryologically, the most likely site of the fistula is the posterior urethra, although fistulization may occur at the base of the bladder.

○ **List at least 3 mechanisms that have been proposed to explain why testicles descend from the abdomen into the scrotum.**

The first is the abdominal pressure theory, which proposes that intra-abdominal pressure forces the testis out of the abdomen. The second is that the process is entirely controlled by hormonal influence. Another theory is that the gubernaculum pulls the testis into the scrotum.

○ **What is the embryologic origin of the appendix epididymis?**

The Wolffian duct.

○ **What is the embryologic explanation for uterus didelphys?**

The müllerian ducts are paired structures that fuse distally to form the upper portion of the vagina and the uterus, the cranial unfused portions forming the fallopian tubes. Failure of fusion may result in one of several anomalies of the uterus, including uterus didelphys and bicornuate uterus.

○ **Explain the embryologic cause of midshaft hypospadias.**

Hypospadias is a result of incomplete formation of the urethra. If the urethral folds fail to fuse in the midline, hypospadias may result.

○ **In cloacal exstrophy, how can an anomaly such as hemiscrotum with hemiphallus come to exist?**

If the cloacal membrane ruptures early, this acts as a wedge to keep the genital tubercles and genital folds widely separate, so each component of the hemiscrotum and hemiphallus develops widely separate from its contralateral mate.

○ **At what stage in gestation is nephron formation completed?**

Nephron formation is usually completed by approximately 36 weeks.

○ **What is the embryologic explanation for communicating hydrocele?**

The explanation is that the processus vaginalis fails to obliterate (persistence of a patent processus vaginalis).

○ **Glomerular filtration rate (GFR) progressively increases during fetal development. At what postnatal age does GFR reach its peak?**

At approximately 4 months.

○ **A male neonate is found to have bilateral hydroureteronephrosis, echogenic renal parenchyma, and bilateral pneumothorax. What is the most likely diagnosis?**

This child is likely to have urethral obstruction secondary to posterior urethral valves.

○ **What is the mechanism of neonatal testicular torsion?**

The mechanism of this type of torsion, that is, extravaginal torsion, is thought to be different from intravaginal torsion seen in adolescents and adults. In extravaginal torsion, the entire spermatic cord and its coverings appear to twist.

○ **In Potter syndrome (bilateral renal agenesis), are the adrenal glands usually absent?**

No. The adrenals are usually normal.

○ **What is the renal anatomic defect found in association with megacalycosis?**

Underdevelopment of the renal medulla.

○ **What is the likely location of a ureter that originates from a higher than normal site on the mesonephric duct?**

According to Mackie and Stephens, the ureter will come to lie more caudal and medial in the bladder than a normal ureteral orifice.

○ **What is the importance of the mesonephric kidney to normal embryonic development of the genitourinary tract?**

The mesonephric kidney never functions in the human, but the mesonephric (Wolffian) duct is key to the genital ducts in the male and to the development of the ureteral bud, and thus the kidney.

○ **Explain one theory for the development of ureteroceles.**

Failure of normal perforation of Chawalla's membrane, which separates the ureter from the bladder, is thought to result in the formation of ureteroceles.

○ **What are the anatomic correlates of the müllerian tubercle in both male and female?**

The verumontanum and the hymen, respectively.

○ **In patients with a thoracic kidney, is a diaphragmatic hernia necessarily present?**

No.

○ **What is a proposed etiology for the formation of calyceal diverticula?**

It is proposed that failure of involution of third- and fourth-order branches of the ureteral bud may result in formation of calyceal diverticula.

○ **Infundibulopelvic stenosis may represent an embryologic midpoint between which 2 congenital renal anomalies?**

Ureteropelvic junction obstruction and multicystic renal dysplasia.

○ **What is the embryologic origin of the seminal vesicle?**

The Wolffian duct.

○ **What is the mechanism by which the cloaca becomes divided into the urogenital sinus and rectum?**

The urorectal septum grows to meet the cloacal membrane, forming the perineal body as it fuses with the cloacal membrane. This divides the cloacal membrane into an anterior urogenital membrane and a posterior anal membrane.

○ **Which portions of the male urethra have their embryologic origin from the urogenital sinus?**

The prostatic and membranous urethra.

○ **As a horseshoe kidney ascends from the pelvis, which vessel may prevent its ascent into the flank?**

The inferior mesenteric artery.

○ **Which embryonic structure, extending from the bladder to the umbilicus, may remain patent and result in urinary drainage?**

The allantois.

○ **For normal gonadal development, the primary germ cells must migrate from the wall of the yolk sac to paired structures along the dorsal portion of the embryo between the dorsal mesentery and the mesonephros. What are these paired structures that will develop into the primitive gonad?**

They are the genital ridges.

○ **There have been 2 general theories to explain the formation of the glanular urethra. Explain each theory.**

The first is that the urethral folds, which fuse to form the pendulous urethra, fuse all the way to the glans. The second theory holds that the pendulous urethra is formed in this manner, while a solid core of ectoderm burrows into the glans to unite with the proximal urethra and then canalize.

○ **Explain the embryologic origins of the labia minora and labia majora.**

The labia minora are formed from the urethral folds, while the labia majora are derived from the genital swellings.

○ **Explain the proposed etiology for exstrophy of the urinary bladder.**

Exstrophy occurs when early rupture of the cloacal membrane causes failure of mesenchymal migration into the area.

○ **Explain the embryogenesis of vasoureteral fusion.**

The ureter forms as a branch (ureteral bud) off of the Wolffian duct. In normal male embryogenesis, as the distal Wolffian duct is assimilated into the trigone during bladder formation, the ureteral bud (ureter) and the Wolffian duct (now the vas deferens) separate. Failure of this distal assimilation and separation may result in vasoureteral fusion, or more precisely, a failure of separation of the 2 structures.

○ **Define Potter syndrome. List its common etiologies and phenotypic (clinical) findings.**

Potter syndrome is the result of oligohydramnios secondary to prenatal kidney disease and renal failure. Bilateral renal agenesis is a common cause of the most severe and fatal form of this disease. Early rupture of membranes, renal cystic disease, and posterior urethral valves are other causes. Pulmonary hypoplasia, sacral agenesis, and various cardiovascular anomalies may also be present.

The common facial characteristics of the syndrome (Potter facies) include low-set ears, prominent inner canthal folds, a flattened or blunted nose, a prominent depression between the lower lip and the chin. In addition, the babies appear prematurely senile and often have bowed legs and clubbed feet. Most of these findings are thought to be deformations resulting from the severe oligohydramnios.

○ **What anomalies of the male internal genital structures may be found in association with unilateral renal agenesis?**

Ipsilateral absence of the vas deferens and hypoplasia or cystic deformation of the seminal vesicle are found most often.

○ **Are congenital anomalies of the urinary tract more likely to occur on the right side or on the left side of the body?**

Left-sided anomalies predominate.

○ **What other congenital anomalies may be found in patients with renal ectopia?**

Genital anomalies are not uncommon: primarily uterine and vaginal anomalies in females and cryptorchidism, hypospadias, or other urethral anomalies in males.

○ **What is one proposed embryologic explanation for the development of megacalycosis?**

A proposed mechanism is nonobstructive enlargement of the calyx caused by hypoplasia or malformation of the renal papilla.

○ **List some of the common histologic findings of renal dysplasia.**

Distorted renal architecture with immature glomeruli, cartilage, and primitive ducts, lined with columnar epithelium and surrounded by fibromuscular collars.

○ **There are 2 predominant theories that aim to explain the development of renal dysplasia. List them.**

The first theory is that dysplasia results from obstruction of the developing nephron. The second, or "bud" theory, proposed by Mackie and Stephens, proposes that abnormal ureteral bud development causes the ureter to join the metanephric blastema abnormally, such that abnormal renal parenchyma results.

○ **What is an Ask-Upmark kidney, what is its clinical significance, and what other urological abnormality is it often associated with?**

An Ask-Upmark kidney is a small kidney with areas of segmental hypoplasia and sometimes dysplasia. Although originally thought to be an embryologic error, there is concern that the histologic changes might be in part because of renal scarring. Ask-Upmark kidneys can be a cause of severe hypertension. Most are associated with vesicoureteric reflux.

○ **What is the most common congenital anomaly of the contralateral kidney in a child with a congenital UPJ obstruction?**

The most common finding is another UPJ obstruction.

○ **List the components of the VATER syndrome.**

They are **V**ertebral defects, imperforate **A**nus, **T**racheoesophageal fistula, and **R**enal and **R**adial dysplasia.

○ **What structures in male and female are formed from the genital swellings?**

Male: the scrotum. Female: the labia majora.

○ **What anatomic structure often herniates into the groin in female inguinal hernia.**

The ovary.

○ **Which specific Y chromosome gene is felt to be responsible for male sex differentiation and where is it located?**

The SRY gene (also known as the testis determining factor), which is located on the short arm of the Y chromosome, is felt to be the gene that initiates differentiation of the indifferent gonad into a testis.

○ **At what stage of gestation does descent of the testis occur?**

Descent of testis into the scrotum occurs in late gestation, usually between 30 and 40 weeks. Descent may not be complete until after birth, especially in premature infants.

○ **What is the percentage of boys with cryptorchidism at birth in full-term male infants?**

Approximately 3%.

○ **What urological finding is associated with cystic fibrosis?**

Agenesis of the vas deferens is found in a high percentage of males with cystic fibrosis.

○ **What urachal anomalies can you name other than patent urachus?**

Anomalies that may be seen as urachal remnant variants include urachal cyst, urachal sinus, urachal diverticulum, and alternating urachal sinus.

○ **Briefly outline a proposed embryologic origin for a communicating hydrocele of the cord, and define how this would differ from the origin of a communicating hydrocele.**

A communicating hydrocele represents a persistence of the patent processus vaginalis, a tongue-like extension of the peritoneum.

A communicating hydrocele of the cord requires a distal occlusion of the processus vaginalis, which must be accompanied by a relative narrowing of the processus proximal to the occluded processus. The area between the occlusion and the partial occlusion then traps peritoneal fluid to form a cystic dilation of the processus. Since the proximal portion of the processus remains open, these cystic structures may change in size.

○ **What is the abdominal wall structure from which the cremasteric muscle and fascia develop?**

They develop from the internal oblique muscle.

○ **Describe the embryologic mishap that would explain why most males with penopubic epispadias have urinary incontinence.**

Epispadias is at the most minimal end of the spectrum of the epispadias–exstrophy complex, with cloacal exstrophy being the most severe example. This complex results when the cloacal membrane ruptures prior to its closure (before the mesoderm surrounding the membrane and the mesoderm of the genital swellings has grown to the midline and closed the anterior abdominal wall). In penile epispadias, the only defect is the dorsal urethral closure, while in penopubic epispadias with incontinence (the most common form), the bladder neck is not completely formed and incontinence results.

○ **A 5-year-old male presented with a symptomatic left inguinal hernia. At exploration, a solid reddish nodule is found in the cord adjacent to the testis. What might this represent?**

This may be an accessory spleen. Accessory spleens are common and may be located in several areas. They may be carried into the scrotum as the developing left testis descends, and may present as an isolated scrotal nodule or multiple nodules, or as splenogonadal fusion, in which a very elongated spleen is attached like a long tongue extending from the spleen into the inguinal canal.

○ **How does vaginal atresia differ from vaginal agenesis?**

Vaginal atresia involves only the distal vagina. The müllerian structures are not affected. The uterus, cervix, and proximal vagina are all normal and intact.

Vaginal agenesis is the absence of a proximal vagina in a normal 46 XX female with normal hormones. A hymenal fringe and a small distal vaginal pouch are usually present.

○ **What is Mayer–Rokitansky–Kuster–Hauser (MRKH) syndrome?**

Another name for vaginal agenesis.

○ **What urological problems are most commonly associated with vaginal agenesis?**

Unilateral renal agenesis or ectopia of one or both kidneys occurs in 74% of patients.

○ **What is penile torsion and how is it treated?**

Penile torsion is the term used to describe the rotation of the penis around the longitudinal axis. It is usually a congenital condition, but it can occur after penile surgery. No treatment is necessary, but in rare cases a surgical correction can be done by degloving and skin realignment. A Dartos flap can be used in severe cases.

CHAPTER 6

Congenital Disorders of the Lower Urinary Tract

Anthony Atala, MD

○ **Describe the formation of trigone during development.**

The common excretory ducts (the portion of the nephric ducts distal to the origin of ureteric buds) dilate and become absorbed into the urogenital sinus. The right and left common excretory ducts fuse in the midline as a triangular area, forming the primitive trigone.

○ **How does the bladder appear in prune belly syndrome?**

The bladder usually appears massively enlarged with a pseudodiverticulum at the urachus. The urachus is patent at birth in 25% to 30% of children. Histologically, the bladder has an increased ratio of collagen to muscle fibers in the absence of obstruction.

○ **Why are indirect inguinal hernias frequent in exstrophy patients?**

This phenomenon is attributed to a persistent processus vaginalis, large internal and external inguinal rings, and the lack of obliquity of the inguinal canal.

○ **What is the rate of occurrence of inguinal hernias in bladder exstrophy?**

In a review of 181 children with bladder exstrophy, Connolly and coauthors (1995) reported inguinal hernias in 81.8% of boys and 10.5% of girls.

○ **What is the primary anorectal defect in exstrophy?**

The perineum is short and broad and the anus is situated directly behind the urogenital diaphragm; it is displaced anteriorly and corresponds to the posterior limit of the triangular fascial defect.

○ **What is the average corporal length defect in exstrophy patients?**

It was found that the anterior corporal length of male patients with bladder exstrophy was almost 50% shorter than that of normal controls.

○ **How does the exstrophy patient's prostate compare with the normal age-matched control's prostate?**

The volume, weight, and maximum cross-sectional area of the prostate appear normal compared with published control values. However, in exstrophy patients, the prostate does not extend circumferentially around the urethra, and the urethra is anterior to the prostate in all patients.

○ **What is the classic picture of a female exstrophy patient?**

The vagina is shorter than normal, hardly greater than 6 cm in depth, but of normal caliber. The vaginal orifice is frequently stenotic and displaced anteriorly; the clitoris is bifid, and the labia, mons pubis, and clitoris are divergent. The uterus enters the vagina superiorly so that the cervix is in the anterior vaginal wall. The fallopian tubes and ovaries are normal.

○ **What is the incidence of reflux after surgical closure of the bladder in exstrophy patients?**

Reflux in the closed exstrophic bladder occurs in 100% of cases, and subsequent surgery is usually required at the time of bladder neck reconstruction. If excessive outlet resistance is gained at the time of either initial closure or combined epispadias and bladder exstrophy closure, and if recurrent infections are a problem even with suppressive antibiotics, ureteral reimplantation is required before bladder neck reconstruction.

○ **What are the most significant changes in the management of bladder exstrophy over the past 2 decades?**

Currently, bladder exstrophy is managed with (1) early bladder, posterior urethral, and abdominal wall closure, usually with osteotomy; (2) early epispadias repair; and (3) reconstruction of a continent bladder neck and reimplantation of the ureters when necessary. Most importantly, however, a definition of strict criteria for the selection of patients suitable for this approach has been created.

○ **What are the advantages incurred by osteotomy at the time of bladder closure?**

Pelvic osteotomy performed at the time of initial closure confers several advantages, including easy approximation of the symphysis with diminished tension on the abdominal wall closure and elimination of the need for fascial flaps. In addition, it allows placement of the urethra deep within the pelvic ring, enhancing bladder outlet resistance. Finally, it brings the large pelvic floor muscles near the midline, where they can support the bladder neck and aid in eventual urinary control.

○ **Why is the combined anterior osteotomy preferred to the classic posterior osteotomy?**

Besides the ease of approximation, combined osteotomy was developed for 3 reasons:

1. Osteotomy is performed with the patient in the supine position, as is the urological repair, thereby avoiding the need to turn the patient.
2. The anterior approach to this osteotomy allows placement of an external fixator device and intrafragmentary pins under direct vision.
3. The cosmetic appearance of this osteotomy is superior to that resulting from the posterior iliac approach.

○ **When can you remove the external fixation device after primary closure?**

When good callus formation is seen on radiography, the fixation device and pins are removed with the patient under light sedation.

○ **In cases of small bladder strip at birth, which is preferable: rapid closure or closure after a reasonable waiting period?**

Ideally, waiting for the bladder template to grow for 4 to 6 months in the child with a small bladder is not as risky as submitting a small bladder template to closure in an inappropriate setting. This may result in dehiscence and allows the fate of the bladder to be sealed at that point.

○ **A young child presents with persistent urinary tract infections (UTI) and apparent high-grade reflux after primary closure of the bladder. What is the proper management?**

Proper management is to begin long-term antibiotic therapy to control the infections. It may also be necessary to dilate the urethra or to begin intermittent catheterization.

○ **When is combined closure of exstrophy and epispadias repair considered?**

Combined closure of exstrophy and epispadias repair is considered in patients who have had closure surgery delayed beyond the newborn period or in patients in whom the initial newborn closure fails.

○ **What is the primary goal of bladder neck reconstruction procedures?**

The primary goal of these procedures is urinary continence, which is defined as a 3-hour dry interval. If this is not achieved within 2 years after bladder neck reconstruction, failure to achieve continence has resulted.

○ **What are the key determinants of management in bladder exstrophy?**

- Size and quality of bladder template.
- Extent of pubic diastasis and malleability of the pelvis.
- Need for osteotomy.
- Length and width of urethral plate.
- Penile size.
- Associated anomalies.

○ **What is the innervation pattern of the corporal bodies and bladder in cloacal exstrophy patients?**

Enervation to the duplicated corporal bodies arises from the sacral plexus, travels through the midline, perforates the interior portion of the pelvic floor, and courses medially to the hemibladders.

○ **What is the rate of occurrence of intestinal tract abnormalities in cloacal exstrophy?**

Omphalocele was reported to occur between 88% and 100% of cases, with most studies reporting omphalocele in more than 95% of cases.

○ **What is the most common müllerian defect in cloacal exstrophy?**

The most commonly reported müllerian anomaly is uterine duplication seen in 95% of patients.

○ **What procedures are performed in the one-stage repair of cloacal exstrophy?**

- Excision of omphalocele.
- Separation of cecal plate from bladder halves.
- Joining and closure of bladder halves followed by urethroplasty.
- Bilateral anterior innominate and vertical iliac osteotomy.
- Gonadectomy in males with un-reconstructible phallus.
- Terminal ileostomy/colostomy.
- Genital revision if needed.

○ **What is the 2-stage repair of cloacal exstrophy?**

First stage (newborn period)

- Excision of omphalocele.
- Separation of cecal plate from bladder halves.
- Joining of bladder halves.
- Gonadectomy in male with un-reconstructible phallus.
- Terminal ileostomy/colostomy.

Second stage

- Closure of joined bladder halves and urethroplasty.
- Bilateral anterior innominate and vertical iliac osteotomy.
- Genital revision if needed.

○ **What is the incidence of vesicoureteral reflux (VUR) in epispadias patients?**

The ureterovesical junction is inherently deficient in complete epispadias, and the incidence of reflux has been reported to be between 30% and 40%.

○ **What are the primary objectives of repair of male epispadias?**

The objectives of repair of penopubic epispadias include achievement of urinary continence with preservation of the upper urinary tract and the reconstruction of cosmetically acceptable genitalia.

○ **What is megacystis?**

The term *megacystis* is often used to describe any condition leading to a distended fetal bladder in utero, without referring to the cause of the dilation. Historically, congenital megacystis was thought to be caused by bladder neck obstruction, leading to massive bilateral VUR and a thin bladder wall.

○ **How sensitive is prenatal ultrasound in the diagnosis of posterior urethral valves?**

Ultrasonography is sensitive in detecting fetal hydronephrosis, but the specific diagnosis of posterior urethral valves is more difficult. Nonetheless, a thickened bladder and a dilated posterior urethra are suggestive of posterior urethral valves.

○ **What is the most important diagnostic study for posterior urethral valves?**

Voiding cystourethrography (VCUG) remains the most important study in diagnosis of posterior urethral valves because it defines the anatomy and gross function of the bladder, bladder neck, and urethra.

○ **What is the gold standard treatment in the management of posterior urethral valves?**

In general, endoscopic primary ablation is the preferred surgical procedure to treat posterior urethral valves. Vesicostomy is reserved for very small infants if the endoscopic equipment is too large for safe intervention.

○ **What are the prognostic indicators of future renal function in patients with posterior urethral valves?**

There are 4 basic predictors of renal function in patients with posterior urethral valves: ultrasound appearance, serum chemistries, age at diagnosis, and presence of reflux.

○ **How is nocturnal polyuria explained in patients with nocturnal enuresis?**

Nocturnal polyuria can be either absolute, which is usually associated with a derangement of the circadian rhythm of antidiuretic hormone secretion, or relative, mainly due to a reduced functional bladder capacity during sleep at night.

○ **What is the definition of hypospadias?**

Hypospadias, in boys, is defined as a group of 3 anomalies of the penis: (1) an abnormal ventral opening of the urethral meatus that may be located anywhere from the ventral aspect of the glans penis to the perineum, (2) an abnormal ventral curvature of the penis (chordee), and (3) an abnormal distribution of foreskin with a "hood" present dorsally and deficient foreskin ventrally. The second and third characteristics are not present in all cases.

○ **What are the current theories explaining congenital penile curvature?**

Currently, 3 major theories are proposed for the cause of penile curvature. These include (1) abnormal development of the urethral plate; (2) abnormal, fibrotic mesenchymal tissue at the urethral meatus; and (3) corporal disproportion or differential growth of normal dorsal corpora cavernosal tissue and abnormal corporal tissue ventrally.

○ **During what gestational week does the foreskin develop?**

At approximately the 20th week of gestation.

○ **Higher maternal serum levels of man-made organochloro compounds (PCBs and similar chemicals) appear to correlate with what congenital urological abnormalities in newborn children?**

Undescended testes and hypospadias. The theory is that the chemical burden in the mother affects her endocrine function.

○ **What is the incidence of cryptorchidism in full-term male newborns?**

Cryptorchidism affects 3% of full-term male newborns. Approximately 75% of cryptorchid testes will spontaneously descend, usually by 3 months of age.

○ **What is the risk for an undescended testis in a newborn male if a family member is already affected?**

The risk is 3.6-fold overall, 6.9-fold if a brother is affected, and 4.6-fold if the father is affected.

○ **What is the risk of infertility in patients with cryptorchidism?**

Although biopsy findings from children with unilateral cryptorchidism typically demonstrate reduced total germ cell counts, paternity has been found to be significantly compromised in men with previous bilateral, but not unilateral cryptorchidism.

○ **Is there an increased risk of testicular malignancy with undescended testes?**

There is an increased risk of testicular malignancy with undescended testes. The higher the position of the undescended testes, the greater the risk of developing malignancy. Almost half the tumors that develop from undescended testes occur in testes located abdominally, 6-fold higher than for inguinal testes.

○ **What is the most common tumor that develops from a cryptorchid testis?**

The most common tumor that develops from an undescended testis is a seminoma.

○ **What role does radiologic testing have in the assessment of undescended testes?**

Radiologic testing does not have a relevant role in the assessment of undescended testes and should not influence surgical management.

○ **Do bilateral nonpalpable testes warrant special assessment?**

Bilateral nonpalpable testes warrant immediate assessment in the newborn period to determine the presence or absence of testes and to rule out an intersex state.

○ **When is the ideal time for surgical intervention for undescended testes?**

Surgical intervention on an undescended testis should optimally be performed between 6 and 12 months of age.

○ **What is the best management if a testicular nubbin is found?**

Viable testicular elements will be present in up to 13% of testicular remnants/nubbins and should therefore be removed.

CHAPTER 7

Congenital Disorders of the Upper Tracts

Megan S. Schober, MD, PhD,
Kevin M. Feber, MD, FAAP, and
Evan J. Kass, MD, FACS, FAAP

○ **What are the features of Potter syndrome?**

Compressed facies, low-set ears, and limb contractures.

○ **What is the etiology of Potter syndrome?**

Potter syndrome, or Potter sequence, is a series of changes that occur in a fetus secondary to extreme oligohydramnios. This can be from an inability to produce urine such as renal agenesis, bilateral multicystic renal dysplasia, or juvenile polycystic kidneys. Another reason for oligohydramnios is an impaired ability to void such as posterior urethral valves.

○ **What is the embryological basis and the characteristic findings of the Mayer–Rokitansky–Küster–Hauser (MRKH) syndrome and how does it usually present?**

Müllerian agenesis, which leads to a congenital absence of the middle and upper third of the vagina with variable uterine and fallopian tube defects. In approximately one-third of these cases, upper tract anomalies can also be found. These include renal agenesis or hypoplasia, renal ectopia, pelvic kidney, and horseshoe kidney. Skeletal abnormalities (usually vertebral) occur in 10% to 20%. There are 2 types of MRKH syndrome. Type A (typical) has symmetric remnant müllerian muscular buds and normal fallopian tubes and Type B (atypical) is associated with asymmetric buds and abnormal fallopian tubes. Although Type B has been deemed "atypical," it is actually more common than Type A. Renal and skeletal abnormalities occur only in Type B MRKH syndrome. The most common presentation is primary amenorrhea.

○ **Patients found to have a missing vas deferens during an infertility workup should be screened for what abnormality and how?**

Ipsilateral renal agenesis that can be confirmed on renal ultrasound.

○ **What is the incidence of unilateral renal agenesis?**

Approximately 1:1400 births.

○ **What is the incidence of bilateral renal agenesis?**

Approximately 1:4000 with a ratio of male to female of 2.5:1. This is a lethal condition associated with a number of genetic syndromes.

○ **What is the long-term prognosis for a baby born with a solitary kidney?**

If there are no other associated anomalies, prognosis is good. However, contralateral reflux is found in one-third of children with renal agenesis and is not uncommon in patients with multicystic dysplastic kidney. Patients with solitary kidneys are at increased risk for developing proteinuria, hypertension, and renal insufficiency over the course of his or her lifetime; however, the patient's life expectancy is normal.

○ **What is the most common additional urologic abnormality associated with a horseshoe kidney?**

The incidence of horseshoe kidney is 1:400 to 1:1800 with a male predominance of 2:1. Up to 35% of patients with a horseshoe kidney have evidence of significant ureteropelvic junction obstruction, more commonly on the left. Patients with a horseshoe kidney are also at a greater risk of vesicoureteral reflux (VUR) with reported rates of 80%.

○ **Is there an increased cancer risk with fused kidneys?**

There is a 1.5-fold to 8-fold increased risk of Wilms tumor in these kidneys. It is unclear at this time if there is an increased risk of adult urologic cancers in fused kidneys; however, some studies demonstrate an increased risk of transitional cell carcinoma in these patients.

○ **The cephalad migration of a horseshoe kidney is limited by what structure?**

The inferior mesenteric artery.

○ **What is the normal direction of rotation of the human kidney as it ascends out of the pelvis?**

The kidney normally rotates 90° ventromedially during ascent. Therefore, the renal pelvis, which was originally directed anteriorly, becomes directed medially.

○ **True/False: Most crossed ectopic kidneys are fused with their mate.**

True. Approximately 90% of crossed ectopic kidneys are fused with a normally placed mate.

○ **What is the incidence of antenatal hydronephrosis?**

In the United States, more than 600,000 fetal ultrasounds are performed. Of these, 0.2% to 2% will detect antenatal hydronephrosis. Postnatal ultrasound demonstrates that 66% to 75% persist after birth.

○ **What is the most common cause of hydronephrosis in the fetal kidney?**

Ureteropelvic junction obstructions are the etiology of 60% to 80% of cases of persistent fetal hydronephrosis. VUR is responsible for 25% to 35% of postnatal hydronephrosis.

○ **True/False: Most cases of prenatally diagnosed ureteropelvic junction obstruction require urgent surgical intervention following delivery.**

False. Debate continues surrounding the management of prenatally diagnosed ureteropelvic junction obstructions. Most often surgery is not necessary or can be performed on an elective basis after an appropriate evaluation and period of observation.

○ **In what percent of patients with ureteropelvic junction obstruction does the contralateral kidney demonstrate evidence of ureteropelvic junction obstruction?**

In patients found to have ureteropelvic junction obstruction, evidence for bilateral obstruction exists in 10% to 40% of cases.

○ **In what percent of patients with ureteropelvic junction obstruction does vesicoureteral reflux coexist?**

Vesicoureteral reflux coexists in 15% of cases.

○ **What is the most common type of renal cystic disease?**

Multicystic dysplastic kidney disease. Incidence is 1:3000 to 1:5000 of live births.

○ **A child is discovered to have a multicystic dysplastic kidney. This patient's contralateral kidney should be screened for what abnormalities?**

The contralateral collecting system should been screened for VUR, which is present in 18% to 43% of cases, and for ureteropelvic junction obstruction, which has been demonstrated in 3% to 12% of cases. Duplex system, agenesis, or ectopia can also been seen in the contralateral kidney.

○ **What is the average amount of renal parenchyma drained by the upper pole of a duplicated collecting system?**

About one-third of total renal parenchyma is drained by the upper pole of a duplicated collecting system.

○ **A ureteric bud arising on the mesonephric duct in an abnormally low position predisposes to what abnormality?**

The ureteric bud will arrive early at the urogenital sinus causing the ureteral orifice to ultimately reside in a more cranial and lateral position within the bladder and be predisposed to VUR.

○ **What can happen if the ureteral bud originates significantly higher than normal on the mesonephric duct?**

The ureter may not incorporate into the bladder and instead open into the urethra or other mesonephric remnants. In the male, an ectopic ureter can end in the epididymis, vas, or seminal vesicle. Because the ectopic ureter always ends above the external urinary sphincter in a male, incontinence is typically not an issue. In a female, an ectopic ureter can end anywhere along the Gartner duct and secondarily rupture into the vagina.

○ **The upper pole ureter of a duplicated collecting system is predisposed to what abnormality?**

Obstruction with subsequent hydronephrosis. The lower pole ureter is predisposed to VUR because of its lateral insertion and shortened submucosal tunnel.

○ **What is the Meyer–Weigert rule?**

In a complete ureteral duplication, the ureter that inserts more caudal and medial is the upper pole ureter.

○ **True/False: Ectopic ureteral orifices in female patients are often associated with duplicated collecting systems.**

True. More than 80% of ectopic ureters in female patients are associated with duplicated collecting systems. If the patient has an ectopic ureter and a duplicated collecting system, the ectopic ureter drains the upper pole.

○ **Do male patients with ectopic ureteral orifices tend to have duplicated collecting systems?**

No. Ectopic ureteral orifices in male patients drain single collecting systems in the majority of cases.

○ **A boy with a duplicated collecting system is found to have an ectopic ureter. Where will the terminal portion of the ectopic ureter most likely be found?**

Ectopic ureters in males terminate in the posterior urethra in approximately 50% of cases and the seminal vesicles in about 30% of cases. In males, the ectopic ureter terminates proximal to the external urinary sphincter, therefore, incontinence is typically not an issue with these patients.

○ **True/False: In a girl with continuous urinary incontinence found to have an ectopic ureter, the ectopic ureteral orifice will most likely be found within the vagina.**

False. The ectopic ureteral orifice will most often be found within the urethra or at the vestibule.

○ **What is Chawalla membrane?**

Chawalla membrane is a 2-cell layer ureteral membrane that transiently divides the ureteral bud from the urogenital sinus at approximately 37 days gestation. Incomplete dissolution of this membrane is believed to be the etiology of ureterocele formation.

○ **Ureteroceles tend to occur in patients of what race and sex?**

Ureteroceles are significantly more common in Caucasians and occur 4 to 7 times more frequently in females than in males. Studies have shown left-side predominance and 10% are bilateral.

○ **What is a pseudoureterocele?**

A radiographic finding in which the distal end of a dilated ectopic ureter coursing behind the bladder elevates the trigone giving the appearance of an ureterocele.

○ **What is the most common cause of urethral obstruction in a young girl?**

A prolapsing ureterocele.

○ **What is the length-to-diameter ratio in a normal nonrefluxing pediatric ureter?**

5:1.

○ **What is the embryology of a circumcaval ureter or preureteral vena cava?**

Circumcaval (or retrocaval) ureter occurs secondary to abnormal embryology of the inferior vena cava (IVC), not the ureter. The IVC develops from a plexus of fetal veins. Normally, the IVC forms from the right supracardinal vein as the right subcardinal atrophies. If the right subcardinal vein fails to atrophy and becomes the IVC, a segment of ureter becomes trapped behind the vena cava. Circumcaval ureter usually occurs on the right; but if it occurs on the left, it is usually associated with duplicated IVC or partial/complete *situs inversus*.

○ **What is the most common etiology of drug-induced renal calculi in children?**

Secondary hypercalciuria as a side effect of long-term use of furosemide, glucocorticoids, or theophylline in premature infants.

○ **What is a pseudotumor of the kidney?**

A hypertrophied column of Bertin that may be sufficiently large to compress and deform the adjacent collecting system.

○ **What is the usual clinical course of classic congenital mesoblastic nephroma?**

Classic congenital mesoblastic nephroma is a benign tumor and treatment is limited to surgical excision. It typically presents as an asymptomatic palpable abdominal mass, but may also present with hypercalcemia or hematuria.

○ **What is a nephrogenic rest?**

A nephrogenic rest is an abnormal focus of embryonal cells within a developmentally normal kidney. Although these cells can be a precursor to Wilms tumor, the majority of nephrogenic rests involute and do not result in tumor formation. They can also mimic Wilms tumor radiographically and histologically in small biopsies or frozen sections.

○ **What hepatic abnormality is associated with autosomal recessive polycystic kidney disease?**

Congenital hepatic fibrosis.

○ **What are the prenatal ultrasound characteristics of autosomal recessive polycystic kidney disease?**

As a result of the enormous number of interfaces created by the tightly compacted, dilated collecting ducts, the kidneys appear large and homogeneously hyperechogenic with loss of corticomedullary differentiation.

○ **What neurological, gastrointestinal, and cardiac anomalies are associated with autosomal dominant polycystic kidney disease?**

Circle of Willis and Berry aneurysms, colonic diverticula, aortic aneurysms, and mitral valve prolapse.

○ **Juvenile nephronophthisis and medullary cystic disease are transmitted by what modes of inheritance?**

Juvenile nephronophthisis is an autosomal recessive disease characterized by renal cysts and fibrosis and is thought to occur from a mutation in 1 of at least 8 genes in the nephrocystin family. Medullary cystic kidney disease is transmitted as an autosomal dominant trait characterized by tubulointerstitial fibrosis and renal cysts.

○ **What are the characteristics of Alport syndrome?**

Hereditary nephritis, high frequency hearing loss, ocular abnormalities, microhematuria, and proteinuria.

○ **What is sirenomelia and what renal defect is associated with it?**

It is a rare congenital syndrome in which the lower extremities are fused together. It occurs in approximately 1 in 60,000 to 100,000 births and is almost always fatal due to the associated renal agenesis. If kidney function is preserved, survival is possible but extremely rare.

○ **Is ureteropelvic junction (UPJ) obstruction in children more common in boys or girls?**

Boys, by a ratio of about 2:1.

○ **In children with UPJ, which side is involved more often or is it a tie?**

It is more commonly found on the left than the right with 60% found on the left. Some series have documented that bilateral obstruction occurs in 10% to 40% of cases of UPJ obstruction.

○ **What is Fraley syndrome?**

Fraley originally described this syndrome in 1966 as a condition where an aberrant crossing vessel causes clinical obstruction and hydronephrosis of the upper pole infundibulum resulting in significant renal pain and/or hematuria. Stones, pain, infection, and hematuria are commonly associated with the syndrome. It requires surgical repair only if symptomatic.

○ **What is Dietl crisis?**

Symptoms of acute bilateral flank pain, nausea, and vomiting after an acute increase in urinary output. It is caused by a secondary obstruction of the UPJ when the renal pelvis cannot tolerate the increased output and "kinking" at the UPJ occurs.

○ **Describe the process of normal renal formation and the defect that may cause the agenesis of a kidney?**

An orderly branching ureteral bud is required for complete formation of the adult kidney. At the end of the 4th week of gestation, the ureteral bud arises from the mesonephric (wolffian) duct. A normal metanephric blastema needs to be present to induce the ureteral bud to branch into major and minor calyces. Agenesis of the kidney results when the ureteral bud fails to develop or the nephrogenic ridge is absent.

○ **In a patient with a normal left kidney and a right pelvic kidney, what is the location of both adrenal glands?**

The adrenal glands are both normally positioned.

○ **What are the 6 potential locations of an ectopic kidney?**

Pelvic (below aortic bifurcation), iliac (between L2 and the iliac crest), abdominal, thoracic (rarest 1:16,000), contralateral, or crossed (1:7000).

○ **In a horseshoe kidney, are the calyces normal in number and orientation?**

The calyces are normal in number, but have an atypical orientation. Since the kidney does not rotate, the calyces are oriented posteriorly and the pelvic axis stays in the obliquely lateral or vertical plane.

○ **Identify 3 specific causes of significant hydronephrosis caused by UPJ obstruction in patients with a horseshoe kidney?**

The obstruction results from one or more of the following:

1. High insertion of the ureter into the renal pelvis.

2. Aberrant course over the isthmus impairing drainage.

3. Anomalous blood supply/crossing vessel.

○ **What is a calyceal diverticulum?**

A transitional epithelium-lined cystic cavity located within the renal parenchyma and connected to an adjacent minor calyx by a narrow channel or infundibulum.

○ **In a patient with a complete ureteral duplication with a refluxing lower pole moiety and a normal upper pole moiety who is undergoing ureteral reimplantation, should the ureters be reimplanted separately or together?**

Near the UVJ, the 2 ureters share a common adventitial blood supply that runs longitudinally between the 2 ureters. Both ureters should be reimplanted together in a common sheath reimplantation to avoid compromise to the vasculature.

○ **In a female, what anomalies may result from incomplete or altered müllerian development caused by mesonephric duct maldevelopment?**

Complete absence of the ipsilateral horn and the fallopian tube with a unicornuate uterus is the most common anomaly. A bicornate uterus with incomplete development of the horn on the affected side can also occur. When there is partial or complete fusion of the müllerian ducts in the midline, a didelphic or septated uterus with a solitary or duplex cervix may result.

○ **What test should be ordered if, during a physical examination, the vas deferens or body and tail of the epididymis are missing? What disorder would be suspected?**

An abdominal ultrasound to evaluate for unilateral renal agenesis.

○ **When does the kidney reach its adult location?**

The kidney reaches its adult location by the end of the 8th week of gestation.

○ **In crossed fused ectopia, how are the 2 renal units joined?**

The inferior aspect of the normal kidney is usually attached to the superior pole of the ectopic kidney. Eighty-five percent of crossed ectopic kidneys are fused. The left kidney is 3 times more likely to cross to the right.

○ **In fusion anomalies, how do the ureters insert into the bladder?**

The ureter from each kidney is usually orthotopic.

○ **The müllerian ducts stop developing at approximately what age of gestational development?**

The müllerian ducts regression begins around 8 weeks of gestation and they are almost completely absent at 10 weeks.

○ **Medullary sponge kidney (MSK) has been associated with what urological problems?**

Recurrent urinary tract infections (UTIs), renal leak-type hypercalciuria, hypocitraturia, hematuria, and nephrolithiasis.

○ **What renal pelvis pressure reading suggests obstruction when performing a Whitaker test?**

Intrapelvic pressure <15 cm H_2O indicates efficient flow, >20 cm H_2 indicates obstruction, and between 15 and 20 cm H_2O is equivical.

○ **What is the most common congenital urinary malformation?**

Ureteral duplication (1:125).

○   **True/False: Symphysiotomy (division of the isthmus) is routinely recommended after pyeloplasty in patients with horseshoe kidney.**

False. Due to the abnormal vasculature, the kidneys tend to resume their previous position, so a symphysiotomy is no longer recommended. It also increases the risk of bleeding, fistula formation, and renal infarction.

○   **What syndromes are associated with horseshoe kidney?**

Turner syndrome (7% incidence) and Trisomy 18 (20% incidence).

○   **Compared to normal kidneys, horseshoe kidneys have a higher incidence of what urologic problems?**

Hydronephrosis, UPJ obstruction, stones, urinary tract infections, and tumors.

○   **What tumor is associated with horseshoe kidney?**

There is a 1.5- to 8-fold increase in Wilms tumor occurrence. Recent studies have shown that although it was previously believed there was an increase in the rate of renal cell carcinoma, transitional cell carcinoma, and oncocytoma in horseshoe kidneys, this is probably not true.

CHAPTER 8 Prune-Belly Syndrome

Mark R. Wakefield, MD, FACS,
Julie M. Riley, MD, and
Elizabeth Malm-Buatsi, MD

○ **What are alternate, perhaps less stigmatizing, names for prune-belly syndrome?**

Prune-belly vividly describes the clinical appearance of most patients with the syndrome. However, many clinicians consider the negative connotations to be stigmatizing and socially undesirable. Thus, several alternatives have been proposed. Eagle–Barrett syndrome recognizes one of the original descriptions of a series of 9 patients in 1950. Abdominal wall deficiency syndrome is a descriptive nomenclature. Triad syndrome emphasizes the 3 components of the classic syndrome. Nonetheless, prune-belly syndrome remains the common terminology, in part because of its intensely descriptive nature.

○ **What are 3 classic features that characterize prune-belly syndrome?**

Triad syndrome refers to the following 3 specific features of prune-belly syndrome:

1. Urinary tract dilation, specifically megaureter.

2. Abdominal wall deficiency.

3. Cryptorchidism.

The defective abdominal musculature gives the typical appearance of a wrinkled prune, with laxity of the anterior abdominal wall. The testes are both nonpalpable. The urinary tract dilation includes tortuous, dilated ureters, as well as varying degrees of an enlarged smooth-walled bladder and dilated prostatic urethra.

○ **What is the approximate incidence of prune-belly syndrome?**

The true incidence is not well known. The estimated incidence is similar to that of bladder exstrophy. The reported range is 1 per 29,000 to 40,000 live births. With increasing prenatal diagnosis and termination, the incidence has been decreasing. The classic triad syndrome only occurs in males. However, variations that include 2 of the 3 features can occur in males and females. The incidence is uncertain for patients with incomplete prune-belly syndrome, but probably is one-fourth as common as the classic syndrome. Furthermore, approximately 15% of patients with incomplete prune-belly syndrome were females. More common in twins, African Americans, and kids born to younger mothers.

○ **What is the incidence of prune-belly syndrome in females?**

Of all prune-belly syndrome cases, 3% to 5% occur in females.

○ **What is the most common genetic karyotype in patients with prune-belly syndrome?**

Normal. However, several genetic defects are associated with prune-belly syndrome. These include Turner syndrome, Monosomy 16, Patau syndrome (trisomy 13), Edward syndrome (trisomy 18), and Beckwith–Wiedemann syndrome.

○ **To what does pseudo-prune-belly syndrome refer?**

Incomplete prune-belly syndrome refers to patients with 2 of the 3 classic findings of the triad. For females, this would include the dilation of the urinary tract and lax abdominal wall musculature, but not the undescended testes. Pseudo-prune-belly syndrome refers to those males with ureteral dilation and undescended testes, but normal abdominal wall. Fifty percent will go on to renal failure often due to delay in diagnosis.

○ **What percent of patients will have atypical presentation of prune-belly syndrome?**

An incomplete form of prune-belly syndrome is present in as many as 25% of patients. Most will have the typical urinary tract finding of dilated ureters, but will have either normal abdominal wall musculature (pseudo-prune-belly syndrome) or descended testes. Females with incomplete prune-belly syndrome are even less common, affecting less than 5% of patients with the syndrome. In females, the urinary tract dilation may be less severe.

○ **How does prune-belly syndrome present in females?**

Prune-belly syndrome is uncommon in females and makes up just 5% of all prune belly syndrome patients. Females don't have gonadal anomalies. They have abdominal wall and genitourinary tract anomalies only. Forty percent have anorectal anomalies and bladder outlet obstruction is common. Forty percent of females with prune-belly syndrome die during the neonatal period.

○ **What are some proposed embryologic etiologies of prune-belly syndrome?**

There are several theories explaining the embryogenesis of prune-belly syndrome. Each theory has both supporting experimental and empiric evidence, but none been proven. These theories are not mutually exclusive.

Urinary tract obstruction may result from a transient urethral membrane at a critical phase of development. Abdominal wall laxity then results from outward compression from the dilated urinary tract. The migration of the testicles is blocked by the enlarged bladder. Primary prostatic maldevelopment with hypoplasia of the prostatic urethra is another possible cause of urinary tract obstruction. A final postulated cause is felt to be due to transient obstruction at the glanular and penile urethral junction. In any case, fetal urinary ascites may or may not occur.

Primary mesodermal maldevelopment may also explain prune-belly syndrome. Failure of myoblast precursors to differentiate and/or migrate appropriately may explain the abnormal development of the abdominal wall. The laxity of the abdominal wall may then be the primary event. The decreased intra-abdominal pressures then result in urinary tract dilation and undescended testicles. However, if the developmental defect occurs early enough (3rd week of gestation), then all of the abnormalities may be explained by a common event in the mesenchymal tissues.

Persistence of the yolk sac has been implicated in the abdominal wall abnormalities resulting in redundant tissues. The allantoic diverticulum becomes overdeveloped and becomes incorporated into the urinary tract as redundant tissues.

○ **Which is the prevailing theory?**

Mesodermal arrest. This is thought to occur between the 6th and the 10th gestational week although it could occur as early as 3 weeks gestation.

○ **Histopathology of the abdominal wall muscles is suggestive of what type of etiology: developmental arrest or muscular atrophy?**

Developmental arrest. The lack of aponeurotic layers supports this etiology.

○ **What are the 3 categories of prune-belly syndrome?**

Category I has marked oligohydramnios secondary to dysplasia or severe bladder outlet obstruction, pulmonary hypoplasia, and Potter features. Prognosis is very poor in this group as most are either stillborn or die within the first few days of life. Little intervention is warranted in this group. A common intervention for this category is catheter drainage. This consists of 20% of the cases.

Category II shows minimal or unilateral renal dysplasia, full triad features without pulmonary hypoplasia. The course tends to be variable from stabilized renal function to progressive azotemia. This would include patients with urethral atresia and a patent urachus. The goal of treatment in this group is to stabilize renal function. The treatment in this category has the most controversies. This consists of 40% of the cases.

Category III consists of patients with mild or incomplete forms of prune-belly syndrome. There is no renal dysplasia or pulmonary insufficiency seen. There is stable renal function. Invasive treatment is necessary in those patients with recurrent infections. This consists of the remaining 40% of the cases.

○ **Fetal ascites may be transient in prune-belly cases. Why?**

It is reabsorbed, usually before birth.

○ **What is the role of prenatal diagnosis with fetal ultrasound in prune-belly syndrome?**

In general, prenatal diagnosis of prune-belly syndrome has not been reliable. There are high false-positive and false-negative rates of prenatal diagnosis. The typical intrauterine appearance of prune-belly syndrome is bilateral hydronephrosis with an enlarged noncycling bladder. Earlier fetal ascites and oligohydramnios may also be suggestive of prune-belly syndrome. However, the differential diagnosis of these findings includes posterior urethral valves, vesicoureteral reflux, bilateral ureteropelvic junction obstruction, neurogenic bladder, and megacystitis/megalourethra syndromes.

○ **When are most cases of prune-belly syndrome diagnosed?**

During the 2nd trimester.

○ **What are the antenatal findings of prune-belly syndrome?**

Bilateral hydronephrosis and hydroureter, distended thin-walled bladder, and oligohydramnios. Oligohydramnios implies renal dysfunction, which leads to pulmonary hypoplasia.

○ **What is the differential diagnosis of antenatal ultrasound findings consistent with prune-belly syndrome?**

Posterior urethral valves and megacystitis microcolon intestinal hypoperistalsis syndrome.

○ **What genetic defects have been associated with prune-belly syndrome?**

Chromosome 17q12 deletion has been associated with prune-belly syndrome. This is the gene for HNF1β, which is a transcription factor regulating mesodermal and endodermal development. However, this has been associated in only a few cases. Moreover, functionally significant HNF1β mutations have been found recently to be quite uncommon in prune-belly syndrome patients (Granberg et al., 2012).

○ **Late presentations of prune-belly syndrome are typified by what characteristics?**

Although the typical appearance of the abdomen in neonates with prune-belly syndrome usually leads to prompt diagnosis, some children present at a later age. These children often have less severe forms of the syndrome. These children may present with difficulty sitting from a supine position as a result of weaker abdominal muscles. Walking may be delayed due to difficulty with standing and balance. Older children will have a characteristic potbelly with loss of wrinkling of the skin due to stretching of the abdominal viscera.

○ **What diagnostic evaluation in patients with prune-belly syndrome should be avoided?**

A voiding cystourethrogram (VCUG) should be avoided in the early prenatal period. Instrumentation of the urinary tract puts the patient at increased risk of infection and sepsis. The diagnosis should be suspected based on physical examination findings. The dilated bladder and ureters are often palpable due to the lax abdominal wall. Although used previously to confirm diagnosis, intravenous pyelogram does not image the urinary tract well due to poor concentrating ability of neonatal kidneys and dilution of contrast in the dilated urinary tract. Abdominal ultrasound can be useful in assessing the degree of urinary tract dilation. Serial assessment of serum electrolytes, renal function, and urine culture are important diagnostic tests. A renal scan is necessary when renal function stabilizes to evaluate renal function and drainage.

Some experts, however, recommend an early VCUG despite the risks because it is the best way to identify reflux and urethral stenosis. Bladder size can be determined as well as the presence of any urachal remnants.

○ **What is the most common nongenitourinary anomaly in patients with prune-belly syndrome?**

Thoracic cage malformations, including pectus excavatum and pectus carinatum, occur in more than 75% of patients with prune-belly syndrome. The chest wall malformations are likely due to the restrictive effects of oligohydramnios. In the most severe form, pulmonary hypoplasia can occur with associated pneumothorax, pneumomediastinum, and high neonatal mortality rate. Most patients, however, have only mild pulmonary dysfunction, often only evident on formal pulmonary function testing. Patients with prune-belly syndrome will have a less forceful cough due to weaker abdominal musculature placing them at increased risk for postoperative respiratory distress, pneumonia, and bronchitis. Other common anomalies include cardiac (10%), gastrointestinal (30%), and orthopedic deformities (50%).

○ **What is the most common anomaly of the musculoskeletal system in patients with prune-belly syndrome?**

Skin dimples on the knee or elbow are the most common abnormality of the musculoskeletal system, excluding the typical abdominal wall defects. The skin dimples occur in 45% of patients. More severe anomalies include varus deformity of the feet (club foot), which occurs in 25% of patients, congential hip dislocation (5%), spinal dysmorphism (5%), and rarely severe lower extremity hypoplasia. Skin dimples are likely a result of compression from oligohydramnios. Other etiologies have been proposed: ischemia from compressed iliac vessels or a common defect in mesenchymal development at 3 weeks gestation.

Cardiac abnormalities occur in 10% of patients with prune-belly syndrome. The most common cardiac abnormalities in prune-belly syndrome are patent ductus arteriosus, ventricular septal defect, atrial septal defect, and tetralogy of Fallot.

Malrotation of the midgut occurs more frequently in patients with severe prune-belly syndrome. Other gastrointestinal anomalies, including gastroschisis, omphalocele, anorectal anomalies, and Hirschsprung have been described in patients with prune-belly syndrome. Chronic constipation and acquired megacolon can be an issue.

○ **In addition to the classic triad of findings, what are the common anomalies of the urinary system in prune-belly syndrome?**

The penile urethra is usually normal, although a megalourethra is associated with prune-belly syndrome. The prostatic urethra is hypoplastic in most patients with prune-belly syndrome. The bladder neck is wide open and tapers to the normal membranous urethra. The prostatic urethra appears dilated as a result of the prostatic hypoplasia. The prostatic utricle and ejaculatory ducts are dilated. The bladder is enlarged, but usually does not have trabeculation. The patent urachus may persist, especially if there is urethral atresia. The ureters are involved with the proximal ureters typically being less dilated. The kidneys are afflicted by varying degrees of hydronephrosis and renal dysplasia.

○ **What is the likelihood of renal failure among patients with prune-belly syndrome?**

One-third or 20% to 30% of patients will progress to renal failure.

○ **What causes renal failure in patients with prune-belly syndrome?**

Renal failure in patients with prune-belly syndrome results from the reflux of infected urine and subsequent pyelonephritis. High-grade obstruction or high-pressure reflux may result in severe renal dysplasia at birth, as seen in some neonatal autopsy studies. However, most patients with prune-belly syndrome have low-pressure vesicoureteral reflux. As long as the urine remains sterile, the risk of renal failure appears to be low, despite the high incidence of reflux and dilation of the upper tract.

○ **What is the role of renal transplantation in patients with prune-belly syndrome?**

Renal transplantation in patients with prune-belly syndrome is as successful as transplantation for other indications in children. Special attention must be directed toward management of the urinary tract prior to transplantation. Adequate bladder emptying with clean intermittent catheterization is often necessary and is preferable to urinary diversion. Acute graft torsion due to abdominal wall laxity is a unique problem to the prune-belly population.

○ **How common is vesicoureteral reflux in patients with prune-belly syndrome?**

Vesicoureteral reflux occurs in as many as 85% of the patients with prune-belly syndrome. The reflux tends to be low pressure. Most children with prune-belly syndrome do not outgrow this reflux. Nonetheless, surgery to correct the reflux is usually reserved for those patients with recurrent pyelonephritis, whose reflux is refractory to more conservative therapies such as vesicostomy. Ureteroneocystostomy is associated with a high risk of ureterovesical junction obstruction and recurrence of reflux in patients with prune-belly syndrome.

○ **What are the typical characteristics of the kidney in patients with prune-belly syndrome?**

Fifty percent of patients with prune-belly syndrome will have dysplastic kidneys. Dysplasia shows either Potter type 2 or 4. Type 2 is more indicative of mesenchymal defect, whereas type 4 is related to obstruction. The renal pelvis is often dilated. The degree of dilation is not proportional to the degree of dysplasia. Renal infection, not the degree of obstruction or reflux, poses the greatest risk.

○ **What are the typical characteristics of the ureters in patients with prune-belly syndrome?**

The ureters in patients with prune-belly syndrome are dilated in 80% of the cases. The proximal ureters tend to be spared with increased dilation and tortuosity in the distal segments. The ureters may have decreased smooth muscle and an altered collagen matrix, which leads to a loss of luminal coaptation and ineffective peristalsis. The proximal ureters are more suitable for reimplantation when indicated because of improved proximal peristalsis. The distal ureters have poor blood supply and show smooth muscle deficiency with fibrous degeneration. Vesicoureteral reflux is present in up to 85%. Ureteropelvic junction obstruction can also occur, but the biggest risk to the kidney is infection and not obstruction.

○   **What are the typical characteristics of the bladder in patients with prune-belly syndrome?**

The bladder in patients with prune-belly syndrome is massively enlarged, but smooth-walled with minimal trabeculation or diverticula. There is an increased ratio of collagen to muscle fibers in the bladder. Dilation of the urachus may result in pseudodiverticulum at the dome of the bladder. The intertrigonal ridge is wide with lateral and superiorly placed ureteral orifices. The bladder neck is open and funnels into the prostatic urethra giving the appearance of an hourglass on VCUG.

○   **What are the urethral abnormalities associated with prune-belly syndrome?**

Dilation of the posterior urethra is seen in patients with prune-belly syndrome that is secondary to prostatic hypoplasia. This prostatic hypoplasia leads to ejaculatory failure and retrograde ejaculation is very common.

Urethral atresia is also associated with prune-belly syndrome. A patent urachus must be present in order for survival. Prune-belly syndrome is also associated with a megalourethra. There are 2 types of megalourethra. A fusiform deformity consists of a deficiency of both the corpus spongiosum and cavernosum. When the patient voids, the entire phallus dilates. A scaphoid deformity is a deficiency of only the corpus spongiosum with preservation of the glans and corpus cavernosum. The ventral urethra is seen to dilate with voiding.

○   **Are posterior valves associated with prune-belly syndrome?**

Occasionally.

○   **What is the significance of a patent urachus in prune-belly syndrome?**

A patent urachus is present in 25% to 30% of patients with prune-belly syndrome. It is frequently found in the setting of urethral obstruction. Early deaths do occur when patients with urethral obstruction do not have a patent urachus so it may allow for survival in some patients.

○   **What does cystometrogram evaluation in patients with prune-belly syndrome typically demonstrate?**

Bladder function in patients with prune-belly syndrome is variable. Initial urodynamic evaluation with cystometrogram will usually demonstrate a high-capacity bladder with normal compliance, decreased sensation, and poor contractility. Bladder pressures during voiding are low. Emptying is often incomplete. Despite this, 50% of patients void spontaneously with normal voiding pressures and flow rate and low postvoid residual. Bladder herniations are common.

○   **What is the typical location of the undescended testicles in patients with prune-belly syndrome?**

The testicles are usually located at the pelvic brim. Early orchiopexy is usually possible. The Fowler–Stephens technique is often necessary for the testicles to reach the scrotum. Testicular autotransplantation with microvascular anastomosis has also been performed.

○   **How are undescended testicles managed in prune-belly syndrome?**

Procedures are used similar to those used in patients without prune-belly syndrome and include single-stage orchiopexy with preservation of the vascular bundle, single-stage Fowler–Stephens, or a two-stage Fowler–Stephens procedure. There is, however, a higher rate of testicular loss in prune-belly syndrome (Zugor et al., 2012).

○ **What is the cause of infertility in patients with prune-belly syndrome?**

Infertility of patients with prune-belly syndrome is multifactorial. Failure of emission or retrograde ejaculation is common. Prostatic and seminal fluids may be insufficient. Spermatogenesis may be altered. Early orchiopexy, electroejaculation, and intracytoplasmic sperm injection may allow for fertility in some patients. Intra-abdominal testes tend to develop progressive tubular fibrosis. Human chorionic gonadotropin (HCG) therapy does not help in these cases.

○ **What are the growth characteristics of patients with prune-belly syndrome?**

In general, the growth of children with prune-belly syndrome depends upon their renal function. With impaired renal function, there is significant growth delay. Nonetheless, growth retardation occurs in more than one-third of patients with normal renal function (Woods, 2007).

○ **Can any treatment be given prenatally?**

Fetuses with prune-belly syndrome may need intrauterine intervention if there is obstruction and concern for pulmonary maturation. A vesicoamniotic shunt may be placed to bypass the obstruction. Criteria for intrauterine surgery is second or third trimester, oligohydramnios, megacystis, advanced hydronephrosis, normal karyotype, urine sodium less than 100 mg/dL, and urine osmolality less than 210 mOsm. Complications include dislodgement, urinary ascites, premature labor, and chorioamnionitis.

○ **What is the initial postnatal management of prune-belly syndrome?**

The initial management of patients with prune-belly syndrome has evolved and now relies upon the recognition of the syndrome and generally involves noninvasive therapies. Stabilization of the associated cardiopulmonary complications is paramount, as they are often more serious in the neonatal period. Usually the child is able to spontaneously void, but this may be facilitated by bladder massage. Prophylactic antibiotics are indicated as vesicoureteral reflux can be assumed to exist. Catheter drainage or other instrumentation should be considered cautiously, as the possibility of urinary tract infection is a significant risk. If the patient has persistent azotemia or acidosis, urinary tract diversion may be necessary. Stomal stenosis appears to be more common in children with prune-belly syndrome; therefore, a large caliber (28F) vesicostomy is advisable. Occasionally, percutaneous nephrostomies are needed in the setting of sepsis. Cutaneous ureterostomies may be necessary if the ureters are obstructed distally due to extreme tortuosity. Urethrotomy to improve urinary drainage is now limited to the few patients with anatomic urethral obstruction. Circumcision is advisable in order to reduce the risk of infection.

○ **What are the long-term treatment options for patients with prune-belly syndrome?**

The treatment of patients with prune-belly syndrome must be individualized. However, in general, most patients can be treated conservatively with delayed surgical reconstruction. Prophylactic antibiotics are indicated in the initial treatment of vesicoureteral reflux, which is present in more than 85% of patients. If recurrent pyelonephritis ensues, a ureteral reimplant may be necessary. The proximal ureters are utilized as their function is less impaired than the distal ureter. If tapering of a redundant ureter is needed, imbrication may be advantageous in order to preserve ureteral blood supply. Reduction cystoplasty is usually limited to excision of urachal remnants. Clean intermittent catheterization with/without mitrofanoff is a better option than reduction cystoplasty. Orchidopexy should be performed early, often with a transabdominal approach. A staged procedure such as a Fowler–Stephens procedure may be needed in order for the testicles to reach the scrotum. Microvascular autotransplantation has also been employed. Abdominal wall reconstruction is primarily a cosmetic procedure, but may improve pulmonary function.

○   **What are the common types of abdominal wall reconstruction?**

The 4 most utilized surgical procedures are the Randolph, Ehrlich, Monfort, and Firlit techniques. The Randolph technique involves a transverse incision from the 12th rib to the pubic symphysis to the opposite 12th rib with a full-thickness removal of the skin, lower abdominal musculature, and peritoneum. Healthy fascia is approximated to the anterior iliac spines, pubic tubercle, and inferior fascia. The Ehrlich technique utilizes a vertical midline incision that allows for preservation of the umbilicus. The skin and subcutaneous tissues are elevated off the muscle and fascial layers and an overlapping, pants over vest, advancement of each side to the contralateral flank is performed, preserving the less affected lateral muscles and fascia. The Monfort technique uses a similar approach as the Ehrlich technique but instead of a straight vertical incision, an elliptical incision is made to remove redundant skin. The underlying tissue and muscle is freed from the fascia and vertical incisions are made on the lateral fascia. These incisions are closed over the medial fascia. This procedure can also be performed laparoscopically. The Firlit procedure stays extra-peritoneal. Skin flaps are created laterally from a midline vertical incision. The lateral fascial layer is plicated in a double-breasted fashion without lateral fascial dissection or incision of the midline fascial plate. This procedure too has been successfully performed laparoscopically.

Abdominal reconstruction has only been shown to improve appearance and there has been no measurable improvement of function of the bladder.

○   **What is the prognosis for patients with prune-belly syndrome?**

The prognosis for patients with prune-belly syndrome has improved. Some infants are stillborn and as many as 25% of patients in some series died in the neonatal period due to urosepsis, renal failure, or most commonly concomitant cardiopulmonary disease. With improvement in neonatal intensive care, the neonatal mortality rate is less than 10%, death is most often due to renal failure as a result of severe renal dysplasia. Despite avoidance of urinary tract instrumentation and the use of suppressive antibiotics, urinary tract infections are common. More than 75% of patients will develop urinary tract infections; however, febrile infections and pyelonephritis are unusual, especially in those patients with good renal function. Renal failure occurs in 25% to 30% of patients with prune-belly syndrome. The presence of early renal insufficiency and urosepsis predicts progression to renal failure. A nadir serum creatinine greater than 0.7 mg/dL predicts the development of renal failure. When needed, renal transplantation can be performed safely (Hassett et al., 2012).

CHAPTER 9

Cryptorchidism: Diagnosis and Management

Jeffrey P. Wolters, MD, MPH,
Neil A. King, MD, and
Harry P. Koo, MD, FAAP, FACS

○ **What is the SRY gene, what does it do, and where is it located?**

SRY stands for Sex determining Region on the Y chromosome. It is located on the short arm of the Y chromosome.

○ **What role does SRY play in testis development?**

SRY is believed to induce Sertoli cell differentiation and testis development. SRY upregulates the expression of **SOX9 gene**, which then promotes further differentiation of Sertoli cells.

○ **What role does SOX9 play in testis development?**

The SOX9 gene is structurally similar to SRY. SOX9 is probably activated by SRY because both genes are expressed by fetal Sertoli cells. SOX9 is believed to (1) further promote the differentiation of the Sertoli cells, and (2) upregulate mullerian-inhibiting substance (MIS) gene expression.

○ **During sexual differentiation of the gonad into a testis, what are the first cells to differentiate in the testis and approximately when does that happen?**

The Sertoli cells differentiate at around 6 to 8 weeks.

○ **What is the primordial hormone of the fetal testis? When and where does it begin to get produced?**

Mullerian-inhibiting substance (MIS) is a glycoprotein that is produced and secreted by Sertoli cells around the 8th week of gestation and is responsible for regression of the mullerian ducts. Evidence for the role of MIS in testicular descent is conflicting.

○ **What 2 structures are the remnants of the regressed mullerian ducts?**

The appendix testis and the prostatic utricle.

○   **What cells in the testes are responsible for the production of testosterone in utero?**

Leydig cells, just like in adults.

○   **Describe the 2 separate stages of testicular descent. Describe the role and actions for insulin-like hormone 3 and calcitonin gene-related peptide. Where are these substances made?**

1. The first stage occurs at 8 to 15 weeks gestation. There is enlargement of the gubernaculum and regression of the **cranial suspensory ligament (CSL)**. Leydig cells produce **insulin-like hormone 3**, which stimulates the caudal gubernaculums to grow and become thicker. Mullerian-inhibiting substance may have a role in stimulating the swelling reaction in the gubernaculum.

2. The second stage occurs between 25 and 35 weeks gestation and requires the migration of the gubernaculum and testis from the inguinal region to the scrotum. This stage is thought to be more androgen dependent. In addition, the genitofemoral nerve releases **calcitonin gene-related peptide**, which may guide the migration of the testis.

○   **What is the CSL and what happens to it in adults?**

The undifferentiated gonad is initially located high in the abdomen, anchored by the CSL. During intra-abdominal descent (1st stage of testicular descent), androgens lead to the regression of the CSL. In females, the CSL persists because of the absence of androgens.

○   **When does testicular descent typically begin and finish?**

Descent typically begins in the 23rd week of gestation when the processus vaginalis elongates into the scrotum. At 24 weeks, descent is complete in 10% of fetuses, at 27 weeks 50%, at 28 weeks 75%, and at 34 weeks 80%.

○   **True/False: Spontaneous descent of an undescended testicle is rare after the first year of life.**

True. Less than 10% of cryptorchid testes will descend spontaneously beyond 6 months of age.

○   **What are the incidences of cryptorchidism in premature, full-term neonates, 1-year olds, and adults, respectively?**

The incidences are 30%, 3%, 1%, and 1%, respectively.

○   **At 1 year of age, what percentage of cryptorchid testes have descended in premature infants and in full-term infants, respectively?**

It is 95% for premature infants and 75% for full-term infants. The majority of all descents will have occurred in the first 3 to 6 months of life.

○   **What is now believed to be the single greatest predisposing factor for cryptorchidism?**

Low birth weight (independent of length of gestation).

○   **What maternal factors contribute to cryptorchidism?**

Endocrine disrupting chemicals (EDC) found in many pesticides have been shown to have antiandrogenic effects on the developing male fetus in both human and animal models. This is thought to cause genital malformations including cryptorchidism, hypospadias, and micropenis. Paternal exposure to EDCs may also be associated with increased risk for cryptorchidism.

○ **What is the relationship between maternal smoking and obesity on the incidence of cryptorchidism?**

Maternal smoking and obesity are not associated with increased incidence of cryptorchidism.

○ **What percentage of cryptorchid testes are bilateral?**

30%.

○ **What percentage of cases of cryptorchidism are accompanied by epididymal anomalies?**

35% to 75%. It is thought that the cranial gubernaculum develops an abnormal embryologic attachment. This can lead to a spectrum of malformations, ranging from simple elongation to aberrant fusion, complete disjunction, or even total absence of the epididymis. Therefore, even in the setting of normal germ cell development, fusion anomalies may have a significant negative impact on fertility.

○ **True/False: Due to the embryologic association of the ureteric bud and the Wolffian duct, an ultrasound of the upper urinary tracts is recommended in patients with true cryptorchidism.**

False. The incidence of upper tract abnormalities in cryptorchidism is no greater than the general population. Therefore, ultrasound evaluation of the upper tracts is only indicated in cases of suspected intersex conditions.

○ **What is the difference between a cryptorchid and an ectopic testis?**

A cryptorchid testis is located along the normal path of descent, but has failed to reach a dependent position in the scrotum. Ectopic testes descend normally through the external inguinal ring, but then migrate away from the normal pathway.

○ **What are some possible locations for an ectopic testis and which of these is the most common?**

Ectopic tests can be found in the perineum, the femoral canal, suprapubic, and transverse scrotal locations. However, the most common location is the superficial inguinal pouch (Denis-Browne pouch), between the external oblique and Scarpa's fascia.

○ **What is a retractile testicle, and how is it different than cryptorchidism?**

A retractile testis is a normal testicle, which can be pulled up, into the inguinal canal during physical examination. It is thought to result from overactive cremasteric muscles. An uncommon phenomenon of delayed testicular ascent has been falsely ascribed to retractile testes. "Testicular ascent" probably represents an undescended testis that appears to be almost completely descended in the infant or young child.

○ **How should a retractile testicle be followed?**

Children with retractile testis should be monitored regularly (annually or biennially) until puberty or until the testes have clearly descended permanently.

○ **What options are available for medical therapy for cryptorchidism?**

Human chorionic gonadotropin (hCG) and luteinizing hormone-releasing hormone (LHRH).

○ **What is the overall efficacy of hormonal/medical therapy?**

Approximately 20%.

○ **What is the mechanism of action of hCG, how is it administered, what is the recommended dosage and the duration of therapy?**

Administration of hCG stimulates Leydig cells, which results in increased plasma testosterone levels, thus promoting testicular descent. The normal dosing of hCG is a total dose of 10,000 to 15,000 units administered by injection twice weekly over 2 to 3 weeks (doses are adjusted for children weighing less than 20 kg). **Above 15,000 IU of hCG, deleterious side effects become more common:** increased rugation and pigmentation of the scrotum, transient increase in penile size, and development of pubic hair. It also can cause changes in testicular histology.

○ **What is the mechanism of action and dosage for LHRH?**

LHRH stimulates the anterior pituitary to release LH, which promotes testicular descent. LHRH, which is preferred in Europe, is administered transnasally at a dose of 1.2 mg daily for 4 weeks.

○ **Can hCG and LHRH be used together?**

Yes.

○ **What percentage of cryptorchid testes are nonpalpable?**

20%.

○ **What percentage of "nonpalpable testes" are actually absent on surgical exploration?**

Approximately 30%.

○ **What is the role of imaging versus physical examination by a urologist with respect to localizing a nonpalpable testis?**

A good physical examination by a urologist is often more valuable and reliable than an ultrasound. While CT and MRI may discern the gonads in older children and young adults, they both have false-negative rates that make them poor choices to verify absence. In addition, CT and MRI require sedation in younger children, and often may not change the eventual management approach. Ultrasound has sensitivities of 60% for a nonpalpable testis, but has been shown to have higher sensitivity for an identifying inguinal testis (95%) that was difficult to palpate due to body habitus.

○ **What is the best approach to locating a nonpalpable testis?**

The first-line intervention is a thorough examination under anesthesia. This will often offer the surgeon a better opportunity to reaffirm or primarily establish testicular position. If the testis(es) remains nonpalpable, a diagnostic laparoscopy is the most reliable technique for localizing a nonpalpable testis or proving its absence.

○ **What are the 3 possible definitive findings that can be appreciated during a diagnostic laparoscopy for undescended testis?**

1. Absent (vanishing) testis (ie, blind-ending vessels above the internal ring).

2. Cord structures entering the internal ring.

3. Intra-abdominal testis.

○ **What is the Fowler–Stephens orchidopexy? In what cryptorchid condition is this technique commonly applied?**

Ligation of the primary testicular blood supply often becomes necessary in the management of intra-abdominal and high inguinal (occasionally) testis. Fowler–Stephens orchidopexy may be performed open, laparoscopically, or as a combined laparoscopic and open procedure; it may be performed in single-stage or 2 stages. The reported success rates are 60% to 97%.

When the spermatic vessels are divided (the primary blood supply), the blood supply to the testis becomes dependent on collateral circulation from the **deferential artery**—a branch of the inferior vesical artery, and the **cremasteric vessels**—a branch of the inferior epigastric artery.

○ **What are the 4 main risks associated with an undescended testis?**

1. Subfertility—approximately 25% of patients with unilateral cryptorchidism and 50% of patients with bilateral cryptorchidism. (Note: The higher the cryptorchid testis, the more significant the degree of dysfunction.)
2. Neoplasia—testicular cancer (risk is up to 10 times greater).
3. Hernia—a patent processus vaginalis is present in approximately 90% of all cryptorchid testes.
4. Testicular torsion—which is more common in undescended testes.

○ **Is orchidopexy protective against subsequent testicular cancer?**

No. The relative risk of cancer in a patient with a history of treated or persistent cryptorchidism is 2.5 to 8. Although it appears that earlier orchidopexy may improve the risk, patients who undergo orchidopexy after puberty are 2 to 6 times more likely to have testicular cancer than those who undergo prepubertal orchiopexy. Patients with bilateral cryptorchidism and associated genitourinary anomalies are also at higher risk for testicular cancer.

○ **What is the most common tumor in an abdominal cryptorchid testis, before and after orchidopexy?**

Patients who have not undergone orchiopexy are more likely to develop seminomatous germ cell tumors (74%), while patients who have undergone orchiopexy are more likely to develop nonseminomatous germ cell tumors (63%).

○ **A 12-year-old boy is noted to have a solitary left testicle on routine physical for the youth basketball league. His mother states that he underwent a diagnostic laparoscopy as a toddler that revealed blind-ending cord vessels on the right side. What are the preferred recommendations to this boy's mother with respect to playing a contact sport and future imaging?**

Contact sports are permissible, but use of a protective cup is recommended. If the exploratory history of blind-ending vessels is accurate, then no further imaging is necessary.

○ **Physical examination under anesthesia performed on a 9-month-old boy reveals a nonpalpable left testis. Diagnostic laparoscopy reveals the left testicular vessels and vas coursing distal to the internal inguinal ring. What is the next course of action and what is the most likely finding?**

The next step is to continue the exploration (either with laparoscopy or through an inguinal incision). The most likely finding at that time would be the presence of a testicular remnant.

○ **In the scenario of the preceding question, if a testicular remnant is discovered what should be done and why?**

The remnant should be excised due to its potential for future malignant degeneration.

○ **What percentage of atrophic remnants have viable testicular elements, and thus potential for malignant conversion? What is the risk of developing carcinoma in the contralateral testis?**

Thirteen percentage of atrophic remnants contain germ cell tissue, placing these patients at a potential risk for malignant conversion. Patients with an atrophic testicle are also at 36% risk for developing carcinoma in situ in the contralateral testicle.

○ **A 4-year-old boy undergoes a left inguinal exploration for a presumed palpable testis at a level just above the external ring. At the time of exploration, the vas deferens is noted to end blindly just past the level of the internal ring. What is the next step and why?**

Laparascopic or extended abdominal exploration. A blind-ending vas is not definitive evidence of an absent testis. Abdominal exploration needs to be performed to identify either an abdominal testis, or testicular remnant, or definitive evidence of blind-ending vessels.

○ **A newborn is being evaluated for proximal hypospadias and bilateral nonpalpable testes. What potentially life-threatening condition needs to be considered and urgently evaluated?**

Congenital adrenal hyperplasia (CAH) from 21-hydroxylase deficiency must be ruled out in newborns with bilateral cryptorchidism and ambiguous genitalia.

○ **What is the most frequent histologic finding in the cryptorchid testis of a 4-year-old boy?**

Decreased number of germ cells.

○ **Elevation of what hormone in previously cryptorchid men has been correlated to eventual decreased paternity rates?**

Elevation in follicle-stimulating hormone (FSH) is associated with decreased paternity rates. Previously cryptorchid patients with significant elevations in FSH have been shown to be more likely to be azoospermic. Patients with bilateral cryptorchidism have significantly higher FSH compared to unilateral cryptorchidism.

○ **A 20-hour-old neonate has a right scrotal mass that does not transilluminate. What is the most likely diagnosis?**

Extravaginal torsion of the spermatic cord.

○ **Carcinoma in situ (CIS) is present in approximately 1.7% to 3% of previously cryptorchid testes and postulated to have originated within the fetal gonocytes. What is the risk for subsequent development of testicular cancer in gonads that harbor CIS?**

Genetic and histologic studies have shown that carcinoma in situ (*also referred to as intratubular germ cell neoplasia or ITGCN*) cells are similar to gonocytes, but do not differentiate to spermatogonia. Instead, they persist in the postnatal cryptorchid testis. Fifty percent of patients diagnosed with CIS of the testis develop invasive testicular cancer within 5 years of diagnosis. It is now generally agreed that nearly all occurrences of testicular cancer are preceded by the presence of CIS, with the exception of 2 rare tumor types (infantile germ-cell tumor and spermatocytic seminoma) which occurs in older men.

CHAPTER 10

Megaureter, Ectopic Ureter, and Ureterocele

Madhu Alagiri, MD

○ **True/False: The ureter during embryologic development undergoes solidification and later recanalization.**

True. In the first 7 to 8 weeks of gestation, the fetal ureter looses its lumen and recanalizes. The reason for this is unknown, but it may help to explain the presence of ureteral dilation especially if the recanalization process is prolonged.

○ **True/False: The mesonephric duct is necessary for the development of the ureter.**

True. The ureteral bud arises from the mesonephric duct to interact with the metanephric blastema to form the future collecting system and renal parenchyma.

○ **What happens if the mesonephric duct is absent or maldeveloped?**

Absence or maldevelopment of the mesonephric duct will lead to ipsilateral renal agenesis along with absence of genital duct structures such as the vas deferens and seminal vesicles.

○ **Define megaureter.**

A megaureter is an antomical term referring to an enlarged ureter typically measuring greater than 1 cm in diameter. It is easily seen on ultrasound. The typical pediatric ureter is less than 5 mm in diameter and is rarely seen on ultrasound examination.

○ **Describe the 4 types of megaureter.**

Megaureters arise from an underlying pathology such as obstruction or vesicoureteral reflux. The 4 types of megaureter are the obstructed megaureter, the refluxing megaureter, the obstructed, refluxing megaureter, and the nonobstructed, nonrefluxing megaureter.

○ **True/False: The nonobstructed, nonrefluxing megaureter requires surgical correction.**

False. The nonrefluxing, nonobstructing megaureter is likely a result of previous reflux and/or obstruction that has resolved. It does not require immediate surgical correction and often resolves spontaneously over time.

○   **True/False: The presence of hydroureteronephrosis on antenatal ultrasound usually indicates obstruction and can be the precursor to an obstructing megaureter.**

False. Hydroureteronephrosis and hydronephrosis are common findings on antenatal ultrasound. The findings are usually benign and are referred to as physiologic hydronephrosis without obstruction. However, true obstruction or high-grade vesicoureteral reflux may be present and further studies such as serial ultrasounds, voiding cystourethrogram, and diuretic renal scans may be necessary.

○   **Describe the surgical options and reasoning for reducing the diameter of a megaureter during surgical reimplantation.**

The infant ureter has an impressive ability to distend in response to obstruction or high-grade vesicoureteral reflux thus creating a megaureter. Successful surgical repair requires tapering of that ureter to allow for efficient peristalsis of urine. Additionally, reducing the ureteral diameter will decrease the need for a longer submucosal tunnel to prevent vesicoureteral reflux. The primary methods for tapering include plication or excision of the redundant ureter.

○   **Define an ectopic ureter.**

An ectopic ureter simply refers to a ureter that does not terminate in the bladder.

○   **What is the most common site for the termination of an ectopic ureter in a male?**

The ectopic ureter can terminate in a variety of places but always proximal to the urethral sphincter. The most common site of termination is the prostatic urethra.

○   **Name 3 potential sites of termination for an ectopic ureter in a female.**

The perineum, vagina, and uterus are common sites of termination for an ectopic ureter in a female. Unlike a male, the female often presents with incontinence without dry periods. Careful examination will sometimes reveal the steadily dripping ectopic orifice in the introitus.

○   **True/False: When considering a heminephrectomy for an atrophic, upper-moiety renal segment associated with an ectopic ureter, small accessory arteries and veins to the lower moiety can be divided with impunity because of the extensive arterial and venous collateral circulation.**

False. While the venous drainage to the kidney is redundant, care should be taken to preserve all accessory arteries to the lower pole segment since arterial collateral circulation is not present. Division of these vessels will result in tissue ischemia.

○   **A newborn child presents with a history of a 3-cm upper pole cyst first noted on routine antenatal ultrasound. What is the likely diagnosis and best course of action?**

The large "cyst" is most likely the hydronephrotic dysplastic remnant of a duplex system. An obstructing ectopic ureter, which has since involuted, may have been responsible for the findings. Serial ultrasounds can help to determine if the cyst is involuting.

○   **Describe an alternative to reimplanting an ectopic ureter in a duplex system and indicate its advantages.**

An ectopic ureter is often dilated and may need to be tapered prior to reimplantation. Additionally, in a duplex system, the ipsilateral ureter would also have to be reimplanted in a common sheath. As an alternative, the ectopic ureter can be connected to the normal ureter or renal pelvis as in ureteroureterostomy or ureteropyelostomy. This approach would avoid the bladder and precludes reimplanting the normal ureter.

○ **Define the "drooping lily" sign seen on a voiding cystourethrogram and describe its clinical significance.**

A drooping lily sign refers to the finding of reflux into a lower moiety of a duplex system. The renal pelvis of the lower moiety is laterally displaced and the calyces are directed laterally and inferiorly giving rise to the appearance of a drooping lily on the radiograph.

○ **True/False: A megaureter with grade V vesicoureteral reflux has minimal chance for spontaneous resolution except for the newborn male infant.**

True. High-grade vesicoureteral reflux in male infants has a markedly increased chance of fully resolving. This subset should therefore be placed on observation protocols rather than considered for immediate surgical correction.

○ **True/False: A duplex system with upper and lower moiety reflux is identified on a screening voiding cystourethrogram. This would indicate that both the upper and lower moieties are completely duplicated and both are refluxing.**

False. Upper and lower moiety reflux is often seen on a voiding cystourethrogram with apparent full duplication. However, full duplication is rarely present. Instead, the bifurcation of the ureters occurs close to the bladder and is easily missed on the radiograph.

○ **Describe the megacystis–megaureter anomaly associated with high-grade vesicoureteral reflux.**

Megacystis–megaureter refers to a large bladder and dilated ureters caused by the yo-yo reflux of urine between the bladder and ureters. During voiding, the bladder contracts and sends much of the urine up into the refluxing ureters. When the bladder relaxes after voiding, the urine rushes back into the bladder. The bladder never truly empties and thus can be quite capacious.

○ **A 6-year-old girl presents with persistent urinary incontinence. A screening ultrasound indicates a left duplex system and upper moiety hydroureteronephrosis. What further radiologic studies need to be considered?**

There should be a high degree of suspicion for an ectopic ureter. A voiding cystourethrogram and diuretic renal scan will help identify vesicoureteral reflux, renal function, and obstruction. If an ectopic ureter is not clearly identified, magnetic resonance urography may need to be considered to clearly identify ureteral anatomy prior to surgical repair.

○ **True/False: To prevent bacterial colonization of the introitus and vagina in a child with an ectopic ureter, nitrofurantoin should be used as antibiotic prophylaxis.**

False. While nitrofurantoin is an excellent choice for antibiotic prophylaxis with its low tissue and intestinal levels, it does not significantly affect introital or vaginal flora. Trimethoprim–sulfamethoxazole would be the preferred choice because it is present in vaginal secretions.

○ **Define a ureterocele.**

A ureterocele is a cystic dilation of the terminal ureter. It may be either obstructing or nonobstructing. It may also be a part of a single system or part of the upper moiety of a duplex system. The presumed etiology is the persistence of a fetal membranous obstruction (Chwalle membrane) that develops into a ureterocele.

○ **Define an ectopic ureterocele.**

An intravesical ureterocele remains completely within the bladder. An ectopic ureterocele arises from within the bladder, but part of the cystic dilation extends into the bladder neck or urethra.

○ **Define a cecoureterocele and its clinical importance. What is the preferred surgical treatment of this entity?**

A cecoureterocele is a ureterocele in which part of the cavity extends submurally into the bladder neck and urethra. It is important to recognize this entity during repair because inadvertent closure of the urethral segment will result in an enclosed cystic space. Marsupialization of the urethral component into the bladder rather than full excision is the preferred surgical management.

○ **Define a prolapsed ureterocele and its clinical significance. What is the preferred surgical management of a prolapsed ureterocele?**

A prolapsed ureterocele occurs in females, and simply means a ureterocele that has extruded through the urethra. It is obvious as an intralabial mass on examination. Ultrasound often will confirm the diagnosis. The prolapsed ureterocele can be of particular concern because it can result in urine outlet obstruction and resultant infection and sepsis. Puncture and decompression of the ureterocele is the first step in surgical management.

○ **True/False: An ectopic ureter may be mistaken for a ureterocele on ultrasound evaluation.**

True. An ectopic ureter and ureterocele can both look like a cystic mass in the bladder on ultrasound. The ureterocele is usually thin walled and the ectopic ureter tends to have a thicker wall, but this may not always be the case.

○ **True/False: Antenatal detection of ureteroceles is the most common mode of diagnosis.**

True. With the advent of prenatal ultrasound as a routine part of perinatal care, the infant is often diagnosed prior to birth. Prior to the use of ultrasound, infants and children would present later in life with infection and obstruction.

○ **True/False: Endoscopic incision of a ureterocele is a common first step in managing this disorder.**

True. Endoscopic incision can often correct the obstruction associated with ureteroceles, but may create a patulous opening allowing high-grade reflux to occur.

○ **Describe the upper tract approach for ureterocele repair in a duplex system and provide its main advantages.**

The upper tract approach involves a heminephrectomy and partial ureterectomy for a nonfunctional renal segment, or in the case of a functioning upper moiety, a ureteropyelostomy. The primary advantages to this approach are that it avoids bladder surgery, can be definitive, and will correct the primary source of morbidity, which is renal obstruction.

○ **Describe the lower tract approach for ureterocele repair in a duplex system and its primary advantages.**

The lower tract approach refers to correction of ureterocele by entering the bladder, removing the ureterocele, and then reimplanting the ureter. The advantages to this approach are that it can be less morbid by reducing the risk to the lower moiety renal segment. A refluxing ipsilateral ureter can be corrected at the same time. The primary disadvantage is that it may still leave a nonfunctioning renal segment that may require further surgery.

CHAPTER 11

Urological Emergencies in the Newborn

Miriam Harel, MD,
Patrick H. McKenna, MD, FACS, FAAP,
Fernando A. Ferrer, MD, FAAP, FACS,
and John H. Makari, MD, MHA, MA

○ **How often does prenatal sonography detect a significant fetal anomaly?**

In 1% of pregnancies.

○ **How many of these are genitourinary, and what is the most common urologic abnormality?**

Twenty-five percent are genitourinary. Hydronephrosis is the most common urologic abnormality found on sonography, representing 50% of all genitourinary fetal anomalies.

○ **What is the significance of bilateral hydronephrosis?**

This may indicate vesicoureteral reflux (VUR), fetal ureteral folds, or megaureters. Posterior urethral valve (PUV) must also be considered in a male fetus, especially if there is evidence of a dilated bladder.

○ **What is the cause and significance of oligohydramnios?**

Abnormal or deficient fetal kidneys will produce less urine, which leads to oligohydramnios. Therefore, a screening ultrasound evaluation of the fetal kidneys is reasonable if oligohydramnios is found. Oligohydramnios may also be caused by rupture of amniotic membranes, inadequate urine production, obstructive uropathy, or post-term gestation. Renal causes of oligohydramnios include renal agenesis or dysplasia, obstruction, or hypoperfusion of the kidneys. Oligohydramnios may lead to pulmonary hypoplasia. The second trimester is the most critical for fetal lung maturation.

○ **Which are potentially more dangerous: obstructive or nonobstructive lesions of the kidneys?**

In association with hydronephrosis, obstructive lesions are more dangerous, especially if bilateral. However, bilateral renal dysgenesis (caused by diseases such as autosomal recessive polycystic kidney disease, multicystic dysplastic kidney) may be lethal.

○ **Renal pelvic diameter measurements can be helpful in determining the significance of hydronephrosis. What measurements would be considered significant?**

Specific measurements are somewhat controversial. An anteroposterior (AP) diameter greater than 7 mm in the second trimester and 10 mm in the third trimester are some guidelines. Smaller is better.

○ **A distended bladder that does not empty suggests which diagnosis?**

Posterior urethral valve, prune-belly syndrome, urethral atresia, or neuropathic bladder (eg, spina bifida).

○ **Which of these is the most dangerous?**

Urethral atresia has the highest mortality rate among these.

○ **Consultation is requested for an otherwise healthy term infant with a palpable right-sided abdominal mass. Prenatal sonography was not performed. How do you proceed with your physical examination?**

A general examination must begin with initial attention to subcutaneous nodules (neuroblastoma) or dehydration, particularly with hematuria (as seen in renal vein thrombosis). The patient should be placed in the lateral decubitus position for kidney palpation by supporting the flank with one hand and palpating the upper quadrant subcostally with the opposite hand. Care should be taken to avoid extensive abdominal manipulation after the initial examination to prevent the rare occurrence of rupture as seen in cases of Wilms' tumor/ mesoblastic nephroma. Transillumination of the flank mass may distinguish cystic from solid lesions. Following a complete physical examination, including careful blood pressure measurements, abdominal sonography is indicated.

○ **A 23-year-old pregnant female presents for evaluation of prenatally detected unilateral hydronephrosis. There is no oligohydramnios. What would be your consideration and recommendation to the patient?**

Prenatal fetal hydronephrosis is the most commonly diagnosed fetal urologic abnormality. While the overall incidence of hydronephrosis on prenatal sonography is between 1% and 1.5%, the incidence of clinically significant hydronephrosis is between 0.2% and 0.4%. With normal amniotic fluid levels, close follow-up throughout the pregnancy and in the neonatal/newborn period as well as through the first year of life are required. It is important to note that a postnatal ultrasound evaluation performed within the first 48 hours of life may underestimate the degree of hydronephrosis due to physiologic oliguria in the newborn. The majority of cases of prenatal low-grade hydronephrosis may stabilize and resolve within the first year of life.

○ **This woman delivered a 7 lb, 3 oz otherwise healthy male infant. Postnatal sonography confirms the presence of unilateral hydronephrosis. What further evaluation do you recommend?**

Careful physical examination with an emphasis on observing the infant's active voiding is an important first step. The infant should be started on antibiotic prophylaxis, as the incidence of urinary tract infection (UTI) is approximately 3% to 4% in the first 6 months of life. A voiding cystourethrogram (VCUG) and nuclear renogram (DTPA or MAG 3) should also be scheduled. Nuclear renography is dependent on glomerular filtration rate (GFR) for excretion of the isotope. Neonatal GFR increases several fold during the first 2 months of life. Therefore, the optimal timing of the renal scan is during the second month of life. Recent work suggests a conservative approach to nuclear renography in patients with mild hydronephrosis.

○ **A 32-week prenatal sonogram of a male fetus followed for hydronephrosis reveals increasing bilateral hydronephrosis, a dilated bladder, and new-onset marked oligohydramnios. What is your recommendation?**

Posterior urethral valve leading to bilateral hydronephrosis with oligohydramnios is the most likely etiology, and this situation potentially represents a rare urologic indication for induction of labor or fetal intervention. Fetal lung maturity should be evaluated with a lecithin/sphingomyelin amniotic fluid ratio prior to a final recommendation. If fetal surgical intervention is considered, fetal renal function should be estimated by the urinary sodium chloride, osmolality, and β_2 microglobulin obtained by fetal bladder aspiration. A high-grade obstruction of a single system also requires a similarly rapid response. The outcomes for fetal intervention with respect to improvement of renal function are mixed.

○ **A male infant delivered at an estimated 34 weeks gestational age without prenatal care demonstrates failure to thrive and neonatal ascites. The infant is noted to have a diminished, dribbling urinary stream. What is the most likely diagnosis?**

The most common cause of bladder outlet obstruction in the male newborn is a PUV. An abdominal mass, failure to thrive, and neonatal ascites are among the most common presenting symptoms. Clearly, the widespread use of prenatal sonography has directed early investigations in patients with PUV.

○ **What prenatal sonographic findings are suggestive of a PUV, and what is the most important information needed to determine further prenatal care?**

Increased bladder wall thickness on prenatal sonography may indicate outlet obstruction, and dilation of the posterior urethra (keyhole sign) is strongly suggestive of PUV. The most important information needed to determine further prenatal care is the presence and timing of onset of oligohydramnios. In the setting of oligohydramnios, increased renal echogenicity is a poor prognostic indicator. Urinary electrolytes have been shown to be a useful indicator of renal salvageability only in the setting of oligohydramnios and in early gestation (18–24 weeks).

○ **Prenatal sonography at 22 weeks reveals bilateral hydroureteronephrosis with a distended bladder consistent with a PUV. Attempts at placement of a vesicoamniotic shunt are unsuccessful. Labor is induced at 32 weeks. What is the initial management at birth?**

Recognition of prenatal hydronephrosis suggests the need for repeat sonography at birth to establish a baseline view of the renal collecting systems. When a suspicion of PUV exists, bladder catheterization should be performed and the patient should be placed on prophylactic antibiotics. A VCUG should be performed when the patient is stable. When a PUV is present, VCUG often demonstrates a thick, trabeculated bladder with a dilated posterior urethra.

○ **A 35-week gestational age male infant with an apparent PUV on VCUG has tense abdominal distension with a fluid wave and a urine output of 0.2 mL/kg/h despite aggressive fluid resuscitation. What is the most likely diagnosis?**

Neonatal urinary ascites occurs in 7% of male infants with PUV. The diagnosis is based on clinical and radiological evidence and can be confirmed by a diagnostic tap of the ascites. When bladder outlet obstruction is suspected, catheter drainage is initiated followed by drainage of ascites only if respiratory compromise is suspected.

○ **Following ablation of PUV, difficulty passing a catheter into the bladder is encountered. What is the most likely cause?**

Hypertrophied bladder neck resulting from bladder outlet obstruction.

○ **A 32-week gestational age infant is delivered after induction of labor for oligohydramnios and hydronephrosis. A cystic mass is noted on the ventral surface of the penoscrotal junction. What finding is expected on the VCUG?**

A cystic mass at the penoscrotal junction especially with dribbling urinary stream is likely the rare finding of an anterior urethral valve. VCUG will likely show a large ventral diverticulum due to a crescentic cusp on the ventral aspect of the urethra. VUR may also be seen with this condition.

○ **What are causes of nonobstructive fetal hydronephrosis?**

VUR (incidence of 15%–20% in white patients and less than 1% in black patients with prenatal hydronephrosis) and fetal ureteral folds are common causes of mild or transient ureteral dilatation noted on prenatal sonography.

○ **A prenatal sonogram detects oligohydramnios and the presence of multiple small cysts (1–2 mm in diameter). Liver sonography demonstrates periportal fibrosis. What is the most likely diagnosis, and what is its prognosis?**

Hepatic fibrosis with a polycystic kidney is consistent with autosomal recessive polycystic kidney disease of the infantile form. Postnatal sonography typically reveals bilaterally large, echogenic kidneys with poor corticomedullary differentiation. (Contrast urography would reveal severely delayed function and a nephrogram with an alternating radially oriented sunray pattern.) Infantile presentation typically leads to death by 2 months of age.

○ **What is the most likely cause of an abdominal mass in a healthy-appearing male infant, and how can it be differentiated from the second most common cause of neonatal abdominal masses?**

Hydronephrosis due to ureteropelvic junction (UPJ) obstruction is the most common cause of a neonatal abdominal mass. Multicystic dysplastic kidney (MCDK) is the second most common cause of the neonatal abdominal mass and can be distinguished from UPJ obstruction by the sonographic findings of multiple noncommunicating cysts, minimal or absent renal parenchyma, and the absence of a central large cyst. The 2 entities can also be differentiated by the ^{99m}Tc DMSA renal scan. The renal scan usually demonstrates some function in the hydronephrotic kidney and nonfunction of the MCDK.

○ **An infant is diagnosed with a right MCDK. What is of concern regarding the contralateral kidney?**

The contralateral kidney and collecting system must be carefully studied in cases of MCDK. Contralateral VUR is the most commonly encountered abnormality with an incidence of 15% to 40%. Contralateral hydronephrosis due to UPJ obstruction occurs in approximately 10% of infants with MCDK.

○ **A 1-month-old female infant is admitted to the neonatal intensive care unit (NICU) with failure to thrive and respiratory distress. Physical examination reveals a large right-sided abdominal mass. Sonography reveals an enlarged right kidney with multiple noncommunicating cystic structures. A renal scan reveals no perfusion to the affected side and normal function of the left kidney. What treatment would you recommend?**

This clinical scenario is consistent with the findings of MCDK. Symptoms including respiratory distress, failure to thrive, hypertension, or hemorrhage are indications for nephrectomy in certain cases of MCDK. However, a subset of these patients may be managed by aspiration of the dominant cyst(s), as the cystic fluid does not tend to reaccumulate. Aspiration can typically be done by sonographic guidance and may provide immediate or even long-term management.

○ **A clinically stable, otherwise healthy term neonate is diagnosed with left MCDK by sonography. The right kidney is noted to be free of reflux with intact renal function. Is there a role for observation?**

In the absence of hypertension, feeding, or developmental problems due to mechanical or obstructive complications, immediate surgical excision is unnecessary. Concern for onset of hypertension, malignant degeneration of the MCDK to Wilms' tumor, or, less commonly, renal cell carcinoma remains an argument for prophylactic removal of these nonfunctioning moieties. The minimal morbidity of a procedure accomplished through a small incision and the freedom from regular follow-up or sonography are additional factors favoring nephrectomy. Noninterventional follow-up and the ability to sonographically follow MCDK, as well as the high incidence of near-complete involution favor observation in these cases. One must remember, however, that while the cystic fluid found within MCDK may be resorbed, the cyst wall is a persistent remnant. MCDK should be followed sonographically until at least age 5; nephrectomy should be performed if there is an increasing solid component.

○ **A term infant is noted to have a fixed, unilateral mass extending to the midline. Also noted are multiple bluish skin nodules. What is the most likely diagnosis and treatment?**

This clinical picture most likely represents neuroblastoma, an embryonal tumor of neural crest origin. Neuroblastoma is the most common solid abdominal mass and the most common malignant tumor in infancy. For low-stage tumors (stage I to II), surgical excision remains the treatment of choice. For stage III and higher disease, chemotherapy and radiation therapy are employed as multimodal therapies. As an exception for higher stage disease, surgical excision is often the standard of care without irradiation or chemotherapy in cases of stage IV-S disease (hepatic metastases, skin nodules, and bone marrow involvement).

○ **A term female infant is oliguric at 48 hours of age. Physical examination reveals a palpable, distended bladder, and an erythematous interlabial mass. Renal sonography reveals hydronephrosis of the left upper pole. What is the most likely diagnosis?**

The most common cause of urethral obstruction in the female infant is an obstructing ureterocele. In addition, 80% of ureteroceles are associated with the upper pole ureter of a minimally functioning duplicated system. The sonographic findings are consistent with a ureterocele arising from a duplicated collecting system.

○ **Antenatal sonography of a 25-week gestational age female fetus reveals right-sided hydronephrosis and an intravesical cystic dilatation consistent with a ureterocele. Follow-up postnatal sonography, however, demonstrates persistent hydronephrosis, but no obvious ureterocele. What technical errors during sonography may confound the diagnosis?**

There are common errors in the sonographic technique that may render the diagnosis of ureteroceles difficult. If the bladder is overdistended, then the ureterocele may become effaced and may not be visible on sonography and even on VCUG. Additionally, if the injected contrast is too concentrated on cystourethrography, the ureterocele may become obscured on radiologic imaging. On the other hand, if the bladder is completely empty during sonography, a large ureterocele can mimic the wall of the bladder, and distinction between the bladder wall and ureterocele may be difficult.

○ **A neonate is noted to have deficiency of abdominal wall musculature, diffuse dilatation of the urinary tract, and hydronephrosis. The patient is clinically stable. Does this patient require acute urological intervention to address the upper tract dilatation?**

Rarely does a case of group 2 prune-belly syndrome as described above require urgent urological intervention. Sonography and serial electrolytes are used to assess parenchymal reserve and extent of uropathy. A diuretic renal scan should be performed. Patients presenting with group 1 characteristics, on the other hand, including oligohydramnios, pulmonary hypoplasia, cardiac anomalies, urachal abnormalities, or pneumothorax require intervention for the cardiopulmonary abnormalities prior to other aspects of care.

○ **The neonate with prune-belly syndrome described in the previous question may be expected to have up to an 85% rate of VUR. Should a VCUG be immediately performed to determine the grade of reflux and subsequent treatment?**

Instrumentation of a neonate with prune-belly syndrome is associated with a high risk of infection and should be performed only with antibiotic prophylaxis.

○ **A lower abdominal mass is palpated in a newborn female. Examination of the perineum reveals a mass in the introitus. The mass persists following placement of a urethral catheter. What is the most likely diagnosis?**

A lower abdominal mass in an otherwise healthy female patient is most likely due to hydrometrocolpos or distension of the vagina and uterus.

○ **What anatomical abnormalities most commonly lead to hydrometrocolpos?**

An imperforate hymen is the most common cause of hydrometrocolpos. A less common etiology is a high transverse vaginal septum, which can be associated with a persistent urogenital sinus. In cases of a high transverse vaginal septum, the external anatomy may appear deceptively normal but sonography of the abdominal mass will reveal a cystic midline structure posterior to the bladder without septation.

○ **On prenatal sonography, the bladder cannot be identified. What condition should be considered?**

Inability to identify the bladder on repeat studies should raise suspicion for bladder exstrophy. Common observations in the fetus with bladder exstrophy include nonvisualization of the fetal bladder, a lower abdominal wall mass inferior to a low-lying umbilicus, diminutive genitalia, and abnormal widening of the iliac crests.

○ **A term male infant is noted to have multiple genitourinary anomalies at birth consistent with the classic bladder exstrophy/epispadias complex. How must the exstrophic bladder be maintained prior to surgical intervention?**

The mucosa of the bladder must be protected while the candidacy for surgery is discussed. Noncontact care may consist of placing the child in an incubator without a diaper and with saline mist to keep the mucosa moist. Alternatively, the bladder mucosa may be protected by a plastic wrap to prevent the mucosa from sticking to clothing or to the diaper. The umbilicus should be ligated with silk suture rather than a plastic umbilical clamp when exstrophy is recognized antenatally or postnatally. Broad-spectrum antibiotics may be started to sterilize the bladder wall prior to surgical intervention.

○ **A term male infant is brought to the emergency department with fever, irritability, and weight loss. The infant is uncircumcised. Until what age is the infant more susceptible to UTI than circumcised male infants?**

Regardless of phimosis, the presence of a foreskin predisposes an infant to UTI until approximately 6 months of age versus age-matched circumcised males. Colonization of the newborn prepuce diminishes as a risk factor beyond 6 months of age.

○ **Three days following Gomco clamp circumcision, a newborn infant develops brisk bleeding from the incision. What is the risk of hemorrhage, and how should it be treated following circumcision?**

Hemorrhage occurs in <1% of cases. The incidence is highest at 3 days after birth due to the physiologic depression of plasma levels of vitamin K-dependent clotting factor. If conservative measures such as compression with an epinephrine-soaked gauze sponge or thrombin application fail, hemostatic suture placement is required.

○ **Consultation is requested approximately 7 days following a neonatal circumcision. Examination of the penis reveals dehiscence of the incision line with complete exposure of the ventral penile shaft. What is the preferred approach?**

Healing by secondary intention is the preferred approach following such a dehiscence. In rare cases, extensive denudation of skin may require skin grafting to prevent secondary chordee or scarring. Other acute complications of neonatal circumcision include infection, laceration, glans amputation, urinary retention, and necrosis. Nonacute complications of neonatal circumcision include excessive residual skin, skin asymmetry, epithelialized skin bridges, epidermal inclusion cysts, skin tethering/chordee, concealed (buried) penis, phimosis, meatal stenosis, urethrocutaneous fistula, and lymphedema.

○ **Consultation is requested for a glans amputation during a neonatal circumcision. How should this be managed?**

As with all acute complications during circumcision, immediate attention and treatment is the best management. Generally, glans amputation is partial. The amputated portion should be wrapped sterilely and kept cool on ice. It should not be submerged in saline. Primary anastomosis with long-lasting absorbable sutures (eg, PDS) should be performed. There are no vessels of sufficient size to permit microvascular re-anastomosis. The urethra should be stented. Viability of the amputated portion is improved when repair occurs within hours of the injury, but it has even been documented in delays up to 18 hours.

○ **A newborn undergoes a circumcision with a Gomco clamp. Three days later, he has 2 separate streams. What is the next step?**

Urethrocutaneous fistula is a rare complication of circumcision. It may occur if the urethra is crushed by the circumcision clamp or if a suture is inadvertently placed into the urethra. This can be repaired if recognized immediately. When the diagnosis is delayed, observation for 4 to 6 months may result in spontaneous closure. Otherwise, formal closure of the fistula will be needed.

○ **During newborn infant circumcision, local anesthetic containing 1:1000 epinephrine is injected. Blanching of the penile skin and glans is observed. Physical exam demonstrates mild peripheral vasoconstriction of the hands and feet, blood pressure of 90/60 mm Hg, and a pulse of 160. What is the next step?**

This patient has primarily local effects of the injected epinephrine. These can be treated with the alpha-adrenergic antagonist phentolamine delivered subcutaneously at the injection site at a dose of 0.1 to 0.2 mg/kg. The patient should be monitored closely for adverse effects.

○ **A 9-day-old infant undergoing a sepsis workup is noted to have a palpable right-sided abdominal mass with associated gross hematuria. What is the most likely diagnosis?**

The most likely diagnosis is renal vein thrombosis (RVT). Sixty to seventy percent of patients with RVT have findings of a palpable mass with associated gross hematuria and proteinuria.

○ **A 2-day-old infant born to a diabetic mother has polyuria (10 mL/kg/h). Is the child at risk for compromised renal function?**

Yes. Infants of diabetic mothers experiencing an osmotic diuresis as well as infants with profuse diarrhea, sepsis, acute hypoxia, and hypotension are at risk for RVT. RVT often occurs due to low renal perfusion pressures and increased blood viscosity secondary to extracellular volume contraction with resultant sludging of blood in renal venules.

○ **A 4-day-old infant with a palpable abdominal mass, gross hematuria, and thrombocytopenia undergoes an abdominal Doppler sonogram that confirms the diagnosis of unilateral RVT without caval thrombus. What does appropriate treatment include?**

Vigorous hydration, electrolyte management, and treatment of the underlying cause are critical. Aggressive anticoagulation and thrombolytic therapy are employed in certain situations. Thrombolytic agents such as urokinase, streptokinase, and tissue plasminogen activator are utilized for bilateral RVT.

○ **Following successful treatment of RVT, what sequelae may develop?**

Fibrosis of the kidney, renovascular hypertension, nephrotic syndrome, and chronic pyelonephritis are all possible sequelae of RVT. Hypertension in association with an atrophic kidney is often renin-mediated, and a nephrectomy is curative.

○ **A 35-week gestation newborn is anuric for 36 hours following birth. Physical examination is unremarkable. Should a workup for acute renal failure commence?**

No. 92% and 99.4% of term newborns void within 24 hours and 48 hours of birth, respectively. Acute renal failure is suspected only if anuria persists more than 48 hours.

○ **The same infant persists with an urine output of 0.7 mL/kg/h and a serum creatinine of 1.1 mg/dL at 72 hours. There is no history of oligohydramnios. What is the most common cause of oliguria in the newborn, and how is it treated?**

Prerenal renal failure secondary to inadequate perfusion is the most common cause of oliguria in the newborn. Hypotension from sepsis, maternal antepartum hemorrhage, or surgical bleeding may lead to renal hypoperfusion. Similarly, congestive heart failure due to cardiac anomalies or dehydration may also lead to renal ischemia. Neonatal intensive care admission with volume expansion will rapidly reverse prerenal renal failure. Oligohydramnios is usually present in infants with anuria or oliguria due to postrenal causes.

○ **A term infant in the neonatal intensive unit has multiple unsuccessful attempts at umbilical artery catheterization. Consultation is requested 24 hours later for apparent new-onset neonatal ascites. What is the likely diagnosis and recommended treatment?**

Urachal laceration due to attempted umbilical arterial catheterization is the most common cause of neonatal intraperitoneal bladder rupture. Evaluation should consist of a VCUG and possibly a diagnostic paracentesis. While management may be conservative for most cases of neonatal ascites, initial operative management is recommended in cases of intraperitoneal bladder rupture.

○ **A 1300-g preterm infant is being treated for respiratory distress syndrome (RDS) in the NICU. Abdominal x-rays reveal bilateral 0.7 mm renal stones. What is the etiology of this condition?**

Furosemide, commonly used in the treatment of RDS and other conditions common to premature infants in the NICU setting, is associated with nephrolithiasis. Furosemide causes a hypercalciuric state with a secondary increased resorption of calcium in the proximal tubule and subsequent renal stone formation. Excessive calcium and glucose intake in specialized formulas for premature infants is another recognized cause of neonatal nephrolithiasis.

○ **A premature infant in the NICU with a patent ductus arteriosus receives furosemide at 2 mg/kg/d for 4 weeks. An abdominal x-ray reveals bilateral nephrocalcinosis. What is the most appropriate treatment?**

Furosemide-induced renal parenchymal stone disease rarely requires surgical intervention. The administration of hydrochlorothiazide, reduced calcium intake, and cessation of furosemide therapy often results in resolution of nephrolithiasis. Nephrocalcinosis may be followed with serial sonography. A baseline calcium-to-creatinine ratio of less than 0.2 portends a higher rate of resolution. In cases of discrete massive calculus formation, shock wave lithotripsy or open surgical intervention may be warranted.

○ **Umbilical artery catheterization is performed on a premature infant in the NICU. Twenty-four hours later, the infant has gross hematuria and hypertension. The hypertension is refractory to aggressive medical management. What is the diagnosis and the most appropriate treatment?**

A recognized complication of umbilical artery catheterization is renal artery thrombosis, either alone or as part of an extensive aortoiliac thrombus. The clinical diagnosis can be confirmed by Doppler sonography and radionuclide imaging, if necessary. Management is dependent on the clinical setting, and unilateral involvement is best managed expectantly, although thrombolytic therapy may be appropriate. Control of hypertension is the most important aspect of management and occasionally requires nephrectomy, as in this life-threatening case.

○ **A 38-week gestational age male infant is delivered following prolonged labor with meconium aspiration. Aggressive resuscitation efforts are successful. On day 3 of life, an abdominal mass is palpated on the right side. What is the likely sonographic finding, and what is your diagnosis?**

Sudden increases in intra-abdominal pressure during prolonged labor may result in adrenal hemorrhage with the observed physical findings. Adrenal hemorrhage typically involves the right adrenal gland, and sonographic findings initially demonstrate a hyperechoic or solid mass over the superior pole of the kidney. With time, the lesion may become hypoechoic and decrease in size. This finding should not be confused with neuroblastoma, the most common adrenal malignancy of infancy, which typically has a solid appearance on sonography but may be cystic or have a mixed echogenic pattern.

○ **A 39-week-old term infant has a firm right scrotal mass at birth. The mass is painless and does not transilluminate. The overlying skin is erythematous and indurated. What is the most likely cause, and what other entities should be considered in the differential diagnosis?**

The most common cause of a scrotal mass at birth is testicular torsion. The differential diagnosis for the described presentation includes hydrocele, incarcerated inguinal hernia, scrotal hematoma, tumor, meconium, trauma, and more rarely ectopic spleen or adrenal tissue.

Neonatal testicular torsion is extravaginal, since the tunica vaginalis is not adherent to the surrounding dartos fascia of the scrotal wall until 4 to 8 weeks of age. Torsion in the neonate, therefore, involves the testis, spermatic cord, and overlying tunica vaginalis. In the adolescent, the tunica vaginalis is fixed to the dartos fascia; therefore, testicular torsion is intravaginal.

○ **An infant with a firm scrotal mass at birth is diagnosed with testicular torsion. The infant is hemodynamically stable, and the contralateral testis is normal. Is surgical exploration and detorsion with orchidopexy necessary?**

It is well known that successful testicular salvage in the event of neonatal testicular torsion is exceedingly rare. Exploration with an intent of salvage alone is not justified. The role of scrotal exploration with contralateral testicular fixation due to the potential for asynchronous torsion until the tunica vaginalis adheres to the scrotal wall remains controversial. Clearly, however, if bilateral torsion is suspected, then exploration despite the low incidence of salvage is necessary.

○   **A term male infant is admitted to the intensive care unit immediately postpartum with hypotension and tachycardia. Physical examination is remarkable for a penis of only 1.5 cm stretched penile length. The external genitalia are otherwise normal. Electrolyte studies reveal hyponatremia, hyperkalemia, and hypoglycemia. What is the most likely diagnosis, and how must the infant be treated?**

This critically ill infant with obvious micropenis (penile length 2.5 standard deviations below the mean or less than 2.0 cm in a newborn male) must be evaluated for panhypopituitarism. Following intravenous glucose and electrolyte replacement, serial serum glucose, sodium, and potassium evaluations are necessary. Serial gonadotropin and testosterone measurements from birth through 3 months of age will eventually document a neonatal luteinizing hormone (LH) surge in normal infants.

○   **On initial examination, a term infant has left-sided cryptorchidism and a midshaft hypospadias. What is the incidence of a disorder of sexual development (DSD) in this patient?**

Phenotypic males with cryptorchidism and hypospadias are estimated to have a 20% to 30% incidence of DSD. Similarly, male phenotype with bilateral nonpalpable testes and perineal hypospadias alone should initiate an investigation for DSD.

○   **What familial risk factors increase risk of DSD in infants?**

Most DSD result from autosomal recessive inheritance, and inquiry regarding siblings with abnormal genitalia, infant death, or abnormal events at puberty is necessary. Maternal ingestion of androgenic medication (eg, Danazol), progestational agents, or drug abuse should also be carefully investigated.

○   **A term infant with severe hypospadias and unilateral cryptorchidism is suspected of having DSD. What is the most common DSD with this presentation?**

The most common DSD in patients with severe hypospadias, a testis on one side, and a nonpalpable undescended testis is mixed gonadal dysgenesis. This patient likely has a testis on one side and streak gonad on the contralateral side.

○   **Physical examination of a 37-week-old infant shows a hypertrophied clitoris and partially fused, rugated labioscrotal folds. The karyotype is 46 XX. What is the diagnosis and the most likely cause?**

The infant likely has a 46 XX DSD, previously referred to as "female pseudohermaphrodite." This group constitutes 60% to 70% of all DSD in the neonatal period. Congenital adrenal hyperplasia (CAH) is the most likely cause in patients with a 46 XX DSD.

○   **An infant is suspected of having CAH. What life-threatening condition must be considered, and how is it diagnosed?**

A potentially lethal metabolic consequence associated with DSD is the salt-wasting form of CAH, which does not typically manifest in electrolyte disturbances until 1 to 2 weeks postnatally. Therefore, the etiology of DSD must be determined prior to discharge. CAH results from 21-hydroxylase deficiency in 95% of cases. The more common form leads to virilization and aldosterone deficiency in three-fourths of patients, while virilization alone is present in approximately one-fourth of patients with 21-hydroxylase deficiency. Salt wasting may also be present in patients with the much rarer causes of CAH, including 11β-hydroxylase deficiency (5% of patients with CAH, salt wasting less common) and 3β-hydroxysteroid-dehydrogenase deficiency (less than 1% of patients with CAH, almost always manifests with salt wasting).

○ **A 2-week-old infant is brought to the emergency department with profound hypotension and hyperkalemia. Genital examination demonstrates virilization. What treatment should be administered?**

The salt-wasting form of CAH should be suspected and must be aggressively treated initially with a bolus infusion of 20 mL/kg normal saline. Cortisol replacement is started with a hydrocortisone sodium succinate bolus at 50 mg/m^2 followed by an infusion of 50 to 100 mg/m^2 added to intravenous fluids. For this critically ill infant, deoxycorticosterone (DOCA) at 1 to 2 mg should be injected intramuscularly every 12 to 14 hours.

○ **A 1-week-old female infant is evaluated in the emergency department for failure to thrive. Physical examination reveals hypertension and virilization of the genitalia with hypertrophy of the clitoris. An arterial blood gas sample is consistent with metabolic acidosis, and the potassium level is 6.5 mg/dL. What is the most likely diagnosis?**

CAH resulting from 11β-hydroxylase deficiency is most consistent with this presentation and constitutes 5% of cases of CAH. A deficiency at this enzymatic level results in accumulation of 17-hydroxyprogesterone and androgens as well as the potent mineralocorticoid DOCA. Hyperkalemic acidosis and hypervolemia with hypertension are presenting features.

○ **An uncircumcised male infant is referred for a clean-catch urine culture revealing 50,000/mL *Staphylococcus epidermidis*. Is a VCUG indicated?**

Further evaluation in this child should not commence until a repeat culture is obtained using urine specimen collected in another manner. While plastic bag collected urine cultures are useful if negative, a confirmation must be sought with a catheterized specimen or suprapubic aspirate. If, however, a single organism with a colony count greater than 100,000/mL in a symptomatic infant is obtained even when collected by a plastic bag, the infant should be treated for UTI.

○ **A 32-week-gestation neonate is found to have candiduria on 2 successive urine cultures. He is voiding spontaneously, and his renal/bladder sonogram is normal. What is the most appropriate therapy?**

Parenteral fluconazole. *Candida* is the most common cause of nosocomial fungal UTI. Indwelling intravascular catheters and broad-spectrum antibiotics increase the incidence of candidal infection, particularly in premature low birth weight infants. Aggressive parenteral treatment is required due to a high incidence of subsequent candidemia occurring in 25% to 85% of neonates with candiduria. Fluconazole is the treatment of choice in premature infants due to significantly fewer side effects when compared to amphotericin. If hydronephrosis and fungus balls are present in the collecting system, percutaneous drainage and irrigation with antifungals may be needed.

○ **A 10-day-old infant boy is hospitalized for failure to thrive. After his umbilical stump fell off, fluid has intermittently drained from the umbilicus. The umbilical fluid has a creatinine of 10 mg/dL and grows >10^5 cfu/mL of *E. coli*. What is the next step?**

Antibiotics and VCUG. The differential diagnosis of a wet umbilicus in the infant includes patent urachus, omphalitis, simple granulation of the healing stump, patent vitelline or omphalomesenteric duct, infected umbilical vessel, and external urachal sinus. An elevated creatinine level in the fluid draining from the umbilical stump suggests a patent urachus. A VCUG will confirm the diagnosis and fully evaluate possible coexisting bladder outlet obstruction.

○   **An infant is found to have an imperforate anus on newborn examination. What urologic evaluation should be performed?**

Urologic anomalies are frequently found in patients with anorectal malformations. Urologic abnormalities are present in 60% of patients with anorectal lesions occurring above the levator muscles ("high" lesions) and in 20% of patients with lesions below the levator muscles ("low" lesions). Rectourethral fistula is present in 25% of all patients with imperforate anus and is found much more commonly in those with high lesions. When a rectourethral fistula exists, urine can flow into the colon leading to electrolyte resorption and recurrent UTIs even after diverting colostomy. Other urologic findings include VUR, neuropathic bladder, renal agenesis or dysplasia, and cryptorchidism. Evaluation should include renal–bladder sonography, VCUG, and urodynamic evaluation in patients with high lesions or those with spinal abnormalities.

○   **A healthy newborn boy has bilateral Grade 4 VUR. What is this most commonly associated with?**

VUR in newborn boys is commonly associated with an infantile filling/voiding pattern characterized by high-grade reflux and associated with uninhibited detrusor contractions during filling, high pressure voiding due to elevated outlet resistance, detrusor-sphincter dyssynergy, and high postvoid residuals. Compliance and contractility are usually normal in these boys. These patients are best managed with prophylactic antibiotics and observation. In most cases, the VUR will resolve as neuro-urologic maturation occurs during the first year of life.

○   **A 2-month-old uncircumcised boy with a sacral dimple undergoes evaluation of a febrile UTI. Sonography shows bilateral hydronephrosis and a conus medullaris at the mid aspect of L4. VCUG shows bilateral Grade IV reflux, slight beaking of the bladder neck, and a normal urethra. What is the next step?**

A cystometrogram (CMG) would be the next step. This infant has a compromised urinary tract, and a neurogenic cause must be considered. Spinal ultrasound is a convenient method of screening in the neonatal period. The conus normally ends above L2. Given this patient's low conus, a CMG would be important to assess filling and storage pressures.

CHAPTER 12 Enuresis

Hyeyoung Lee, MD, MS and
Sang Won Han, MD, PhD

○ **A normal 7-year-old boy suddenly develops daytime urinary frequency every 20 minutes without incontinence. His symptom is limited to daytime only, and no enuresis was reported. Medicosurgical history, physical examination, urinalysis, and brief ultrasound of the kidneys and bladder are normal. What is the most appropriate management option?**

The daytime urinary frequency is a benign, yet extremely common condition, which occurs in otherwise normal children who have no associated daytime incontinence or nighttime symptoms. The etiology is generally unknown and a conservative approach is not unreasonable. Symptoms quite often occur in association with psychological stress or environmental changes. It usually resolves in 2 to 4 months and is characteristically unaffected by anticholinergic drugs. However, urinalysis should be performed for the differential diagnosis of symptomatic cystitis.

○ **An otherwise normal 6-year-old boy wets his bed 2 or 3 times a week at night. He has no urinary symptoms during the daytime. What is the most likely cause of his nocturnal enuresis?**

Primary nocturnal enuresis can be multifactorial but is commonly explained to occur from nocturnal urine output that is in excess of the bladder reservoir capacity during sleep at night. Nocturnal polyuria, whether it is absolute in association with deranged antidiuretic hormone secretion or relative due to reduced functional bladder capacity during sleep, results in a mismatch between urine production and nocturnal bladder capacity. Decreased arousal to the sense of bladder fullness during sleep is also considered as one of the causes.

○ **Urinary overproduction in enuretic children would be due to what?**

- Abnormal circadian secretion of vasopressin.
- Increased natriuretic factor secretion.
- Increased dietary sodium.
- Defect in renal aquaporin-2 receptors in the kidney.

○ **What percentage of nocturnal enuresis patients have a significantly smaller functional bladder capacity than age-matched normal children?**

Approximately 20%. Functional capacity meaning that the bladder is not anatomically small, but tends to contract before it is full.

○ **What percentage of nocturnal enuresis patients have a problem with arousal from sleep?**

Approximately one-third. Enuretic children are universally regarded as deep-sleepers who do not wake up in response to bladder distension or detrusor contractions which are strong arousal stimuli. This high arousal threshold may have brainstem explanations or may be caused by chronic arousal stimuli itself.

○ **True/False: Treatment of nocturnal enuresis with overactive bladder with an anticholinergic is no better than placebo.**

True. But adding an anticholinergic to other remedies in difficult cases may be helpful. A buzzer alarm alone will cure approximately two-thirds.

○ **A 7-year-old boy has been taking imipramine for 3 months due to enuresis. What is the most potent pharmacologic effect of imipramine on the lower urinary tract?**

The antienuretic mechanism of tricyclic antidepressant imipramine is not absolutely clear, but it is most likely linked to noradrenergic action in the brainstem. Its actions in the urinary tract are direct inhibition of bladder smooth muscle, and analgesic effect. Imipramine is only considered in severely therapy-resistant individuals due to the relatively high rate of side effects and the potential for overdose.

○ **True/False: A 4-year-old boy with nighttime bed wetting should be actively evaluated and treated for enuresis.**

False. The diagnosis of enuresis can only be made after 5 years of age.

○ **A 6-year-old girl has been suffering from marked urinary frequency and urgency for 2 weeks. Physical examination is normal, and her urinalysis and culture are normal. The next step should be?**

Observation. In the case of a pediatric benign condition, evaluation should be minimal if no significant complication is eminent. In most cases, spontaneous improvement is the rule.

○ **The mother of a 5-year-old boy who still wets his bed at night was concerned about the chance of recovery by the age of 15. What is the percent of recovery you can tell this mother?**

Ninety-nine percent.

○ **The parents of a 6-year-old girl who still wets her bed at night tell the pediatrician that her older brother was also an enuretic. What percentage of children at age 5 are enuretic?**

Approximately 15% of normal children will still wet at night at 5 years of age. Enuresis is defined as an involuntary discharge of urine. The term is often used alone, imprecisely, to describe wetting that occurs only at night during sleep. It is more accurate, however, to refer to nighttime wetting as nocturnal enuresis and to distinguish it from daytime wetting or diurnal enuresis. The age at which enuresis becomes inappropriate depends on the statistics of developing urinary control, the pattern of wetting, and the sex of the child. Nocturnal enuresis occurring after the age of 5 or by the time the child enters grade school is generally considered a cause for concern.

○ **What is the spontaneous resolution rate for nocturnal enuresis without treatment?**

The spontaneous resolution rate is approximately 15% per year.

○ **Parents of an infant boy are curious about enuresis, since both of the parents were enuretic themselves. What percentage of patients with nocturnal enuresis have a positive family history for the same condition?**

Between 50% and 75%.

○ **What is the first event in the development of bowel and bladder control?**

In terms of continence, children develop nocturnal bowel continence before daytime bowel or bladder continence. The enuretic seldom exhibits an abnormality in bowel function or bladder function during the day and control of bladder function at night is the last event to occur. The usual sequence of development is (1) nocturnal bowel continence, (2) daytime bowel continence, (3) daytime bladder continence, and (4) after several months, nocturnal control of bladder function.

○ **A pediatrician consulted urology for a urodynamic evaluation of a 6-year-old boy with primary nocturnal enuresis. What is the finding you are most likely to find?**

It is stated that many enuretic children wet their beds not because their bladders are full, but because they suffer from nocturnal detrusor overactivity. There is great overlap between nocturnal enuresis and urgency or urge incontinence. Ambulatory cystometries of children with therapy-resistant enuresis provide direct proof of this overlap. A significant proportion of children with severe nocturnal enuresis show a marked reduction in functional bladder capacity when compared with age-matched controls. This may be related to the high prevalence of underlying bladder dysfunction, particularly of detrusor overactivity at night, in enuretic children. It has also been shown that other types of bladder dysfunctions, notably dysfunctional voiding and marked detrusor overactivity with extremely high voiding pressure suggestive of an obstructive pattern, are not uncommon in enuretic children.

○ **An otherwise normal 6-year-old boy wets his bed 2 or 3 times a week at night. What may be some of the contributing factors in his condition?**

Enuresis is caused by nonorganic disturbances affecting normal development, such as social factors and stress, which can modify urinary control. An increased prevalence of enuresis has been found in children from deprived environments and retardation in skeletal maturation, which may reflect delayed maturation of regulatory central nervous system functions.

○ **True/False: Nocturnal enuresis is generally considered a sleep disorder.**

False. It has been proposed that enuresis is a sleep disorder, but recent studies indicate that although objective arousal thresholds are high in enuretics, the sleep electroencephalogram (EEG) of enuretic children is not necessarily different from that of dry children.

○ **Enuretic children are known to have normal bladder capacity under anesthesia, but exhibit decreased functional capacity. What is the predicted average bladder capacity in an 8-year-old boy and what is the formula used to estimate pediatric bladder capacity?**

The most widely accepted formula for the predicted bladder capacity in children is:

Bladder capacity (mL) = [age (years) + 2] × 30.

Thus, if a child is 8 years old: (8 + 2) × 30 or 300 mL.

However, bladder capacity (mL) = 30 + [age (years) × 30] is also used.

○ **A 6-year-old boy with enuresis, frequency and urgency, uninhibited detrusor contractions, and decreased functional capacity had been taking various remedies for his enuresis. After a thorough evaluation of his condition, the physician recommended anticholinergics. For which of his conditions has anticholinergic therapy proven most effective?**

Anticholinergic therapy has the greatest chance of success in the child with signs of detrusor overactivity such as low daytime volume, urgency, and urge incontinence. However, constipation and residual urine must be checked before starting any anticholinergic medication.

○ **A 6-year-old boy had been taking various remedies for his enuresis. He has evidence of bladder hyperactivity, frequency and urgency, detrusor instability, day and night incontinence, as well as nocturnal enuresis. For which of his conditions has anticholinergic therapy been proven most ineffective?**

Nocturnal enuresis. Anticholinergic drug therapy has been effective for enuresis in only 5% to 40% of patients. However, since anticholinergics eliminate uninhibited bladder contractions and increase bladder capacity, this therapy may be effective selectively for enuretic patients with symptoms of bladder hyperactivity, such as urgency, frequency, and day and night incontinence, while it is most effective in patients with proven uninhibited bladder contractions.

○ **Is limiting fluid intake before bedtime a reasonable first step in controlling enuresis?**

The first step can be nighttime fluid restriction, which can minimize the nocturnal urine output. Simply limiting fluids to reduce urine output is not generally effective. However, the importance of antidiuretic hormone (ADH) levels is now elucidated. Measurements of urinary and serum ADH demonstrate an absence or reversal of the normal circadian rhythm in enuretics who have lower than normal excretion of nocturnal ADH > desmopressin (DDAVP), a synthetic analog of ADH, became available. It has an effect lasting 7 to 10 hours. DDAVP has been shown to be more effective than placebo in treating enuresis, with effective rates up to 60%, especially in older children. Patients on DDAVP are 4.5 times as likely to say dry overnight as controls. Limitations are the relatively high cost of the drug and the potential for recurrence upon discontinuation.

○ **An 8-year-old boy had been taking imipramine before camping for 2 years and is very satisfied. How does imipramine work in controlling enuresis and would you expect imipramine to have an antidepressant effect at antienuretic doses?**

Imipramine taken at antienuretic doses will have impact on REM and light NREM sleep. It will also have anticholinergic effects as well as change the sympathetic input to the bladder, but there will not be any significant antidepressant action. The medication is known to be a weak anticholinergic agent with direct antispasmodic activity, alpha sympathetic inhibitory action, and norepinephrine reuptake inhibition.

○ **How well does imipramine work in the treatment of enuresis and how frequently is it used?**

Imipramine, a tricyclic antidepressant, is the most widely used antienuretic agent worldwide, but it's currently recommended only as a secondary agent in the United States. Enuresis can be eliminated in more than 50% of children and will be improved in another 15% to 20%; however, up to 60% of patients will relapse upon discontinuation. Its peripheral effects increase bladder capacity by (1) weak anticholinergic activity (ineffective in abolishing uninhibited detrusor contractions); (2) direct antispasmodic activity (not apparent at clinically effective antienuretic doses); and (3) complex effect on sympathetic input to the bladder (prevents norepinephrine action on alpha receptors and enhances its effect on beta receptors by inhibiting norepinephrine reuptake). Imipramine's effects on the central nervous system include its antidepressant activity and its action on sleep. Imipramine significantly alters sleep patterns by decreasing the time spent in REM sleep and increasing the time spent in light NREM sleep. It is unlikely that the effect of imipramine against enuresis is related to antidepressant activity, because such an effect requires much higher dosages and its onset would be significantly delayed.

○ **What is the most effective treatment for enuresis currently available?**

Management of enuresis has been divided into pharmacologic therapy and behavior modification. Behavioral modification has been quite successful, but only for the very motivated parents and child. Bladder training was developed to increase functional bladder capacity, but has not seen much success. Another method of alternative behavior modification is responsibility reinforcement, such as reward and motivation. This also requires active and willing participation of the child to succeed.

It has been reported that the most effective therapy of treating enuresis is conditioning therapy, as in the bell alarm (buzzer alarm) method. Superior results have been reported with this method compared to other forms of behavioral therapy, as well as pharmacologic therapy with DDAVP. Imipramine is used as a second-line therapy.

○ **A 20-year-old army recruit was referred to an Army hospital after his confession of enuresis. He had not been free of bed-wetting throughout his life. What advise can you give him regarding diet to help minimize his problem?**

This patient has primary nocturnal enuresis. Enuresis is found in approximately 1% of the adult population, often with overt abnormalities on urodynamic studies such as uninhibited bladder activity. The extent of the investigation is usually more thorough than those carried out in younger enuretics. Cessation of compounds that might increase nocturnal urine output, such as caffeine, and behavioral modification, such as nighttime fluid restriction, should be strongly advised before recommending other forms of treatment.

○ **A 6-year-old girl is being evaluated for both nocturnal and diurnal enuresis. Workup with history and physical examination, neurologic examination, urinalysis, and urine culture are normal. What is the next appropriate step?**

Most children with enuresis do not have a definite lesion. A careful history, physical examination, and urinalysis with culture are needed for all children with bed-wetting and are usually sufficient. In patients with diurnal enuresis, normal history and physical examination, no evidence of neuropathy and a negative urine examination, the urinary tract anatomy should be screened. This can be accomplished noninvasively and satisfactorily with an ultrasound examination of the kidneys, ureters, and bladder before and after voiding.

○ **A 7-year-old girl with urgency and diurnal incontinence wets her bed about 3 times a week. Workup with history and physical examination, neurologic examination, urinalysis, and urine culture are normal. Radiographic imaging studies including abdominal ultrasonogram and voiding cystourethrogram are negative. What is the primary treatment?**

Diurnal enuresis occurs in 5% of 7-year-old children. In most children, the underlying problem is infrequent voiding. Timed voiding programs alone will be successful in the majority of children, but require several months to be effective. Anticholinergics such as oxybutynin can be tried along with timed voiding.

○ **A 6-year-old girl with diurnal enuresis also has severe constipation and fecal soiling. However, radiographic studies of her spine and neurologic examination are normal as well as urinalysis and no residual urine is noted. What is the most appropriate treatment?**

This girl presents typical findings of dysfunctional elimination syndrome. It has been observed that a large fecal impaction may induce significant detrusor instability and other bladder dysfunctions, which in turn will result in urgency, urinary tract infection (UTI), and reflux. A high incidence of enuresis in children with UTIs and constipation has been reported. The evidence available so far strongly suggests that there is an important relationship between constipation, detrusor instability, reflux, UTIs, and enuresis. With neurologic abnormalities and UTI ruled out, timed voiding along with treatment of constipation can improve not only fecal soiling but also diurnal enuresis. Anticholinergics in this condition are not recommended as they are likely to aggravate constipation and may cause UTIs.

○ **A 4-year-old girl who is toilet-trained complains of urinary incontinence. She says her underwear becomes wet right after she finishes voiding. What is the most likely diagnosis?**

The most likely diagnosis is vesicovaginal reflux. This best describes postvoid dribbling, which is typically when urine gets trapped in the vagina during voiding and dribbles out soon after standing in otherwise normal toilet-trained girls with no other associated urinary symptoms. Vesicovaginal reflux itself is harmless and tends to resolve with age, but it can create a damp environment prone to infection. Therefore, the child may be taught to empty her vagina by simply voiding with her thighs apart and leaning forward after voiding before getting up.

○ **What percentage of secondary nocturnal enuresis is due to psychological factors and what specific disorder is involved most often?**

Secondary enuresis defined as reoccurrence of enuresis after at least 6 months of symptom-free period is related to psychological factors in about 50%, usually anxiety provoking factors. However, enuretic children suffer from low self-esteem as long as they wet their beds. Enuresis is more common among children with neuropsychiatric disturbances, such as attention deficit hyperactivity disorder (ADHD). Approximately 15% among children with enuresis have ADHD and vice versa.

○ **How significant is the benefit of treating the psychological factors to improving the outcome over just treating the nocturnal enuresis directly?**

There is no significant proven benefit in treating the underlying anxiety disorder compared to just treating the enuresis.

○ **What percentage of children with ADHD also have nocturnal enuresis and is it reasonable that they would occur together?**

Approximately 15% of ADHD cases also have enuresis. Both problems are believed to involve the same brain stem area abnormality, so it's likely they would occur together.

○ **What percentage of ADHD children with nocturnal enuresis will have urodynamic evidence of overactive bladder dysfunction?**

Approximately 50%.

○ **Overactive bladder associated with nocturnal enuresis responds best to which therapy?**

Enuresis alarm behavioral therapy works best, except in children who also have ADHD.

CHAPTER 13

Disorders of Sexual Development

Richard N. Yu, MD, PhD and
David A. Diamond, MD

○ **What structure undergoes condensation and shortening to promote descent of the testis?**

The gubernaculum anchors the testis to the genital region condenses to allow descent.

○ **How many attachments does the gubernaculum have and what are they called?**

The gubernaculum typically has 5 attachments, which are called slips.

○ **What transcription factor is associated with testicular descent from the abdominal cavity to the inguinal canal (transabdominal)?**

INSL3 (insulin-like 3) is expressed by testicular Leydig cells. Production of this protein rises in the second trimester of gestation and works in conjunction with testosterone to promote testicular descent.

○ **What transcription factor is critical for gonadal differentiation toward the male lineage?**

SRY (sex determining region on the short arm of the Y chromosome), also known as the testis determining factor (TDF). SRY directly binds to specific DNA loci and regulates the differentiation of the bipotential gonad toward testicular development. Thus far, the SRY protein is considered the "master switch" that initiates testicular development.

○ **What happens if the TDF is not expressed or mutated in a genotypic male (46 XY)?**

The bipotential gonad differentiates toward the ovarian lineage. Sertoli and Leydig cells do not form; Mullerian inhibiting substance (MIS) and testosterone are not produced. Thus, Mullerian duct development is promoted and Wolffian duct development is suppressed.

○ **At what time point in fetal development does the gonad differentiate to become a testis or ovary?**

Between the 6th to 8th week of gestation, the indifferent (bipotential) gonad differentiates into either a testis or an ovary.

○   **What cell type is responsible for producing MIS?**

The fetal Sertoli cells produce MIS.

○   **What soluble factor superfamily does MIS belong to?**

Transforming growth factor beta (TGFβ).

○   **Which active steroid hormone is important for Wolffian duct induction and proliferation?**

The presence of testosterone results in the proliferation of the Wolffian duct system and the development of the efferent ductules, rete testis, epididymis, vas deferens, and seminal vesicles.

○   **What enzyme converts testosterone into dihydrotestosterone (DHT)?**

The conversion is mediated by 5-alpha-reductase.

○   **How does DHT influence male sexual development?**

DHT is the active form of testosterone that induces virilization of the genitals. DHT influences the elongation of the genital tubercle to form the penis, tubularization of the urethra, and fusion of the labioscrotal folds.

○   **MIS suppresses the development of which female reproductive structures?**

MIS prevents the development of the oviduct, uterus, cervix, and upper third of the vagina.

○   **What is the most common cause of disorders of sexual development (DSD) in children in North America and Europe and how common is it?**

The most common cause is Klinefelter syndrome (incidence in the United States is approximately 1:500 live births).

○   **What physical findings are most suggestive of disorders of sexual development (DSD)?**

Ambiguous genitalia; nonpalpable gonads and severe hypospadias.

○   **What laboratory tests are most often used to confirm the presence of congenital adrenal hyperplasia?**

The most appropriate tests include fluorescence in situ hybridization (FISH) or karyotype analysis, and plasma 17-hydroxyprogesterone >500 mg/dL.

○   **What are the 2 most common enzyme defects resulting in congenital adrenal hyperplasia?**

21-hydroxylase deficiency (90% of cases) and 11-beta hydroxylase deficiency (5% of cases). Both enzyme defects result in elevated plasma levels of 17-hydroxyprogesterone. 11-beta hydroxylase deficiency specifically results in elevated plasma levels of 11-deoxycortisol and 11-deoxycorticosterone.

○   **What imaging studies are the most helpful in defining the anatomy associated with a DSD?**

Use of the abdomino-pelvic ultrasound (to look for the presence of a uterus) and a fluoroscopic genitogram to look for a vaginal connection to the urogenital sinus are extremely helpful.

○ **What is the typical appearance of a patient with complete androgen insensitivity syndrome (CAIS) and why?**

These patients appear as normal phenotypic females with normal development of secondary sexual characteristics. Development of the external male genitalia does not occur due to the lack of androgen receptor activation.

○ **What is the typical development of the internal genitalia in patients with CAIS?**

On examination, these patients have a short, blind-ending vagina with no internal Mullerian duct structures. Since MIS is present during embryogenesis, the Mullerian duct structures do not develop.

○ **What is the most common demonstrable defect seen in patients with CAIS?**

The most common finding is the absence of high-affinity binding of **DHT**.

○ **What are the common clinical presentations that most often lead to the diagnosis of CAIS?**

Primary amenorrhea (peripubertal) and female patients with bilateral inguinal hernias. Approximately 2% of females presenting with these findings will have CAIS. Females with clinically significant hernias may benefit from vaginoscopy at the time of surgery to confirm the presence of a cervix.

○ **What is the most common karyotype in patients with ovotesticular DSD (true hermaphroditism)?**

The most common karyotypic finding is 46XX.

○ **What are the most common gonadal malignancies associated with a dysgenetic gonad and the presence of a Y chromosome?**

The most common malignancies are gonadoblastomas and dysgerminomas.

○ **What is the most common karyotypic finding in Klinefelter syndrome?**

One additional X chromosome (47, XXY).

○ **What is the histopathologic finding in patients with pure gonadal dysgenesis?**

Bilateral streak gonads and underdeveloped Mullerian structures are found.

○ **During development, when does the gonad develop into a testis?**

During the second month.

○ **What is anti-Mullerian hormone (AMH)?**

AMH is the same as MIS.

○ **True/False: An ovotesticular DSD often has a degree of Wolffian development near the testicular tissue even when joined to an ovary.**

True. The gonad contains both ovarian and testicular elements. The paracrine effect of the testicular element on the Wolffian duct results in the development of this tissue to varying degrees.

○ **The external genitalia of both sexes are identical through how many weeks of gestation?**

Seven weeks.

○ **What is the incidence of a DSD condition when 2 impalpable testes are found on examination?**

Fifty percent.

○ **Congenital adrenal hyperplasia is associated with what potentially lethal condition?**

Salt-wasting nephropathy occurs in 75%. If not recognized, the resulting hypotension can cause vascular collapse and death.

○ **A perfectly normal-appearing, phenotypic male presents with an inguinal hernia on one side and an impalpable testis on the other. Karyotype is 46XY. What DSD problem is most likely?**

Isolated deficiency of MIS.

○ **What is the controversy regarding management of CAIS?**

Whether or not to leave the gonads in situ until the child completes pubertal development.

CHAPTER 14

Neurogenic Voiding Dysfunction

Leonard Glickman, MD and George P. H. Young, MD, FACS

○ **What are the pathways and influences involved in normal micturition?**

Voluntary control is exerted by the cerebral cortex by release of tonic inhibitory signals to the pontine micturition center (PMC). The PMC initiates voiding by stimulation of parasympathetics at S2-S4 causing detrusor contraction. The PMC also inhibits sympathetic fibers T11-L2 causing relaxation of the bladder neck and proximal urethra. Finally, the PMC inhibits the somatic fibers of the pudendal nerve causing relaxation of the external sphincter.

○ **Neurogenic control of the bladder in infants is by what part of the central nervous system also known as the primitive voiding center?**

Sacral reflex center.

○ **Where does the pudendal nerve originate?**

Nucleus of Onuf. This nucleus is a collection of sacral somatic nerve cells that originate from the lateral border of the ventral horn of the sacral spinal cord (S2-S4).

○ **Explain the functions of the pudendal nerve.**

It controls the external urethral sphincter. The pudendal also innervates the penis as well as the ischiocavernosus and bulbocavernosus muscles. The pudendal and pelvic nerves also receive postganglionic axons from the caudal sympathetic chain ganglia.

○ **Overstimulation of the pudendal nerve produces what urological problem?**

Urinary retention.

○ **What can cause overstimulation of the pudendal nerve?**

Trauma to the suprasacral–infrapontine spinal cord.

○   **What cord segment is evaluated with the bulbocavernosus reflex?**

This test evaluates the integrity of the S2-S4 segments.

○   **Briefly summarize the parasympathetic innervation of the bladder?**

Parasympathetic efferents originate from the pelvic nerves S2-S4. The ganglions are located near the organ and the neurotransmitter is acetylcholine. The receptors are muscarinic (M2/M3) and stimulation results in bladder contraction.

○   **Where are the parasympathetic postganglionic neurons located?**

In the detrusor wall as well as the pelvic plexus.

○   **What is the most common type of muscarinic receptor in the bladder?**

The M2 type is the most common type as it accounts for approximately 80% of the bladder's muscarinic receptors. Its exact function in the bladder is unknown, but it is thought to be involved with the neuromodulation of bladder compliance. The M2 receptors are primarily cardiovascular where they help mediate heart rate and cardiac output.

○   **Which muscarinic receptor is most involved with cholinergic stimulation of the detrusor?**

M3, even though it only represents about 20% of the total muscarinic receptors in the bladder. M1 receptors are primarily located in the central nervous system and salivary glands. They deal with cognition and saliva production. This is why a selective M3 antimuscarinic agent should theoretically have fewer central nervous system and dry mouth side effects than nonselective agents. The M5 receptors are primarily located in the ciliary muscle of the eye.

○   **What is the pathway of the sympathetic innervation of the bladder?**

Sympathetic preganglionic nerves exit from the lumbar spinal cord to synapse in the sympathetic chain ganglia. The postganglionic sympathetics then travel through the inferior splanchnic nerves to the inferior mesenteric ganglia. They finally travel in the hypogastric nerve to the pelvic plexus and the urogenital organs.

○   **What is the role of sympathetic innervation of the bladder and outlet?**

Together they promote bladder storage via the hypogastric nerve (T10-L2). Alpha (bladder base and prostate) and beta (bladder body) receptors exist on the bladder and alpha receptors are on the prostatic capsule. Beta activation results in inhibition of muscle contraction. Alpha activation results in increased outlet resistance.

○   **What types of afferent fibers exist in the bladder?**

Myelinated (Aδ) and unmyelinated (C) axons.

○   **How do they differ?**
- Aδ bladder afferents are finely myelinated axons located in the detrusor smooth muscle and sense bladder fullness (tension).
- C bladder afferents have unmyelinated axons, are located in the detrusor mucosa, and most are mechanoinsensitive (hence the term "silent C fibers"). These fibers can be recruited after injury/inflammation to form new functional afferent pathways (becoming mechanosensitive) that can cause pain and urge incontinence.

○ **What is capsaicin?**

A vanilloid, capsaicin stimulates and desensitizes unmyelinated C fiber axons to produce pain and release neuropeptides. Resiniferatoxin (RTX) is an ultrapotent analog of capsaicin.

○ **How is capsaicin involved with spinal cord injuries?**

Although normal micturition is associated with myelinated Aδ afferent fibers, after spinal cord injury a capsaicin-sensitive unmyelinated C fiber-mediated spinal reflex may develop, resulting in detrusor overactivity (DO).

○ **What is the distinction between the smooth and the striated urinary sphincters?**

The smooth sphincter refers to a physiological rather than an anatomic sphincter. It is located at the smooth musculature of the bladder neck and the proximal urethra. Control is involuntary. In contrast, the striated sphincter is anatomic and includes the skeletal muscle surrounding the membranous urethra in men and the middle segment of the urethra in females. This sphincter also includes the striated muscle surrounding the urethra in both men and women. The outer portion of this sphincter is under voluntary control.

○ **The rhabdosphincter contains what specific type of muscle fiber?**

Striated, slow-twitch (type 1) muscle fibers.

○ **Which neurotransmitter is involved in urethral smooth muscle relaxation during voiding?**

Nitric oxide (NO) has been identified as the neurotransmitter responsible for urethral smooth muscle relaxation. Pelvic parasympathetic nerves are responsible for mediating the release of NO.

○ **According to Wein, what are the 3 factors necessary for (A) normal bladder and urine storage to occur, and (B) normal bladder emptying to occur?**

The factors necessary for urine storage:

1. Accommodation of urine at low pressure with appropriate sensation.
2. A closed outlet at rest and one that remains so with increases of intra-abdominal pressure.
3. No involuntary bladder contractions.

Requirements for normal emptying:

1. A contraction of adequate magnitude and duration.
2. Lowering of outlet resistance when this contraction occurs.
3. No anatomic outlet obstruction.

○ **What is the guarding reflex?**

A reflex pathway that functions during the filling phase. As the bladder fills with urine, low-level vesical afferent activity via the pelvic nerve causes external sphincter contraction through somatic pathways. In turn, the somatic afferents from the sphincter inhibit parasympathetic efferent signals suppressing bladder activity and allowing urine to be stored in the bladder. It is thought that alterations in these primitive reflex pathways contribute to neurogenic bladder dysfunction.

○ **What properties of the bladder allow for normal low pressure filling?**

In general, the bladder contains viscoelastic properties that allow the bladder to maintain a low pressure of 10 cm H_2O throughout the filling phase. This property is known as compliance. Compliance (C) is defined as the change in bladder volume divided by the change in intravesical pressure, $C = \Delta V / \Delta P$. Along with smooth muscle, approximately 50% of the bladder wall contains collagen and 2% elastin. As the collagen content of the bladder wall increases, the compliance decreases. Injury, denervation, and obstruction can all cause increases in collagen content of the bladder wall.

○ **What is the order of processes in micturition?**

Afferent activity from the bladder activates the PMC, which first acts to inhibit the spinal guarding reflex. The pudendal nerve mediates relaxation of the striated external sphincter. This is followed by relaxation of the bladder neck/proximal urethra by sympathetic fibers from T11-L2. Almost simultaneously the detrusor contracts and detrusor pressure rises via the S2-S4 parasympathetic efferents.

○ **The first recordable event of the micturition reflex is?**

Cessation of sphincter EMG activity.

○ **Injury to which parts of the brain causes voiding dysfunction?**

Voluntary voiding is dependent on intact neuronal pathways between the frontal cortex and the septal-preoptic region of the hypothalamus as well as intact connections between the paracentral lobule and the brainstem. Injury to these areas of the cortex results in increased bladder activity due to loss of cortical inhibitory signals.

○ **How do bladder reflexes change from an infant to an adult?**

It is important to remember that by definition the infant and the toddler will have DO. Children younger than 2 to 3 years of age lack the cerebral maturity to emit inhibitory signals to prevent voiding reflexes. As the infant's bladder fills with urine and reaches its functional capacity the bladder will reflexively contract and empty. These neonatal pathways that cause detrusor overactivity do not disappear with age. They are, however, controlled by higher cortical function that develops with age. Neurologic disease and advanced age can cause these primitive reflexes to reemerge and cause urgency and urge incontinence.

○ **Define "detrusor hyperreflexia" and explain how it differs from "detrusor instability."**

Detrusor hyperreflexia is defined as DO due to a disturbance of the neural control mechanisms. Without evidence of a relevant neurological disorder, the term "detrusor hyperreflexia" cannot be used, and instead the term "detrusor instability" is used.

○ **What are the 3 hypotheses that explain DO?**

1. Neurogenic—DO may arise from generalized, nerve-mediated excitation of the detrusor muscle from various sources. Cerebral damage can reduce suprapontine inhibition. Spinal cord lesions can damage axonal pathways allowing primitive spinal bladder reflexes to occur. New reflexes secondary to C fiber bladder afferent neurons can disrupt normal sacral activity. Over time, sensitization of peripheral afferents in the bladder can trigger DO.

2. Myogenic—DO contractions result from a combination of an increased likelihood of spontaneous contraction and enhanced propagation of activity between muscle cells. Patchy denervation commonly occurs in DO, which can affect smooth muscle cell spontaneous contractions, and ultimately propagation over a wider area of detrusor.

3. Peripheral autonomous activity—This hypothesis suggests that increased bladder sensation results from increased localized detrusor contraction and that DO is due to enhanced coordination of modular activity through the myovesical plexus.

○ **What is overactive bladder (OAB)?**

OAB is a symptomatic diagnosis that is usually secondary to DO. DO is a diagnosis that requires urodynamic testing. The quantification of OAB symptoms should be by frequency–volume chart and validated questionnaires.

○ **From cranial to caudal, explain how neurological lesions typically effect voiding dysfunction.**

- CNS lesions typically result in detrusor hyperreflexia. Normally, the CNS inhibits reflex contraction of the detrusor. Loss of this tonic detrusor inhibition (due to stroke, Parkinson disease [PD], **multiple sclerosis** [MS], and brain tumors) results in DO with normal coordination of detrusor and sphincter, and normal sphincter tone and sensation. (Please note MS can have ANY manifestation depending on the location of the lesion.)
- Pontine micturition center (PMC)—lesions above the PMC are described above, with coordinated DO. Below the PMC, the detrusor and external urethral sphincter become uncoordinated, resulting in detrusor–sphincter dyssynergia (DSD).
- Spinal cord lesions above S2 are upper motor neuron (UMN) lesions and result in DSD. All spinal cord injuries can result in spinal shock. Spinal cord injuries above T6 may result in autonomic dysreflexia.
- Neurological lesions below S2 can be due to spina bifida, MS, surgeries (APR), myelodysplasia, disc herniation, and results in an acontractile detrusor, and therefore retention.

○ **In addition to anticholinergic agents, which class of oral medications can be used to treat DO?**

The sympathetic efferents that effect bladder function are known to cause detrusor relaxation during the filling phase of the micturition cycle. It has been shown that β-3 adrenoceptor activation leads to detrusor relaxation. Therefore, a β-3 adrenoceptor selective agonist drug can be used to prevent detrusor activity.

○ **What are the side effects and precautions in using this class of medication? Can it be used together with anticholinergics?**

Mirabegron (Myrbetriq) is currently available. Side effects include an increase in blood pressure and there has been an increased incidence of urinary tract infection (UTI) noted with its use so far. Special precautions involve an increase in digoxin levels and 2D6 pathway issues. Use with anticholinergics is not currently recommended.

○ **What is the bladder ice-water test?**

A test that can be performed to check for the reemergence of primitive neonatal voiding reflexes. It is performed by instilling 100cc of sterile normal saline at 4°C in the bladder. In a normal adult a cold sensation will be felt but there will be no bladder instability. In an infant, or in an adult with voiding pathology, the cold saline will induce an involuntary detrusor contraction. The reflex is initiated by temperature-sensitive receptors that are supplied by unmyelinated c-fibers afferents.

○ **The sacral spinal cord begins at what level and ends at which spinal cord level?**

It is important to distinguish between spinal column segment (bone level) and the corresponding cord level. The sacral spinal cord actually begins at the column level of T12-L1. It terminates as the cauda equina at spinal column level L2.

○ **After the cerebral shock phase wears off, what type of bladder condition is found most often?**

Detrusor hyperreflexia with coordinated urethral sphincter activity. This occurs because the PMC is released from cerebral inhibitory control. Clinically, this causes frequency, urgency, and urge incontinence.

○ **How is the above situation treated?**

Foley catheter or intermittent catheterization during cerebral shock phase. Anticholinergic medications afterward.

○ **Spinal shock typically lasts how long?**

6 to 12 weeks.

○ **What is the voiding pattern observed in a complete cord injury above the sacral reflex?**

Most commonly, these lesions result in urge incontinence from detrusor hyperreflexia, absent sensation below the level of the lesion, smooth sphincter synergy, and striated sphincter dyssynergia. Lesions above the sympathetic outflow tract T7 or T8 (spinal column level of T6) may also result in smooth sphincter dyssynergia.

○ **A diver suffers from a complete spinal cord injury at the level of T8. What pattern of voiding would be expected immediately following the accident?**

The immediate result is a period of spinal shock. There is generally bladder areflexia and acontractility. Some EMG activity may be present at the external sphincter, but there is no voluntary control. Urinary retention is the most common finding initially, and is typically managed with a Foley catheter. The areflexic period generally lasts 6 to 12 weeks, but may persist up to 1 to 2 years.

○ **A construction worker falls from a rafter on the job site and suffers a sacral spinal cord injury. After spinal cord shock has resolved, what are his expected neurological and urodynamic findings?**

In general, the patient can be expected to have depressed deep tendon reflexes with varying degree of flaccid paralysis below the level of the complete lesion. Detrusor areflexia with normal or high bladder compliance is the norm. Classically, the bladder outlet is found to have a competent but nonrelaxing smooth sphincter with a striated sphincter that retains some fixed tone, but is not under voluntary control.

○ **How would you manage the patient in the above question?**

The main goal of treatment is to maintain low bladder storage pressures to prevent upper tract damage from occurring. This is best achieved with the use of CIC in patients who have the dexterity necessary for self-catheterization.

○ **Which drugs have been used to treat outflow obstruction at the level of the striated sphincter?**

Baclofen, benzodiazepines, and dantrolene have all been investigated for their efficacy in treating outlet obstruction secondary to a tonically closed striated sphincter. Unfortunately, none of these medications have been shown to satisfactorily inhibit sphincter spasticity.

○ **What percent of patients with spinal cord injury have vesicoureteral reflux (VUR)? What contributing factors may influence this?**

Reported incidence is 17% to 25%. Contributing factors include elevated filling and voiding pressures, as well as infection. Potential treatments depend on the specific clinical circumstance and include pharmacotherapy, urethral dilation, neuromodulation, deafferentiation, augmentation cystoplasty, or sphincterotomy.

○ **While performing cystoscopy on a patient with a high cervical cord injury, he develops hypertension, flushing, sweating, headache, and bradycardia. What is the problem, what causes it and what should be done to correct it?**

This is a classic description of autonomic hyperreflexia. It arises from massive autonomic discharge in patients with cord injuries above the sympathetic outflow tract (T6). Prevention is based on the use of spinal anesthesia in susceptible patients and administering oral nifedipine (10 mg) 30 minutes prior to the procedure. Initial management of symptoms is immediate withdrawal of the bladder stimulus, alpha blockade, and bladder decompression with Foley catheter.

○ **Who first described autonomic dysreflexia (aka hyperreflexia) and when?**

Anthony Bowlby in 1890.

○ **Can autonomic dysreflexia occur during the spinal shock period?**

Usually not. It generally occurs only when reflexes begin to return.

○ **Which patients are most at risk for autonomic dysreflexia?**

Those with cervical injuries as well as those who have had this symptom complex previously and are known to be prone to it.

○ **What is the key symptom in a spinal cord injured patient that should alert caregivers to a possible autonomic dysreflexia problem?**

Sudden, severe headache should alert caregivers to the possibility of an autonomic dysreflexic episode.

○ **Why is autonomic dysreflexia dangerous?**

The combination of proximal (cranial) vasodilation with severe hypertension can cause a cerebral hemorrhage or stroke if not recognized and treated quickly.

○ **What is the level of spinal injury that can lead to autonomic dysreflexia?**

Injuries at T6 or higher can lead to autonomic dysreflexia.

○ **What is the rate of autonomic dysreflexia in individuals with a T6 or higher injury?**

Usually about 50% to 90%.

○ **Autonomic dysreflexia not caused by bladder distension is most likely from what cause?**

Fecal impaction.

○ **What immediate pharmacological therapy should be started in autonomic dysreflexia?**

Immediate release nifedipine and nitroglycerine paste. The nifedipine should be the bite-and-swallow rather than sublingual form.

○ **Is terazosin useful in the prevention of autonomic dysreflexia?**

Yes, but other agents are preferred.

○ **What diseases result in peripheral neuropathy resulting in urinary retention?**

Diabetes, AIDS, polio, Guillain–Barre syndrome, tabes dorsalis, and pernicious anemia.

○ **After a stroke, what percentage of patients develop acute urinary retention?**

25%.

○ **A female patient recently underwent surgery for rectal cancer and now presents with urinary complaints. What surgery did she most likely have and what urinary complaints is she most likely to present with? How often is such dysfunction permanent?**

Radical pelvic surgery can cause collateral damage to the pelvic nerves resulting in vesicourethral dysfunction. Voiding dysfunction after radical pelvic surgery is most commonly seen after abdominoperineal resection with a reported incidence of 20% to 68%, but is also seen very commonly with abdominal hysterectomies, low anterior resections, and proctocolectomies. Voiding dysfunction is permanent in approximately 15% to 20% of these patients. Urodynamics typically show an areflexic bladder with obstruction secondary to a sphincter with a fixed tone not subject to voluntary relaxation. The bladder neck is often open and nonfunctional. Patients also typically present with urinary incontinence due to overflow incontinence.

○ **Describe the effects on voiding following a cerebrovascular accident.**

The effects on micturition are divided into acute and long term. The initial period of shock may be associated with urinary retention secondary to detrusor areflexia. The most common long-term sequela is detrusor hyperreflexia. Sensation and compliance are generally intact.

○ **What effect does Alzheimer disease (AD) have on voiding?**

Alzheimer dementia involves the loss of gray and white matter in the frontal lobes. Incontinence may ensue and may be secondary to detrusor hyperreflexia with voluntary sphincter activity or may be due to loss of awareness to void.

○ **What is normal pressure hydrocephalus (NPH) and what urologic abnormality can be seen?**

NPH is a condition typified by a rise in cerebrospinal fluid in the brain causing abnormally enlarged ventricular size with a normal opening pressure on lumbar puncture. These patients often present with the classic triad of dementia, ataxia, and urinary incontinence. In general, incontinence in these patients is caused by DO and with sphincter synergia.

○ **Does outlet obstruction exist in patients with PD?**

Voiding dysfunction exists in 35% to 70% of patients with PD. The most common symptoms are urgency, frequency, nocturia, and urge incontinence. The most common finding on urodynamics is detrusor hyperreflexia with smooth sphincter synergy. In contradistinction to patients post-CVA, those patients with PD generally do not have outlet obstruction and subsequently respond poorly to prostatectomy. This may be due to poorly sustained bladder contractions and poor sphincter relaxation.

○ **In what way is PD different from a stroke urodynamically?**

Both demonstrate detrusor hyperreflexia, but PD patients usually have a weakened sphincter as well.

○ **What is multiple system atrophy (MSA)?**

MSA is a progressive neurodegenerative disorder of unclear etiology characterized by parkinsonism, as well as cerebellar, autonomic, and pyramidal cortical dysfunction. Initial symptoms include urgency, frequency, urgency incontinence, and erectile dysfunction. As the disease progresses patients begin to experience difficulty initiating and maintaining voiding. This likely occurs due to pontine and sacral cord lesions. VCUG may reveal an open bladder neck consistent with intrinsic sphincter deficiency (ISD). EMG studies may also show striated sphincter denervation, which predisposes patients to sphincteric incontinence.

○ **How do you differentiate MSA and PD?**

MSA generally has the following features:

1. Urinary symptoms precede or present with parkinsonian symptoms.

2. Urinary incontinence.

3. Significant postvoid residual volume.

4. Initial erectile failure.

5. Abnormal sphincter EMG.

○ **How does MS affect voiding and what is the most common finding?**

MS is a demyelinating disease that most commonly involves the posterior and lateral columns of the cervical spinal cord. Fifty to ninety percent of these patients have voiding dysfunction at some point. The most common finding is detrusor hyperreflexia. Thirty to sixty-five percent of these patients have striated sphincter dyssynergia.

○ **In MS, how often is detrusor areflexia found?**

20% to 50%.

○ **What parameters predispose patients with MS to significant urologic complications?**

Men with (1) detrusor-sphincter dyssynergia, (2) detrusor filling pressures > 40 cm H_2O, and (3) indwelling catheters.

○ **What is diabetic cystopathy?**

This is a term that describes the effects of diabetes on the urinary bladder. The most recent evidence points to both a sensory and motor dysfunction. Urodynamically, these bladders demonstrate impaired sensation, increased capacity, decreased contractility, and impaired flow patterns. Pressure/flow studies can differentiate poor bladder emptying from outlet obstruction. Timed voiding plays a pivotal role in therapy.

○ **Diabetic cystopathy typically occurs how long after the onset of diabetes?**

10 years.

○ **What is Shy–Drager syndrome and what urodynamic findings are associated with it?**

This disorder results from cell loss and gliosis in the cerebellum, substantia nigra, intermediolateral columns of the spinal cord, and Onuf nucleus. Clinically, patients demonstrate orthostatic hypotension, anhidrosis, and certain degrees of parkinsonian symptoms plus autonomic dysfunction. Diagnostically, these individuals are identified by the uncommon findings of an open bladder neck (in contrast to PD patients) and striated sphincter denervation on EMG.

○   **Patients with Shy–Drager syndrome should avoid what type of urological surgery?**

TURP, because the rate of total incontinence is high.

○   **TURP should generally be avoided in what disease states?**

In addition to Shy–Drager syndrome, TURP should be avoided if possible in PD patients due to high rates of incontinence.

○   **What kind of voiding disorder would a patient with syphilis present with?**

Syphilitic myelopathy is an increasingly rare entity in the world today, especially in developed countries. However, patients with untreated syphilis can develop tabes dorsalis, which causes dysfunction of the dorsal columns and posterior sacral roots. This causes loss of bladder sensation resulting in large residual urine volumes (sensory neurogenic bladder).

○   **What is Fowler syndrome?**

Urinary retention in a young woman without anatomic cause or obvious neurological dysfunction, occurring intermittently with normal voiding in between. It is characterized by retaining urine for over a day but without urgency despite a bladder capacity of 1 L. MRI of the brain and the entire spinal cord is normal. Diagnosis is based on EMG abnormalities of the striated urethral sphincter.

○   **Name and define the 4 types of incontinence.**

1. Stress urinary incontinence manifests as leakage secondary to increased intra-abdominal pressure due to weak pelvic support.
2. Urge incontinence is leakage with the urge to void, usually associated with advanced age, neurological diseases (MS, stroke, UMN diseases, and brain tumors), and idiopathic.
3. Overflow incontinence patients leak when they have a full bladder, with constant leaking or dribbling. These are commonly associated with grade III or IV prolapse, previous surgeries (APR), and lower motor neuron diseases (detrusor areflexia).
4. Global incontinence is a constant leakage requiring extensive workup.

○   **In patients with neurogenic voiding dysfunction, what urodynamic finding has the highest correlation with the development of upper tract damage?**

DSD correlates highest with the upper tract damage.

○   **A finding of detrusor-sphincter dyssynergia implies injury to which neurologic pathway?**

Coordinated, synergistic voiding requires an intact neural axis between the pontine-mesencephalic reticular formation and the sacral spinal cord.

○   **In patients with bladder outlet obstruction, what is the typical opening pressure on pressure-flow studies?**

These patients have opening pressures greater than 80 cm H_2O.

○ **What is ALPP and what is it used to determine?**

ALPP is the abdominal leak point pressure and is defined as the intravesical pressure at which urine leakage occurs due to increased abdominal pressure in the absence of a detrusor contraction. The ALPP is used to determine urethral sphincteric strength. In general, an ALPP < 60 cm H_2O signifies ISD. An ALPP between 60 and 90 cm H_2O is indeterminate for ISD, and an ALPP > 90 cm H_2O suggests there is little or no ISD.

○ **Name 3 risk factors for female ISD.**

1. Prior urethral or periurethral surgery such as anti-incontinence surgery or excision of a urethral diverticulum.
2. Neurologic insult affecting parasympathetic, sympathetic, and/or somatic nerves.
3. Pelvic radiation that can affect mucosal coaptation of the female urethra and cause associated nerve damage.

○ **What are the general factors that contribute to urinary incontinence in women?**

Predisposing factors such as anatomy and collagen status. Inciting factors such as childbirth and previous surgery. Promoting factors such as infection and obesity. Decompensating factors such as aging.

○ **How do Kegel exercises reduce incontinence?**

These exercises not only produce a direct physical obstruction to urinary leakage, but they also can help abolish uninhibited detrusor contractions. This is accomplished by stimulation of afferent sacral nerves at low frequencies (below the pain threshold of C fibers). This causes inhibition of efferent pelvic nerve firing thereby reducing detrusor activity.

○ **Kegel exercises stimulate the activity of which pelvic nerve?**

Pudendal nerve.

○ **What is the failure (attrition) rate of pelvic floor biofeedback and what is the most important factor in successful therapy?**

Biofeedback works by bringing to conscious control that which was previously unconscious. The most important factor in the success of therapy is a well-motivated patient. In fact, attrition rates remain as high as one-third even in well-established centers.

○ **Why is pharmacotherapy using acetylcholine-like drugs not clinically useful in facilitating bladder emptying?**

These drugs are rapidly hydrolyzed by cholinesterases thereby limiting their efficacy.

○ **What are the urodynamic parameters used to diagnose bladder neck obstruction in women?**

While validated nomograms do not exist, the following findings are highly suggestive of obstruction: sustained detrusor contraction of normal or high pressure, poor flow of urine, and lack of bladder neck funneling on fluoroscopy. All of these findings must be accompanied by a synergic external urethral sphincter for bladder neck obstruction to exist.

○ **What are some of the causes of urinary retention in females?**

Etiologies of retention in women include MS, spina bifida occulta, viral sacromyeloradiculitis, lumbar disc protrusion, cauda equina syndrome, bladder neck obstruction, pseudomyotonia, and reflex sympathetic dystrophy.

○   **What factors may contribute to urinary incontinence following radical prostatectomy?**

Any one or combination of the following may contribute to incontinence:
- Residual outlet obstruction.
- Detrusor instability.
- Sphincter incompetence.
- Preexisting neurologic disease.

○   **Two days following a lumbar laminectomy, a 61-year-old male is in urinary retention. What is the recommended initial treatment?**

Disc disease is commonly associated with voiding dysfunction. The most common finding is that of detrusor areflexia. Generally, patients present with symptoms of poor emptying. Interestingly, laminectomy may not improve the bladder dysfunction. Treatment in this male would consist of catheter placement and urodynamic studies.

○   **When evaluating incontinence in geriatric patients, what does the mnemonic DIAPPERS refer to?**

Delirium, **I**nfection, **A**trophic vaginitis, **P**sychological problems, **P**harmaceuticals, **E**xcess urine output, **R**estricted mobility, **S**tool impaction.

○   **What is the most common type of urinary incontinence in the elderly?**

Urge incontinence is the most common cause of urinary incontinence in the elderly. Many conditions that are prevalent in this population predispose them to this type of incontinence including CVA, PD, spinal cord injury, MS, and BPH.

○   **Is urinary incontinence a normal consequence of aging?**

While age-related changes are present in the elderly and predispose them to incontinence, this should not be considered a normal part of aging and a thorough evaluation is indicated.

○   **What broad categories of medications may be associated with urinary incontinence?**

ACE inhibitors, alcohol, β-adrenergic agonists and antagonists, calcium channel blockers, diuretics, narcotics, sedatives and hypnotics, and vincristine.

○   **What are the indications for urodynamics testing in the incontinent patient?**

Any patient who reports a history of a failed incontinence procedure or previous radical pelvic surgery, patients with mixed symptoms (including both stress and urge), history of a neurologic disorder, failed medical therapy, and most importantly any patient in whom stress incontinence is not demonstrated on physical examination.

○   **What are common therapies designed to treat bladder storage deficits of bladder etiology in order of invasiveness?**

Behavioral therapy/biofeedback, pharmacological therapy (anticholinergics, TCAs, calcium antagonists, potassium channel openers, prostaglandin inhibitors, α-adrenergic agonists, β-adrenergic antagonists, DMSO, capsaicin, resiniferatoxin, botulinum toxin), bladder overdistension, electrical stimulation/neuromodulation, interruption of innervation (selective sacral rhizotomy), and augmentation cystoplasty.

○ **What are common therapies designed to treat bladder storage deficits due to bladder outlet related issues in order of invasiveness?**

Behavioral therapy/biofeedback, electrical stimulation, pharmacological therapies (β-adrenergic agonists, TCAs, β-adrenergic agonists/antagonists), vaginal supportive devices (pessaries), periurethral bulking agents (collagen, synthetics), vesicourethral suspension, sling procedures (both with prolapse repair if needed), artificial urinary sphincter, bladder outlet reconstruction, and myoplasty.

○ **What are common therapies designed to aid in bladder emptying due to bladder contractility problems in order of invasiveness?**

Valsalva/credé, bladder training, pharmacological therapies (parasympathomimetics, prostaglandins, α-adrenergic antagonists, and opioid antagonists), electrical stimulation (neuromodulation), reduction cystoplasty, and bladder myoplasty.

○ **What are common therapies designed to aid in bladder emptying due to bladder outlet problems in order of invasiveness?**

- *At the site of obstruction*: pharmacological therapies (α-adrenergic antagonists, 5a-reductase inhibitors, LHRH agonists/antagonists, antiandrogens), prostatectomy, bladder neck incision/resection, urethral stricture repair, urethroplasty.
- *At the smooth sphincter*: pharmacological therapies (α-adrenergic antagonists, β-adrenergic agonists), transurethral resection/incision, Y-V plasty.
- *At the striated sphincter*: behavioral therapy/biofeedback, pharmacological therapy (benzodiazepines, baclofen, dantrolene, α-adrenergic antagonists, botulinum toxin injection), urethral overdilation, surgical sphincterotomy, pudendal nerve interruption.

○ **How does neuromodulation work on both storage and emptying functions?**

Two theories:

1. Inhibition of afferent fibers from the bladder that affects sensation and micturition reflex arcs in the spinal cord.
2. Direct stimulation of efferent fibers via the pudendal nerve to the external sphincter causes sphincter closure and reflexive detrusor relaxation.

○ **In theory how would sacral neuromodulation aid in treating urinary retention?**

In patients with spinal cord injuries who have alterations in their suprasacral pathways, the guarding and urethral reflex may be constitutively active causing urinary retention. Neuromodulation may inhibit the excitatory flow from the urethral outlet and allow for bladder emptying.

○ **Where is the lead for a sacral nerve stimulator (SNS) placed, and how does it work?**

Sacral nerve stimulators (eg, InterStim) are used for refractory urge incontinence, OAB, and idiopathic urinary retention for patients who have failed conservative therapy. The lead is placed in the S3 foramen, where both the pelvic plexus and pudendal nerve run.

○ **How is the correct placement of a sacral stimulator lead determined clinically and what is the appropriate response that is observed?**

The lead is tested by a clinical nerve stimulation test. The appropriate motor response is dorsiflexion of the great toe and bellows contraction of the levator muscles in the perineal area (anal wink).

○ **What are the clinical indications for a SNS?**

SNS can be used for both storage dysfunction (eg, urgency–frequency and urge incontinence) and emptying dysfunction (nonobstructive urinary retention). There are no defined preclinical factors, such as urodynamic findings, that can predict which patients will respond to sacral neuromodulation.

○ **How often do the nerves from the S2-S4 sacral foramina differ?**

The detrusor is innervated primarily by S3 and to a lesser extent by S2 and S4. Rectal stimulation is by means of all 3 roots equally. Erectile stimulation is mainly by S2 with a small contribution from S3 but none from S4.

○ **What are the contraindications to sacral neuromodulators?**

Contraindications include significant bone abnormalities in the spine or sacrum that may prohibit access to the foramen, inadequate mental capacity of patients who could not manage the device, physical limitations that prevent voiding (functional incontinence), future need of MRI, and noncompliance. SNS are not contraindicated and can be used in specially selected patients with MS, spinal cord injury, and chronic cystitis, and even in certain pediatric cases.

○ **What is the most common complication associated with SNSs?**

The InterStim device is relatively new; however, pain at the neurostimulator site was the most common complaint (15% of patients) after 1 year of follow-up. Lead migration occurs in roughly 12% of SNS procedures performed previous to the newer InterStim device with its tined leads. Surgical revision was required in 33.3% of InterStim cases to resolve an adverse event. Explantation for lack of efficacy occurred in 10.5%. Infection of the battery site warrants explantation of the entire system.

○ **How does botulinum toxin (Botox) work?**

Botox blocks the release of acetylcholine and other transmitters from presynaptic nerve endings. Injection into the detrusor impairs contractility, and results in temporary muscle atrophy at the injection sites. The desired chemical denervation is a reversible process, and axons are regenerated in about 3 to 6 months. Botox is efficacious for at least 3 to 4 months, and has been shown to be effective for up to 1 year. Additional injections of Botox are required over time because the effect of Botox does decline over time. However, there does not seem to be a reduction in response with additional injections. Moreover, Botox has also been shown to suppress afferent nerve activity by inhibiting the release of substance P and CGRP from sensory terminals.

○ **When can Botox be used?**

There are a number of potential uses for Botox. Careful workup is necessary to determine when it will be most efficacious. With DO, Botox can result in improvements in symptoms of frequency, urge incontinence, and the sense of urgency. Botox can also improve bladder capacity, volume at first reflex detrusor contraction, bladder compliance, and decreases in detrusor pressures during bladder filling and voiding. Recently, Botox has been used to treat pelvic floor spasticity as well as patients with nonneurogenic OAB and even interstitial cystitis. Its efficacy has also recently been shown in benign prostatic hyperplasia, where injections into the prostate can induce prostatic atrophy by inducing apoptosis, inhibiting proliferation, and downregulating α_{1A}-adrenergic receptors.

○ **How is Botox administered for treatment of DO?**

While the optimal dose of Botox for treatment of DO has yet to be determined, the widely used dosage is 200 U, which is administered transurethrally at 20 to 30 sites around the bladder with sparing of the trigone and bladder dome.

○ **What are some of the differences between SNSs and Botox injections?**

The FDA has approved neuromodulation for use in urge-incontinence, urge-frequency syndrome, and idiopathic urinary retention. As of August 2011 Botox has been approved for use in the treatment of neurogenic detrusor overactivity only. Some patients may prefer a trial of Botox injections. Its advantages include a lower initial cost, simpler procedure, and no need for permanent implant or possible revisions. Its main disadvantage is that it only lasts 3 to 9 months, requiring repeat administration. Currently, long-term response to neuromodulation is better established than Botox, as there is no direct comparison study.

○ **What is required for bladder control to mature from the infant voiding pattern to the adult voiding pattern?**

Along with an intact nervous system the following 3 events need to occur simultaneously for the maturation of the micturition cycle to occur:

1. Progressive increase in functional bladder storage capacity.

2. Maturation of voluntary control over the urethral sphincter.

3. Development of direct volitional control over the bladder-sphincter unit in order to initiate voluntary voiding.

○ **What is Hinman syndrome?**

Initially known as nonneurogenic neurogenic bladder or subclinical neurogenic bladder. It describes a form of bladder–sphincteric dysfunction in children that was characterized by a combination of bladder decompensation with incontinence, poor emptying, and recurrent urinary infections. Most children also have significant bowel dysfunction, including encopresis, constipation, and fecal impaction.

○ **What is Ochoa (urofacial) syndrome?**

Children with this syndrome exhibit all the classic features of dysfunctional voiding, including urinary incontinence, recurrent UTIs, constipation, reflux, and upper tract damage, but they also have a peculiar painful or apparently crying facial expression during smiling. It has autosomal recessive inheritance and has been located on chromosome 10. Urodynamic studies characteristically showed a sustained contraction of the external sphincter during voiding. The resulting severe bladder–sphincter dysfunction is often associated with a dismal outcome.

○ **What is dysfunction elimination syndrome in children?**

It is a term used to recognize that many children with dysfunctional voiding and recurrent UTIs often have associated bowel dysfunction, including constipation, fecal impaction, and encopresis. Any gross distention of the rectum by impacted feces can result in mechanical compression of the bladder and bladder neck, leading to urinary obstruction. In addition, it has been observed that large fecal impaction may induce significant detrusor instability and other bladder dysfunctions, which in turn will result in the urge syndrome, UTI, and reflux.

○ **What percentage of clinical problems seen in pediatric urology are the result of neurologic lesions that affect lower urinary tract function?**

25%.

○ **What is the most common cause of neurogenic bladder dysfunction in children?**

Abnormal development of the spinal canal and internecine spinal cord. Myelomeningocele accounts for more than 90% of all open spinal dysraphic states, with a spectrum of neurologic lesions depending on which neural elements have everted with the meningocele sac.

○   **Where is the most common location of a meningocele?**

The bony vertebral level provides little information regarding the exact neurologic level or lesion produced. The most common site of meningocele is the lumbosacral spine (47%), followed by lumbar (26%), then sacral (20%).

○   **What are the most common abnormalities of the lower urinary tract found to coexist with VUR in children?**

Detrusor overactivity and uncoordinated detrusor–sphincter function during micturition. These abnormalities may occur secondary to urinary infection or can be acquired during the period when voluntary control of micturition is being established. Remember, reflux from incompetence of the ureterovesical junction may be worsened by detrusor instability, and patients with this dysfunction often have bilateral high-grade reflux and injured upper renal tracts.

○   **What medications are used to treat children with OAB?**

- Antimuscarinic agents, such as oxybutynin, are the gold standard and act by reducing the frequency and intensity of involuntary contractions, resulting in an increase in the functional bladder capacity. The nonselective pattern of activity and penetration of the blood–brain barrier are known to induce systemic and central side effects.
- α-adrenergic blockers are used in patients with evidence of bladder neck dysfunction for relaxation of the bladder neck.
- Tricyclic antidepressants, such as imipramine, have been found to be effective for increasing urine storage by both decreasing the detrusor contractility and increasing outlet resistance. They should be used judiciously in children because of the high incidence of side effects.

○   **How can the expected bladder capacity be measured in the pediatric population?**

- For young infants the following formula can be used: Bladder capacity (mL) = 38 + 2.5 × age (months).
- For older children the Koff formula can be used: Bladder capacity (mL) = (age [years] + 2) × 30.

CHAPTER 15 Urodynamics

Gamal M. Ghoniem, MD, FACS

○ **True/False: A high postvoid residual urine volume correlates with both the symptoms and urodynamic findings associated with bladder outlet obstruction (BOO).**

False. A high postvoid residual volume does not necessarily mean BOO. This condition can be present in association with any physical BOO or it can be present in association with a poorly contracting bladder. Conversely, this condition may not be present in patients with severe BOO if they have enough detrusor function to overcome the outlet obstruction. Elevated postvoid residual volumes when present do not necessarily lead to infection.

○ **A 40-year-old female with incontinence had a uroflow with Q_{max} of 50 mL/s, a mean of 25 mL/s, and a configuration that looks like a bread loaf standing on end. The most likely single diagnosis is?**

Sphincteric incontinence with low outlet resistance.

○ **What are the 2 events most likely to produce a similar electromyographic (EMG) pattern?**

Striated sphincter dyssynergia and Valsalva voiding both produce similar EMG patterns of increased activity. Patients with these conditions void in the absence of coordination between the detrusor muscle and the external urethral sphincteric unit.

○ **During the act of volitional voiding what would you expect a normal EMG pattern to look like?**

During the act of normal volitional voiding there is increase of detrusor pressure and decrease of EMG activity.

○ **At initiation of normal voiding, which event happens first?**

The initial measurable event upon voiding is decreased EMG activity. This precedes an increase in detrusor pressure and a decrease in maximum urethral pressure.

○ **What is the relationship between pressure and flow during normal micturition in men and women?**

Normal urinary flow in young healthy males should be 15 to 25 mL/s and the associated detrusor pressure should be of less than 40 cm H_2O. Women typically void with similar or slightly higher peak flow rates, but the associated detrusor pressures are lower and usually approximately 20 cm H_2O. Interestingly, identical results on repeated measurements are difficult to obtain with repeated pressure flow studies in the same healthy individual.

○ **What does an intermittent flow pattern in an individual with normal deep tendon and bulbocavernosus reflexes and normal perineal sensation most likely indicate?**

Intermittent flow in an otherwise normal individual is most suggestive of abdominal straining. The neurologically intact patient cannot have neurogenic detrusor overactivity (NDO) or detrusor sphincter dyssynergia (DSD).

○ **A patient with incontinence shows evidence of low compliance by urodynamics. The Valsalva leak point pressure is 20 to 30 cm H$_2$O. What would you tell the patient her risk of upper tract deterioration is?**

Valsalva leak point pressures less than 40 cm H$_2$O will actually protect the upper tracts from pressure-induced hydronephrosis and subsequent deterioration in renal function. The lower the leak pressure, the less likely upper tract deterioration will happen, when bladder compliance is low.

○ **In phase 2 (the tonus limb) of the cystometrogram, bladder compliance is most dependent upon which factor?**

Viscoelastic properties of the detrusor. Other neural factors like cerebral inhibition of reflex bladder activity and intact thoracolumbar spinal cord are more active in the final phase.

○ **What is the most important parameter in uroflowmetry with volumes between 150 and 350 mL: maximum flow rate or average flow rate?**

Maximum flow rate is most indicative of normal detrusor function.

○ **A patient, with no evidence of neurologic disease, has evidence of involuntary detrusor contractions during the filling phase of a CMG. What is your diagnosis? Idiopathic detrusor overactivity or poor compliance?**

Idiopathic detrusor overactivity (IDO). In the presence of neurological disease, identical findings on a cystometrogram (CMG) would lead to the diagnosis of NDO.

○ **What is the Valsalva leak point pressure (VLPP)?**

The Valsalva leak point pressure is the pressure at which passive urethral resistance is overcome by increasing abdominal pressure during straining and urine leaks through an otherwise closed sphincter. This is not a measure of detrusor function and the result can be affected by the presence of a large cystocele.

○ **How is detrusor pressure (P_{det}) calculated?**

$P_{ves} - P_{abd}$ (vesical pressure − abdominal pressure). The detrusor pressure is important in recognizing pressure increases due to abdominal and not true vesical pressure, eg, straining.

○ **What does high bladder compliance relate to?**

Bladder accommodation. High compliance does not relate to high leak pressure.

○ **What does the static infusion urethral pressure profile most accurately predict?**

Intrinsic sphincter deficiency (ISD). It does not predict striated sphincter dyssynergia or urethral obstruction.

○ **What is the most common urodynamic findings seen in patients with cerebrovascular accident (CVA)?**

Neurogenic detrusor overactivity, normal compliance, smooth sphincter synergia, and striated sphincter synergia.

○ **True/False: In patients with cerebral infarction, the upper tracts are at minimal risk of deterioration.**

True. Immediately following the injury, these patients often manifest detrusor areflexia. As they convalesce, patients with cerebral lesions (CVA, subdural hematoma, closed head injuries, brain tumors, etc) most commonly develop NDO. They can have uninhibited motor neurogenic bladders with NDO. The bladder activity in these patients is characterized as complete coordinated incontinence. These patients void at normal pressures, but in an uninhibited manner with coordination between the detrusor muscle and sphincter mechanism. In these cases, there is no detrusor sphincter dyssynergia, and high-pressure voiding is not a common finding.

○ **When do you most likely see pseudodyssynergia?**

In a patient with a CVA. In these patients, the sensation is intact.

○ **A 72-year-old male develops urgency, frequency, and urge incontinence following a CVA. Prior to his CVA, he complained of a decreasing stream and hesitancy. His postvoid residual is 130 mL. What is the most likely cause of his high residual?**

Benign prostatic hyperplasia with BOO would be the most likely explanation for his elevated postvoid residual volume. CVA causes NDO.

○ **Are suprapontine lesions (stroke, dementia, etc) usually associated with detrusor sphincter dyssynergia?**

No. They are usually associated with NDO or detrusor areflexia, phasic idiopathic detrusor overactivity, or detrusor overactivity.

○ **A 21-year-old male patient with cerebral palsy and severe mental retardation has day and night incontinence. What is the most practical and informative urodynamic evaluation?**

A postvoid residual plus renal ultrasound. In this situation, with an uncooperative patient, video urodynamic studies, pressure-flow studies, or even simple cystometry are not likely to impact your management.

○ **What are the urodynamic findings in a complete spinal cord transection at cord level T10 after spinal shock has disappeared?**

Neurogenic detrusor overactivity, striated sphincter dyssynergia, and smooth sphincter synergia.

○ **What are the fluorourodynamic findings in patients with voiding dysfunction secondary to Shy–Drager syndrome?**

Shy–Drager syndrome or multiple system atrophy (MSA) has distinct fluorourodynamic findings. An open bladder neck at rest, decreased detrusor compliance, striated sphincter denervation resulting in incontinence. Other autonomic features include orthostatic hypotension, dry mouth, and constipation. Other manifestations are parkinsonism and cerebral ataxia.

○ **Are uninhibited detrusor contractions diagnosed by filling CMG always due to BOO?**

No. They can be caused by neurologic diseases that affect upper motor neuron function or BOO, or idiopathic.

○ **What are the urodynamic findings generally associated with autonomic hyperreflexia?**

Neurogenic detrusor overactivity, striated sphincter dyssynergia, and smooth sphincter dyssynergia. Lesions above T6 are usually associated with smooth sphincter dyssynergia.

○ **Which condition is detrusor striated sphincter dyssynergia most frequently associated with?**

Suprasacral spinal cord injury. It is absent in Parkinson disease, stroke, myelomeningocele, and radical pelvic surgery.

○ **What is the most common urodynamic abnormality in patients with voiding dysfunction secondary to multiple sclerosis?**

Neurogenic detrusor overactivity. The second most common dysfunction is striated sphincter dyssynergia.

○ **At approximately which vertebral column level does the sacral spinal cord begin and end?**

T12-L2.

○ **Two weeks after an abdominoperineal resection, a 70-year-old male with minimal voiding symptoms prior to his surgery has a postvoid residual of 400 mL. What are the most likely urodynamic abnormalities and what is the preferred management strategy?**

Detrusor areflexia and low compliance will result from pelvic nerve injury, and the best management would be clean intermittent catheterization (CIC) with or without anticholinergics.

○ **What is the most common cause for upper urinary tract deterioration in the spinal cord injury (SCI) patient?**

Striated sphincter dyssynergia. This results in elevated detrusor pressures, high residual urine, hydronephrosis with secondary urinary infections, and renal failure.

○ **What is the best treatment for a T10 paraplegic with type 1 striated sphincter dyssynergia, grade 1 reflux, a postvoid residual of 250 mL, no hydronephrosis, normal compliance, and unsustained detrusor contractions?**

Intermittent catheterization. The description fits a safe reservoir; only CIC is indicated.

○ **A C5-6 SCI female patient has low bladder compliance, an incompetent bladder neck, urethral erosion, and grade 1 hydronephrosis. What would be the best treatment?**

A bladder neck closure or obstructive sling with ileovesicostomy.

○ **A C5-C6 male SCI patient has no change in postvoid residual urine following external sphincterotomy. What is the most likely reason?**

Impaired bladder contractility (hypocontractility). Less common conditions such as inadequate sphincterotomy, smooth muscle dyssynergia, and urethral stricture can cause large residuals.

○ **During cystoscopy, a C7 quadriplegic patient complains of sweating and headache. His blood pressure has rapidly risen to 210/120. What is the best initial management?**

Raise the head of the bed and empty the bladder. In this emergency situation, the offending cause, ie, distention, should be treated immediately, and usually this is enough to control the autonomic hyperreflexia. Other measures, such as nitroglycerine patch, oral nifedipine, or even phentolamine intravenously, are not effective enough in controlling this serious situation. Unattended, serious complications such as stroke can occur.

○ **A C5 quadriplegic on external condom catheter drainage has recurrent episodes of autonomic dysreflexia (AD). Urodynamic evaluation shows high-pressure detrusor contractions and prolonged external sphincter dyssynergia. What is the best option for management?**

External sphincterotomy will minimize the future morbidity in this individual. If it fails, urinary diversion should be considered.

○ **What is the main indication for pressure–flow studies?**

To help distinguish detrusor hypocontractility from urethral obstruction low-flow conditions, with or without large residual urine, which can result from any of these conditions.

○ **What percent of men with symptoms of prostatism are found to have urodynamically proven outlet obstruction?**

30%.

○ **What study yields a definitive diagnosis of BOO?**

Detrusor pressure/flow study is the gold standard for the diagnosis of BOO.

○ **What is the clinical presentation of tethered cord syndrome?**

Patients typically present in infancy with detrusor areflexia and urinary retention.

○ **What are the characteristics of diabetic cystopathy?**

An increased bladder capacity, impaired detrusor contractility, hypocontractility, and decreased bladder sensation with diminished urinary stream.

○ **What are the factors that lead to a favorable outcome following prostatectomy in patients with Parkinson disease?**

Normal intravesical voiding pressures with decreased flow rate, voluntary urethral sphincter contractions, which can interrupt the urinary stream, adequate voluntary detrusor contractions, and perceived urgency. However, decreased detrusor contractility is not favorable. Alternative minimally invasive measures using thermotherapy, radiofrequency, or laser may be considered.

○ **What are the strong indications for a urodynamic evaluation?**

Multiple sclerosis (MS), spina bifida, sacral agenesis, high imperforate anus, and monitoring of a patient with spinal cord injury are all indications for a urodynamic evaluation.

○ **What is the estimated bladder capacity of a healthy 2-year-old male?**

120 mL. A simple formula to use is age in years + 2 = capacity in ounces.

○ **What is the initial management of the newborn with myelodysplasia?**

The initial management should include serum electrolytes, BUN, serum creatinine, measurement of residual urine, renal sonogram, and VCUG. The urodynamic studies the day prior to spinal closure are not indicated.

○ **When should urodynamic studies be performed for myelomeningocele patients?**

Urodynamics are helpful in the newborn period as a baseline study. This is important in order to assess the relative risk of the upper tracts based upon the bladder dynamics and to monitor any changes during the course of the disease.

○ **Why has vesicostomy been demonstrated to be effective in initial management in infants born with posterior urethral valves?**

A vesicostomy is a simple and safe procedure in infancy, bringing the dome of the bladder to the skin. This results in upper tract decompression in 90% of the cases. Reflux is not a problem because voiding pressures are eliminated. The risks of urethral injury are avoided, since valve ablation may be delayed. In addition, vesicostomy doesn't cause a permanent reduction in bladder capacity.

○ **A 3-year-old boy received a vesicostomy at 4 months of age secondary to posterior urethral valves. He now presents with progressive hydronephrosis and a serum creatinine of 2.5 mg/dL. A CMG revealed low bladder compliance. What is the next best step in management?**

A high urinary diversion would be appropriate. Other management strategies, such as augmentation cystoplasty and vesicostomy closure or CIC, are usually not effective.

○ **To further characterize the cause of a 350-cc residual urine in a 60-year-old, non–insulin-dependent diabetic, what is the most informative study?**

A simultaneous detrusor pressure/flow study.

○ **A 50-year-old female with urgency and frequency following a suspension procedure voids with a detrusor pressure of 50 cm H_2O at a peak flow of 12 mL/s. The most likely diagnosis is:**

Urethral obstruction. Storage (irritative) bladder symptoms with high voiding pressures are indicative of outlet obstruction after a suspension procedure.

○ **A 53-year-old female underwent midurethral sling 1 year ago. She complains of continuous urinary incontinence in upright positions. Seventeen years ago, she underwent abdominal hysterectomy and retropubic suspension. Videofluorourodynamics show an open bladder neck with minimal hypermobility, no involuntary contractions, and good bladder capacity, with low Valsalva leak pressure. What is the best operative option?**

A pubovaginal sling procedure at bladder neck level or urethral bulking agent (UBA) injection. The patient has ISD and would not benefit from repeat suspension midurethral sling.

○ **A 55-year-old man has had a detubularized right colon orthotopic continent diversion. He has done well for 1 year, but now complains of increasing incontinence. Pouch urodynamics revealed several pressure spikes. What is the mechanism most likely responsible for his incontinence?**

A return of coordinated bowel contractions.

○ **Why is nocturnal enuresis common with orthotopic diversions?**

Because of loss of the spinal reflex arc recruiting external sphincter contraction.

○ **How can you best describe cecal contractions?**

Intermittent high-pressure contractions. They are usually massive contractions and not peristaltic.

○ **What is the new classification of detrusor activity?**

According to the International Continence Society updated terminology, "detrusor overactivity" is now classified as "idiopathic detrusor overactivity" (replacing detrusor instability term), or "neurogenic detrusor overactivity" (replacing detrusor hyperreflexia term).

○ **How can you differentiate between striated external sphincter and smooth muscle internal sphincter dyssynergia in SCI patients?**

Using fluorourodynamics. In the case of internal sphincter dyssynergia, the bladder neck will be closed and detrusor pressure will be high with possible trabeculations, diverticula, and reflux. Similar findings can be found in external sphincter dyssynergia with the exception of an open bladder neck and dilated posterior urethra.

○ **Identify the name and site of the spinal cord micturition center.**

Onuf's nucleus in the sacral spinal cord (S2-3 anterior horn).

○ **What are the most likely urodynamic and videourodynamic findings in a 42-year-old woman with urinary incontinence, high residual urine volume, hydronephrosis, and urinary tract infection 18 months after a low anterior resection for rectal cancer?**

Detrusor hypoactivity, decreased compliance, open bladder neck, and fixed external sphincter tone. These changes are secondary to peripheral detrusor denervation involving both sympathetic and parasympathetic nerve fibers as a result of her surgery.

○ **A neurologically normal 40-year-old woman with no previous anti-incontinence surgery presented with lower urinary tract symptoms (LUTs) and urge incontinence. Her urodynamic study showed P_{det} of 55 cm H$_2$O and corresponding Q_{max} of 8 mL/s. She has 150 mL residual urine. What is her diagnosis and best management?**

The patient has functional BOO. Alpha blocker medication.

○ **What is the reason for not obtaining a leak pressure measurement in a postprostatectomy incontinence (PPI) patient who demonstrated stress incontinence on physical examination?**

Such patients often have scarred urethras that won't leak with the relatively large urethral catheter used. The leakage can only be demonstrated conclusively when the catheter is removed.

○ **What percent of overactive bladder (OAB) patients in clinical practice remain on antimuscarinic therapy beyond 1 year?**

Less than 30%. The reasons are side effects, cost, and lack of efficacy.

○ **At what point does nocturia significantly affect quality of life (QOL) scores?**

It begins to have an effect at 2 times per night. At 3 or more episodes, it's considered a major bother.

○   **What percent of urology residents have never actually personally performed a full urodynamics examination?**

Approximately 70%.

○   **True/False: Antibiotic prophylaxis should be given to all patients undergoing urodynamic testing?**

False. Only if the patient has other risk factors; eg, urethral disease, neurogenic bladder, history of urethral manipulation/trauma.

○   **What happens to the intraluminal ureteral pressure during bladder filling?**

The ureteral intraluminal pressure increases and the frequency of ureteral contractions increase.

○   **C4-5 Quadriplegic male is found to have AD with a blood pressure of 195/110 during urodynamic testing in a supine position. You stopped filling and let the catheter drain the bladder. What would be your next step in his management?**

The first step to treat acute AD regardless of the cause is to sit the patient in the upright position thus producing orthostatic decrease in blood pressure.

○   **Which parameter determines the treatment of neurogenic dysfunction?**

Detrusor leak point pressure (DLPP) when exceeds 40 cm H_2O, upper urinary tract damage is probable. DLPP primarily assesses bladder compliance; however, it is partially related to outlet resistance.

CHAPTER 16 Urethral Strictures

Jeremy B. Myers, MD, FACS, William O. Brant, MD, FACS, and Tom F. Lue, MD, ScD (Hon), FACS

○ **What portions of the urethra make up the anterior versus the posterior urethra?**

The designation of the anterior and posterior urethra refers to a developmental division between the distal and proximal urethra. The anterior urethra is composed of the meatus, fossa navicularis, the pendulous (penile urethra), and the bulbar urethra. The pendulous urethra is bounded distally by the meatus and proximally by the penile scrotal junction. The bulbar urethra begins at the junction of the pendulous urethra and is proximally defined by the urogenital diaphragm. The posterior urethra is composed of the short membranous urethra, starting at the urogenital diaphragm and ending at the prostate, and the prostatic urethra, which travels through the prostate to the bladder neck.

○ **What is the arterial blood supply to the anterior urethra?**

There are 2 arteries that supply blood to the anterior urethra. The bulbar artery arises from the internal pudendal artery and enters the urethra at the proximal bulb. The second artery is the dorsal penile artery, which also arises from the internal pudendal artery. This artery courses along the dorsal aspect of the corporal bodies giving off penetrating arteries to the urethra along its course.

○ **How is the distal urethra perfused when the urethra is transected during trauma or an anastomotic urethroplasty?**

If the bulbar artery is transected, the blood supply to the distal urethra is maintained by penetrating arteries from the dorsal penile artery as well as retrograde flow via the connection or arborization between the distal bulbar artery and the dorsal penile artery located in the glans of the penis.

○ **What is the blood supply for a pedicled penile skin flap?**

The dorsolateral and ventrolateral artery arise from the external pudendal artery, which in turn arises from the femoral artery.

○ **What is the blood supply to the scrotal skin?**

Superiorly, it is also supplied by branches of the external pudendal artery arising from the femoral artery. Inferiorly, a posterior scrotal artery arises from the perineal artery, which in turn arises from the internal pudendal artery, and ultimately the hypogastric artery.

○ **Increased urinary pressure behind a tight urethral stricture can have what effect on the urethra?**

Spongiofibrosis, which is the scarring process in the corpus spongiosum underlying the visually evident stricture, may develop for a considerable distance both proximally and distally due to cracking of the epithelium and underlying scar tissue as high-pressure urine is forced by the strictured area.

○ **Where is a dorsal onlay graft or flap placed versus a ventral onlay graft or flap?**

Dorsal refers to the dorsum of the urethra, similar to the dorsum of the penis. So a dorsal onlay graft or flap would rest against the ventral aspect of the corpora cavernosa; these corporal bodies serving as its roof and vascular bed of the graft. A ventral onlay graft or flap lies on the ventral aspect of the urethra. If a free graft is used, the corpora spongiosum is often closed below it to provide a vascular bed to nourish the graft.

○ **What process occurs after a graft placement which allows for survival of the graft?**

There is a 2-step process, lasting approximately 96 hours, called imbibition and inosculation. In the first step, imbibition, which lasts about 48 hours, the graft absorbs its nutrients passively from the graft bed or "imbibes" these nutrients. The second step is called inosculation and is the process of connection of vessels from the graft bed to the graft and ingrowth of capillaries.

○ **True/False: Congenital urethral strictures are common etiologies of stricture disease.**

False. Congenital urethral strictures are rare and are probably overestimated. Histopathologically they differ from acquired strictures in that their walls consist of smooth muscle rather than scar tissue. They form as a result of inadequate fusion of the anterior and posterior urethra.

○ **True/False: Urethral stricture development secondary to gonorrhea tends to result in discreet lesions within the bulbar urethra.**

False. While infectious strictures tend to develop within the bulbar urethra, they also tend to involve considerable length of the urethra and underlying spongiosum.

○ **Urethral stricture following cardiothoracic surgery with bypass may occur in up to 22% of cases. Which portion of the urethra is most at risk for stricture development?**

Pendulous urethra. Etiology may be related to local tissue ischemia/hypoxia during the bypass portion of the operation.

○ **Prior to repair of a completely obliterative urethral stricture, optimal radiographic evaluation includes which studies?**

In addition to a retrograde urethrogram, a voiding cystourethrogram is essential to identify the proximal extent of the stricture.

○ **True/False: Substitution urethroplasty tends to fail earlier than anastomotic repair.**

False. Anastomotic repair tends to fail within the first year, while substitution urethroplasty has been shown to fail at a rate of 5% per annum with a 60% successful outcome rate after 10 years.

○ **In substitution urethroplasty, what factors lead to increased restenosis rates?**

Tubularized flaps have a higher restenosis rate than patch flaps. In addition, the use of scrotal skin has a higher failure rate when compared to penile shaft or preputial skin.

○ **When treating a urethral stricture with progressive weekly dilations, what is the largest caliber dilator that should be used?**

Current recommendation: do not exceed a 24F dilator.

○ **When treating a urethral stricture with visual urethrotomy, the 12-o'clock position incision was made too deep. What specific complication can occur?**

Peyronie-like reaction resulting in chordee and erectile dysfunction.

○ **Is there any difference between internal urethrotomy and simple dilation outcomes in the treatment of urethral strictures?**

There is no proven efficacy difference between the 2 methods of treatment.

○ **What is the reported success rate of urethral dilation or internal urethrotomy and does it decrease with successive similar treatments?**

Recent studies show that the success rate of internal urethrotomy is much lower than previously thought. Contemporary studies report success rates as low as 10%, compared to older studies showing up to a 40% to 60% success. After the first internal urethrotomy fails, success declines further and is virtually 0% with subsequent procedures.

○ **What factors predict stricture recurrence postdilation or internal urethrotomy?**

Long strictures >2 cm are unlikely to be cured. Prior dilation or internal urethrotomy lowers success rates substantially, as well as the presence of lichen sclerosis (balanitis xerotica obliterans) or a history of pelvic radiation therapy. Pendulous strictures are also more resistant to successful urethrotomy or dilation excepting thin fossa navicularis or meatal strictures occurring after instrumentation.

○ **What is the optimal time for a urethral catheter after internal urethrotomy?**

Three to five days. Longer periods of catheterization have not been shown to help. Self-catheterization for dilation does seem to improve outcomes but is often not tolerated.

○ **Why is anastomotic urethroplasty generally inappropriate for treating pendulous urethral strictures?**

The resulting urethral shortening is sufficient to cause ventral chordee.

○ **What is the disadvantage of using scrotal skin for urethral reconstruction?**

A high incidence of dermatitis, which can lead to restenosis. Also, the genital skin is hair bearing, which can lead to stone formation and encrustation within the neourethra.

○ **What role does placement of a urethral metal stent have in management of urethral strictures?**

There is a very limited role for urethral stenting in the treatment of urethral strictures due to an unacceptably high rate of restenosis, worsening of stricture disease, pain, and urinary tract infection. In addition, subsequent urethroplasty is very difficult after failed urethral stent placement.

○ **Which type of bulbar urethral stricture lends itself best to anastomotic urethroplasty?**

Short strictures usually <3 cm in length and those that are due to trauma.

○ **What are the signs of a traumatic urethral injury from pelvic fracture during the acute evaluation in the emergency department?**

Blood at the meatus, inability to void, failure to pass a catheter, perineal and scrotal hematoma, and a high ballotable prostate all are signs of urethral injury or disruption.

○ **What is the potential advantage of endoscopic realignment of the urethra after a traumatic disruption injury?**

When a catheter is placed successfully across a urethral injury, some injuries, especially partial injuries may heal without needing subsequent urethroplasty. Excessive manipulation or misplacement of catheters in attempting realignment can dramatically worsen injuries and if realignment of the urethra is not possible with reasonable efforts a suprapubic tube should be placed without further manipulation.

○ **When should repair of pelvic urethral distraction injury be undertaken?**

Three months is generally considered to be a sufficient period of time to allow for resolution of tissue edema, periurethral hematoma, and "stabilization" of the injury. Immediate repair is associated with recurrent stricture and a higher rate of erectile dysfunction.

○ **What maneuvers can gain length for an anastomotic repair of a long posterior urethral defect?**

Maneuvers that can aid in bringing together the urethra for long posterior urethral defects are extensive mobilization of the bulbar urethra, separation of the proximal corporal bodies, partial pubectomy, and possibly rerouting the urethra around one of the corporal bodies.

○ **Retrograde urethrography may exacerbate a urethral stricture by what mechanism?**

Excessive pressure may cause extravasation of contrast material and lead to worsened periurethral fibrosis.

○ **When performing substitution urethroplasty over fibrosed spongiosum, which is considered superior: graft or flap substitution?**

Flap substitution. In cases where the underlying blood supply is in question, a flap, which carries its own blood supply, has a more predictable outcome.

○ **Meatal and fossa navicularis strictures associated with lichen sclerosis (balanitis xerotica obliterans) are best managed with what approach?**

Urethral reconstruction is usually necessary as dilation in this condition rarely results in a long-term success.

○ **Which has a higher success rate and why: skin island onlay flap or a tubularized flap?**

The skin island flap is better. Tubularized flaps tend to form anastomotic strictures.

○ **How should a stricture of the membranous urethra be managed in a patient who has had a previous trans urethral ressection of the prostate (TURP)?**

Unfortunately, membranous urethral strictures are common after TURP. Direct vision internal urethrotomy (DVIU) or urethral reconstruction carries a high risk of incontinence since there is no bladder neck sphincteric mechanism. Therefore, management is usually serial self-intermittent catheterization if tolerated. If this fails, patients can undergo urethroplasty with staged placement of artificial urinary sphincter in the future to manage the predictable incontinence that will develop after urethroplasty.

○ **What is the incidence and treatment of bladder neck contractures after radical prostatectomy?**

The incidence is 5% to 15% and the initial treatment of choice is dilation or internal urethrotomy. For recurrent strictures of the bladder neck, men may need further procedures such as formal repair and reanastomosis.

CHAPTER 17 Prostatic Hyperplasia

Zachary Klaassen, MD,
W. Bruce Shingleton, MD, and
Stephen W. Leslie, MD, FACS

○ **The development of the transition zone of the prostate begins at what week of embryologic development?**

This occurs at week 16 of development of the fetus.

○ **The transition zone constitutes what percent of the prostate?**

The transition zone comprises 4% to 5% of the glandular prostate.

○ **What is the average weight of the prostate in an adult male at 40 years of age?**

At this age, the mean weight of the prostate is approximately 20 g.

○ **The prostate is in contact with how many and what fascial layers?**

The 3 fascial layers, which abut the prostate, include Denonvilliers posteriorly, the endopelvic fascia cranially, and the lateral pelvic fascia.

○ **What artery provides the major source of blood for the prostate?**

The prostatovesicular artery arising from the inferior vesical artery is the main source of arterial blood to the prostate.

○ **The plexus of Santorini drains into what major veins?**

This venous complex drains into the hypogastric veins.

○ **The urethra divides the prostate into what areas?**

The urethra demarcates the prostate into the fibromuscular (ventral) and glandular (dorsal) areas.

○ **What is the largest zone of the prostate?**

Typically, the peripheral zone is the largest zone accounting for approximately 75% of the prostate gland.

○ **The outer zone of the prostate is of what embryologic origin?**

The endoderm gives rise to the outer (peripheral) zone of the prostate.

○ **What is the anatomic female equivalent to the prostate gland?**

The Skene glands in the female urethra are the homolog to the male prostate.

○ **What typical female malignant neoplasm can arise in the prostate?**

Endometrial carcinoma can occur at the prostatic utricle.

○ **Where are Cowper's glands located?**

They are located within the urogenital diaphragm.

○ **Lymphatic drainage of the prostatic urethra is primarily to which lymph nodes?**

The obturator and external iliac lymph nodes are the main lymphatic drainage group.

○ **What effect do finasteride and dutasteride have on serum testosterone levels?**

There is no change in serum testosterone levels. Dutasteride may lower serum dihydrotesterone.

○ **What percent of the ejaculate arises from the prostate gland?**

Prostatic secretions constitute 15% of the total ejaculate volume.

○ **The fibromuscular stroma is composed of mainly what type of tissue?**

Smooth muscle fibers are the main component of the fibromuscular stroma.

○ **What cell types are present in the acinar epithelium?**

There are 2 cell types: glandular cells and basal cells.

○ **Dutasteride and finasteride have what effect on prostatic tissue levels of 5 alpha-DHT?**

Both decrease 5 alpha-DHT prostatic tissue levels.

○ **Dutasteride and finasteride produce what side effects in regard to sexual function?**

The side effects include decreased libido, decreased ejaculatory volume, and erectile dysfunction.

○ **The majority of alpha-1 adrenoceptors are located where in the genitourinary (GU) tract?**

The alpha-1 receptors are located mainly in the bladder neck and prostate.

○ **Define the respective temperature ranges for thermotherapy and hyperthermia of the prostate.**

Temperatures >44.5°C constitute thermotherapy and temperatures <44°C are termed hyperthermia.

○ **How many isoenzymes exist for 5-alpha-reductase?**

There are 2 isoenzymes: type 1 and type 2, with type 2 being the major isoenzyme in the prostate.

○ **What 2 growth factors are important in the development of BPH?**

Transforming growth factor alpha and epidermal growth factors have been identified as the major growth factors in the development of BPH.

○ **Describe the effect of androgen ablation on the cell populations of the prostate.**

Epithelial cells are mainly affected by a decrease in androgens and show varying degrees of atrophy as compared to stromal cells.

○ **What alpha-receptor subtype is most numerous in the prostate?**

Alpha 1A is the most prevalent alpha-receptor subtype in the prostate.

○ **Prostatic secretions include what element?**

A high level of zinc is present in prostatic secretions.

○ **What drugs penetrate into the prostatic fluid?**

Trimethoprim–sulfamethoxazole and fluoroquinolones are the only drugs that achieve therapeutic levels in the prostatic parenchyma.

○ **What is the average age at which men develop symptomatic BPH?**

Sixty-nine years.

○ **Does prostate doubling time normally increase or decrease with age?**

Decreases.

○ **What portion of the male population develops a prostate of 100 g or more?**

4%.

○ **On an average, how much does the prostate grow each year?**

0.6 cc/y with a mean decrease in urinary peak flow rate of 2 mL/s/y.

○ **How many patients with BPH present with some degree of renal failure?**

10%.

○ **Where in the prostatic cell is testosterone converted to 5-alpha-dihydrotestosterone?**

This conversion occurs in the cytoplasm.

○   **What specific receptor does tamsulosin work on?**

Alpha 1A.

○   **What are the main side effects of alpha-blockers?**

Dizziness and asthenia.

○   **What specific side effect does tamsulosin tend to produce more than other alpha-blockers?**

Tamsulosin is more likely to cause ejaculatory problems than other alpha-blockers so patients should be warned about this before starting therapy especially if sexually active.

○   **What is the mechanism of action for BPH phytotherapeutic agents such as saw palmetto?**

It is unknown at this time.

○   **What is the known effect of saw palmetto on symptomatic BPH in randomized controlled trials?**

No significant difference has been found between placebo and saw palmetto in controlled trials.

○   **When were the technical improvements to create the modern resectoscope first completed and by whom?**

In 1932 by Dr. Joseph McCarthy.

○   **Who first described the prostate anatomically and who named it prostate?**

Vesalius described it in 1538. Caspar Bartholin named it "prostate" in 1611.

○   **What advances to the resectoscope were designed by Dr. Theodore M. Davis?**

Thicker cutting loop, insulated outer sheath, and the dual foot pedal control.

○   **Who provided the first correct and detailed description of the prostatic blood supply and when?**

Ruben Flocks in 1937.

○   **Who is credited with the first description of modern transurethral resection of the prostate (TURP) technique?**

Reed M. Nesbit who published his technique in 1943 in his landmark book *Transurethral Prostatectomy.*

○   **What is the difference between the Stern–McCarthy and Iglesias resectoscopes?**

The Stern–McCarthy uses a rack and pinion lever action while the Iglesias uses a spring-loaded thumb control.

○   **What percent of patients with BPH will have symptom improvement or stabilization without treatment?**

Up to 50% of patients with BPH will have symptom stabilization or improvement regardless of whether treatment is started.

○ **BPH is the most common cause of what urologic symptom?**

Gross painless hematuria. BPH is commonly associated with gross painless hematuria in men older than 60 years. When present, one must still perform a complete evaluation to rule out neoplasm and stones as an etiology.

○ **What percent of men develop symptoms secondary to BPH?**

Fifty percent of men with BPH will have symptoms as they age.

○ **What is the relationship between symptom score and degree of obstruction as determined by pressure flow study?**

Various studies have shown no correlation between symptom score and pressure study regarding degree of obstruction.

○ **Where are prostatic calculi located within the prostate?**

The calculi are located between the prostatic adenoma and the surgical capsule.

○ **Do they have any clinical significance?**

No.

○ **What are they made of?**

Usually calcium phosphate.

○ **Is BPH an inherited, genetic disorder?**

Although not usually thought of as being a genetic disorder, BPH clearly shows inheritable characteristics. Patients with a positive family history tend to develop symptoms at an earlier age and they tend to have larger prostate glands (82 vs 55 g).

○ **True/False: Proscar (finasteride) reduces the risk of acute urinary retention more than Avodart (dutasteride)?**

False. The risk reduction is reportedly the same for both (57%).

○ **What are the significant differences between finasteride (Proscar) and dutasteride (Avodart)?**

Dutasteride is both a type 1 and type 2 inhibitor of 5-alpha reductase. Finasteride affects only type 2. Dutasteride has a 5-week half-life, while finasteride is just 8 hours. The average reported shrinkage of the prostate with dutasteride is 27%, but only 18% with finasteride.

○ **Of the two, is dutasteride or finasteride more effective clinically?**

They are essentially equivalent. Dutasteride might be effective in slightly smaller prostates than finasteride.

○ **What is the mechanism of action for silodosin (Rapaflo)?**

Silodosin is a new selective alpha-blocker therapy with a high pharmacologic selectivity for the alpha(1A)-adrenoreceptor.

○ **How does silodosin compare to tamsulosin?**

Silodosin is well tolerated for relief of both voiding and storage symptoms in patients with lower urinary tract symptoms (LUTS) associated with BPH. It has comparable efficacy to tamsulosin and alfuzosin.

○ **True/False: Exposure to tamsulosin within 14 days of cataract surgery may be associated with serious ophthalmic adverse events.**

True. The alpha-adrenergic receptor blockade associated with tamsulosin may increase the intraoperative difficulty of cataract surgery. Adverse events do not appear to be linked to tamsulosin use >14 days prior to cataract surgery.

○ **Nocturnal urinary overproduction is an etiological factor in what percentage of men with nocturia?**

Up to 70%.

○ **True/False: Evaluation of a patient for BPH requires a prostate digital rectal examination (DRE) examination and PSA.**

True. It is necessary to determine if there is evidence of prostate cancer in the patient.

○ **What is the most common cause of LUTS?**

Benign prostatic hyperplasia.

○ **True/False: Postvoid residual urine volume should be monitored regularly if a patient elects medical therapy for treatment.**

True. The patient may develop significant elevated volumes without clinical symptoms.

○ **Is medical or surgical therapy indicated for the initial treatment of uncomplicated BPH?**

Medical therapy is the recommended first option.

○ **True/False: LUTS are not specific for BPH.**

True. As men age, different diseases can cause voiding symptoms but BPH remains the most common.

○ **True/False: A patient with BPH who develops an elevated serum creatinine should have a renal US.**

True. Renal insufficiency is rare in patients with BPH, but can occur and requires radiographic evaluation. Bilateral symmetrical hydronephrosis in patients with azotemia is strongly suggestive of urinary retention.

○ **True/False: Finasteride substantially reduces the risk of incident clinical BPH in healthy older men.**

True. Data from the Prostate Cancer Prevention Trial showed that the rate of clinical BPH was 19 per 1000 person-years in the placebo arm and 11 per 1000 person-years in the finasteride arm ($P < 0.001$). Finasteride reduced the risk of incidental clinical BPH by 40%.

○ **What is the role of tadalafil (Cialis) for treatment of LUTS?**

In an international, randomized, parallel, placebo-controlled clinical trial, monotherapy with tadalafil or tamsulosin resulted in clinical improvements versus placebo in LUTS/BPH; but only tadalafil also improved erectile dysfunction.

○ **Does increasing the dose of saw palmetto improve effectiveness for treatment of LUTS attributed to BPH?**

No. A double-blind, multicenter, placebo-controlled randomized trial of men 45 years of age or older, with a peak urinary flow rate of at least 4 mL/s and an AUASI score of between 8 and 24 did not show a reduction in LUTS more than placebo with 3 times the normal dose of saw palmetto.

○ **What percent of men older than age 50 will someday develop symptomatic BPH?**

At least 50%.

○ **True/False: Transurethral incision of the prostate (TUIP) is useful regardless of the size of the prostate?**

False. Success with this technique is typically limited to a prostate 30 g or less in size.

○ **What alternative minimally invasive treatment modalities are available for use in anticoagulated patients?**

Laser prostatectomy and transurethral electrovaporization (TUVP) have been successfully used in anticoagulated patients for the treatment of BPH.

○ **What is one disadvantage of Nd:YAG or "Green light" laser prostatectomy versus TURP?**

There is no tissue specimen available for histologic examination in patients treated by laser.

○ **Does treating BPH with hyperthermia cause a temporary rise in serum PSA?**

In a review of clinical trials of hyperthermia treatment, post-treatment PSA was not significantly elevated following hyperthermia treatment for BPH.

○ **True/False: Electrovaporization of the prostate (TVP) requires a longer operative time than TURP?**

True. During TVP, only a small segment of the prostate is treated at a given interval versus a larger surface area covered by each pass of the loop of the resectoscope resulting in longer operative time for TURP.

○ **What is the danger of using distilled water during transurethral surgery?**

Intravascular hemolysis will occur with the use of distilled water.

○ **What is the danger of increasing the height of irrigation fluid during transurethral surgery?**

Fluid absorption during TURP has been estimated at 20 cc/min of resection time. The height of the irrigant will cause increased fluid absorption across open venous sinuses.

○ **True/False: Saline is safe and effective to use for irrigation during transurethral surgery.**

False. Saline irrigation results in dissipation of electric current and renders the resectoscope useless, unless a bipolar unit is used.

○ **The average TURP removes how much tissue?**

It removes 22 g.

○ **What is the only absolute indication for an open prostatectomy?**

Need for an additional open bladder procedure.

○ **What is the usual maximum operating time limit for TURP to minimize complications?**

Ninety minutes is the maximum resecting time, but less than 60 minutes is best.

○ **What is the maximum size prostate that can be treated by TURP?**

There is no arbitrary size limit. It depends on the skill and experience of the surgeon and the 90-minute resecting time limit.

○ **Contraindications to TURP are:**

Active anticoagulation, recent MI, dysfunctional external sphincter, recent radiation therapy to the prostate, and active urinary tract infection. Shy–Drager syndrome and Parkinson are relative contraindications.

○ **Where is the external sphincter muscle closest to the bladder neck?**

At the 12-o'clock position. This is why you should be careful doing the resection in this area to stay proximal to the verumontanum.

○ **What is the danger if the verumontanum is accidentally resected?**

While ejaculatory duct obstruction is possible, the main danger is loss of the distal urethral landmark.

○ **What is the maximum recommended height of the irrigating fluid above the bladder during TURP?**

It is 60 cm. Fluid absorption substantially increases beyond this height.

○ **What technique can be used to perform a TURP when contractures, penile prostheses, or deformity prevent access through the penis?**

A perineal urethrostomy.

○ **Where is the prostate tissue thinnest?**

At the 12-o'clock position.

○ **What is the main advantage of Bipolar TURP?**

It can be used with normal saline irrigation.

○ **What are the most common mistakes made in TURP surgery?**

- Failure to do a perineal urethrostomy when indicated.
- Elevation of irrigating fluid to over 60 cm in height above the bladder.
- Not quitting early if it appears clear that finishing the resection would take much longer than 90 minutes. These partial resections usually do quite well if at least one side of the prostate has been completed.
- Continuing to attempt to cauterize bleeding sites where the surgical capsule has been perforated. If this is not successful, continuing cautery will usually result in more rather than less bleeding.

○ **What should be done if the seminal vesicles are opened or perforated during a TURP?**

Nothing. They will usually heal without incident.

○ **What should be done at the end of the TURP just before placing the catheter?**

Carefully inspect for bleeding vessels. Lowering the irrigation flow and pressure will allow additional bleeding sites to become visible. Make sure all prostate chips have been evacuated. Carefully check any bladder diverticula for chips. Finally, inspect the ureteral orifices and external sphincter muscle to make sure there was no inadvertent injury. Also make sure your resectoscope is inspected to make sure there are no missing pieces. There are reported cases of the resectoscope tips coming loose and remaining in the patient, sometimes for years.

○ **True/False: The most difficult procedure for an urologist to learn to do well is the TURP.**

True.

○ **Many TURP techniques begin the resection at the 12-o'clock position. Is this a good practice?**

Probably not. The intention is to allow the lateral lobes to fall down into the prostatic urethra making the resection easier. However, the prostate tissue is thinnest here, which allows early perforation. Also, there is no direct visualization of the key distal landmark, the verumontanum, and so there is a greater risk of an inadvertent injury to the external sphincter muscle, which is most proximal at this position. Starting at the median lobe or lateral lobes would be safer.

○ **What anatomical structure is immediately external and adjacent to the prostate at the 12-o'clock position?**

Batson's plexus, which is a highly vascular venous pexus. This is why we recommend carving of the tissue in the lateral and posterior lobes, but usually only straight line resecting for the roof of the prostate at the 12-o'clock position.

○ **What is the role of intraprostatic stents in the management of BPH?**

At the present time, it is a useful temporary treatment for urinary retention.

○ **True/False: Radiofrequency ablation of the prostate (TUNA) can deliver an improvement in symptoms up to at least 1 year.**

True. However, long-term results from studies are lacking.

○ **True/False: Transurethral microwave therapy should not be used in patients with prostate size >100 g.**

True, although clinical studies have been done showing a benefit in those patients.

○ **What percent of men with BPH will ultimately undergo surgery for it?**

29%.

○ **What is the minimal average percentage amount of tissue removal by TURP needed to alleviate BPH symptoms?**

Approximately 30%.

○ **True/False: Holmium laser ablation and photoselective laser vaporization of the prostate have similar efficacy.**

True.

○ **What are the expected reductions in PSA and prostate volumes in holmium laser ablation and photoselective laser vaporization of the prostate?**

Each is expected to demonstrate a 35% to 40% reduction in both PSA and prostate volumes.

○ **How do the outcomes differ between plasmakinetic resection of the prostate (PKRP) and conventional TURP?**

PKRP is associated with a shorter operative time, duration of bladder irrigation, duration of catheter use, and blood loss. At 2 years of follow-up, both procedures have comparable international prostate symptom score (IPSS) and PSA levels.

○ **How do the outcomes differ between photoselective vaporization of the prostate (PVP) and conventional TURP?**

PVP is associated with a decreased catheterization time and length of hospital stay; operative time is longer with PVP. Postoperative blood transfusion and frequency of clot retention are less common with PVP; however, no difference was noted in intermediate-term functional outcomes. There may be more irritative symptoms in the immediate postoperative period with PVP. TURP is associated with a lower reoperative risk.

○ **Postobstructive diuresis is thought to be due to what factor?**

The obstruction results in altered function of the collecting duct cells manifested as a loss of renal concentrating ability with resultant diuresis. The ability to acidify the urine is also often impaired with an obstructive process. The ensuing postobstructive diuresis will resolve once the collecting ducts have regained their ability to conserve a fluid load and the renal medullary interstitium has regained its osmotic gradient.

○ **What is the reported incidence of urethral stricture after TURP?**

Urethral strictures have a reported incidence of 2.7% to 20% following TURP.

○ **During a TURP a large venous sinus is opened. What are the next steps to be performed?**

Lower the height of the irrigation fluid to decrease further fluid absorption. Diligent efforts to endoscopically gain control of the bleeding should be undertaken, but can be difficult. Therefore, it may be necessary to quickly finish the resection and place a Foley catheter with appropriate traction, which will usually tamponade the bleeding. Serum electrolyte studies are appropriate to monitor for TUR syndrome (dilutional hyponatremia), and intravenous Lasix should be administered to help minimize the dilutional hyponatremia that can be associated with the unroofing of a large venous sinus.

○ **The treatment of TUR syndrome includes:**

Symptomatic dilutional hyponatremia must be managed aggressively. The total body sodium deficit is calculated using the following formula: (0.6 × weight in kilograms) × (desired serum sodium − the measured serum sodium) = total body sodium deficit. This value divided by 513 mOsm/L gives the liters of 3% saline that must be administered to correct the total body sodium deficit. One-half the total body deficit should be corrected in the first 2 hours and the remainder over the next 6 hours. Failure to correct the sodium deficit can have lethal results.

○ **Bacterial prostatitis is caused by what gram-positive organism?**

The gram-positive organism is *Enterococcus*.

○ **What is the 5-year risk for reoperation after TURP?**

Approximately 5%. This increases to 13% at 10 years.

○ **Symptoms of dilutional hyponatremia generally do not occur until the serum sodium reaches what level?**

Until serum sodium reaches 125 mEq or less.

○ **What percent of patients develop some degree of dilutional hyponatremia?**

Approximately 2%.

○ **What should be done if bleeding is encountered during a TURP and the bleeding source cannot be found?**

Check the opposite side of the prostate capsule. Many bleeding vessels will "Ricochet" off the opposite sidewall. Next, do a careful, methodical inspection of the lining of the prostate and bladder neck. Fill the bladder. This will tilt the inferior bladder neck and distal trigone forward and expose additional potential bleeding points.

○ **Is there a role for angiography in managing hematuria after TURP?**

Yes, if the hematuria is not well controlled by other means and is severe enough to warrant a more aggressive approach. Superselective unilateral arterial embolization has been reported to be highly successful in selected cases of severe hemorrhage after TURP that could not be controlled otherwise.

○ **A 72-year-old male presents with urinary retention and a TURP is performed. During the surgery, despite your exemplary technique, excessive bleeding is encountered. The entire prostatic fossa is oozing heavily and the patient is bleeding from various places including the IV sites, lips, mouth, and nose indicating some type of coagulopathy. The platelet count is normal and stable, but the fibrin split products are extremely high. What is going on and what's the treatment?**

The patient has primary fibrinolysis, probably from prostate cancer. Fibrinolysins from the cancer are released during the TURP and resulted in the coagulation disorder. The lack of any thrombocytopenia suggests the diagnosis. Treatment is with intravenous Amicar.

CHAPTER 18

Female Incontinence and Vesicovaginal Fistula

Forrest Jellison, MD and Ja-Hong Kim, MD

○ **Define urinary incontinence.**

Urinary incontinence is the complaint of any involuntary leakage of urine and is considered to be a *storage* symptom. This is often socially embarrassing and impacts *negatively* on a patient's *quality of life*. It is important to *confirm* the fluid lost as *urine* and *rule out* fluid from *another source*, that is, peritoneal or uterine. Furthermore, one must *identify* the urine is *per urethra* and not from a *urinary fistula* or *ectopic ureter*. In addition, urinary leakage may need to be distinguished from sweating or vaginal discharge.

○ **What are other storage symptoms as defined by the International Continence Society?**

- Frequency is the complaint by the patient who considers that he/she voids too often by day. Although variable in nature (fluid intake, comorbidities, and hours of sleep), frequency can be defined as *voiding > 8 times* in a 24-hour period.
- Nocturia is the complaint that the individual is *interrupted from sleep* to void *one or more times*.
- Urgency is the complaint of a sudden compelling *desire to pass urine*, which is difficult to defer. It can be difficult to measure.
- It is important to further characterize these symptoms with a 1- or 3-day *bladder diary* recording of micturition episodes, voided volumes, and fluid intake.

○ **Describe the symptoms associated with the various types of urinary incontinence.**

- Urge urinary incontinence is the complaint of involuntary leakage accompanied by or immediately preceded by urgency.
- Stress urinary incontinence is the complaint of involuntary leakage on effort, exertion, sneezing, or coughing.
- Mixed urinary incontinence is the complaint of involuntary leakage associated with urgency in addition to exertion, effort, sneezing, or coughing.
- Continuous urinary incontinence is the complaint of continuous involuntary loss of urine.
- Nocturnal enuresis is the complaint of involuntary loss of urine that occurs during sleep.
- Postvoid dribble is the term used to describe involuntary loss of urine after voiding, usually after rising from the toilet.
- Overflow incontinence is any involuntary loss of urine associated with overdistension of the bladder.

○ **Can stress incontinence induce urge incontinence?**

Yes. Urgency may result from *compensatory responses* initiated in the incontinent patient. For example, once the initial symptom of stress incontinence is noticed, the patient may *urinate frequently* to keep the bladder empty, thus reducing the chance of stress-related incontinent episodes. As the *bladder accommodates* to these lower volumes, *decreased bladder capacity* and/or *compliance* may ensue. Subsequently, when the bladder distends beyond its reduced functional capacity, the patient experiences sensory urgency, frequency, and urinary incontinence.

Alternatively, urgency as a physiologic response may be a product of *urine passage* into the *proximal urethra*. This *activates somatic afferent nerves* in the pudendal nerve that produce a *detrusor contraction* by activating the pontine micturition center through the *micturition reflex* and the resultant stress leakage, termed "stress-induced detrusor overactivity." Correction of the stress incontinence may eliminate the urgency.

○ **List the components of normal urinary continence in response to increases in abdominal stress.**

Normal continence in the female is a product of several forces working together. These forces include the proper *anatomic location* of the sphincteric unit, the critical functional and anatomic *urethral length*, the *mucosal coaptation* of the urethral surface, and the increased urethral pressure generated by *reflex pelvic contractions* at the time of stress. Failure of one of the components of this delicate balance will not invariably produce stress incontinence because of the compensatory effect of the other forces.

○ **Describe the urethral "washer effect."**

The female urethra consists of a 4-cm tube of inner epithelium and outer muscularis. The infolded epithelium is enclosed by a rich vascular sponge, which in turn is surrounded by a fibromuscular and smooth muscle coat. This *submucosa*, consisting of loosely woven connective tissue scattered throughout with smooth muscle bundles and an elaborate vascular plexus, provides a *compressive "washer effect" vital to the mechanism* of continence. The effectiveness of this washer is thought to be *estrogen dependent*.

○ **List the structures that compose the female sphincteric unit.**

The sphincteric unit has an internal and external sphincter. The *internal sphincter*, involuntary **smooth** muscle, is located at the bladder neck. The *external sphincter* is located at the midurethral complex which consists of **skeletal** muscle (slow and fast twitch) that is under voluntary control.

○ **List the structures that provide normal pelvic support.**

- The fascia of the pelvic floor may be collectively referred to as the *levator fascia or endopelvic fascia*. Although the fascia works in an integrated fashion to provide pelvic support, certain areas of the fascia have been separately described because of their importance in supporting individual female pelvic structures.
- The *pubourethral ligaments* connect the midportion of the urethra with the inner surface of the inferior pubis. Laterally, this midportion of the urethra is supported by segments of the levator fascia just below their attachments to the pubis. Collectively, these may be referred to as the *midurethral complex*.
- The *urethropelvic ligaments* (periurethral fascia) connect the proximal urethra and bladder neck laterally to the tendinous arch of the obturator muscle.
- The *vesicopelvic ligaments* (pubocervical fascia) connect the bladder base laterally to the tendinous arch of the obturator muscle.
- The *cardinal-sacrouterine ligaments* connect the uterine cervix and isthmus to the sacral vertebrae.
- The *broad ligaments* connect the uterine body to the pelvic sidewall.

○ **Describe outlet abnormalities associated with urinary incontinence.**

Urethral hypermobility: The pelvic floor fails to support the vesical neck and proximal urethra. This results in either the vesical neck and proximal urethra being situated *below* the inferior margin of the symphysis pubis at rest or they descend from a position situated *above* the inferior margin of the symphysis pubis during *strain*.

Intrinsic sphincter deficiency (ISD): The internal urethral sphincter fails to maintain continence even at low detrusor pressures (0–60 cm H_2O) with resultant leakage of urine per urethra.

○ **Define detrusor overactivity.**

Detrusor overactivity is a urodynamic observation characterized by involuntary detrusor contractions during the filling phase, which may be spontaneous or provoked. It can be further classified as either *neurogenic detrusor overactivity* when there is a relevant neurological condition (previously termed "detrusor hyperreflexia") or *idiopathic detrusor overactivity* when there is no defined cause (previously termed "detrusor instability").

○ **Is urge incontinence the same as detrusor overactivity?**

Sometimes. Urge incontinence implies involuntary bladder contractions that may or may not be associated with urine leakage. These may not be identifiable on urodynamics given that patients can suppress involuntary contractions.

○ **What is bladder compliance?**

Bladder compliance describes the relationship between bladder volume and detrusor pressure and is dependent upon the *viscoelastic properties of the detrusor*. Compliance is calculated by dividing the *change in volume* by the *change in detrusor pressure* during 2 specific points at the time of filling cystometry: (1) at the start of the bladder filling and (2) at cystometric capacity or immediately before the start of any detrusor contraction that causes significant leakage. The result is expressed in mL/cm H_2O.

○ **Distinguish between abdominal, Valsalva, and detrusor leak point pressures (LPP).**

Abdominal/Valsalva LPP: Intravesical pressure at which urine leakage occurs due to increased abdominal pressure in the *absence* of a *detrusor contraction*. In the normal patient, urine loss should never occur during abdominal straining even at high pressures.

Detrusor LPP: Lowest detrusor pressure at which urine leakage occurs in the *absence* of either a *detrusor contraction or increased abdominal pressure*. In the normal patient, urine exits the urethra at relatively low bladder pressures during voiding. A detrusor LPP greater than **40 cm H_2O** has been used to identify patients with neurologic abnormality who may be at risk for upper tract damage. Detrusor LPP can be measured during involuntary detrusor contraction in patients with detrusor overactivity.

○ **What is the role of the history?**

Because urinary symptoms may be similar despite disparate etiologies, the history is often nondiagnostic when considering female urinary incontinence. There is a 30% error in diagnosing stress urinary incontinence if only the history is used. Evaluation of the incontinent female must include a history, physical examination, and adjuvant testing. However, because more than one symptom is often present, it is essential to determine the relative severity of each complaint. It is important to focus on the *chief presenting symptom* in deciding the next diagnostic or therapeutic step.

○ **Describe the key components of an initial evaluation of female urinary incontinence.**

- Q-tip test: Assesses mobility of the urethra. With stress, the tail of the applicator will transcribe an arc of 0° to 30° in most women. Movement of *greater than 35°* suggests *urethral hypermobility*.
- Stress testing: Assesses urethral leak with stress. With the bladder full (ie, at least 200–300 mL), the patient is asked to cough or strain. The patient with stress incontinence will immediately lose urine as a brief, small squirt associated with the stress. The position is variable. *Eighty percent* of patients will leak in the *lithotomy* position; an additional *10%* of patients will leak at an *incline* of 45°, while the final *10%* of patients will only leak in the *standing* position.
- Speculum examination: Assesses concomitant pelvic floor defects. Urethral hypermobility may be measured with a Q-tip, but a speculum exam is necessary to evaluate the anterior vaginal wall, the vaginal apex, an enterocele, a rectocele, the anal sphincter, and the perineal body.
- Bladder or voiding diary: Measures the voided volumes, daytime frequency, incontinence episodes, pad usage, and other information such as fluid intake, degree of urgency, and leakage during a defined period (ie, 1- or 3-day interval).
- Pad testing: Assesses the quantity of urine lost during incontinence episodes; methods range from a short provocative test to a 24-hour pad test. Increase of >15 g in pad weight gain is considered abnormal.
- Postvoid residual: Assesses volume of urine left in bladder after voiding by either an ultrasound bladder scanner or straight catheterization.

○ **What are the AUA guidelines for initial evaluation for female stress incontinence?**

- Standards: Focused history and physical, *objective demonstration of SUI, PVR*, U/A C/S if indicated.
- Recommendation: Characterization of incontinence (stress, urge), frequency and severity, impact on lifestyle expectations of treatment, and additional diagnostic testing if indicated (pad test and/or voiding diary, urodynamic, cystoscopy, and imaging).

○ **What are the indications for urodynamic testing?**

- When there is mixed urinary incontinence and the component of stress incontinence is not predominant to the urge incontinence. (A randomized control trial, the VALUE study, suggests that **preoperative urodynamics** *does not affect outcomes or the surgical approach* for *uncomplicated stress predominant incontinence*.)
- When initial *evaluation* and results of simpler *diagnostic tests* have been inconclusive.
- When *empirical treatments* have proved unsuccessful.
- When the patient complains of *incontinence* but it *cannot be **demonstrated*** clinically.
- In symptomatic patients who have *previously* undergone corrective *surgery*.
- In patients with an *elevated postvoid residual*.
- In patients with a history of *prior radical pelvic surgery or radiation*.
- In patients with known or suspected *neurologic disorders* to rule out upper tract damage.
- When assessing *urethral function* (ISD).
- When *Grade III* or greater *pelvic organ prolapse* (POP) is present.
- In patients where *voiding dysfunction* is suspected.

○ **During urodynamic testing of a female with clinically demonstrable stress incontinence, you find that she does not leak with a catheter in place. What should be done next?**

The catheter should be *removed* as there is a 50% chance that the patient will *leak* during urodynamic testing.

○   **What are the indications for cystoscopy?**

In all patients with *urgency* as a complaint, bladder pathology such as bladder stone, bladder diverticula, bladder cancer, and carcinoma in situ must be ruled out. All patients with *hematuria* or *sterile pyuria* should undergo cytologic examination, cystoscopy, and upper tract evaluation. It is more controversial, but patients with pure stress urinary incontinence may undergo preoperative cystoscopy to evaluate for incidental coexisting disease if suspected, especially those with history of *radiation, prior pelvic, or incontinence surgery.*

○   **Describe several radiographic evaluations useful in assessing female urinary incontinence.**

- Cystogram with voiding films (VCUG): Often obtained videourodynamics, these tests are useful in comparing resting and straining films. *Lateral* films are helpful in identifying urethral position at rest and hypermobility with straining. These standing lateral films are also useful in assessing the degree of cystocele if present. Urinary leak may be observed on the lateral straining films.
- Ultrasound: Useful in identifying urethral mobility and prolapse, ultrasound can be performed transabdominally, transrectally, or transvaginally. The quality of the examination is highly dependent upon the skills of the ultrasonographer.
- MRI: Usually reserved for cases of more severe prolapse, the dynamic MRI of the pelvis is very helpful in identifying cystocele, uterine prolapse, and rectocele. It is also useful in revealing any concomitant pelvic pathology when hysterectomy is being considered as part of pelvic repair. Use of the HASTE sequence MRI is particularly helpful in identifying urologic pathology.

○   **What is the role of Kegel exercises and estrogens in female urinary incontinence?**

- Kegel exercises: If performed properly and diligently, Kegel exercises can strengthen the levator musculature, which can lead to an increase in urethral pressure, better urethral reflex response to stresses, reduction of cystocele, and improved cough-urethra pressure transmission in stress urinary incontinence. These exercises are also useful for urge incontinence. By increasing pudendal activity to the sphincter muscles, this may in turn stimulate a reflexive inhibitory input to the detrusor, thereby suppressing involuntary bladder contractions.
- Estrogens: Lack of estrogen causes the urethral mucosa and underlying blood vessels to atrophy, leading to a decreased compressive washer effect. Estrogen causes hypertrophy and thickening of the urethral mucosa and engorgement of the blood vessels beneath. Estrogen should be given vaginally for optimal improvement of OAB symptoms and urge incontinence. Studies have failed to show an improvement of SUI with estrogen replacement.

○   **Identify several behavioral modifications which should be offered as first-line standard treatments for a woman with urge incontinence.**

- Kegel exercises or pelvic floor muscle training: see above.
- Timed voiding: Instruct the patient to void on a timed schedule. The specific interval should be based on voiding before the development of urgency. Increase the interval after several weeks without urgency.
- Prompted voiding: Instruct the patient not to delay voiding. Additionally, the patient must concentrate on completely relaxing and emptying the bladder during the void.
- Fluid restriction: Limit the fluid intake for patients to 4 to 6 glasses per day. Avoid caffeine-containing beverages and fluid consumption after dinner.
- Avoidance of bladder irritants: Eliminate bladder irritants such as alcohol and caffeine, which can exacerbate lower urinary tract symptoms and have a diuretic effect.

○ **List the various pharmacologic treatments for a woman with urge incontinence.**

- Anticholinergics: AUA guidelines recommend anticholinergics as a (**standard**) treatment with *extended release* preferred over *immediate release* to minimize side effects. They antagonize the muscarinic receptors of the bladder resulting in increased total bladder capacity, decreased amplitude of bladder contraction, and increased bladder volume before first bladder contraction.
- B3 agonists (Mirabegron): Selectively activates the B3 receptor in the dome of the bladder that causes the *detrusor muscle to relax* and increases bladder capacity. Side effects include an increase in blood pressure, nasal congestion, fatigue, constipation, and tachycardia. It received FDA approval June, 2012. This may offer more treatment options to those that have intolerable side effects or contraindications (closed angle glaucoma) to anticholinergics.
- Antispasmodics: Primarily cause relaxation of detrusor smooth muscle in addition to anticholinergic effects and local anesthetic effects.
- Tricyclic antidepressants: Unique in the ability *to increase urethral outlet resistance* due to *adrenergic stimulation* on the smooth muscle of the bladder neck and proximal urethra in addition to *anticholinergic effects, direct detrusor relaxation*, and a sedative action that may be related to *antihistaminic* properties (eg, imipramine hydrochloride and amitriptyline hydrochloride). Due to multiple effects of TCA they may be useful in treating mixed urinary incontinence.
- Calcium channel blockers: Uncommon as first-line agents, calcium channel blockers inhibit the inflow of calcium after membrane depolarization and have the potential of relaxing the smooth muscle of the bladder (eg, nifedipine).

○ **What are the treatment options in patients with refractory urge incontinence?**

- Botox injection: *Inhibits acetylcholine release from presynaptic cholinergic nerve terminals* to suppress unstable contractions (only FDA approved for refractory neurogenic OAB). This occurs by interfering with the docking of vesicles at presynaptic nerve ending by targeting of SNARE protein formation through cleaving of SNAP-25.
- Sacral neuromodulation: Uses electrical stimulation of the sacral nerve root of S3, which results in *afferent inhibition* of sensory processing in the spinal cord. Studies suggest that it has a conditioning effect on neural excitability and can restore neural equilibrium between facilitatory and inhibitory influences. Although, the exact mechanism of action in each of these conditions may be different.
- Percutaneous tibial nerve stimulation: Electrical stimulation of the *posterior tibial nerve* transmits the electrical pulse to sacral plexus which *modulates afferent sensation* and may have a conditioning effect on the bladder. This exact mechanism is uncertain, but is believed to function similarly to sacral neuromodulation. This involves intermittent weekly treatments for 3 months and then monthly thereafter. There are other alternative treatment schedules and these must be continued to have benefits.
- Bladder augmentation: Allows for increased total bladder capacity and physical interruption of the overactive detrusor muscle. It is used as a last resort after exhausting all possible pharmacologic interventions for urge incontinence.

○ **Surgical implanted sacral neuromodulation devices or sacral nerve stimulation is targeted at which sacral nerve and how successful is it?**

Optimally, the S3 sacral nerve root. Only one side is typically treated. Stimulation of S3 results in *bellows* and *plantar flexion of the great toe*. Approximately 75% of otherwise intractable cases of urge incontinence report significant improvement with this therapy. Approximately 50% are completely dry.

○ **Is sacral nerve stimulation useful in urinary retention? Can it be used in men?**

Yes to both.

○ **Tricyclic antidepressants like imipramine are reasonably effective in what proportion of patients with incontinence?**

Improvement is reported in approximately 60% and may be especially useful for those with mixed urinary incontinence by increasing the outlet at the bladder neck and relaxing the detrusor, as explained previously.

○ **How does capsaicin work?**

Intravesical capsaicin desensitizes unmyelinated (c-fibers) afferent nerves. It is most useful in patients who demonstrate bladder hypersensitivity on an ice water test. Improvement of 40% to 100% has been reported.

○ **Describe the nerve control of bladder function.**

It is much more effective than oral forms. Plasma and tissue levels are higher and side effects are low as hepatic metabolism is avoided.

○ **How effective is intravesical oxybutynin?**

It is much more effective than oral forms. Plasma and tissue levels are higher and side effects are low as hepatic metabolism is avoided.

Sympathetic stimulation causes bladder relaxation and tightens the sphincter (think storage). Innervation comes mostly from the **hypogastric nerve: T11-L2.**

Parasympathetic stimulation causes bladder contractions and relaxation of the internal sphincter (think voiding). Innervation comes through the **pelvic nerve** from the **S2-4 sacral plexus.** Overactive bladder anticholinergic medications typically work here.

Somatic (voluntary) control of the external sphincter and pelvic floor muscles is provided by the **pudendal nerve** which also comes from the **S2-4 sacral plexus**. When stimulated, it tightens the sphincter.

○ **What is the current role for needle suspension for stress urinary incontinence?**

Needle suspension prevents urethral descent with stress. It has been effective in the treatment of urethral hypermobility but does not affect incontinence due to ISD.

○ **What is the role for urethral bulking agents for stress urinary incontinence?**

Various materials have been injected in the urethra either through the periurethral or transurethral methods as a bulking agent to treat urinary incontinence. The ideal injectable agent should be biocompatible, nonantigenic, noncarcinogenic, and nonmigratory. It is effective in the treatment of *intrinsic sphincter deficiency*, but does not affect incontinence due to urethral hypermobility.

○ **What is the role for suburethral sling surgery for stress urinary incontinence?**

Suburethral (pubovaginal) sling procedures effectively prevent urethral descent with stress and improve the urethral washer effect. Therefore, slings are equally effective for urethral hypermobility and ISD. However, there are increased postoperative risks of retention with detrusor overactivity.

○ **An elderly woman presents with urinary urgency and frequency. Ultrasound evaluation determines her postvoid residual to be 350 mL. What is the diagnosis?**

This patient has *detrusor overactivity with impaired contractility*, which generally presents commonly in the elderly patients. Treatment is difficult since pharmacologic treatment of the detrusor overactivity often exacerbates the retention. This optimally requires clean intermittent catheterization that is often difficult in the elderly population. It is important to rule out large cystocele or other co-existing anatomic abnormalities, which can "kink" the urethra and cause increased bladder outlet resistance.

○ **A 46-year-old woman, gravida 4, para 4, presents with urgency, frequency, and urinary incontinence. Physical examination is normal, Marshall test is negative, and urodynamic evaluation reveals a normally compliant bladder without involuntary bladder contractions. What is the diagnosis?**

This patient has classic *urge incontinence*. It is important to focus on the chief presenting symptom in evaluating a patient with urinary incontinence. Despite the obstetrical history and the lack of involuntary bladder contractions, the diagnosis remains urge incontinence. The *absence* of **detrusor overactivity** on a *single urodynamic* study does *not exclude* its diagnosis.

○ **A woman presents with complaints of urgency and precipitous voiding shortly following a cough or sneeze. What is the diagnosis?**

This patient has *stress-induced urge incontinence*. Stress incontinence is the involuntary loss of urine during coughing, sneezing, or increases in intra-abdominal pressure. The described patient loses urine after the intra-abdominal pressure has returned to normal and continues to empty her bladder precipitously. This suggests an involuntary bladder contraction occurring due to the stress stimulus.

○ **A woman presents with urodynamically demonstrated stress incontinence with urinary urgency. What is the treatment of choice?**

First treat the stress incontinence. Urgency may result from compensatory responses initiated by the incontinent patient. Alternatively, urgency may be a product of urine passage into the proximal urethra with stress leakage. In 65% of patients with mixed stress and urge incontinence, correction of the stress incontinence will resolve the urgency. However, if the urgency component is successfully treated medically, many patients are satisfied without the surgery.

○ **A woman presents with urinary incontinence immediately following a repair of a large cystocele. What is the diagnosis?**

Occult stress urinary incontinence. The full bladder contributes to normal continence by creating a valvular effect through limited posterior rotation of the bladder base against a well-supported urethra during stress. Cystoceles exacerbate this valvular effect and may mask underlying urethral dysfunction. Correction of a large cystocele in this setting leads to incontinence due to either urethral hypermobility or ISD.

○ **A woman with stage 2 symptomatic POP without incontinence is scheduled to have vaginal prolapse repair. Should she undergo a concomitant midurethral sling?**

Yes. Placement of a midurethral sling will *reduce* her odds of developing *occult stress incontinence* based on one randomized control trial (OPUS). Potential for increased *complications* from placement of the sling include UTI, major bleeding, bladder perforation, and incomplete bladder emptying which should be *discussed* in preoperative counseling. The number needed to treat (NNT) is 6 to prevent 1 episode of occult SUI.

○ **What are the differences between the retropubic (TVT) and transobturator (TOT) midurethral slings?**

In the majority of the trials, both treatments had equivalent outcomes for SUI. The complications differed with **TOT** having more *chronic thigh and groin pain* and the **TVT** has more *bladder perforation and voiding dysfunction*. In patients with ISD, TVT may improve outcomes.

○ **A woman complains of incomplete emptying and straining to void 4 weeks after a retropubic (TVT) is performed. What is her diagnosis during the voiding UDS and what should be her treatment?**

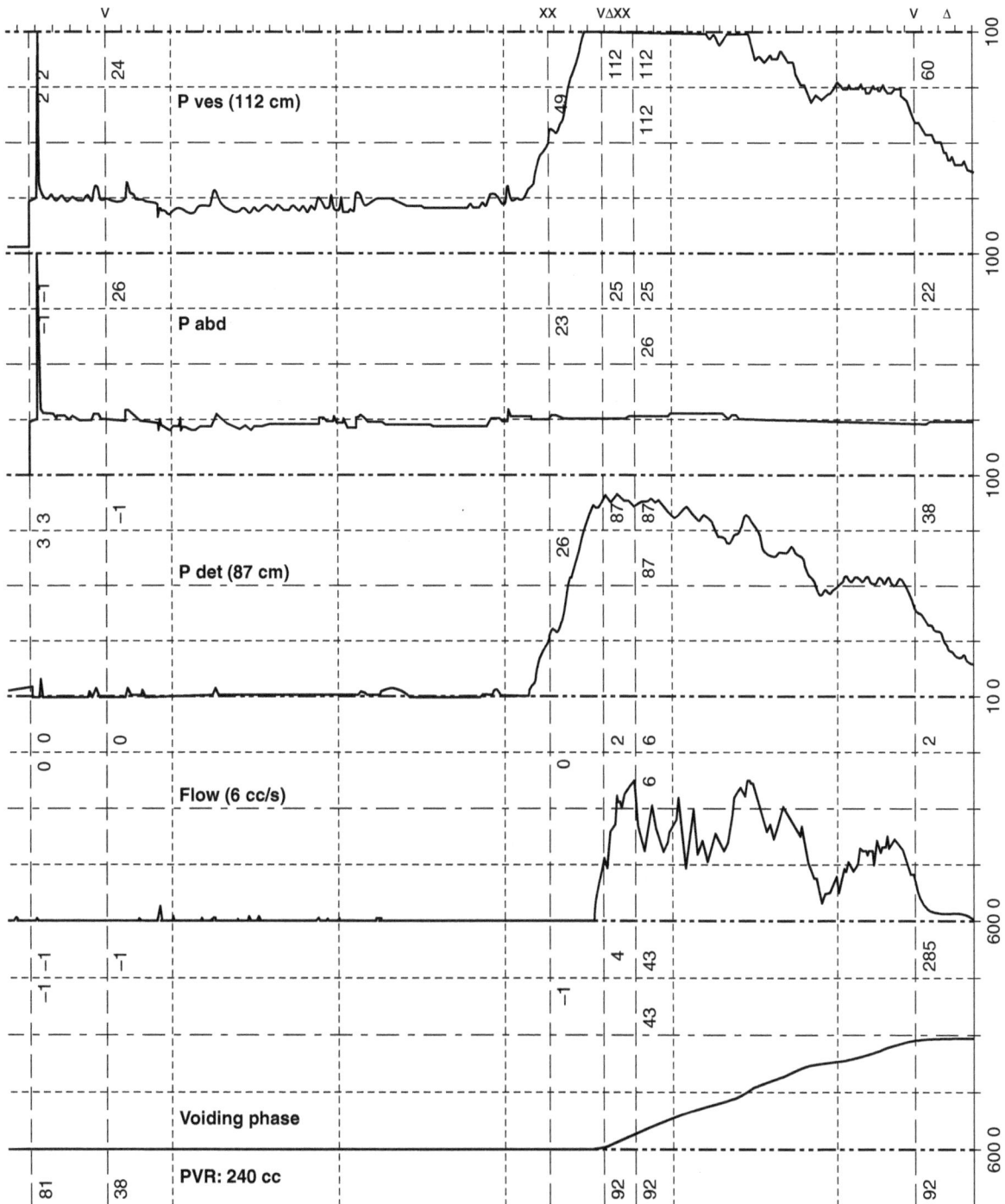

The UDS demonstrates high pressure voiding with decreased flow rate. In addition, it has elevated PVR. These findings show that she is *obstructed* from the retropubic midurethral sling. The sling may be revised by *transection or partial excision*. An attempt to loosen the sling may be attempted, but this would likely be unsuccessful as the sling has become fixed into the surrounding tissue.

○ **Immediately following a needle bladder neck suspension, a woman complains of persistent stress urinary incontinence. What is the diagnosis?**

Intrinsic sphincter deficiency. Needle suspension corrects urethral hypermobility, but is ineffective against intrinsic sphincter deficiency. Bulking urethral injections correct intrinsic sphincter deficiency but are ineffective against urethral hypermobility. Suburethral sling procedures correct both deficiencies.

○ **When performing a sling procedure, where should the mesh be located?**

At the mid to distal urethra, not the proximal urethra.

○ **Does vaginal surgery for stress incontinence have a significant impact on postoperative sexual function in women?**

When measured with a validated tool and compared with preoperative assessments, it does not appear that vaginal surgery for stress incontinence has any significant negative impact on sexual function in women.

○ **What is transient urinary incontinence?**

It is acute incontinence caused by a nonurological problem such as a change in medication.

○ **True/False: The only true cause of urinary stress incontinence is intrinsic sphincteric deficiency (ISD), which may or may not be associated with vesicourethral hypermobility?**

True. Sphincteric dysfunction may be caused by neurological factors, muscular degeneration, or trauma. Congenital problems may also be present.

○ **A 44-year-old woman leaks urine with exercise, cough, and has elevated PVR. What type of incontinence is seen during the filling phase of urodynamics?**

Vesical

Abdominal

Detrusor 4 cm H$_2$O

Flow

10

0

2

Valsalva

Urodynamic *stress urinary incontinence* is demonstrated by urinary leakage during the Valsalva with equivalent rise in abdominal and vesical pressure during the filling phase. It is important to notice that the vesical and abdominal pressures are being equally transduced, which helps to confirm the validity of the study.

○   **A healthy 55-year-old female complains of frequency and urinary incontinence that have not improved with anticholinergics. What are the important findings on the filling UDS?**

This patient demonstrates *detrusor overactivity* that is associated with urinary leakage or *urge incontinence*. It is important to notice that there is similar rise in detrusor and vesical pressure with no change in abdominal pressure. Since she has no neurologic causes for these findings, she has *idiopathic detrusor overactivity with associated urge incontinence*.

○ **A 50-year-old female with multiple sclerosis has urinary incontinence and is evaluated with during the filling phase by urodynamics. Is she incontinent?**

Since this patient has neurologic disease, this explains her findings of *neurogenic detrusor overactivity* that is associated with *urge incontinence.*

○ **What is the classic presentation of a vesicovaginal fistula?**

Continuous urinary leakage after pelvic surgery.

○ **What are the predisposing factors for vesicovaginal fistula?**

Prior pelvic surgery or malignancy are the majority (75%) of cases with other factors such as radiation therapy, endometriosis, prior cervical conization or vaginal fulguration procedures, use of pessaries, steroid use, lack of estrogen effect, congenital deformities of any of the pelvic structures, and history of voiding problems or neurogenic bladder.

○ **What other symptoms may present in the immediate postoperative period if a vesicovaginal fistula is present?**

Excessive abdominal pain, extravasation with distension, hematuria, UTI, and excessive drainage from the wound or vagina are common complaints.

○ **True/False: A painless, watery discharge of varying amounts from the vagina developing 7 to 14 days after pelvic surgery suggests a vesicovaginal fistula.**

True. This is another way in which vesicovaginal fistulae may present.

○ **True/False: Excision of the fistulous tract and interposition of a well-vascularized tissue flap are important considerations in vesicovaginal fistula repair.**

False. It is not necessary to excise the fistulous tract as it provides a strong anchoring tissue and in most cases heal well without it. If excision of the fistula would cause too much collateral damage to the surrounding tissue or blood supply, it is OK to leave it. In the case of a fistula near the ureteric orifice, excision of the tract may necessitate the ureter to be reimplanted. Interposition of a tissue flap is necessary only in cases of previous surgery, radiation therapy, or obstetrical injury.

○ **True/False: The preferred surgical repair for vesicovaginal fistula is transabdominal.**

False. The transvaginal route is preferred for most fistula repairs. Only the most complex repairs will need a different approach. The surgeon's experience largely influences the approach as some surgeons prefer abdominal approach with large fistulas, narrow introitus (nulliparous) with no prolapse, history of radiation, ureteric injury, or a small bladder capacity requiring a bladder augmentation.

○ **What is the optimal timing of formal vesicovaginal repair?**

That depends on the risk factors and etiology of the fistula. In uncomplicated cases caused by iatrogenic injury, a period of 2 to 3 weeks may be sufficient; 3 to 6 months is recommended for injuries caused by obstetrical trauma; and 12 months is needed in cases of radiation therapy.

○ **What is the preferential side to base an omental flap?**

The right branch of gastroepiploic artery is usually larger and more caudal, although the flap may be based on either pedicle.

○ **What is the blood supply to a martius flap?**

It is based on the inferior blood supply from the posterior labial branches of the internal pudendal artery. Superiorly the external pudendal artery and laterally the obturator artery are transected so that the flap can be mobilized and be based on its inferior blood supply.

○ **What findings must be present on a VCUG for it to be an adequate test?**

Lateral and *post void* films must be performed. *Voiding* images with the patient in lateral position may be necessary to demonstrate a small fistula.

○ **What percent of surgical vesicovaginal fistulas have ureteric involvement?**

12% of vesicovaginal fistulas have ureteric involvement, which emphasizes the importance of preoperative upper tract imaging.

Upper Urinary Tract Obstruction

Udaya Kumar, MD, FRCS Urol, Dip Urol (Lon) and David M. Albala, MD

○ **In evaluating upper tract obstruction, which is the radiopharmaceutical of choice?**

^{99m}Tc-mercaptoacetyltriglycine (MAG3). It is more efficiently excreted by the kidney than DTPA, delivers a lower dose of radiation to the kidney than OIH, and provides better visualization of the anatomy of obstruction than other agents.

○ **What is the basis of the Whitaker test?**

It provides urodynamic evidence of mechanical obstruction of the upper tract at a given flow rate. As it is an invasive test, it is only used in cases with extreme dilatation of the upper tract or when renal function is too poor for adequate diuretic response.

○ **What are the phases in pressure changes in the ureter after unilateral occlusion of the ureter?**

Following unilateral occlusion, there is a rise in both ureteric pressure and renal blood flow for 1 to 1.5 hours. Then in phase 2, there is a continued rise in ureteric pressure while renal blood flow declines (5 hours). In the final phase, both renal blood flow and ureteric pressure fall.

○ **What are the causes of postobstructive diuresis?**

Postobstructive diuresis occurs after relief of bilateral ureteric obstruction or obstruction of a solitary kidney. It may be classified as physiologic, when caused by retained urea, sodium, and water, or pathologic when caused by impaired concentrating ability or sodium absorption.

○ **What is the embryological basis of the retrocaval ureter?**

The persistence of the posterior cardinal vein as the major portion of the inferior vena cava causes medial migration of and compression of the right ureter.

○ **What are the types of retrocaval ureter?**

There are 2 types. Type 1, or the "low loop type," is the most common and the dilated proximal portion assumes a reverse J shape. Type 2 or the "high loop" is rarer. In this case, the ureter passes behind the vena cava at the level of or just above the UPJ.

○   **How common is hydronephrosis in pregnancy?**

Unilateral or bilateral hydronephrosis occurs by the third trimester of pregnancy in 90% to 95% of asymptomatic patients. In more than 80% of patients, right-sided hydronephrosis predominates.

○   **True/False: In the treatment of ureteric obstruction due to endometriosis, hormonal therapy is the treatment of choice.**

False. Surgery is more likely to be successful. The choice of surgery depends on the extent of ureteric involvement and the patient's desire to have more children. Ureterolysis with unilateral or bilateral oophorectomy and hysterectomy may be required. In severe cases, nephrectomy may be needed.

○   **How common is ureteral injury following hysterectomy?**

In routine hysterectomy, the incidence varies from 0.5% to 3% and is bilateral in one of every 6 cases. After radical hysterectomy, the incidence varies from 10% to 15%.

○   **How is ureteral involvement in Crohn disease treated?**

Rarely is ureterolysis required for ureteral involvement in Crohn disease. Medical or surgical therapy for Crohn disease is usually effective in resolving ureteral involvement. It may also be indicated in some cases of severe retroperitoneal fibrosis (RPF) with encasement of the ureter.

○   **What are the causes of RPF?**

Two-thirds of cases are idiopathic. Other causes include prolonged use of methysergide and other ergot derivatives. RPF can occur secondary to other disease processes of the retroperitoneum such as hemorrhage, urinary extravasation, trauma, perianeurysmal inflammation, radiation therapy, surgery, inflammatory, bowel disease, collagen disease, and fat necrosis.

○   **What are the symptoms of RBF?**

In approximately 90% of cases, there is a characteristic pain with a girdle-type distribution. The pain is dull and noncolicky. Later it becomes severe and unrelenting. The pain may be relieved by aspirin and not by narcotics. Rarely, there may be features of compression of the great vessels. Uremia is a late feature.

○   **What are the features of RBF on intravenous urography?**

There is medial deviation of the ureters on IVU. Although this finding is present in up to 20% of normal studies, in RPF the displacement extends higher than the normal variant. There is usually associated obstruction and hydronephrosis. CT or MRI is most useful in establishing a diagnosis.

○   **How is RBF treated?**

Any suspected medication like methysergide is withheld. If the patient is uremic, renal drainage should be established with ureteral stenting or nephrostomy tube placement. Steroid therapy may be useful in some but bilateral ureterolysis is required in most cases.

○   **What is pelvic lipomatosis?**

Pelvic lipomatosis is a proliferative disease of unknown etiology involving the mature fatty tissues of the pelvic retroperitoneum. It occurs exclusively in men in the third to sixth decade of life and is more common in African American men. This benign condition may lead to compression of the pelvic viscera including the ureters.

○ **What conditions may be associated with pelvic lipomatosis?**

It may be associated with cystitis cystica, cystitis glandularis, adenocarcinoma of the bladder, chronic UTI, hypertension, superficial thrombophlebitis, VU reflux, RPF, nontropical chyluria, and Proteus syndrome.

○ **How is pelvic lipomatosis diagnosed?**

Plain KUB x-ray may show the radiolucent area in the bony pelvis. On IVP, the bladder base is noted to be elevated and the bladder itself takes on a pear shape. CT is useful to confirm the diagnosis.

○ **How common is bilaterality in UPJ obstruction?**

Bilateral UPJ obstruction is seen in 10% to 40% of cases.

○ **True/False: UPJ obstruction occurs more commonly in males and on the left side.**

True. The ratio of male to female is more prominent in infancy (2:1). Left-sided lesions are more common. In infancy, about two-thirds of UPJ obstructions are on the left.

○ **How common is the finding of an aberrant lower polar vessel in UPJ obstruction?**

The incidence varies from 15% to 52%. Although some cases are no doubt caused by aberrant vessels, especially in adults, in most cases it is felt to be a concomitant finding rather than the cause.

○ **Vesicoureteric reflux and UPJ obstruction are found together in what proportion of cases?**

In approximately 10% (minor degree of reflux has been quoted in up to 40%). Severe cases of VU reflux can cause marked tortuosity of the ureter and secondarily give rise to UPJ obstruction.

○ **What are the congenital anomalies associated with UPJ obstruction?**

UPJ obstruction in the contralateral kidney (10%-40%), renal dysplasia, and multicystic disease of the contralateral kidney, unilateral renal agenesis, duplicated collecting system, VU reflux, and the VATER complex.

○ **What is the investigation of choice for UPJ obstruction?**

A diuretic renogram is one of the best noninvasive methods to determine if a dilated upper tract is obstructed or not. The conventional renographic criteria for obstruction that warrant surgical repair are a flat or rising washout curve after furosemide administration, a half-time greater than 20 minutes and differential function less than 40%. Dynamic contrast MR urography is the newest imaging modality for UPJ obstruction. It provides anatomic and functional detail without the radiation exposure. A transit time (time between enhancement of renal cortex and appearance of contrast in the ureter) longer than 590 seconds is felt to indicate obstruction on MR urography.

○ **What test is useful to determine whether a hydronephrotic kidney is salvageable or not?**

A quantitative renal scan using ^{99m}Tc–DMSA is useful in determining whether a patient will benefit from pyeloplasty or not. If a kidney contributes less than 10% of the overall renal function, it should probably be removed.

○ **How is resistive index (RI, on ultrasound examination) defined?**

(Peak systolic velocity – lowest diastolic velocity)/peak systolic velocity.

○ **What is the basis for the use of RI in the diagnosis of obstructive uropathy?**

A decrease in renal blood flow and an increase in renovascular resistance are hallmarks of obstructive uropathy. There is more reduction in diastolic than systolic blood flow, causing a rise in RI.

○ **What conditions other than obstructive uropathy can cause RI to be elevated?**

Values above the normally accepted 0.70 may be found in children, especially infants, in medical renal diseases, dehydration, hypotension, and in patients with a low heart rate.

○ **What are the determinants of the curve obtained during diuretic renography?**

The curve depends on the tracer used, the patient's hydration status, the dose and timing of the administration of the diuretic, and the overall renal function. The shape, size, and distensibility of the renal pelvis, its outlet resistance, gravity, and bladder filling also influence the curve.

○ **What are the patterns of curves described on the diuretic renogram?**

Type 1 (normal), type 2 (obstructed), type 3a (dilated unobstructed), and type 3b (equivocal).

○ **Can urinary biochemical markers be used in the diagnosis of upper tract obstruction?**

Epidermal growth factor, the renin–angiotensin system, monocyte chemoattractants, and transforming growth factors ($TGF-\beta_1$) have been implicated in patients with UPJ obstruction. Transforming growth factors ($TGF-\beta_1$) is elevated in patients with UPJ obstruction. There was 80% sensitivity for obstruction reported in pediatric patients undergoing pyeloplasty. The utility of these markers is yet to be determined.

○ **What are the ultrasound findings of UPJ obstruction in the neonate?**

The pelvis is seen as a large medial sonolucent structure, surrounded by smaller, rounded sonolucent structures representing the dilated calyces. Sometimes, the infundibular communications between the dilated calyces and the renal pelvis may be seen.

○ **True/False: It is difficult to distinguish antenatally between severe hydronephrosis and multicystic dysplastic kidney (MDK).**

True. The ultrasound findings of MDK are lack of reniform shape of the kidney, multiple cysts of varying size, and no evidence of a collecting system. In severe hydronephrosis, the distinction may be difficult.

○ **What are the indications for intervention in UPJ obstruction?**

The presence of symptoms from obstruction, impairment of renal function, the development of infection, or stones. Patients with solitary kidneys and bilateral UPJ obstruction should have intervention. The timing of repair in infants is controversial, as it is difficult to determine which kidneys are at risk.

○ **A dismembered pyeloplasty is not suitable for which UPJ obstruction cases?**

When the UPJ obstruction is associated with lengthy or multiple proximal ureteral strictures or when the renal pelvis is small, intrarenal, and relatively inaccessible.

○ **When is preoperative drainage of a kidney with UPJ obstruction indicated?**

When there is infection associated with obstruction, uremia due to obstruction in a solitary kidney or bilateral disease, and rarely in the patient with severe unrelenting pain.

○ **How is UPJ obstruction treated in the adult?**

Until recently, open surgery (ie, pyeloplasty) was the only option. Minimally invasive alternatives now available include endopyelotomy (antegrade or retrograde), cautery wire balloon incision (Acucise device), and laparoscopic pyeloplasty.

○ **When an endopyelotomy is performed, where is the incision made?**

If a direct endoscopic incision is performed, a direct lateral cut is the safest. This appears to have the least likelihood of encountering a crossing vessel. In one study, a posterior-crossing vessel was found in 6.2% of cases, whereas no vessels were found crossing the UPJ laterally.

○ **What factors predict a poor outcome after endopyelotomy?**

Poor renal function, massive hydronephrosis, and the presence of a crossing vessel result in a reduced success rates.

○ **What are the possible complications of endopyelotomy?**

Hemorrhage is the most commonly encountered problem. Rarely ureteral avulsion, ureteral necrosis, arteriovenous fistula formation, hematoma, urinoma, and urinary infection have been reported.

○ **When hydronephrosis is noted in a horseshoe kidney, what is the likely cause?**

The obstruction is usually due to a UPJ obstruction and not due to pressure on the ureter from the isthmus.

○ **What are the basic techniques used in open pyeloplasty?**

There are 2 fundamental techniques; a pelvic flap is used in Culp and de Weerd, Scardino and Prince, and Foley Y-V plasty operations. An Anderson–Hynes pyeloplasty is the dismembered type.

○ **Which part of the nephron is most resistant to damage from hydronephrosis?**

The glomerulus. Glomerular changes are not evident until 28 days of obstruction. In contrast, distal tubular and proximal tubular atrophy are seen at 7 and 14 days, respectively.

○ **How does urine exit the kidney in complete obstruction?**

In acute obstruction with high pressures, such as ureteral calculi, urine exits through a rupture in the fornices. In low-pressure obstruction, urine exits via lymphatic channels and in chronic hydronephrosis, it is mostly into the renal venous channels.

○ **What is the incidence of UPJ obstruction?**

Urinary dilatation is detected in utero in 1 in 100 pregnancies; of these, significant uropathy is seen in 1 in 500. UPJ obstruction is responsible for 40% of these, placing the incidence of UPJ obstruction at 1 in 1250 births.

○   **What is the crescent sign on the excretory urogram in a patient with UPJ obstruction?**

The calyceal crescents represent transversely oriented collecting ducts and signify recoverable renal function.

○   **What are the causes of UPJ obstruction?**

Intrinsic:

- Congenital–adynamic muscular segment.
- Ureteral mucosal folds.
- High insertion of ureter into renal pelvis.

Extrinsic:

- Aberrant lower pole vessel.
- Retroperitoneal fibrosis.
- Retroperitoneal tumors.

Secondary:

- Renal calculi.
- Fibroepithelial polyps.
- Tumors.
- Failed pyeloplasty.

○   **Which is the most common cause of UPJ obstruction?**

Intrinsic causes are the most common, with an adynamic muscular segment (congenital) occurring frequently.

○   **Where is the most common site for ureteral strictures to occur?**

Ureteral strictures occur most commonly at the ureteropelvic junction. The second most common area of stenosis is at the ureterovesical junction.

○   **What is the appropriate treatment for failed endopyelotomy for UPJ obstruction?**

An open or laparoscopic pyeloplasty (including robotic assisted) are appropriate options depending on experience and expertise available.

○   **What is the appropriate treatment for a failed laparoscopic or open pyeloplasty?**

Endopyelotomy is a reasonable option after failure of pyeloplasty. However, long strictures, severe hydronephrosis, and poor renal function predict a poor outcome.

○   **What is the basis of endopyelotomy?**

Endopyelotomy uses the concept of a full-thickness incision of a narrow segment of ureter allowed to heal over a stent. The concept was first described in open surgery by Albarran in 1903 and popularized by Davis as intubated ureterostomy in 1943. Wickham and Kellett described endoscopic pyelolysis using the percutaneous approach.

○   **What approaches are available in performing endopyelotomy?**

Endopyelotomy can be performed antegrade using the percutaneous approach. Alternatively, it can be performed retrograde either using ureteroscopy (with laser or electrocautery) or using the Acucise balloon electrocautery. Unlike ureteroscopy or percutaneous approaches that are done under direct vision, Acucise endopyelotomy is performed using fluoroscopic guidance. The risk of a hemorrhagic complication is greater with the latter approach.

CHAPTER 20

Intestinal Segments in Urology

David Margel, MD and
Laurence Klotz, MD

○ **True/False: Ileal conduit is the standard form of urinary diversion.**

True. The ileal conduit was described in 1950 by Bricker and has remained a standard urinary diversion against which others are judged (Bricker, 1950).

○ **Which type of surgical urinary diversion is considered the "optimal" form of urinary reconstruction?**

Currently centers of excellence recommend that an orthotopic bladder be offered to most patients as the primary form of urinary reconstruction. Patients with advanced age or comorbidity should generally have an ileal conduit (Hautmann et al., 2007). Patients with prostatic urethral involvement should be considered for a conduit or a continent abdominal diversion.

○ **List the contraindications to an ileal conduit.**

Short bowel syndrome, inflammatory small bowel disease, and previous extensive radiation to the ileum.

○ **List the 3 types of diversion.**

- Abdominal diversion such as ureterocutaneostomy, ileal or colonic conduit, and various forms of a continent pouch.
- Urethral diversion which includes various forms of gastrointestinal pouches attached to the urethra as a continent, orthotopic urinary diversion (neobladder, orthotopic bladder substitution).
- Rectosigmoid diversions, such as uretero(ileo-)rectostomy.

○ **Does the type of urinary diversion affect outcome for muscle invasive bladder cancer?**

No. In a recent study Yossepowitch et al. (2003) compared cancer control and patterns of disease recurrence in neobladder and conduit patients. No cancer-specific survival difference could be identified between the 2 groups when adjusting for the pathological stage.

○ **Does the type of diversion affect the chance of a urethral recurrence following cystectomy for bladder cancer?**

Stein et al. demonstrated that at long-term follow-up urethral tumor recurrence occurs in approximately 7% of men following cystectomy for bladder cancer. Involvement of the prostate with tumor and the form of urinary diversion were significant and independent risk factors for urethral tumor recurrence. Patients undergoing orthotropic diversion have a lower incidence of urethral recurrence (4%) compared with those undergoing cutaneous diversion (8%). These results maybe confounded by selection bias since those at higher risk of urethral recurrence were offered a cutaneous diversion compared to those with orthotopic diversion.

○ **What is/are the absolute contraindication(s) to continent urinary diversion?**

Absolute contraindications to continent urinary diversion are compromised renal function with serum creatinine levels above 1.50 to 2.00 mg/dL, severe hepatic dysfunction, and patients in whom urethrectomy is indicated (usually because of urethral involvement by transitional cell carcinoma (TCC)) (Studer et al., 1998).

○ **A patient is considered for a continent diversion. His serum creatinine exceeds 2.0 mg/dL. How should he be evaluated to determine whether he is a candidate?**

Criteria for candidacy for a continent diversion include the ability to achieve a urine pH of 5.8 or less following an ammonium chloride loading test, a urine osmolality ≥600 mOsm/kg in response to water deprivation, a glomerular filtration rate >35 mL/min, and no more than minimal proteinuria. These tests are helpful in patients desiring continent diversion with borderline renal functions (ie, serum creatinine between 1.50 and 2.00 mg/dL).

○ **Does extensive pelvic disease, a palpable mass, or positive lymph nodes preclude the use of neobladder because of the high propensity for pelvic recurrence or distant relapse?**

No. Convincing evidence suggests that a patient with an orthotopic diversion tolerates adjuvant chemotherapy less well. Local recurrence may be more problematic with a neobladder, but conversion to an ileal conduit if this occurs is a reasonable option. Patients can anticipate normal neobladder function until the time of death (Hautmann and Simon, 1999).

○ **True/False: Continent urinary diversions are better than incontinent diversions in terms of quality of life (QOL).**

False. Published evidence does not support an advantage of one type of reconstruction over the others with regard to QOL (Hautmann et al., 2007). Although the QOL studies have not demonstrated an advantage of orthotopic bladder replacement, many urologists believe that the QOL is improved. Patients usually prefer this option when offered.

○ **What are the surgical principles for bladder reconstruction?**

- High volume
- Low pressure
- Continence mechanism
- Anti reflux mechanism

○ **List the 8 most common complications specific to continent urinary diversions.**

- Stomal stenosis: The incidence of stomal stenosis in continent cutaneous urinary diversions is determined by the different continence mechanisms employed. The incidence of stomal stenosis as defined by difficulty catheterising may be as low as 1.5% for plication anti reflux mechanisms to as much as 54% in Mitrofanoff conduits.
- Incontinence: The incidence of incontinence is hard to report since its definition varies significantly between studies. If assessed strictly as the presence of ANY leakage, incontinence rates of up to 28% are reported but such strict criteria are seldom used. Daytime continence rate is generally 5% to 10% greater than the nighttime continence rate. Studer et al. (2006) report that the continence rate is 92% during the day and 79% during nighttime after 1 year.
- Calculi: These are a frequent encounter in urinary diversions and augmentations and are related to the presence of infection, stasis, mucus, and exposed staples.
- Anastomotic urinary leakage: It ranges between 2% and 10%.
- Anastomotic strictures: These can occur secondary to excessive tension, ischemia, recurrent malignancy, radiation, and failure to achieve mucosal coaptation during surgery. In addition to these factors, the creation of an anti reflux mechanism also increases the risk of stricture at the uretero-bowel anastomosis.
- Incomplete voiding: All forms of continent diversion carry with them an inherent risk of incomplete voiding requiring the utilization of clean intermittent self-catheterisation (CISC).
- Tumor formation: Current evidence, although low level and limited to small case series and case reports, suggests that ureterosigmoidostomy urinary diversion increases the risk of malignancy. This risk is difficult to quantify and appears related to time, being almost unheard of in the first 15 years following diversion. Following ileocystoplasty, continent cutaneous urinary diversion, and orthotopic neobladder formation, there have been isolated reports of malignancy at the anastomotic site but these are almost universally found in patients having had surgery for chronically inflamed or tuberculous bladders. The intrinsic risk of malignancy in patients undergoing surgery for noninflammatory, benign condition, for example detrusor overactivity appears to be no greater than for the age-matched population; however, patients should be warned regarding possible symptoms of malignancy (hematuria) and appropriately investigated whether these can occur. Annual surveillance has been advocated by some although the time of initiation remains a matter for debate.
- Mucus production

○ **Describe several surgical techniques of maintaining continence in a pouch.**

- Nipple valve principle where the valve protrudes into the reservoir cavity and as the reservoir fills, the valve is compressed preventing incontinence.
- The Flap valve technique relies on the proximal segment of the continence channel running on the inner wall of the reservoir. As the reservoir fills, the channel is compressed preventing incontinence. The most popular type of flap valve is the appendix implanted into the reservoir (Mitrofanoff principle).

○ **Is a continent diversion better than conduit diversion for maintaining upper tract function?**

Not necessarily. The only prospective randomized trial is reported by Kristjansson et al. (1995a, b). In this trial, 2 types of conduit diversions (ileal [$n = 18$] and colonic [$n = 20$]) and cecal continent diversion ($n = 8$) were used for the treatment of patients. For the statistical analysis, the combined outcome measures of the ileal and colonic conduit diversions ($n = 38$) were compared to the outcome measures of the cecal continent diversion. There were no statistically significant differences in the relative risks of upper urinary tract infection, number with uretero-intestinal stenosis, incidence of glomerular filtration rate deterioration (of more than 25%), and renal scarring. The confidence intervals were all wide, however, and did not rule out clinically important differences.

○ **In terms of metabolic consequences, what bowel segment is preferably used for bladder reconstruction and why?**

Ileum is preferred to colon for bladder reconstruction. Chloride absorption and bicarbonate excretion are more pronounced in the colon, which leads to a higher risk of hyperchloremic metabolic acidosis, particularly in the presence of renal impairment (Davidsson et al., 1994).

○ **What is the advantage of stomach over other intestinal segments for urinary diversion?**

Stomach is less permeable to urinary solutes, it acidifies the urine, it has a net excretion of chloride and protons rather than a net absorption of them, and it produces less mucus.

○ **True/False: The jejunum is a good option as an intestinal segment for urinary intestinal diversion.**

False. The jejunum is usually not employed for reconstruction of the urinary system, because its use often results in severe electrolyte imbalance.

○ **What are the preferred methods of urinary diversion in patients with history of pelvic irradiation and why?**

In patients with pelvic irradiation, it is preferable to avoid using the ileum because it is the bowel segment that is most affected by pelvic radiation. The preferred method of diversion is either a colon conduit or a continent cutaneous pouch using the colon (eg, Indiana or Mainz pouch) (Leissner et al., 2000; Ravi et al., 1994).

○ **Which part of colon is the most appropriate segment as a colon conduit in patients undergoing a total pelvic exenteration?**

Sigmoid colon. No bowel anastomosis needs to be made.

○ **What is the contraindication to the use of sigmoid colon in addition to disease of the segment and extensive pelvic irradiation?**

If the internal iliac arteries have been ligated and the rectum has been left in situ, use of the sigmoid colon is contraindicated. It may result in sloughing of the rectum or its mucosa.

○ **What are the contraindications to the use of colonic segments?**

Inflammatory large bowel disease and severe chronic diarrhea.

○ **Which part of the gut is most suitable for bladder replacement?**

Unclear. Two randomized trials (Chen 2009; Khafagy, 2006) compared between 2 different bowel segments (ileal and ileocolonic; Chen 2009 and ileal and ileocaecal; Khafagy, 2006) in the treatment of patients with bladder replacement. A Cochrane Meta analysis did not show any difference in daytime incontinence or nighttime incontinence, renal function deterioration, or any other complication. Thus at present no conclusion can be drawn.

○ **What are the main advantages of an ileocecal pouch (Indiana pouch)?**

The main advantage is, clearly, continence. In addition, the terminal ileum remains in the fecal stream (with the exception of the distal 15 cm), and it is avoided, especially following pelvic radiation.

○ **Where are the 3 vulnerable points involving the vascular supply to the colon located?**

Sudeck critical point is located between the junction of the sigmoid and superior hemorrhoidal arteries with the midpoints between the middle colic and right colic arteries. Between the middle colic and left colic arteries are tenuous anastomotic areas. If the colon were transected in these regions, the anastomosis might be at risk because of compromised blood supply.

○ **What are the most common aerobic organisms in the bowel?**

Escherichia coli and *Streptococcus faecalis.*

○ **What are the most common anaerobic organisms in the bowel?**

Bacteroides species and *Clostridium* species.

○ **True/False: A mechanical bowel preparation reduces the concentration of bacteria as well as the total number.**

False. The mechanical preparation reduces the amount of feces, whereas the antibiotic preparation reduces the bacterial concentration.

○ **What are the common adverse effects of antibiotic bowel preparation?**

Diarrhea. Pseudomembranous enterocolitis, monilial overgrowth resulting in stomatitis, malabsorption of protein, carbohydrate, and fat are the other disadvantages.

○ **True/False: The main reason for detubularization of the bowel segment used in urinary diversion is altering the shape of the reservoir from spherical to ellipsoid.**

False. Detubularized bowel segments provide greater capacity at lower pressure and require a shorter length of intestine than do intact segments; shape is of secondary importance (Colding-Jorgensen et al., 1993).

○ **Is the use of an anti reflux ureterointestinal anastomotic technique better than a freely refluxing anastomosis in bladder replacement?**

No. Studer et al. (1996) compared an antireflux mechanism (nipple valve) against a freely refluxing mechanism (afferent ileal tubular segment) in bladder replacement. No differences were noted in upper urinary tract infection, daytime incontinence, nighttime incontinence, and ureterointestinal anastomotic strictures. There was a marginally statistically significant difference in the incidence of upper tract dilatation, suggesting a higher rate after nipple value treatment, but this was based on only 11 cases and the confidence interval was wide (RR 0.22; 95% CI: 0.05 to 0.96, analysis 12.4). Shaaban et al. (2006) compared refluxing and antirefluxing techniques of uretero-enteric anastomosis in different renal units for the same patient. Unfortunately they did not report a paired analysis. Of the 53 renal units allocated to direct ureteroileal anastomosis technique, one was obstructed compared to be 5 among those with an antirefluxive anastomosis. This difference was not statistically significant.

○ **True/False: The pressure within the renal pelvis in refluxing conduit diversions is elevated above normal.**

False. Peristaltic ureteral contractions dampen pressure transmission from the intestine to the renal pelvis. As a result it is not elevated above normal.

○ **Which of the small bowel antirefluxing procedures has the lowest incidence of stricture as an ureterointestinal anastomosis?**

The LeDuc procedure (mucosal trench). It has also the highest success rate in preventing reflux.

○ **Is ureteral stenosis in a patient with a ureterointestinal anastomosis more common on one side than the other and why?**

Ureterointestinal anastomotic strictures occur more commonly with the left ureter. Blood supply to the ureter may be compromised where the ureter crosses over the aorta beneath the inferior mesenteric artery. Additionally, aggressive stripping of adventitia and angulation of the ureter at the inferior mesenteric artery can result in ischemia and subsequent stricture formation.

○ **What technical steps are used to avoid ischemia to the distal ureter in order to decrease the chance of ureteroenteric strictures? And what would be the options of management in case they develop?**

Mobilization of the ureter should be limited and the distal pelvic portion discarded. If placement of the left ureter under the free edge of the left colonic mesentery causes angulation against the inferior mesenteric artery, the ureter may be brought through a higher avascular window within the colonic mesentery. The options of management for ureteroenteric strictures include retrograde or antegrade endoscopic or percutaneous dilatation, or dilation and incision. Stents are left routinely. Success rates are 20% to 50% versus 44% to 63% for incision-based techniques. Open surgical repair is a more invasive procedure, but it has a success rate >90% (Hautmann et al., 2007).

○ **How long are patients at risk for ureterointestinal strictures?**

Late strictures (>10 years) are not uncommon. Patients are at risk for ureterointestinal strictures for the life of the anastomosis.

○ **What is the optimal site for a stoma in a jejunal conduit?**

Left upper quadrant. The portion of jejunum to be utilized should be as distal as possible.

○ **Which type of abdominal stoma is preferable when a collection device is worn?**

A protruding stoma. It has a lower incidence of stomal stenosis and fewer peristomal skin problems.

○ **What is the potential complication of the abdominal stoma placed lateral to the rectus sheath?**

Parastomal herniation. Ideally, the stoma should be placed through the belly of the rectus muscle.

○ **Which stomas are associated with an increased likelihood of parastomal hernias?**

The incidence of parastomal hernias for end stomas is 1% to 4%, compared to 4% to 20% for loop stomas.

○ **What are the options if an ileal conduit won't reach the skin?**
- Turnbull stoma (ie, loop ileostomy).
- Excise mesentery from the terminal part of the loop.
- Mobilize the base of mesentery.
- Redo the loop.

○ **Which part of colon is the most appropriate segment for a conduit in patients requiring an intestinal pyelostomy?**

Transverse colon. It is an excellent segment when an intestinal pyelostomy needs to be performed.

○ **Which part of colon is the most appropriate segment to use as a colon conduit in patients who have received extensive pelvic irradiation.**

Transverse colon. This segment of bowel typically lies outside the treated field in patients undergoing pelvic irradiation. The isolated segment will be well supplied by the middle colic artery.

○ **True/False: Routine postoperative use of nasogastric decompression is necessary in all patients following intestinal urinary diversion.**

False. The routine use of nasogastric decompression is unnecessary. Several studies showed that patients who did not receive a routine nasogastric tube fared better in terms of complications such as fever, atelectasis, and pneumonia, and advanced more quickly to a regular diet (Inman et al., 2003).

○ **True/False: In the early postoperative period, irrigation of the continent urinary reservoir is essential.**

True. In the early postoperative period, indwelling catheters must be carefully irrigated to prevent initial mucous buildup within the diversion. After removal of the indwelling catheter, patients with good spontaneous voiding and complete emptying usually pass the mucus spontaneously in the urine. In contrast, patients with incomplete emptying and those performing clean intermittent catheterization (CIC) may need to irrigate to remove retained mucous (Varol and Studer, 2004).

○ **What is the etiologic agent of pseudomembranous enterocolitis?**

Clostridium difficile. C. difficile elaborates cytotoxin A and cytotoxin B that cause diarrhea and enterocolitis.

○ **What are the most common causes of the bowel obstruction following construction of intestinal anastomoses?**

Adhesions and recurrent cancer.

○ **True/False: The incidence of postoperative bowel obstruction in patients who have segments isolated from the colon is less than that occurring with ileum.**

True. Postoperative bowel obstruction occurs in approximately 10% of patients who have bowel segments isolated from the ileum for urinary tract reconstruction compared to 4% of patients who have bowel segments isolated from colon.

○ **What are the complications of intestinal anastomoses?**

Stenosis, obstruction, pseudo-obstructions (Ogilvie syndrome) (acute colonic pseudo-obstruction characterized by massive colonic dilatation in the absence of mechanical cause), intestinal leak, hemorrhage, fistulas, wound infections, pelvic abscesses, and sepsis. One percent of these complications requires operations.

○ **Which factors contribute to a potential anastomotic breakdown?**

Poor blood supply, local sepsis, drains placed in direct contact with an anastomosis, and performance of an anastomosis on previously irradiated bowel. Poor blood supply and local sepsis cause ischemia, whereas drains placed on the anastomosis increase the likelihood of an anastomotic leak.

○ **What are the most commonly isolated bacterial species from intestinal urinary reservoirs? Should they ever be treated?**

They are *E. coli, Pseudomonas, Klebsiella, Proteus,* and *Enterococcus* species (Mansson et al., 1986). They should not be treated as long as they are asymptomatic (Akerlund et al., 1994).

○ **Which patients with asymptomatic bacteriuria and an intestinal diversion should be treated?**

Only patients with predominant cultures of *Proteus* or *Pseudomonas* should be treated. Other bacteria should not be treated unless symptomatic.

○ **What are the consequences of persistent infection in intestinal segments?**

Strictures and renal deterioration. Persistent infection of the intestine exposed to urine may result in strictures, bacterial seeding of the upper tracts, and renal deterioration.

○ **What is the most common cause of stone formation in conduits and pouches?**

Foreign bodies such as staples or nonabsorbable sutures. Persistent infection, lowered pH, stasis, enteric hyperoxaluria, and hypercalciuria are the other factors.

○ **What are the rates of spontaneous pouch rupture and how should they be managed?**

Spontaneous pouch ruptures occur in approximately 1.5% to 4.3% cases. It should be considered in all patients with continent urinary diversion who present with acute abdominal pain. The pouch should be catheterized to check for urinary retention or hematuria and a CT scan is the preferred radiological investigation (Mansson et al., 2003; Nippgen et al., 2001). The overall clinical features of the patient dictate the choice between conservative treatment with drainage and antibiotics versus surgical exploration (Baseman et al., 1997; Choong et al., 1998).

○ **What are the most common complications of an ileal conduit and how frequent are they?**

Stomal and peristomal complications include skin lesions, stenosis, and retraction of the stoma. These were reported to occur in up to 31% of cases. Parastomal hernia is seen in 10% to 15% of cases (Iborra et al., 2001). Upper urinary tract deterioration is seen in 34% of cases. This is caused by chronic bacteriuria, reflux, and obstruction (Singh et al., 1997).

○ **True/False: Continent urinary diversions have a higher overall complication and reoperation rates in contrast to ileal conduits.**

False. There is no difference between continent urinary diversions and ileal conduits in terms of overall complication and reoperation rates (Parekh et al., 2000; Gburek et al., 1998).

○ **What should the maximum upper level of sustained bladder pressure be in a patient with a continent neobladder?**

40 cm H_2O. Sustained pressures over 40 cm H_2O put the upper tracts at risk.

○ **What is the most common complaint of a patient with an orthotopic diversion?**

Nocturnal enuresis. The loss of native bladder and its reflexes and the production of an increased urine volume are responsible for this complaint.

○ **What are the patterns of day time incontinence following orthotopic urinary diversion? How would you manage patients with a persistent, severe form of daytime incontinence?**

Daytime continence is achieved earlier postoperatively compared with nighttime continence and 85% to 90% of patients with orthotopic bladder will be continent during the day at 1 year from surgery, those rates may decrease 4 to 5 years postoperatively, in part because of decreased tone of the urethral sphincter with advanced age (Madersbacher et al., 2002). Persistent severe incontinence after orthotopic urinary diversion may be treated by periurethral collagen injection, definitive placement of a urethral sling, or an artificial urinary sphincter (Tchetgen et al., 2000).

○ **What are the patterns of nighttime incontinence following orthotopic urinary diversion? And how would you manage persistent forms of nighttime incontinence?**

Nighttime continence requires a 6- to 12-month postoperative interval to reach maximum levels as the capacity and the compliance of the diversion increase. The reported prevalence of persistent nighttime leakage is between 27% and 50% at 1 year from surgery. The treatment of persistent enuresis includes limiting fluid intake after the evening meal, voiding before going to sleep, and timed voiding once or twice during the night. Use of imipramine hydrochloride 25 mg at bedtime is reported to decrease nighttime leakage in up to 25% of patients (El Bahnasawy et al., 2000).

○ **Which is the most common electrolyte abnormality in patients who have an ileal conduit and how often is it found?**

Hyperchloremic metabolic acidosis. It is seen as a late complication in 13% of patients.

○ **What is the mechanism of hyperchloremic acidosis in patients with ileal diversions?**

Ionized transport of ammonium is responsible for hyperchloremic acidosis in patients with ileal diversions. When ammonium substitutes for sodium in the Na/H antiport, NH_4 is coupled with the exchange of bicarbonate for chloride. So, NH_4 is absorbed across the lumen into the blood in exchange for H_2CO_3. In addition, potassium channels in bowel lumen may contribute to ammonium entry to the blood.

○ **What are the symptoms of the electrolyte abnormality that occurs with ileal and colonic diversions?**

Easy fatigability, anorexia, weight loss, polydipsia, and lethargy. Exacerbation of diarrhea is often seen in patients with a ureterosigmoidostomy.

○ **True/False: Normal serum pH and bicarbonate exclude metabolic acidosis in patients with intestinal urinary diversions.**

False. Normal serum pH and bicarbonate do not exclude severely compensated metabolic acidosis, blood gas analysis and body weight measurement are required. If possible, these patients should not be given hydrogen antagonists and/or proton pump inhibitors, because these contribute to systemic acidosis by preventing hydrogen excretion with subsequent bicarbonate preservation on the cellular side (Mills and Studer, 1999).

○ **What is the optimal management of hyperchloremic metabolic acidosis in a patient with intestinal urinary diversion?**

The key to successful management is proper diagnosis by exclusion of urinary infection and sepsis, as well as awareness of the salt-losing syndrome. Proper treatment includes catheter reinsertion to insure good drainage and to minimize further chemical reabsorption, rehydration with intravenous normal saline, and correction of acidosis with sodium bicarbonate at a dose of 1.3 g tid. Potassium citrate may also be used to avoid too high a sodium load and prevent hypokalemia. Patients with incomplete emptying and those with reduced renal function are most vulnerable to these metabolic problems (Racioppi et al., 1999).

○ **What is the consequence of the treatment of metabolic acidosis by $NaHCO_3$ alone?**

Severe hypokalemia. The treatment must involve both correction of the acidosis with bicarbonate and replacement of potassium. Potassium citrate may be helpful.

○ **What is the treatment of persistent hyperchloremic metabolic acidosis in patients with ileal conduits if an excessive sodium load is undesirable?**

It has been shown in animal models that both chlorpromazine and nicotinic acid result in inhibition of cyclic adenosine monophosphate (AMP), which impedes chloride ion transport, so HCO_3 levels increase (Koch and McDougal, 1985). These agents used alone do not correct the acidosis in humans, but they limit its development and thus reduce the need for alkalinizing agents. Chlorpromazine may be given in a dose of 25 mg tid and should be used with care in adults because there are many untoward side effects, including tardive dyskinesia. Nicotinic acid may be given in a dose of 400 mg tid or qid and should not be used in patients with peptic ulcer disease or significant hepatic insufficiency (Dahl and McDougal, 2007).

○ **Which kind of urinary diversion has the highest possibility of hypokalemia?**

Ureterosigmoidostomies. Ileal segments reabsorb some of the potassium when exposed to high concentrations of potassium in the urine whereas colon does not.

○ **What are the causes of hypokalemia in patients with intestinal urinary diversion and what would be the treatment?**

The potassium depletion is probably owing to renal potassium wasting as a consequence of renal damage, osmotic diuresis, and gut loss through intestinal secretion. Treatment with potassium citrate is often effective especially for patients with colonic reservoirs (Koch et al., 1990).

○ **What kinds of electrolyte abnormalities are seen in patients with a jejunal conduit?**

Hyponatremic, hypochloremic, and hyperkalemic metabolic acidosis. Sodium chloride replacement and thiazides are the treatment of choice.

○ **What is the likely diagnosis of a patient with a jejunal conduit who has lethargy, nausea, vomiting, dehydration, muscular weakness, and an elevated temperature?**

Metabolic disturbance. Hyponatremia, hypochloremia, hyperkalemia, azotemia, and acidosis are seen in patients with jejunal conduits.

○ **How effective is IV hyperalimentation for the treatment of the metabolic disturbances in a patient with a jejunal conduit?**

Administering hyperalimentation solutions may exacerbate the syndrome.

○ **Which electrolyte abnormalities are seen when the stomach is used for urinary diversion?**

Hypochloremic, hypokalemic metabolic alkalosis. This is a more significant problem if the patient has concomitant azotemia.

○ **True/False: Hypergastrinemia may occur following gastric pouch orthotopic bladder formation.**

True. Hydrochloric acid produced by the parietal cells in the body of the stomach has a negative feedback on antral gastrin secretion. When the body of the stomach is removed, this negative feedback mechanism may be impaired.

○ **What are the most likely causes of altered sensorium in a patient with a urinary diversion.**

Magnesium deficiency, drug intoxication, hyperammonemia, or diabetic hyperglycemia (this is not a consequence of the intestinal diversion).

○ **What are the causes of magnesium deficiency in patients with intestinal urinary diversion.**

Magnesium deficiency is usually due to nutritional depletion, but it may result from renal wasting, altered calcium metabolism, acidosis, and sulfate metabolism (McDougal and Koch, 1989).

○ **In which type of urinary diversion is altered sensorium most commonly found?**

Ureterosigmoidostomy. It has been reported for those with ileal conduits as well.

○ **True/False: Acute changes in ammonia load result in significant changes in serum ammonia levels when hepatic function is normal.**

False. The hepatic reserve for ammonia clearance is immense, and it is unlikely that acute changes in ammonia loads would result in significant changes in serum ammonia levels when hepatic function is normal. Patients who have ammonia-induced coma accompanied by normal liver functions generally have a significant infection with a urease-producing bacterium. Often, the infection is associated with obstruction of the urinary tract. Direct access of bacteria and endotoxin to the liver via the portal circulation results in altered hepatic metabolism without significant alteration in hepatic enzyme concentrations (McDougal, 1992).

○ **What is the treatment of ammoniagenic coma?**

Draining the urinary intestinal diversion to prevent urine exposure to the intestine for extended periods of time, administration of neomycin to reduce the ammonia load from the enteric tract, and limitation of protein consumption should be done to limit the patient's nitrogen load. In severe cases, arginine glutamate 50 g in 1000 mL of 5% dextrose in water intravenously to complex the ammonia in the gut and to prevent its absorption. Additionally, lactulose may be given orally or per rectum.

○ **True/False: Serum concentrations of urea and creatinine are less accurate measures of renal function after enteric diversion.**

True. Urea and creatinine are reabsorbed by both the ileum and the colon.

○ **What is the most accurate means of determining renal function in patients with a urinary diversion?**

Measurement of renal function with serial serum determination of ^{51}Cr–EDTA after bolus injection is the most accurate method of determining renal function. This agent crosses the intestinal mucosa in negligible quantities.

○ **Which classes of drugs can be problematic in patients with urinary intestinal diversion regarding drug toxicity?**

Drugs that are absorbed by the gastrointestinal tract and excreted unchanged by the kidney. This includes phenytoin, certain antibiotics, and methotrexate.

○ **What is the mechanism of hypocalcemia in intestinal urinary diversion?**

Hypocalcemia is a consequence of depleted body calcium stores and excessive renal wasting. Chronic acidosis is buffered by carbonate in the bone, with subsequent release of calcium into the circulation. The kidneys clear the released calcium, resulting in a gradual decrease in body calcium stores. Renal tubular absorption of calcium is also inhibited directly by sulfate and enhanced by acidosis. Treatment consists of calcium therapy (McDougal and Koch, 1989).

○ **What is the cause of bone demineralization in intestinal urinary diversions and how can it be prevented?**

The cause is complex, but long-term changes in acid–base balance are likely the major contributory factor. Other causes are vitamin D resistance and excessive calcium loss by the kidney. It has been shown in animals with urinary diversions that oral supplementation with bicarbonate can prevent demineralization even in the absence of significant systemic acidosis (Inman et al., 2003). Some institutions now recommend oral sodium bicarbonate at a dose of 1.3 g tid when base deficit is >2.5 mmol/L (Stein et al., 1997).

○ **A patient with urinary diversion has hip pain, lethargy, and proximal myopathy. What is the diagnosis?**

Osteomalacia.

○ **What are the abnormalities in serum chemistry in a patient who develops osteomalacia?**

The calcium is either low or normal, the alkaline phosphatase is elevated, and the phosphate is low or normal.

○ **In a patient with osteomalacia, you've corrected the acidosis and provided dietary calcium. What is the next step?**

1-α-hydroxycholecalciferol (alfacalcidol) should be administered. This is a vitamin D metabolite that is more potent than vitamin D_2.

○ **Loss of which bowel segment may cause vitamin B_{12} and bile salt malabsorption?**

Terminal ileum.

○ **What is the effect of vitamin B_{12} deficiency?**

Vitamin B_{12} deficiency results in macrocytic anemia and neurological degeneration.

○ **What length of time is required for the depletion of vitamin B_{12} stores in the complete absence of absorption in a patient who has an extensive terminal ileum resection?**

Three to four years. Partial malabsorption may take up to 30 years to become clinically manifest.

○ **What are typical neurological manifestations of vitamin B_{12} deficiency?**

Peripheral neuropathy, optic atrophy, subacute combined degeneration of the spinal cord, and dementia.

○ **Loss of which segment of bowel is associated with folic acid malabsorption?**

Jejunum. In addition, malabsorption of fat and calcium may be seen.

○ **True/False: In patients with ileal neobladder, vitamin B_{12} and folic acid levels should be measured on a regular basis starting 2 years after surgery.**

True. According to a recent recommendation by a WHO consensus conference on bladder cancer, vitamin B_{12} and folic acid levels should be routinely measured starting from year 2 after surgery (Hautmann et al., 2007).

○ **What is the lipid profile effect of a patient in whom 60- to 100-cm ileum are removed from the fecal stream?**

Serum cholesterol decreases, while triglycerides increase.

○ **What are the major consequences of lipid malabsorption seen in patients with ileal resection?**

A deficiency of the fat-soluble vitamins (A, D, E, and K) and an increase in incidence of gallstones and renal stones.

○ **In which part of the intestinal segments used for urinary diversion does the least net water movement occur?**

Stomach. It is followed by the colon, ileum, and jejunum, respectively.

○ **What is the most common histologic type of cancer seen in association with urinary intestinal diversion?**

Adenocarcinoma, especially following ureterosigmoidostomy. These patients should be followed by stool occult blood and/or colonoscopy after 5 years postdiversion.

○ **A 27-year-old male with spina bifida undergoes an ileal conduit undiversion. How should the defunctionalized intestinal conduit segment be managed?**

Excision of the segment is appropriate. If left in situ, it has malignant potential.

○ **A patient is diagnosed with a recurrent invasive lesion in the urethra following radical cystectomy and neobladder construction. What is your treatment?**

Urethrectomy. Convert to a continent diversion, if possible, or remove the reservoir and convert to a conduit.

○ **Which kind of neobladder is the most amenable for conversion of a patient to a conduit?**

Studer neobladder. It has a 15- to 20-cm isoperistaltic proximal ileal limb.

○ **What is the preferred method of delivery in pregnant women with intestinal urinary diversion?**

Elective cesarean section before the onset of labor is the preferred method of delivery in patients with urinary diversion, especially with an orthotopic bladder substitution. Vaginal delivery may result in damage to the pelvic floor muscles and subsequently affect continence mechanisms. Cesarean section should be preformed through a high incision. The mesentery of the reservoir is usually pushed away from the gravid uterus. An experienced reconstructive urologist should be involved and have time to review thoroughly the patient's reconstructed anatomy before the case (Hensle et al., 2004).

CHAPTER 21

Urinary Diversion and Undiversion

Christopher L. Coogan, MD, FACS and Michael P. Hoeh, MD

○ **What is the electrolyte abnormality most commonly seen when stomach is used in the urinary tract? What are signs and symptoms that result from these electrolyte disturbances and how is this often treated?**

Hypochloremic metabolic alkalosis. This is secondary to the HCl secretion by the stomach segment, involving the H^+/K^+ ATPase secretory mechanism of the gastric mucosa.

When it is fully manifested, lethargy, respiratory insufficiency, seizures, and ventricular arrhythmias may occur. These manifestations are typically preceded by vomiting resulting in dehydration.

Patients are generally successfully treated with an H_2 blocker to reduce proton secretion by the gastric segment and rehydration. In life-threatening circumstances, arginine hydrochloride infusion has been employed to rapidly restore acid–base balance. When H_2 blockers are ineffective, proton pump inhibitors (PPIs) have been successfully used. In rare cases when PPIs are ineffective and the life-threatening metabolic alkalosis persists, the gastric segment must be removed.

○ **What is the electrolyte abnormality most commonly seen when jejunum is used in the urinary tract?**

Hyponatremic, hypochloremic, and hyperkalemic metabolic acidosis. This has been termed the "jejunal conduit syndrome." These disorders result from an increased secretion of sodium chloride and water leading to dehydration and increased reabsorption of potassium and hydrogen from both the conduit and kidneys (due to increased renin–angiotensin system from hypovolemia). This syndrome can be quite debilitating, resulting in nausea, anorexia, lethargy, fever, and even death. The more proximal the segment used, the more likely the syndrome is to develop, secondary to the increased surface area available, due to increased villi and microvilli. The jejunum should be used only when there are no other acceptable segments available for use.

○ **What is the electrolyte abnormality most commonly seen when ileum or colon is used in the urinary tract? What are signs and symptoms that result from these electrolyte disturbances and how is this often treated?**

Hyperchloremic metabolic acidosis. This is caused by the substitution of ammonium for sodium in the Na/H transport. Therefore, ammonium chloride is absorbed into the bloodstream in exchange for carbonic acid (CO_2 and H_2O).

Common signs and symptoms include easy fatigability, anorexia, polydipsia, and lethargy. Those with ureterosigmoidostomies also may have an exacerbation of diarrhea.

Alkalinization with oral sodium bicarbonate is effective in restoring normal acid–base balance though it may produce significant intestinal gas. Oral citrate may also be used. Chlorpromazine and nicotinic acid inhibit cAMP and thereby impede chloride transport.

○ **What is the cause of the altered sensorium occasionally associated with intestinal conduits?**

Magnesium deficiency, drug intoxication, or abnormalities of ammonia metabolism. This should be treated with drainage of the urinary intestinal diversion (foley or rectal tube), administration of neomycin (to reduce the enteric ammonia load), minimizing protein intake, and treating the underlying condition.

○ **What commonly used drugs can be reabsorbed in intestinal diversions after excretion from the kidneys and result in toxic serum levels?**

Phenytoin, methotrexate, lithium carbonate, and theophylline may be reabsorbed in their original form from intestinal diversions and lead to toxic serum levels.

○ **True/False: Incontinent urinary diversions are generally associated with fewer metabolic abnormalities.**

True. Given the longer dwell time of urine in contact with the intestinal segment used, both neobladders and continent urinary diversions are associated with a higher risk of electrolyte and metabolic abnormalities.

○ **True/False: Mechanical bowel preparation results in a reduction in bacteria per gram of enteric contents.**

False. Mechanical bowel preparation will reduce the total number of bacteria in the gut, but not their concentration.

○ **Which portion of the small intestine is typically used for ileal conduit formation?**

An ileal segment is selected 10 to 15 cm from the ileocecal valve, which is usually 20–25 cm in length.

○ **Which portions of the small intestine should one avoid using for diversion in patients with history of pelvic radiation?**

The last 2 inches of the terminal ileum, which is often fixed in the pelvis by ligamentous attachments, and the 5 feet of small bowel beginning approximately 6 feet from the ligament of Treitz, the mesentery of which is the longest of the entire small bowel. As such, this portion of the small bowel can descend into the pelvis.

○ **What is the most common stomal complication following urinary diversion?**

Stomal stenosis. The incidence is reported to be 20% to 24% for ileal conduits and 10% to 20% for colon conduits. Other complications include bleeding, bowel necrosis, dermatitis, parastomal hernias, and stomal prolapse.

○ **Which segment of bowel is most suitable for nonrefluxing ureterointestinal anastomoses?**

Colon. Numerous anastomoses (Leadbetter and Clarke, Goodwin, Strickler, and Pagano) employ the seromuscular strength of the tenia to create a backing for the submucosal tunnel needed for the antireflux procedure.

○ **What type of ureteroileal anastomosis carries the highest risk of ureteral stricture?**

Antirefluxing ureteroileal anastomosis. In general, antirefluxing anastomoses carry a higher risk of stricture that persists for the life of the conduit. Although open and endourological methods of repair have been successful, open repair carries a higher success rate (approximately 75% vs 60% for endourological methods).

○   **What is the most common site of ureteral stricture after ileal conduit formation not at the ureteroileal anastomosis?**

The left ureter as it crosses over the aorta. As the left ureter crosses over the aorta and underneath the inferior mesenteric artery, it is both extrinsically compressed and angulated, which may result in stricture formation. In addition, aggressive stripping of the periureteral adventitia may result in vascular compromise at this level, also predisposing to stricture.

○   **Briefly describe the Bricker ureterointestinal anastomosis.**

The Bricker anastomosis is a refluxing end-to-side anastomosis. It involves spatulating the distal end of the ureter, and stitching the full thickness of the bowel to the full thickness of the ureter. This anastomosis boasts both technical ease as well as a low complication rate (see the figure).

○   **Briefly describe the Wallace ureterointestinal anastomosis.**

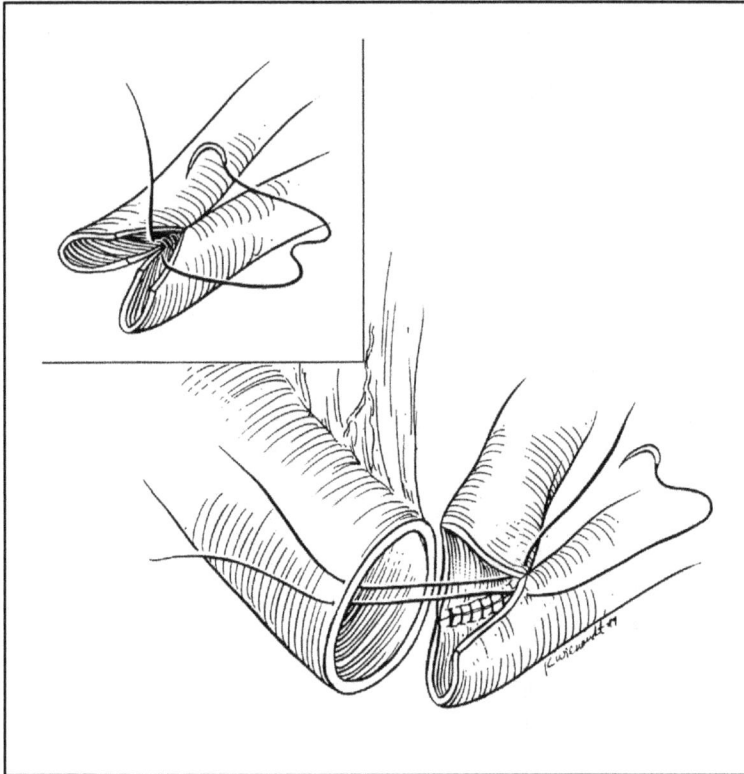

The Wallace anastomosis is a refluxing end-to-end anastomosis. Different techniques are described, but the concept is that the ureteral ends are spatulated and sewn together into a common opening. This "common ureter" is then anastomosed to the end of the intestinal segment used. It has a lower stricture rate due to the wide anastomosis, but is not recommended for patients with extensive carcinoma in situ or a high likelihood of recurrence in the ureter. Recurrence in the distal aspect of one ureter could block the egress of both ureters, causing bilateral obstruction (see the figure).

○   **What is the generally accepted cut-off value of serum creatinine at which continent diversions and orthotopic neobladders are no longer considered?**

2.0 mg/dL. Due to the extended dwell time of urine in contact with the intestinal segments used, continent diversions and orthotopic neobladders should be considered only for those patients with good renal function.

○   **What renal parameters must be met to consider continent diversion in a patient with serum creatinine greater than 2.0 mg/dL?**

Urine pH 5.8 or less after ammonium chloride load, urine osmolality of 600 mOsm/kg or greater with water deprivation, glomerular filtration rate (GFR) greater than or equal to 35 mL/min, and minimal protein in the urine.

○ **What percent of patients with normal preoperative creatinine and GFR who undergo conduit diversion develop renal deterioration?**

Approximately 18% of patients with ileal conduit diversion will have progressive renal deterioration, which may lead to death from renal failure in approximately 6% of patients. 13% of patients with nonrefluxing colon conduits will show progressive deterioration.

○ **What long-term effects can urinary intestinal diversion have on the bony skeleton?**

Osteomalacia. Osteomalacia (or renal rickets) has been reported most commonly with ureterosigmoidostomy, but also with colon and ileal conduits, and ileal ureters. It is thought to be secondary to acidosis, vitamin D resistance, and excessive calcium loss by the kidney.

○ **What type of reservoir requires nocturnal emptying?**

Ureterosigmoidostomy. Although all continent reservoirs may require nocturnal emptying to prevent overdistention, the increased risk of metabolic acidosis from ionized transport of ammonium via the Na^+/H^+ antiport in ureterosigmoidostomy necessitates nocturnal emptying.

○ **True/False: Approximately 75% of urine specimens from ileal conduits are infected.**

True. Intestine, in contrast to urothelium, generally lives symbiotically with bacterial flora. Most patients have no sequelae from their chronic bacteriuria, and are not treated unless they develop symptoms.

○ **What bacterial infections from conduits or continent diversions should be treated?**

Cultures dominantly positive for *Proteus*, *Pseudomonas*, or *Klebsiella* species should be treated. *Proteus* and *Pseudomonas* infections have been linked to upper tract deterioration, and all 3 organisms are urea-splitting, making patients infected with these organisms more likely to form stones.

○ **What is the urinary diversion procedure that puts the patient at the highest risk for development of carcinoma of the intestinal segment?**

Ureterosigmoidostomy. Following ureterosigmoidostomy, as many as 40% of patients will develop tumors at the ureterosigmoid anastomosis given sufficient time. About half of the tumors are adenocarcinoma and the rest are benign polyps. The mean latency period between ureterosigmoidostomy and the diagnosis of tumor is 26 years.

○ **If performing undiversion following ureterosigmoidostomy, what must be done to minimize the risk of tumorigenesis?**

The distal ureteral stumps must be removed from contact with the colonic epithelium. Adenocarcinoma has been reported to occur when the ureterointestinal anastomoses were left in situ, even when the diversion is defunctionalized.

○ **Briefly describe the Mitrofanoff procedure.**

The Mitrofanoff procedure is the creation of a continent, catheterizable urinary diversion. It is usually performed with the appendix, which is anastomosed to the conduit (or bladder) in a tunneled fashion (similar to a ureteroneocystostomy). The other end of the appendix is brought out to the anterior abdominal wall, and is utilized for clean intermittent catheterization.

○   **In patients who have received extensive pelvic radiation, which intestinal segment is preferred for creation of a conduit?**

The transverse colon. Given its position within the abdominal cavity, it is the most likely unaffected by previous pelvic radiation.

○   **What is the blood supply of the appendix?**

The appendiceal artery, a branch usually off of the ileocolic artery, which arises from the superior mesenteric artery.

○   **What is the source of continence for orthotopic neobladders?**

In both the male and female, the preserved striated external sphincter is the source of continence. Daytime continence rates of greater than 95% can be expected if this mechanism is surgically spared.

○   **What are the 2 phenomena thought to be responsible for nocturnal enuresis following orthotopic neobladder procedures?**

First, the spinal reflex arc that recruits external sphincter contraction is gone, as the native bladder (and therefore the afferent nerves) has been removed. The other hypothesis is that there is a significant re-absorption and re-circulation of urinary constituents and metabolites that stimulate increased urinary volume, resulting in nocturnal enuresis.

○   **Briefly describe the ureterointestinal anastomosis described by Studer and colleagues.**

The Studer ileal neobladder incorporates a novel approach to prevent reflux. The proximal limb of small bowel is left intact for a length of 20 to 25 cm, and the neobladder is constructed from the distal 35 to 40 cm of ileum. The ureters are then anastomosed to the intact proximal limb in a standard (Bricker) ureterointestinal refluxing anastomosis. This proximal limb of ileum retains its peristaltic integrity, effectively dampening back-pressure on the upper urinary tract (see the figure).

○ **What tumor location in women is a contraindication to orthotopic neobladder formation after radical cystectomy?**

Bladder neck involvement. Patients with bladder neck involvement often have involvement of the anterior vaginal wall, and orthotopic neobladder formation could compromise the margins of resection.

○ **What tumor location in men is a relative contraindication to orthotopic neobladder formation after radical cystectomy?**

The prostatic urethral stroma. In a multivariate analysis, any prostate tumor involvement (superficial or invasive) is an independent and significant predictor of a urethral tumor recurrence. Carcinoma in situ and tumor multifocality are not individually associated with a significant risk for anterior urethral recurrence.

Patients with documented prostatic mucosal, ductal, or stromal invasion should be counseled about the increased risk of urethral recurrence if the urethra is left in situ and to help them weigh that risk against any perceived advantage of an orthotopic diversion. If an orthotopic diversion is still preferred, the intraoperative frozen section of the urethral margin should be used to make the final decision.

○ **What are the 4 basic methods of achieving continence in a urinary diversion?**

The Mitrofanoff principle, the ileocecal valve, the nipple valve, and the hydraulic valve.

○ **What is the continence mechanism in an Indiana pouch?**

The buttressed ileocecal valve. Neourethral pressure profiles show that the continence zone is confined only to the area of the ileocecal valve, rendering imbricating sutures necessary only for this area.

○ **True/False: The appendix is removed during formation of the Indiana pouch?**

True. The buttressed ileocecal valve is the continence mechanism of the Indiana pouch. The appendix is removed, as it may serve as a nidus for infection and abscess formation.

○   **Describe the Benchekroun hydraulic ileal valve.**

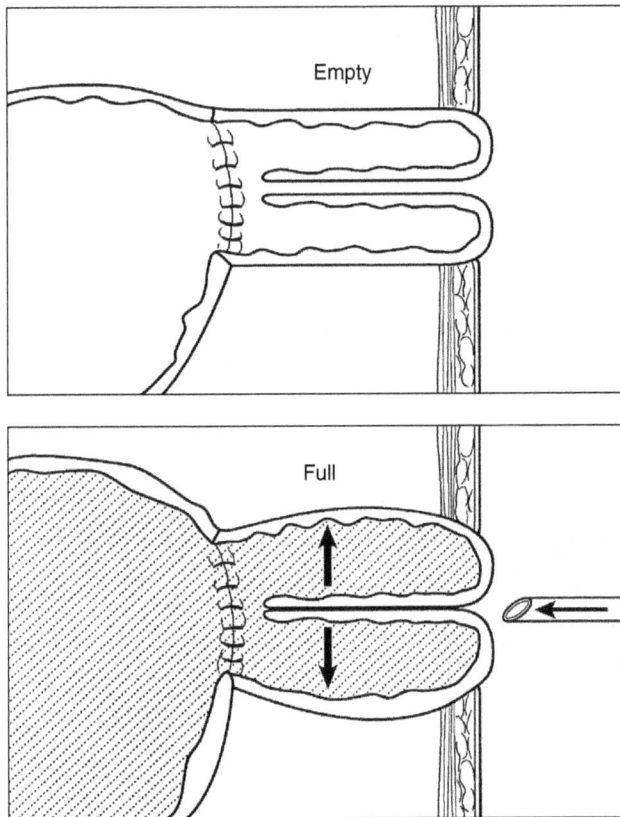

12 to 14 cm of ileum is selected, and reverse intussusception is performed, such that serosa covers the entire segment and mucosa apposes mucosa. The ends are then sutured in position, allowing space between sutures to allow the mucosal surface to fill with urine as pouch pressures increase. The blunt serosal end is secured to the abdominal wall, and catheterization is done so that the catheter passes through a serosally lined channel into the conduit. When pressures rise in the conduit, urine flows into the mucosal space of the valve, coapting the serosal surface, ensuring continence (see the figure).

○   **What is the most common complication of the Benchekroun hydraulic ileal valve?**

Stomal stenosis. Stomal stenosis requiring surgical revision has been reported in up to 73% of patients undergoing this procedure. Devagination of the valve is another complication, with a reported incidence of up to 36%.

○   **What is the "pipe stem" deformity of the ileal conduit, and what is the cause?**

The "pipe stem" deformity of an ileal conduit is the radiographic appearance on loopogram of strictured areas along the course of the loop. This results in a thin, noncompliant loop with decreased peristalsis and propulsion of urine with subsequent deterioration of the upper urinary tracts. The cause is vascular insufficiency. Treatment usually requires replacement of the entire loop.

○ **What is the incidence of stones in patients with ileal conduits?**

Approximately 20%. The etiology of stone formation is multifactorial. Staples and nonabsorbable sutures may act as a nidus for stone formation. There is an increased incidence of bacteriuria following intestinal diversion, which may also cause stone formation.

○ **True/False: Patients with continent diversions are at increased risk of reservoir stones.**

True. This is secondary to the increased urinary excretion of calcium, magnesium, and phosphate in continent diversions as compared to ileal conduits. Also, patients with long segments of ileum used for reconstruction (continent diversions and orthotopic neobladders) may have secondary hyperoxaluria.

○ **What is "pouchitis"?**

Pouchitis is a condition described in continent urinary diversions that is manifested by pain in the region of the pouch and increased pouch contractility. This may result in temporary failure of the continence mechanism. Antibiotic treatment usually results in resolution of these symptoms.

○ **What is the continence mechanism of the Kock pouch?**

The surgical principle used in achieving continence by the Kock pouch is the intussuscepted nipple valve. This surgical procedure is felt to be the most technically difficult to perform of all of the continence mechanisms.

○ **What are the most common complications of the Kock pouch?**

Nipple failure resulting in loss of continence is the most common complication following Kock pouch formation. This can be expected in 10% to 15% of cases even in the hands of the most experienced surgeons.

○ **What is the continence mechanism of the Penn pouch?**

The Mitrofanoff principle. The Penn pouch was the first conduit to utilize the Mitrofanoff principle, using the appendix tunneled into the tenia of the ascending colon.

○ **What is a potential drawback to the use of the appendix as a continence mechanism?**

The appendix has a small luminal diameter, allowing catheterization only with a 12 or 14 Fr coudé catheter. Since intestinal reservoirs produce large amounts of mucus, this often makes irrigation and emptying difficult. Also, the appendix may be surgically absent or of insufficient length for use.

○ **What are the contraindications to ureterosigmoidostomy?**

Hydronephrosis, pelvic radiation, neurogenic bladder, renal, or hepatic dysfunction. Dilated upper tracts are more subject to reflux and obstruction, which can be deleterious to renal function. Previous pelvic radiation will likely involve both the sigmoid and the pelvic ureters. Patients with neurogenic bladder usually have associated functional bowel abnormalities as well. Renal insufficiency is a contraindication to any continent diversion. Patients with hepatic dysfunction should not undergo ureterosigmoidostomy because of the risk of ammonia intoxication.

○   **What is essential in the preoperative evaluation of patients selected for rectal bladder urinary diversion or ureterosigmoidostomy?**

Anal sphincter integrity testing. Patients should be required to retain an enema solution of liquid and solid material in an upright and ambulatory position without soilage for a specified amount of time. Some investigators recommend a 500-mL mixture of thin oatmeal that the patient is asked to retain for 1 hour.

○   **Which patients should undergo routine urinary cytology after continent urinary diversion?**

All patients undergoing continent diversion. Malignancy has been reported in all bowel segments exposed to urine. Thus, urinary cytology should be monitored in all patients undergoing continent diversion regardless of whether or not diversion was performed for a malignant condition.

○   **Which patients should undergo routine colonoscopy after continent urinary diversion?**

All patients whose urine and fecal streams are mixed. In addition to routine cytology in all patients whose urine stream is diverted via an intestinal segment, patients whose urine and fecal streams are mixed should undergo routine colonoscopy to evaluate for intestinal malignancies.

○   **True/False: Renal insufficiency is a contraindication to urinary undiversion.**

False. Many candidates for undiversion will likely have renal insufficiency, either secondary to their underlying pathology or the diversion itself. If transplantation becomes necessary in these patients, it is better done into a functioning lower urinary tract than a urinary diversion.

○   **With what intestinal segment is the "hematuria-dysuria" syndrome associated?**

Stomach. Following gastrocystoplasty, the urine is markedly acidic, which can lead to bladder pain, dysuria, and hematuria, and skin erosion in approximately 30% of patients.

○   **What is the gastrointestinal consequence of the loss of the ileocecal valve?**

In the short-term, this results in frequent bowel movements and diarrhea. Most patients recover bowel regularity following intestinal adaptation or pharmacologic therapy, but some patients have steatorrhea or diarrhea refractory to medical management following loss of the ileocecal valve.

○   **True/False: Refluxing ureterointestinal anastomoses have a higher incidence of renal deterioration than nonrefluxing anastomoses following conduit formation in patients with normal ureters.**

False. In patients with normal peristaltic contractions of the ureter, there does not seem to be detrimental pressure transmission to the renal pelvis in patients with refluxing anastomoses. Additionally, the presence of nonrefluxing anastomoses does not prevent bacterial colonization of the renal pelvis.

○   **What are the contraindications to ileal conduit formation?**

The contraindications to ileal conduits are short bowel syndrome, inflammatory disease of the small intestine, and previous radiation to the pelvis.

○ **What type of continent diversion has the smallest immediate postoperative capacity?**

Ileal pouches. Ileal pouches (eg, Kock or T-pouches) have immediate postoperative volumes of approximately 150 mL. In contrast, right colon pouches routinely have immediate postoperative capacity of approximately 300 mL. This information is essential for patients to catheterize themselves with appropriate frequency during the initial postoperative period.

○ **What is the most common composition of stones formed in urinary diversions?**

The stones are usually of mixed composition, and may be made up of struvite, calcium oxalate, calcium phosphate, and uric acid. Foreign materials may act as a nidus for stone formation within the diversion.

○ **What is the most common type of continent reservoir to form stones?**

The Kock pouch. Another complication of the Kock pouch that is unique is the higher incidence of stones, secondary to the use of staples on the intussuscepted nipple valve.

CHAPTER 22 Male Infertility

Howard H. Kim, MD, Akanksha Mehta, MD, and Marc Goldstein, MD, DSc (Hon), FACS

NUMBERS TO REMEMBER

○ **What are the WHO reference values for count, concentration, motility, and morphology on semen analysis?**

According to the recently revised WHO reference values (2010), a total sperm count ≥39 million per ejaculate, sperm concentration ≥15 million/mL, motility ≥40%, progressive motility ≥32%, and 4% or more normal forms define the lower limits for normal fertility.

○ **What percentage of couples are infertile, and how often is a male factor present?**

Fifteen percent of couples are infertile. A male factor is present in 50% of cases.

○ **What percentage of infertile men have varicoceles?**

30% to 45%.

○ **What percentage of infertile men have no known cause for their infertility even after a thorough workup?**

25% to 30%.

○ **What percentage of infertile men have azoospermia, including obstructive or nonobstructive azoospermia?**

Azoospermia is present in approximately 1% of the general male population, and in up to 10% to 15% of infertile men. Obstruction accounts for 40% of all cases of azoospermia, with the remaining 60% having a nonobstructive etiology.

○ **What percentage of infertile men have chromosomal abnormalities?**

6% to 7%.

○ **What is the most common chromosomal abnormality in men?**

Klinefelter syndrome (1 in 500 men).

○ **What percentage of men with nonobstructive azoospermia have Y chromosome microdeletions?**

Up to 13% of men with azoospermia have Y chromosome microdeletions.

○ **What are the indications for performing a karyotype or Y chromosome microdeletion analysis?**

A karyotype analysis in indicated in men with sperm concentration below 10 million/mL. Men with sperm concentration below 5 million/mL should undergo Y chromosome microdeletion testing in addition to karyotype analysis.

○ **What percentage of men with unilateral and bilateral cryptorchidism have oligozoospermia on semen analysis?**

Thirty percent of men with unilateral cryptorchidism, and 50% of men with bilateral cryptorchidism have oligozoospermia on semen analysis.

○ **A couple has one 4-year-old child and is now having difficulty conceiving again. The male partner has oligoasthenozoospermia and normal hormonal testing. What abnormality can be expected on physical examination?**

A varicocele is found in up to 80% of men with secondary infertility. Varicoceles have been shown to cause progressive worsening of semen parameters.

○ **What percentage of patients undergoing varicocelectomy for infertility can expect to have improvement in semen parameters, and which parameters are most often improved?**

Approximately 70% of patients have improvement in semen parameters after varicocelectomy. Sperm motility is most often improved followed by count and then morphology.

○ **What is the live birth rate for in vitro fertilization (IVF) with intracytoplasmic sperm injection (ICSI) for male factor infertility?**

Approximately 30% to 40% per cycle.

○ **What is the most important predictor of IVF/ICSI outcomes?**

Age of the female partner.

○ **What percentage of men develop significant antisperm antibodies after vasectomy?**

60%.

○ **What percentage of men who have undergone vasectomy eventually seek reversal?**

6% to 10%.

ANATOMY AND PHYSIOLOGY

○ **The pituitary hormones follicle stimulating hormone (FSH) and luteinizing hormone (LH) act on which cells in the testis and what are the specific mediators of feedback inhibition from these cells to the pituitary gland?**

FSH acts on the Sertoli cell to promote spermatogenesis, while LH acts on Leydig cells to stimulate testosterone production. Inhibin, produced by Sertoli cells, provides negative feedback at the pituitary level to inhibit FSH production. Estradiol and testosterone provide negative feedback at the hypothalamic and pituitary levels to inhibit LH production.

○ **Which cells in the testis form the blood–testis barrier and exclude sperm from recognition by the immune system?**

Tight junctional complexes between adjacent Sertoli cells create the blood–testis barrier making the seminiferous tubule an immunologically privileged site.

○ **Autonomic innervation of the testis is provided by which nerve or nerves?**

The superior spermatic nerve and the inferior spermatic nerve.

○ **A germ cell undergoes how many meiotic divisions before producing a mature sperm?**

Germ cells undergo mitotic division to produce numerous primary spermatocytes, which then undergo meiosis I to secondary spermatocytes (2N), and meiosis II to produce spermatids (1N).

○ **Aside from sperm transportation, what is the most important function of the epididymis?**

Sperm maturation occurs along the length of the epididymis, resulting in mature sperm capable of fertilizing oocytes.

○ **What role does prostate-specific antigen (PSA) play in male fertility?**

The protein secreted by prostatic epithelium is a protease enzyme involved in semen liquefaction.

○ **Which substance produced in the seminal vesicle is the major energy source for sperm metabolism?**
Fructose.

○ **What is the role of the acrosome and where is it located?**

The acrosome forms a cap on the sperm head and contains the enzymes necessary for drilling into the zona pellucida of the oocyte.

○ **Do the testis, epididymis, and vas deferens share the same embryological origin?**

No. The testis develops from coelomic epithelium of the genital ridge and underlying mesenchyme. Primordial germ cells migrate to this area. The epididymis and vas deferens, however, develop from the Wolffian (mesonephric) duct.

○ **What is the normal adult testicular size?**

Testes measure 15 to 25 cm³ in volume and 4.5 to 5 cm in longitudinal length in young healthy men. A length of less than 4 cm is considered abnormal.

○ **When evaluating the ejaculatory ducts by transrectal ultrasound (TRUS), what is their normal size?**

They are usually 2- to 8-mm wide and 2- to 3-cm long.

○ **In performing a subinguinal varicocelectomy, the internal spermatic artery is inadvertently ligated and divided. By what blood supply might the testis still survive?**

The deferential artery and the cremasteric artery also supply blood flow to the testis.

○ **A patient develops retrograde ejaculation after retroperitoneal lymph node dissection (RPLND) for testis cancer. Which nerves were likely injured and which class of medications may be used to treat the problem?**

Thoracolumbar sympathetic nerves control closure of the bladder neck during seminal emission via norepinephrine. Alpha-adrenergic agonist drugs have been used to stimulate closure of the bladder neck.

○ **Prolactin release is restricted by what natural chemical?**

Dopamine (from the hypothalamus) inhibits the release of prolactin. Dopamine agonists (cabergoline, bromocriptine, etc) are the treatment of choice for prolactinomas.

○ **What is the effect of thyrotropin-releasing hormone and vasoactive intestinal peptide on prolactin secretion?**

They stimulate prolactin release.

○ **What is the total length of the seminiferous tubules of a normal testis?**

250 m. Seminiferous tubules also comprise 85% of total testicular volume.

○ **At what age do men lose 50% of their Sertoli and Leydig cells?**

Age 50 for Sertoli cells and age 60 for Leydig cells.

○ **What are the glands of Littre?**

Another name for the periurethral glands.

○ **What is the average length of the vas deferens?**

The average length is 30 to 35 cm.

○ **What is the origin of the deferential artery?**

The internal iliac (hypogastric) artery or its branches, the superior or inferior vesicle artery.

○ **Blood entering the testis is 2°C to 4°C lower than rectal (body) temperature as a result of what mechanism?**

Countercurrent heat exchange system of the testicular vasculature.

DIAGNOSIS

○ **What physical finding is most predictive of active sperm production in the testis?**

Testicular size and consistency.

○ **What is the most common finding, on physical examination, which is suggestive of infertility in men?**

Varicocele.

○ **A patient presents with azoospermia, low ejaculatory volume, and a semen pH of 6.5. Postejaculation urine is negative for sperm. The vasa deferentia are palpable. What is the next test that should be performed and what is the most likely diagnosis?**

Transrectal ultrasound of the prostate should be performed to rule out ejaculatory duct obstruction.

○ **When is a testis biopsy indicated in men with azoospermia?**

Normal serum FSH level, normal testicular volume, palpable vasa on physical examination, and a negative serum antisperm antibody assay.

○ **Men with nonobstructive azoospermia can have DNA microdeletions in which genes on which chromosome?**

The AZF (AZoospermia Factor) genes on the Y chromosome.

○ **Which AZF deletion has the best prognosis for successful testicular sperm extraction in men with nonobstructive azoospermia?**

AZFc. Men with complete AZFa or AZFb deletions have never had sperm successfully retrieved from their testes.

○ **Men with congenital absence of the vas deferens (CAVD) can have mutations in which gene?**

The cystic fibrosis transmembrane conductance regulator (CFTR) gene on the long arm of chromosome 7. Men with bilateral CAVD are presumed to be carriers for at least one cystic fibrosis mutation.

○ **A patient is found to have unilateral CAVD. The presence of which organ needs to be confirmed?**

The ipsilateral kidney may be absent due to lack of development of the mesonephric duct.

○ **A patient with primary infertility is found to have a normal sperm count, but zero motility. Viability staining shows that the sperms are alive. Semen culture and antisperm antibody testing are negative. Which syndrome or disease should be suspected?**

Immotile cilia syndrome. If the patient also has chronic sinusitis, bronchiectasis, and situs inversus, he has Kartagener's syndrome.

○   **A patient seen for infertility complains of a new onset right varicocele. What pathological entity should be suspected?**

An imaging study should be obtained to rule out a right-sided retroperitoneal mass.

○   **A patient with Klinefelter syndrome has a small number of sperm in his ejaculate. What would his karyotype most likely reveal?**

46,XY/47,XXY mosaic.

○   **A patient with azoospermia has extremely small testicular size (6 cm³ volume) and an FSH of 26. What is the most likely diagnosis?**

Primary testicular failure or hypergonadotropic hypogonadism, leading to nonobstructive azoospermia.

○   **A patient with a history of unilateral testicular torsion presents with primary infertility. A semen analysis reveals normal volume and count, but significantly low motility, and sperm agglutination. There is no evidence of infection. What condition should be suspected?**

Antisperm antibodies should be suspected in a patient with the above-noted semen parameters and a history of either torsion, cryptorchidism, infection, obstruction, or trauma.

○   **A patient presents with primary infertility. On examination, he has normal male secondary sex characteristics and slightly decreased testicular size. Semen analysis reveals normal volume and pH, but azoospermia. FSH is slightly elevated; LH and testosterone are normal. What are the most likely histologic findings on testis biopsy?**

The 3 most likely histologic findings are (i) germ cell aplasia, (ii) Sertoli cell-only syndrome, in which the seminiferous tubules are lined by Sertoli cells but no germ cells are present, and (iii) maturation arrest, in which germ cells are present but do not progress to mature spermatozoa.

○   **A patient with azoospermia is found to have very low levels of FSH, LH, and testosterone. He also reports anosmia. What is the diagnosis?**

This patient with hypogonadotropic hypogonadism has Kallmann syndrome. Differential diagnosis (especially in the absence of anosmia) would include prolactinoma.

○   **A patient with primary infertility reports having had the mumps at age 6. Is this a clinically significant factor in his infertility?**

No. Prepubertal mumps does not appear to affect the testis while postpubertal mumps orchitis can result in significant testicular damage and atrophy.

○   **A bodybuilder who abuses anabolic steroids presents with azoospermia. What is the mechanism for this failure of sperm production, and is it reversible?**

Exogenous androgenic steroids suppress gonadotropin secretion and interfere with spermatogenesis. This form of hypogonadism is usually reversible after discontinuation of steroid use, but in some cases it is permanent.

○ **A tall, thin patient presents for infertility evaluation. He is found to have gynecomastia. What is the most likely underlying cause for his condition? What will his testicular examination reveal and what will his semen analysis show?**

This patient probably has Klinefelter syndrome. He will therefore have small, firm testes on physical exam and azoospermia on semen analysis. His karyotype of 47,XXY results from nondisjunction of the meiotic chromosomes of the gametes of either parent.

○ **Do men with Klinefelter syndrome have a worse prognosis with microsurgical testicular sperm extraction and ICSI compared to men with nonobstructive azoospermia and normal karyotypes?**

Although the fertilization rate was lower for men with Klinefelter syndrome, sperm recovery and pregnancy rates were similar.

○ **What commonly inhaled controlled substance is associated with infertility, and by what mechanism?**

Marijuana can lead to a decrease in sperm concentration, motility, and abnormal morphology as well as decreased serum testosterone levels and gynecomastia. The drug alters the hypothalamic–pituitary–gonadal axis.

○ **How long does the process of spermatogenesis take? How long does it take for mature sperm to appear in the ejaculate?**

It takes 74 days for spermatozoa to develop from a primitive germ cell or spermatogonia. Including ductal transit time, the time from spermatogenesis to ejaculation is approximately 3 months.

○ **A 13-year-old boy is found to a have a grade II left-sided varicocele on a school sports physical examination. His testes are of equal, normal size, and consistency. Gonadotropin releasing hormone (GnRH) stimulation test reveals a normal LH and FSH response. Would you recommend elective varicocelectomy at this time?**

Fifteen percent of all males have a varicocele and only a small percentage of these men will have difficulties with fertility. With no evidence of decreased testicular volume and no exaggerated FSH release in response to GnRH, elective surgery would not be indicated at this time.

○ **A patient with primary infertility is found to have increased numbers of WBCs in the semen. What is this called and what are the possible causes? What needs to be tested for? Can seminal WBCs have an adverse affect on sperm function?**

Pyospermia (or leukocytospermia) may be due to either a genital tract infection or an inflammatory immunologic response. Cultures to rule out urinary and genital tract infection should be performed. The etiology may never be determined and pyospermia can resolve without specific treatment. Antibiotic therapy is indicated if there is a history of sexually transmitted infections. Increased ejaculation is sometimes suggested. Seminal WBCs can produce reactive oxygen species (ROS) that adversely affect sperm function.

○ **How does testicular radiation exposure lead to infertility? How long after radiation therapy can it take for spermatogenesis to recover? How long after gonadal exposure to radiation should a patient wait before trying to conceive?**

Ionizing radiation is lethal to sperm because it increases free radical formation. It also alters sperm head morphology and damages sperm chromatin structure. It can take up to 5 years for spermatogenesis to recover. Direct effects on DNA can result in numerical and structural chromosomal abnormalities; therefore, conception should ideally be avoided for 2 years following therapy.

○   **Describe the underlying cause of male infertility in Prader–Willi syndrome and Laurence–Moon–Biedl syndrome.**

Both cause hypogonadotropic hypogonadism.

○   **What causes a fertile eunuch, and how is this condition treated?**

The "fertile eunuch syndrome" is due to isolated LH deficiency. FSH is usually normal. Physical examination findings include large testes, low ejaculate volumes, and eunuchoid body habitus. Treatment is human chorionic gonadotropin (hCG) therapy.

○   **When is transrectal ultrasound used in the evaluation of male infertility?**

Men with azoospermia or severe oligozoospermia, palpable vasa deferentia, and low semen volume should undergo TRUS to rule out ejaculatory duct obstruction. Midline cysts or dilation of the seminal vesicles on TRUS are indicative of ejaculatory duct obstruction. Sperm aspirated from dilated seminal vesicles using TRUS guidance can be used for assisted reproduction.

○   **A 15-year-old boy is referred to you with a grade III left varicocele, an 18-cm^3 volume right testis, and a 12-cm^3 volume left testis. What do you recommend?**

Left varicocelectomy. Grade III varicoceles are found in 20% of all men with varicoceles (3% of postpubertal boys) and pose the greatest risk for future infertility. Catch-up growth occurs in 80% of boys after varicocele repair.

○   **Which test should be performed on the female partner of a man with CAVD?**

Screening for cystic fibrosis CFTR gene mutations.

○   **Men with obstructive azoospermia usually have what blood abnormality?**

Circulating antisperm antibodies.

○   **A low serum testosterone level is most often associated with what subjective/clinical disorder?**

Decreased libido.

○   **What are the prognostic indicators for a successful pregnancy after a vasectomy reversal?**

Prognostic indicators include (i) partner age and fertility status, (ii) presence or absence of sperm granuloma, and (iii) duration of obstruction. Shorter duration of obstruction and presence of a sperm granuloma are favorable factors.

SEMEN ANALYSIS AND LABORATORY ASSAYS

○   **Using Kruger strict criteria, what is the clinically significant threshold of normal forms that predicts good fertilization without ICSI?**

4%.

○   **Define oligozoospermia.**

Less than 15 million sperm per mL.

○ **What morphologic semen characteristics comprise the "stress pattern" often seen in patients with a varicocele?**

Increased numbers of sperm with tapered heads, immature germ cells, and amorphous sperm cells.

○ **The laboratory reports an increased number of round cells on semen analysis. What do these cells represent?**

Round cells are either prematurely released immature germ cells or white blood cells representing inflammation or infection. Immunohistochemical staining and the Endtz test can distinguish between the two.

○ **A patient is found to have a normal sperm count and zero motility. Which 2 laboratory tests can help distinguish between immotile and dead sperm?**

The hypoosmotic swelling test and the viability staining can be used to differentiate between immotile and dead sperm. Living sperm experience bulging of the plasma membrane and curling of the tails from fluid absorption under hypoosmotic conditions. In traditional viability staining tests, washed sperm are exposed to dyes, which are taken up by dead but not live cells. Both these tests reflect the integrity of the plasma membrane in living versus dead sperm.

○ **What semen parameters suggest the eventual need for ICSI?**

Less than 5% motility, less than 4% normal morphology, and less than 2 million sperm per mL suggest the need for ICSI. Patients with sperm extracted directly from the epididymis or testis proceed directly to ICSI.

○ **How much binding in an immunobead test would be considered a positive test for antisperm antibodies?**

More than 15% to 20%.

○ **What is CASA?**

Computer **A**ided **S**emen **A**nalysis. It is quite labor intensive and expensive. Also, it is less useful with very low or very high counts. It is most useful as a research tool.

TREATMENT

○ **A patient is undergoing a vasectomy reversal. Fluid expressed from the proximal end of the vas is thick and pasty and no sperm are seen on microscopy. What is the next step the surgeon should undertake?**

Perform a vasoepididymostomy instead of a vasovasostomy.

○ **An azoospermic patient who had a hernia repair as a child resulting in obstruction of the inguinal vas deferens and a normal ipsilateral testis has an atrophic opposite testis with a normal vas deferens. What surgical procedure may restore sperm to the ejaculate?**

A crossover vasovasostomy or vasoepididymostomy.

○ **An azoospermic patient who previously underwent surgery for a pituitary tumor is found to have undetectable levels of FSH and LH. What form of therapy may restore spermatogenesis?**

Treatment with intramuscular hCG and recombinant FSH can replace absent LH and FSH, and initiate spermatogenesis.

○ **A patient with azoospermia is found on transrectal ultrasound of the prostate to have a midline cystic structure causing dilation of the ejaculatory ducts and seminal vesicles. What is the origin of this structure and what procedure may restore sperm in the ejaculate?**

The cyst is likely a Mullerian duct remnant. Transurethral resection of the ejaculatory ducts (TURED) may unroof the obstructing cyst and allow sperm to be present in the semen.

○ **A patient with neuropathy secondary to diabetes mellitus develops anejaculation. If he fails sympathomimetic oral therapy, what is the next option to obtain sperm?**

Electroejaculation. If unsuccessful, then microsurgical vasal or epididymal sperm aspiration may be considered, to obtain sperm for use with IVF.

○ **A patient with azoospermia and bilateral varicoceles underwent a testicular biopsy that revealed late maturation arrest. What treatment option may result in the appearance of sperm in the ejaculate?**

Bilateral varicocelectomy has been reported to reverse late maturation arrest in some cases, resulting in completion of spermatogenesis and appearance of adequate sperm in the ejaculate to allow for IVF/ICSI.

○ **A couple presents with primary infertility. The male partner has normal semen parameters. The female partner's evaluation is also negative. A postcoital test on 2 occasions, however, reveals no sperm in the cervical mucus. What assisted reproductive procedure may increase this couple's chance of conceiving?**

Intrauterine insemination (IUI) is a useful form of treatment for bypassing cervical female factor infertility.

○ **A patient with primary infertility and oligoasthenoteratozoospermia has low normal levels of FSH, LH, and testosterone. What form of empirical medical therapy may help improve his semen parameters?**

Clomiphene citrate (Clomid) has been used in these cases. While most patients experience an increase in FSH, LH, and testosterone, only a small subset of patients will achieve an improvement in semen parameters.

○ **A paraplegic with a cervical spinal cord injury has anejaculation. What is the preferred treatment option for sperm acquisition?**

Vibratory stimulation applied to the frenulum of the penis can result in antegrade ejaculation via the ejaculation reflex arc. If this fails, electroejaculation or microsurgical vasal or epididymal sperm aspiration can be used to obtain sperm.

○ **A patient who has undergone a vasectomy wishes to have a reversal. On examination, he has bilateral sperm granulomas and the sites of the vasectomy are high in the straight segments of the scrotal vasa deferentia. Are these findings more indicative of the need for vasovasostomy or vasoepididymostomy at the time of surgical exploration?**

Vasovasostomy. Sperm granuloma and longer vasal length proximal to the site of obstruction are associated with a lower incidence of secondary epididymal obstruction.

○ **A patient with primary infertility is found to have severe oligozoospermia with only 100 motile sperm in his ejaculate on repeat evaluations. Evaluation reveals no correctable or treatable conditions and empirical medical therapy fails to improve his count. What option is available for this patient to conceive his own biological child?**

Small numbers of sperm can be used to fertilize ova in an IVF cycle employing ICSI; individual sperm are directly injected into an individual ovum.

○ **A patient receives 4 courses of cisplatin-based chemotherapy for testicular cancer. Immediately after treatment he is azoospermic. What are the chances that spermatogenesis will recover and how long can it take?**

His chances for recovery of spermatogenesis are 50% after 2 years and 80% after 5 years. It may take up to 1 year after treatment for sperm production to begin and several years to reach steady-state levels.

○ **When doing a diagnostic testis biopsy, should the procedure be performed unilaterally or bilaterally?**

While one side may be sufficient for diagnosis, there is a 40% incidence of diagnostic discrepancies between the 2 sides, so bilateral biopsies are often recommended. Cryopreservation of some tissue may allow for IVF or ICSI to be performed later.

○ **What is the significance of palpable dilated veins with palpable reflux on valsalva 1 month after varicocele repair?**

Probably nothing. Ligated veins may remain enlarged due to thrombosis, which can take weeks to resolve.

○ **When would you first expect to see improvement in the semen parameters after varicocele ligation?**

By 3 months.

○ **Should a vasectomy and a varicocelectomy be done together?**

Yes, but only if magnification is employed to preserve the internal spermatic arteries and deferential arteries and veins, because after varicocelectomy, the deferential veins provide the only testicular venous return. However, at least one study has demonstrated good results for simultaneous vasectomy and varicocelectomy, using a microsurgical technique to preserve the testicular arteries as well as the deferential veins and arteries to prevent testicular atrophy.

○ **When should consideration be given to IVF/ICSI rather than IUI?**

IVF/ICSI should be considered when the postcoital test indicates no sperm, very few sperm, or in those with unexplained infertility despite only a mild abnormality in semen parameters and 3 or more failures of IUI.

○ **How do clomiphene and tamoxifen work in male infertility and which patients are likely to benefit most?**

Clomiphene and tamoxifen are antiestrogens. They work best in men with low-normal testosterone levels and normal estradiol levels.

○ **Do men with nonobstructive azoospermia and hypogonadism respond to hormonal therapy?**

These men often respond with an increase in testosterone levels, but overall sperm retrieval, clinical pregnancy, or live birth rates are not affected.

○ **Which medication commonly used by young men is linked to sexual and libido dysfunction and infertility?**

Finasteride (Propecia).

○ **Do assisted reproductive technologies increase the risk of birth defects?**

- IVF was not associated with increased risk of birth defects after adjustment for parental factors.
- ICSI was associated with increased risk of birth defects even after adjustment for various factors.

○ **In addition to infertile men with clinical varicoceles, who else may benefit from varicocele repair?**

Men with nonobstructive azoospermia, scrotal pain, androgen deficiency, and progressive testicular dysfunction.

○ **How do human papillomavirus (HPV) infections affect couples undergoing IVF procedures?**

Positive HPV DNA testing in the pale partner may increase the risk for pregnancy loss during assisted reproductive (ART). Conventional semen washing procedures do not eliminate HPV sperm infection.

○ **Are benefits of varicocele surgery limited to younger men?**

No. Older age is associated with similar improvements in semen parameters and testosterone after microsurgical varicocelectomy.

○ **What component in fish oil and tree nuts may potentially improve semen quality?**

Polyunsaturated fatty acids are involved in membrane function as well as sperm maturation.

○ **What are some barriers to fertility treatment?**

In one study, 13% of couples did not pursue any form of fertility treatment after initial consultation. Age, education, diagnosis and intensity of treatment, financial concerns, and depressive symptoms were important factors.

CHAPTER 23

Male Sexual Function and Dysfunction

Alan W. Shindel, MD and
Tom F. Lue, MD, ScD (Hon), FACS

○ **What is the anatomic arrangement of the penis?**

The dorsal penis contains 2 erectile bodies, the corpora cavernosa. Each corpus cavernosum contains a central cavernosal artery that is principally responsible for penile engorgement during erection. There is a single erectile body (the corpus spongiosum) on the ventral portion of the penis that contains the urethra. Each corporal body is enclosed in a sheath of tough connective tissue called the tunica albuginea.

○ **What is Buck's fascia?**

Buck's fascia is the layer of connective tissue that covers both corpora cavernosa and the corpus spongiosum in separate fascial compartments. The dorsal artery, deep dorsal vein, and dorsal nerves of the penis lie beneath Buck fascia.

○ **From which artery is the deep penile blood supply derived?**

The cavernous arteries responsible for erection of the corpora cavernosa receive blood from the internal pudendal artery, which in turn is a branch of the hypogastric artery, which is a branch of the internal iliac artery.

○ **What is the anatomic relationship of the cavernous nerves to the prostate?**

The cavernous nerves, which are branches of the pelvic plexus, travel posterolateral to the apex of the prostate at the 5-o'clock and 7-o'clock positions.

○ **What is the mechanism of penile erection?**

During sexual stimulation, the neurotransmitter nitric oxide (NO) is produced by the action of neuronal nitric oxide synthase (nNOS) and released from the cavernous nerves to smooth muscle in the cavernous arteries and the corpora cavernosa. NO activates guanylate cyclase, which cleaves cellular guanosine triphosphate (GTP) into cyclic guanosine monophosphate (cGMP). Through a complex cascade of events including activation of protein kinase G (PKG), cGMP leads to decreased intracellular concentration of calcium ions; this prompts smooth muscle relaxation in cavernosal arteries and the corpora cavernosa.

With smooth muscle relaxation, the cavernous arteries and erectile tissues dilate, leading to increased penile blood flow and engorgement of the corpora. Shear forces with vasodilation stimulate the production of NO from the endothelium by action of endothelial nitric oxide synthase (eNOS). Engorgement of the corporal bodies with blood compresses the emissary veins (which drain the corpora) against the tunica albuginea. Compression of these veins prohibits blood from escaping the corpora, producing a firm penile erection (full erection phase). With increasing sexual excitement, there is concomitant contraction of the bulbospongiosus and bulbocavernosus muscles. This leads to a pressure increase in the distal corpora cavernosa which may exceed systolic blood pressure. Blood is also forced into the corpus spongiosum, causing engorgement of the ventral shaft and glans of the penis (rigid erection phase).

The NO/cGMP/PKG pathway is the best understood factor in promoting penile erection, but other pathways also play a role. Norepinephrine, endothelin, and sympathetic stimuli tend to promote vasoconstriction. Acetyl choline, vasoactive intestinal peptide, and prostaglandins tend to promote vasodilation. Calcium sensitization via the RhoA/ROCK pathway modulates responsiveness of the actin/myosin contractile proteins in vascular smooth muscle. These other pathways may become increasingly important in future treatments for erectile dysfunction (ED).

○ **What is the mechanism of penile detumescence?**

After sexual excitement has passed NO release from the cavernous nerves and endothelium declines. Concomitantly, the enzyme phosphodiesterase type 5 (PDE5) cleaves cGMP into 5′ GMP, which is not metabolically active. Sympathetic tone is restored, which tends to further promote arterial constriction. With the decline in cGMP concentration, intracellular calcium levels in the vascular smooth muscle rise and contraction occurs, leading to reversal of arterial dilation and drainage of blood from the corpora.

○ **What is the physical sequence of events of ejaculation and which portion of the nervous system controls it?**

Ejaculation is divided into 2 phases, emission and ejection.

Emission is the phase during which the bladder neck closes and seminal fluid (from the prostate and seminal vesicles) is mixed with sperm from the epididymis in the posterior urethra. This phase of ejaculation is under sympathetic nervous system control and may be disrupted by injury to sympathetic nerves (most commonly from retroperitoneal surgery or injury), sympatholytics, and/or bladder neck surgery.

Ejection is expulsion of semen from the penis by rhythmic contractions of the bulbospongiosus muscle. Ejection is mediated by the somatic nervous system. The force of ejection may decline with muscle weakness/age.

○ **Which areas in the brain control erection and ejaculation?**

The medial preoptic area and the paraventricular nucleus of the hypothalamus have been identified as important supraspinal centers for erection and ejaculation. In the central nervous system, the neurotransmitter serotonin typically has an anti-ejaculation effect whereas dopamine typically has a pro-ejaculation effect. Our current understanding of the neurophysiology of sexual function is poor.

○ **What is erectile dysfunction (ED)?**

ED is the persistent/recurrent inability to attain and/or maintain a penile erection rigid enough for satisfactory sexual intercourse.

○ **According to data from the Massachusetts Male Aging Study, ED affects how many men older than 50 years?**

More than 50%. The prevalence of ED increases with age. Less than 10% of men in their 20s and 30s complain of ED, but the condition has been reported in men of all ages.

○ **What are the most common risk factors for ED?**

ED may be divided into organic, psychogenic, or mixed. Vascular risk factors (hypertension, hypercholesterolemia, diabetes, tobacco use, and coronary artery disease) are the greatest risk factors for ED in the Western world. Nerve injury from pelvic surgery and/or neuropathic conditions may also contribute to ED. Deficiency of testosterone may lead to tissue atrophy in the penis as well as diminished libido. Certain medications are also known to increase risk of ED by a variety of mechanisms.

Psychogenic ED may result from depression, anxiety, relationship stress, or other nonorganic factors. Psychogenic factors frequently occur in men with organic ED and may complicate medical treatment. Attention to nonorganic factors is important in management of ED of any etiology.

○ **What classes of antihypertensive medication are most often associated with ED?**

β-Blockers and thiazides. While all anti-hypertensives have been asosciated with some degree of ED, there is some evidence that angiotensin converting enzyme (ACE) inhibitors calcium channel blockers, and angiotensin receptor blockers may have a neutral or even positive effect on erectile function in some hypertensive men.

○ **Are there subtypes of vasculogenic ED?**

Yes. Arterial insufficiency is defined as inadequate arterial response to sexual stimulation, leading to inadequate blood flow into the penis. This may be due to inadequate arterial vasodilation or occlusion of the arteries themselves with atherosclerotic plaques. Venous leak is a failure of the occlusive mechanism in which the emissary veins are compressed between the corporal body and the tunica. Mixed vascular ED is the coexistence of both venous leak and arterial insufficiency.

○ **Why is diabetes a particularly severe risk factor for ED?**

Neuropathy and vascular disease are common in men with diabetes. Diabetes is also associated with decreased levels of circulating testosterone and damage to endothelial and smooth muscle cells. Ergo, diabetes impacts many of the biological processes necessary for penile erection.

○ **Spinal cord injury patients may have reflex erections from tactile stimulation or psychogenic erections. What cord level of injury separates the 2 groups?**

Patients with injuries above T12 may have reflexogenic erections. These erections are mediated by efferent tactile signals transmitted from the penis via the pudendal, pelvic, and hypogastric nerves and afferent signals carried from the sacral spine cord via the pelvic nerve to the pelvic nerve and then the cavernous nerves. However, disruption of transmission via higher spinal cord segments may limit signaling regions of the brain responsible for interpreting and responding to erotic stimuli.

Patients with a level of injury below T12 may experience psychogenic erections (brought on by erotic stimuli processed in the brain) mediated by suppression of sympathetic tone (which promotes vasoconstriction) from the thoracolumbar spinal cord. These patients may however have disruption of the sacral reflex arc described above.

○ **What other sexual problems may be confused with and/or associated with ED?**

Premature ejaculation (PE): Persistent and/or recurrent ejaculation before or shortly after penile penetration associated with a lack of feeling of control over the process and leading to significant patient and/or partner distress. This condition may be lifelong or acquired. PE has been associated with differences in brain processing of serotonin, thyroid hormone disturbances, lower urinary tract symptoms, and/or psychosocial issues.

Hypoactive sexual desire disorder: Decreased interest or receptivity to sexual activity. This condition has been associated with hypogonadism, relationship stress, and psychological issues.

Retarded/delayed ejaculation: Persistent and recurrent difficulty ejaculating and/or attaining orgasm despite ostensibly sufficient sexual stimulation. This condition may be related to neuropathy, changes in sexual activities, and/or psychological issues.

○ **Which commonly used drugs have been associated with impairment in ejaculation and orgasm?**

Alcohol, tricyclic antidepressants (amitriptyline and imipramine), and selective serotonin reuptake inhibitors (SSRI) are the mostly commonly used drugs associated with impairment in ejaculation and orgasm. SSRI have been used with some success as a treatment for PE.

○ **What is an appropriate initial evaluation for a man with ED?**

The timing and nature of the concern must be explicitly confirmed. An assessment should be made for vascular and/or neurological risk factors as well as psychological comorbidities. Medications should be reviewed. A basic electrolyte panel, hemoglobin A1c, resting blood pressure, and serum lipid profile are adequate for initial evaluation in most cases. An AM serum testosterone (free and total) should be considered, particularly if there are other symptoms of hypogonadism and/or if the patients has previously failed oral erectogenic therapy.

○ **What are the Princeton criteria?**

The Princeton criteria are a set of algorithms for stratifying ED patients with respect to their cardiac risk factors. Men with severe cardiac disease should undergo cardiac optimization prior to initiation of any therapy for ED. Men with no or mild cardiac disease may safely start ED therapy without further investigation. Men in the intermediate category may need further evaluation by a cardiologist prior to starting ED therapy.

○ **What is dynamic infusion cavernosometry (DIC)?**

DIC is a procedure to diagnose venous leak as a cause of ED. A needle is placed into the corpora to inject a vasodilating agent. After 10 minutes and/or after a penile erection has developed, sterile saline is infused. The rate of inflow necessary to maintain a set degree of axial rigidity in the penis is a measure of the integrity of the veno-occlusive mechanism of the penis; a high flow rate implies greater leak and suggests venous leak ED.

○ **Normal veno-occlusive function is suggested by what maintenance flow rate on DIC testing?**

A maintenance flow rate of 6 mL/min or less represents normal veno-occlusive function if maximal smooth muscle relaxation has been achieved.

○ **What is the role of cavernosography in the evaluation of ED?**

In a patient in whom venous leak is clinically suspected, contrast injection into the corpora demonstrates the sites of abnormal leaking veins. This test is seldom indicated in the modern era but still is useful for preoperative planning if venous surgery for the treatment of ED is contemplated in carefully selected young patients.

○ **What is nocturnal penile tumescence (NPT)? When do nocturnal erections occur and how is the rigidity of these erections measured?**

NPT is the normal cycle of nighttime erections that occur during rapid eye movement (REM) sleep in healthy males of all ages. Testing for NPT can be performed using a pressure monitor that fits around the penis. NPT testing is typically utilized to determine whether ED is psychogenic or organic; if normal nocturnal erections occur in a patient with ED it somewhat more likely that there is a psychological component to ED. NPT may have some utility in assessment of ED; men with normal NPT and ED should consider psychosexual therapy as an alternative or adjunct to medical treatment options.

○ **What role does penile color Doppler ultrasound play in the diagnosis of ED?**

Color Doppler ultrasound after administration of a vasodilating agent permits accurate assessment of peak systolic velocity (PSV) and end diastolic velocity (EDV) in the cavernosal arteries. A PSV less than 30 to 35 cm/s is indicative of arterial disease while a persistent EDV greater than 5 cm/s predicts patients who may have venous leak. This is the Gold Standard test for vasculogenic ED in the modern era.

○ **A 35-year-old male with ED due to a pelvic fracture and a 65-year-old male with ED secondary to long-standing hypercholesterolemia and hypertension undergo pelvic angiography. What are the expected findings?**

The younger man would likely have a focal stenosis or occlusion of the penile or cavernosal arteries from trauma. The older man would likely have diffuse stenotic plaques of these same arteries.

○ **A patient is seen for a complaint of decreased libido. Physical examination is normal. What is an appropriate initial endocrine evaluation?**

TSH, Free T4, and a morning (between 8 and 11 a.m.) free and total testosterone level are good initial screening tests. If testosterone levels are abnormally low, they should be repeated along with testing for prolactin, luteinizing hormone (LH), and follicle stimulating hormone (FSH) to assess for pituitary dysfunction as a potential cause of hypogonadism.

○ **What is a "low" testosterone level?**

There is controversy about what constitutes an abnormally low testosterone level; however, a serum total testosterone of less than 320 ng/dL (11 nmol/L) OR a serum-free testosterone of 64 pg/mL (220 pmol/L) has been associated with increased risk of "hypogonadism" symptoms (Wu et al., 2010).

○ **What FDA-approved formulations of testosterone supplementation are available in the United States?**

Testosterone can be administered by depot intramuscular injection, transdermal patch, transdermal gel, a transbuccal system, or slow release subcutaneous pellets. Oral testosterone pills are not FDA approved for use in the United States, but are available in other countries.

○ **What evaluation is required before starting a man on supplemental testosterone?**

It is essential to obtain basic electrolytes, liver function tests, a complete blood count, and a serum PSA. A digital rectal examination should be performed to rule out occult prostate cancer. Men with prostate or breast cancer, lower urinary tract symptoms referable to an enlarged prostate, severe heart failure, severe sleep apnea, and/or polycythemia should be cautioned that testosterone may exacerbate these problems although definitive data on the extent of these risks are lacking.

○ **How does hyperprolactinemia cause hypogonadism? How is it treated?**

Hyperprolactinemia leads to suppression of the normal pulsatile secretion of GnRH by the hypothalamus. This in turn leads to decreased LH and FSH secretion by the pituitary gland, which removes the stimulus for testicular production of testosterone. Dopamine agonists such as bromocriptine or cabergoline are used to treat hyperprolactinemia. If a prolactin-producing tumor is present, surgical resection may cure the disorder.

○ **What is PDE5?**

Phosphodiesterase refers to an enzyme that breaks phosphodiester bonds. PDE5 is a specific phosphodiesterase, found at high concentration in the penile tissues, which is responsible for breaking down cGMP.

○ **What is the mechanism of action of PDE5 inhibitors (sildenafil, vardenafil, tadalafil, and avanafil)?**

These drugs inhibit the breakdown of cGMP by PDE5, thereby prolonging smooth muscle relaxation in the cavernosal arteries and corporal bodies.

○ **What are the most common side effects of PDE5 inhibitors?**

Side effects from PDE5 inhibitors are in most cases due to cross-reactivity of the drug with other phosphodiesterase isoforms in other parts of the body. The most common side effects are headache, congestion, dyspepsia, facial flushing, back pain, and visual disturbances; side-effect profiles differ between drugs. Severe side effects such as vision loss from Non-arteritic Ischemic Optic Neuritis (NAION) or cardiac events have been reported but the association between PDE5 inhibitors and these events has not been fully elucidated.

○ **What are contraindications to the use of PDE5 inhibitors?**

PDE5 inhibitors should not be used in patients taking nitrates as this may cause severe hypotension. PDE5 inhibitors should also not be taken within 4 hours of α-blocker medications as this may also lead to hypotension. Men with moderate to severe liver insufficient or severe renal insufficiency should use lower doses due to impairment of drug metabolism.

○ **What are some ways to optimize the efficacy of PDE5 inhibitors?**

Sildenafil and vardenafil should be taken no less than 1 hour before planned sexual activity; tadalafil should be taken up to 2 hours before planned sexual activity. Patients should be instructed that the medication augments but does not cause penile erection. Sexual stimulation is required for these drugs to work. Sildenafil and vardenafil should not be taken after a high-fat meal, as this will slow absorption of the drug.

All PDE5 inhibitors may be taken on demand for the treatment of ED. Tadalafil may be taken daily at a low dose for the management of ED.

○ **Which drugs are most commonly used alone or in combination for intracavernosal pharmacologic injection therapy for ED?**

Prostaglandin El, phentolamine (an α-blocker), and papaverine (a nonselective phosphodiesterase inhibitor). Prostaglandin is the only one of these that is FDA approved, although it may be used in combination with the other 2 after compounding by a pharmacist. Unlike PDE5 inhibitors, these medications are effective irrespective of sexual stimulation and are less impacted by neuropathy.

○ **What are the risks/side effects of intracavernosal injection therapy for ED?**

Fear of needles and penile pain limit the acceptability of this therapy for many patients, although many others find it highly satisfactory. Bleeding, pain, and infection are minor side effects that can be obviated with instruction of a good injection technique. Priapism and corporal fibrosis are more serious complications, which may result from overdose and/or recurrent long-term use.

○ **What is MUSE™? How is it administered?**

MUSE (medicated urethral suppository for erections) is prostaglandin E1 in a small pellet form for intraurethral placement. The patient is instructed to urinate, after which an applicator is placed into the distal urethra and the pellet is dislodged. The pellet dissolves and is absorbed into the corpus spongiosum. Venous channels then transfer the drug to the corpus cavernosum.

○ **What are the side effects of MUSE™?**

Urethral burning and pain are the most common side effects of MUSE™.

○ **What is the vacuum erection device?**

The vacuum erection (or tumescence) device (VED or VTD) is any apparatus placed around the penis which creates a negative pressure environment thus forcing blood into the corporal spaces. These devices are often combined with penile constrictive rings which are applied to the base of the phallus to keep blood trapped within the corpora after the device is removed.

○ **What are the reported side effects of vacuum erection device use?**

Pain is the most common side effect, followed by penile bruising and numbness. The penis may become cold, the ejaculate may be trapped in the urethra by the constriction band, and the base of the penis proximal to the band may pivot during intercourse. The constrictive band should not be left in place for more than 30 to 60 minutes.

○ **What are the advantages/disadvantages of vacuum erection devices?**

Vacuum erection devices carry no risk of medication interactions and are one-time expenditures. They can work in any type of ED. If successful, vacuum devices are highly reliable and reproducible but may take some practice to obtain optimal results. Some men find the device uncomfortable/cumbersome to use and the erection produced may be less rigid than with other modalities.

○ **What is a penile prosthesis?**

A penile prosthesis is any mechanical device placed in the corpora cavernosa for purposes of treating ED. Prostheses may be malleable or semi-rigid rods, 2-piece inflatable devices (one cylinder in each corpora with a reservoir in the rear tip of each cylinder), or 3-piece inflatable models (one cylinder in each corpora with a separate reservoir placed elsewhere in the body, typically retropubic).

○ **What are the relative advantages/disadvantages of different penile prostheses?**

Malleable and semi-rigid devices are easy to operate and have a low risk of failure due to a lack of moving parts. The penis is always firm to touch and thus are somewhat less cosmetically acceptable for many patients.

Inflatable devices produce a more natural flaccid appearance to the penis and permit some expansion with inflation. Given greater complexity and more working parts they have a higher failure rate although modern devices typically last for many years before mechanical failure.

○ **What are the potential complications of penile prosthesis placement?**

Penile pain, damage to adjacent structures (bladder, urethra, and vascular structures), penile foreshortening, and infection. Infection of the device is one of the most dreaded complications and typically necessitates removal of the device although salvage techniques have been effective in patients with mild infections.

○ **A patient experiences undesired inflation of his 3-piece inflatable penile prosthesis. What is the most likely cause?**

Autoinflation occurs when pressure around the reservoir is high enough to force fluid back through the pump into the cylinders at a time when inflation is not desired. This may occur due to inadequate dilation of the reservoir space during prosthesis placement or by formation of a compressive scar around the reservoir during healing. Most modern 3-piece penile prosthetics are equipped with a lockout valve to eliminate or at least reduce this complication.

○ **What is the penile prosthesis SST deformity and how is it corrected?**

Downward bowing of the glans after penile prosthesis implantation is called the SST deformity (named after the supersonic jet's characteristic "nose"). It is the result of either distal corporal underdilation, cylinder undersizing at the time of implantation, or postoperative anatomic changes that leave the glans unsupported. Surgical options for correction include redilating the corpora and resizing the device or glans fixation over the device tip.

○ **Which patients are at highest risk of penile prosthesis infection?**

Patients with poorly controlled diabetes and/or compromised immune function. Patients with spinal cord injury are also at higher risk for infection as they may not have sensation to detect occult erosion of the implant.

Increased risk of infection is also associated with repeat implant operations and surgical revisions. This is thought to be due to the presence of biofilm on explanted components of the old implant. Copious irrigation with antibiotic solutions is recommended during revision/replacement procedures.

○ **After placement of a 3-piece inflatable penile prosthesis a patient has bloody urine. There was no evidence of urethral injury during surgery. What may have occurred and how is this complication best avoided?**

The patient may have sustained a bladder injury during reservoir placement. This type of injury is prevented by draining the bladder completely with a catheter prior to retropubic dissection. Hematuria after penile implant should prompt assessment with cystoscopy and possible open exploration.

○ **During distal dilation of the corpora for placement of an inflatable penile prosthesis, a tear is made in the urethra with the dilator at the level of the urethral meatus. What is the best form of management?**

A cylinder should not be placed in the injured corpora. No attempt should be made to close the urethral tear. A urethral catheter should be left in place. After the urethral tear has healed, a cylinder can be placed on that side (typically at least 4–6 weeks later).

○ **A patient with a 3-piece inflatable penile prosthesis is explored for suspected periprosthetic infection. At surgery, gross pus is found around the cylinders. What is the best form of management?**

The standard of care is to remove all components of the device and irrigate the wound thoroughly. The wound can be closed primarily with drains left in place. Prosthesis reimplantation can be attempted in 4 to 6 months, although there is likely to be significant corporal fibrosis after this much time. Successful salvage procedures have been developed that permit immediate replacement of a prosthesis in the case of low-grade infection or simple prosthetic erosion but should not be attempted in the setting of gross purulence and/or sepsis.

○ **What is penile venous ligation surgery?**

Penile venous ligation surgery is occlusion (by ligation) of some segment(s) of the corpora cavernosa through which a discrete area of venous leak is noted at cavernosography.

○ **Which patients are candidates for penile venous ligation surgery?**

Young patients with a history of primary (lifelong) ED, venous leak without arterial insufficiency on Doppler ultrasound, and a discrete area of venous leak demonstrated by cavernosography are potential candidates for venous ligation surgery. The procedure is unlikely to be effective in cases of diffuse venous leakage. The most recent AUA guidelines on ED (2005–2006) do not recommend use of this technique. It may be considered as an option in carefully selected patients by well trained providers.

○ **What is penile revascularization surgery?**

Penile revascularization surgery is anastomosis of a fresh blood supply to an occluded cavernosal artery distal to the area of obstruction. It is similar in principle to bypass graft surgery in other vascular structures.

○ **Which patients are candidates for penile revascularization surgery?**

Young, healthy patients with a history of traumatic disruption of the pelvis and/or pudendal artery circulation with no evidence of distal penile vascular disease. Older patients with vascular disease typically have too much small vessel disease to make revascularization technically feasible or effective.

○ **Which artery is most commonly used as the source of new arterial blood to bypass obstruction in a penile artery during revascularization surgery?**

The inferior epigastric artery is the most commonly used source of new arterial inflow.

○ **What is penile rehabilitation?**

Penile rehabilitation is the concept of promoting blood flow and/or tissue stretch with the intent of restoring normal erectile function and penile length after some physiological insult, typically radical pelvic surgery.

○ **What are some forms of penile rehabilitation?**

The most common form of penile rehabilitation is routine dosing of PDE5 inhibitors. Penile injection therapy, vacuum erection devices, and/or penile stretching devices may also be used to promote blood flow and/or tissue stretch.

○ **Is penile rehabilitation effective?**

Studies have indicated superior recovery of penile hemodynamics in rats treated with PDE5 inhibitors after cavernous nerve injury compared to similarly injured rats treated with placebo. This recovery was associated with greater smooth muscle content, less collagen fibrosis, greater endothelial integrity, and reduced oxidative stress in penile tissues.

○ **What about penile rehabilitation in humans?**

Several small, single center, and/or nonrandomized studies have suggested superior erectile recovery in men treated with penile rehabilitation after radical prostatectomy compared to men who did not have penile rehabilitation. However, the largest placebo controlled randomized study to date did not demonstrate any difference in erectile function recovery between men treated with daily or on-demand PDE5I and those men treated with placebo only after the washout period. During the treatment phase patients using on-demand PDE5I had higher intercourse success rates compared to the other 2 groups (Montorsi et al., 2008).

○ **What medical therapies are available for the treatment of PE?**

There are no US FDA-approved treatments for PE. Serotonin has an antiorgasmic effect on the central nervous system; for this reason SSRI have been used to treat PE. SSRI have been proven to increase ejaculatory latency in placebo-controlled trials. An on demand SSRI (dapoxetine) has been approved for treatment of PE in some European nations but was not approved by the FDA in the United States. Side effects may include mood changes, nausea, decreased libido, and ED.

Topical application of an anesthetic ointment (cream or spray) to the penis has also been demonstrated to be more effective than placebo in the treatment of PE. The theory behind this treatment is to lessen but not completely abolish penile sensitivity. Side effects may include excessive penile numbness, ED, and genital irritation for the man and/or his sexual partner.

○ **What medical therapies are available for the treatment of sexual desire disorders?**

Testosterone supplementation in hypogonadal men is the most common means of treating decreased libido. For men who are eugonadal or cannot take testosterone supplements, assessment of other health conditions that may contribute to generalized fatigue and/or anhedonia, relationship counseling, and/or treatment of psychiatric comorbidities may be beneficial.

○ **A man hears a "pop" as his penis buckles during intercourse. This is followed by pain, penile bruising, and swelling. What has occurred and how is it treated?**

The patient may have sustained a penile fracture due to rupture of the tunica albuginea of the corpus cavernosum followed by blood extravasation and subcutaneous hematoma formation (the eggplant sign). The preferred management is expeditious penile exploration and repair of the tunica tear.

○ **A patient with clinical evidence of a penile fracture and a ventral hematoma also has urethral bleeding. What concurrent injury should be suspected? How is it diagnosed and treated?**

This patient may have sustained an injury to the urethra as well as a cavernosal tear. He should have a retrograde urethrogram and/or flexible cystoscopy to diagnose the site and extent of the urethral injury. Surgical exploration should follow and the cavernosal, spongiosal, and urethral injuries repaired.

○ **A patient with sickle cell anemia presents to the emergency department with a 8-hour history of prolonged painful erection. What is this condition?**

Ischemic (formerly known as low-flow) priapism. Ischemic priapism may be conceptualized as compartment syndrome of the penis and occurs when arterial inflow is restricted due to venous occlusion. Blood gas testing in ischemic priapism typically reveals acidosis and hypoxia consistent with venous blood.

Importantly, ischemic priapism involves only the corpora cavernosa; the corpus spongiosum is seldom if ever involved. Because of this, the dorsal penile shaft is very rigid but the glans penis and ventral penile shaft are typically soft.

○ **What is the underlying mechanism of priapism?**

The most common cause of priapism in the modern era is use of prescription erectogenic drugs, particularly penile injection agents. Some prescription drugs (such as trazodone) and illicit drugs (such as cocaine) have also been associated with priapism. Priapism may also occur in hematological malignancies and in advanced solid malignancies of the pelvis.

Sickle cell disease is commonly associated with priapism. The traditional belief has been that sludging of sickled red blood cells in the corpora leads to prolonged erection in men with sickle cell associated priapism. New evidence suggests that there may be an underlying defect of endothelial function and/or PDE5 activity in sickle cell disease.

○ **What is the preferred management of priapism?**

Corporal aspiration and irrigation with normal saline through a large bore needle. Oftentimes injection of an α-adrenergic agent (typically phenylephrine) is employed to bring about detumescence by constricting cavernous arteries and reducing compression on emissary veins. A patient being treated with phenylephrine should be placed on a cardiac monitor as phenylephrine may lead to hypertension and reflex bradycardia.

In sickle cell associated priapism, treatment at the underlying sickle cell crisis should be initiated but management of priapism should not be delayed. In patients with priapism associated with malignancy, appropriate therapy for the underlying condition should proceed.

○ **A patient with ischemic priapism fails to respond to repeated corporal aspiration, irrigation, and injection of an α-adrenergic agonist. What is the next appropriate form of treatment?**

Patients who fail conservative therapy need surgical intervention by penile vascular shunting with diversion of corporal blood into an adjacent uninvolved vascular structure (typically but not always the glans or the corpus spongiosum). In cases of prolonged penile erection (greater than 24 hours), significant tissue damage has likely occurred and some degree of ED from prolonged ischemia is to be expected. In these situations, the shunt is undertaken for relief of pain from compartment syndrome more than for erectile function preservation. There are a variety of shunt procedures, discussion of which is beyond the scope of this chapter.

○ **What is stuttering priapism and how is it treated?**

Stuttering priapism is the condition of recurrent priapism. It generally responds to intracavernosal vasoconstrictors and the patient may be instructed on self-administration of this therapy. When this is insufficient or the problem fails to resolve, a 6-month or greater treatment with luteinizing hormone releasing hormone (LHRH) agonists to decrease serum testosterone has been effective. Alternatives include ketoconazole with concomitant corticosteroid supplementation. In many cases, these men maintain normal erectile function despite being on androgen suppression therapy.

Low dose daily PDE5 inhibitors have been used to treat stuttering priapism in a single small case series; the theorized mechanism is upregulation of PDE5 expression. While this may be effective in some cases, there is some concern that this treatment may predispose sickle cell patients to pain crises.

○ **A patient reports nonpainful, persistent partial penile erection after blunt perineal trauma. What is this condition?**

This patient likely has nonischemic (formerly known as high flow) priapism. Nonischemic priapism is typically not painful and the resulting erection is not as firm as what is observed in ischemic priapism. Blood gas testing in nonischemic priapism typically reveals no acidosis and a high oxygen content consistent with arterial blood.

○ **What is the most likely mechanism of nonischemic priapism?**

Nonischemic priapism is typically caused by a cavernosal artery to cavernosal tissue fistula after trauma. This leads to increased filling of the corpora with blood but typically the increase is not sufficient to increase intracorporal pressure to the point that venous outflow is restricted. This may present in a delayed fashion. This can be diagnosed by history, blood gas testing, and/or penile color Doppler ultrasound.

○ **How is nonischemic priapism managed?**

Nonischemic priapism is typically not painful and does not contribute to penile ischemia. Some men with nonischemic priapism report preservation of erectile capacity. Conservative management with observation ± compression can be considered although long term data are scant. Selective arterial embolization or surgical ligation of the fistula may also be considered, but carry a risk of ED by disruption of arterial inflow. Some authors have reported good results using androgen ablation as a noninvasive management strategy for nonischemic priapism, but research has been scant.

○ **What is Peyronie disease?**

Peyronie disease is a term used to refer to nearly any acquired deformity of the erect penis. Classically Peyronie disease is described as curvature of the phallus; however, penile shaft waist defects, septal fibrosis between the corporal bodies, and presence of a palpable plaque in the absence of curvature have also been described as Peyronie variants.

Peyronie disease is distinct from chordee, a congenital curvature (typically ventral) of the penis.

○ **What causes Peyronie disease?**

The etiology of Peyronie is unclear, but TGF-beta and related cytokines appear to play a role in generating scar tissue and resulting plaque/deformity. It is currently believed that trauma (minor or major) to the penis (typically during sexual activity) may lead to accumulation of scar tissue in certain genetically predisposed men.

○ **What conditions are associated with Peyronie disease?**

Men with Peyronie disease have been reported to have a higher rate of Dupuytren contractures of the hands, tympanosclerosis in the inner ear, and Lederhosen syndrome (formation of nodules of fibrotic tissue in the feet). It is apparent from these associations that Peyronie is often associated with fibrotic conditions in other body regions.

○ **What conservative nonsurgical options exist for the treatment of Peyronie disease?**

There are currently (as of January 31, 2013) no US FDA-approved therapies for Peyronie disease. Numerous oral medical therapies have been proposed. Examples include vitamin E, arginine, carnitine, colchicine, pentoxifylline, tamoxifen, and potassium *para*-aminobenzoate. Use of a penile stretching device or vacuum device to mold the penis has also been recommended by some authors. Unfortunately, none of these have emerged as consistently and universally effective. Intralesional injection of verapamil, interferon, and/or collagenase is advocated by some investigators and has some support in the literature.

○ **What surgical options exist for the treatment of Peyronie disease?**

Surgical options for Peyronie disease may be divided into 3 categories.

1. Plication procedures: Placement of sutures (with or without tissue excision) on the convex side of penile curvature to force the penis into a straight alignment.

2. Patch graft procedures: Excision or incision of plaque/tunica on the concave side of penile curvature or over an area of waist defect with subsequent coverage using a graft material (autologous or nonautologous).

3. Penile prosthesis placement: Placement of a penile prosthesis. Typically produces some straightening of deformity, which may be enhanced by modeling or adjunctive plication/plaque incision. Particularly useful for management of Peyronie in the setting of concomitant ED.

CHAPTER 24 Peyronie Disease and Penile Fractures

Stephen W. Leslie, MD, FACS

PEYRONIE DISEASE

○ **What is Peyronie disease?**

Peyronie disease is a fibrotic disorder of the penis in which a tough fibrous plaque forms in the tunica albuginea. These plaques may become calcified. Peyronie disease is often but not always associated with penile pain and progressive deformity, either curvature or narrowing, during the "acute" phase. The "chronic" phase involves resolution of pain with stabilization of the deformity.

○ **What is the incidence of Peyronie disease?**

Approximately 9% of the adult male population and increasing.

○ **Describe the pathophysiology of Peyronie disease.**

While the pathophysiology of the disorder is not entirely clear, it is thought to be due to abnormal wound healing in men with some minimal level of penile trauma or injury, most often from sexual activity.

○ **Is Peyronie disease genetic?**

There appears to be a genetic component as it tends to occur more frequently in relatives with the condition.

○ **Peyronie disease is related to what other conditions associated with abnormal wound healing?**

It is associated with several other conditions related to abnormal wound healing such as Dupuytren contractures and tympanosclerosis.

○ **What percentage of men with Peyronie also have depression?**

Approximately 50%.

○ **How often is ED associated with Peyronie disease?**

Approximately 30% of the time.

○ **What is the natural history of Peyronie? How many patients will improve spontaneously, remain stable, or worsen over time?**

Approximately 12% to 13% will improve spontaneously, 40% to 50% will tend to remain stable, and the remainder will tend to get worse.

○ **What is the specific critical cytokine involved in Peyronie disease, where is it normally found, and how does it work?**

Transforming growth factor-β1 (TGF-β1). It is an activator of collagen synthesis released by neutrophils and macrophages during wound healing.

○ **What is the differential diagnosis of Peyronie? (Name at least 5)**

- Penile fracture.
- Sarcoma (very rare).
- Fracture of the penile septum—with or without hematoma formation.
- Congenital curvature.
- Dorsal vein thrombosis.
- Cavernosal fibrosis.
- Leukemic infiltrate.

○ **Name 3 oral agents that were used for Peyronie but are no longer recommended by most experts.**

Vitamin E, potaba, tamoxifen, and colchicine are no longer recommended. Vitamin E and tamoxifen do not appear to be effective, while potaba and colchicine have significant side effects with little or no benefit consistently reported.

○ **Name at least 5 other promising medical treatments for Peyronie other than intralesional injections and surgery.**

Promising therapies currently include

- Arginine
- Carnitine
- Trental
- Medical-grade penile extenders such as Fastsize (www.fastsize.com)
- PDE5 inhibitors (Viagra, Levitra, and Cialis)
- Iontophoresis (with verapamil and dexamethasone)

○ **Name 3 intralesional agents that appear to be potentially useful for Peyronie disease.**

1. Verapamil
2. Interferon
3. Clostridial collagenase

○ **Which intralesional agent appears to be the most effective and what is the dosing regimen?**

Verapamil has shown the most benefit. Typically, verapamil is injected in 10-mg doses twice a week for 12 weeks. If no benefit is seen after 6 weeks, the dose is increased to 20 mg.

○ **How does Verapamil work in Peyronie?**

Verapamil theoretically works by inhibiting the exocytosis of collagen, fibronectin, and glycosaminoglycans. This effectively interferes with collagen production and ultimately results in reduced scar formation.

○ **What is the role of oral verapamil in the treatment of Peyronie disease?**

Currently, oral verapamil plays no role in the treatment of Peyronie disease. The reason is that the local concentration of verapamil necessary to inhibit fibroblast activity is many times greater than any safe level potentially possible with oral therapy.

○ **What is the optimal role of intralesional or oral steroids in this disorder?**

Steroids are not effective in this disease.

○ **What is the benefit of shock wave lithotripsy and radiation therapy in Peyronie?**

Shock wave lithotripsy has not been effective. Low-dose radiation therapy has shown some benefit in relieving pain when used early in the disease, but it has no effect on the outcome.

○ **How effective is verapamil 15% topical gel for Peyronie?**

There are conflicting reports, but the majority suggest that it has little activity due to poor tissue penetration. Most experts do not recommend it currently.

○ **Which type of treatment, other than surgery, appears to be the most effective in treating Peyronie?**

Intralesional verapamil injections have shown the best results of all nonsurgical therapies. However, the optimal combination of nonsurgical therapies is not yet clear.

○ **What is the rationale for using verapamil to treat Peyronie?**

Verapamil appears to increase collagenase activity, decrease fibroblast proliferation in Peyronie plaques, and affect cytokine expression. It is also thought that it can interfere with collagen and fibronectin transport, which are calcium-dependent processes.

○ **Peyronie most commonly involves what aspect of the penis (dorsal, ventral, or lateral) and why?**

The dorsal midline is involved most often, probably from delamination during sexual activity. This causes an upward curvature.

○ **What surgical treatment options exist for a patient with symptomatic Peyronie disease?**

Patients with a stable, nonpainful plaque and difficulty with penetration due to penile angulation are surgical candidates. Surgical options include penile plication, plaque incision or excision with grafting, and/or implant of a penile prosthesis. The more severe the curvature, the more aggressive the surgical procedure is likely to be.

○ **What is the most common location of the Peyronie plaque: dorsal, ventral, or lateral?**

The dorsal location is the most common.

○ **Is calcification a significant predictor of eventual progression to surgery in Peyronie?**

No. Only men with significantly (Grade 3) calcified plaques are more likely to require surgery. (Grade 3 is defined as greater than 1.5 cm wide or the presence of 2 plaques or plaques more than 1 cm thick.)

○ **Plaque excision and dermal grafting is an appropriate option in which types of patients with Peyronie?**

Plaque excision and dermal grafting are recommended only for patients with good erectile ability where the Nesbit plication technique may not be suitable for some reason. It is also reasonable in patients who will not accept any degree of penile shortening. It is feasible if the penile length is adequate and the expected tunica defect will be 3 cm or less.

○ **Describe the Yachia procedure.**

The Yachia procedure is a modification of the Nesbit plication for Peyronie disease. Instead of excising a wedge of tissue from the tunica, the Yachia procedure uses longitudinal incisions in the tunica, which are then closed horizontally in a Heineke–Mikulicz fashion. (Simple plication procedures without incisions or wedge resections have demonstrated good results in patients with relatively mild curvatures. When doing these plications, a minimal amount of tissue in the actual plication seems to provide better patient satisfaction.)

○ **When is the placement of a penile prosthesis most appropriate in Peyronie patients?**

When there is significant preexisting ED and relatively severe curvature. In many cases, placement of a penile prosthesis alone is sufficient to provide adequate straightening. Manual modeling, where the penis is manually bent in the opposite direction of the curvature during surgery, sometimes provides durable improved straightening. If this is insufficient, then incisions and/or plaque excision with possible grafting will be needed.

○ **Besides ED, what 2 additional disorders are associated with Peyronie disease?**

Dupuytren contractures and tympanosclerosis.

○ **What is Van Buren disease?**

Another name for Peyronie disease. W.H. Van Buren published an early account in English of Peyronie Disease in the *New York Medical Journal* in 1874.

○ **What is the Space of Smith?**

The Space of Smith is the area between the erectile tissue and the tunica albuginea. It is usually obliterated in Peyronie disease.

○ **What is different about the scar tissue in Peyronie disease compared to scar tissue elsewhere in the body?**

The scar tissue in Peyronie retains fibrin within the mature scar. This does not occur elsewhere in the body. Peyronie scar tissue tends to have less elastin and collagenase than most bodily scars and the collagen deposition is more disorganized.

○ **Who first described Peyronie disease and when? (Hint: It wasn't Peyronie!)**

Peyronie disease was first described by Gabriel Fallopius in 1561 and first written about by Guilio Cesare Aranzi in 1587.

○ **Who was Peyronie and when did he write about Peyronie disease?**

Francois Gigot de la Peyronie, the personal physician of King Louis XV of France, did not write about "his" disease until 1743. When he did, he wrote an authoritative treatise on it and his name has been associated with the disorder ever since.

PENILE FRACTURES

○ **What is the average thickness of the tunica albuginea of the penis when flaccid and during an erection?**

It averages 5 mm in thickness when flaccid, and 2 mm when erect.

○ **What is the "rolling sign" and when does it occur?**

The "rolling sign" occurs when the clot within the torn tunica overlying a penile fracture is palpable as an immobile, firm, tender swelling over which the penile shaft skin can be gently rolled.

○ **What structure needs to be intact for the "rolling sign" to occur?**

Buck fascia needs to be intact.

○ **In penile fractures, is Buck fascia usually torn or usually left intact?**

Buck fascia is usually intact.

○ **What is the "eggplant sign" and what problem does it indicate?**

This is the typical appearance of the penis immediately after a penile fracture with extensive hematoma formation and extravasation of blood.

○ **How does the clinical appearance of a penile fracture differ if Buck fascia is torn compared to if it is intact?**

When Buck fascia is intact, the hematoma from the fracture occurs deep to Buck fascia and is relatively contained. When Buck fascia is ruptured, blood will leak into the scrotum, perineum, and lower abdominal wall.

○ **What is the most common site for a penile fracture?**

The most common site of the tear is proximal, near the base of the penis.

○ **Describe the appearance of the actual defect in the tunica.**

The tears are almost always solitary, transverse, and unilateral.

○ **What is the expected incidence of urethral ruptures associated with penile fractures?**

Between 14% and 33%.

○ **What type and direction of force is most likely to cause a urethral rupture in association with a penile fracture?**

When the urethra is stretched during tumescence, it becomes vulnerable to rupturing from an angular force with dorsal bending.

○ **What predisposing factors lead to a greater risk of an associated urethral rupture?**

Periurethral fibrosis and urethral strictures.

○ **What is the most common cause of penile fractures?**

Bending during intercourse with forcible thrusting that misses the introitus and encounters bone. In the Middle East, the most common cause is forceful manipulation (65%).

○ **True/False: A penile fracture cannot generally occur in the flaccid penis.**

False. In approximately 3% of patients, the penile rupture occurs in the flaccid state, usually from direct blunt penile trauma.

○ **True/False: After a penile fracture, the angulation or deviation of the penis is generally toward the side of the tear in the tunica.**

False. The angulation is usually toward the side opposite the tear.

○ **When should a urethral injury be suspected in a penile fracture?**

When there is blood at or from the urethra, difficulty in voiding, inability to pass a catheter, and in the presence of factors predisposing to urethral injury as mentioned earlier. In actuality, every case of penile fracture should be suspect for a urethral rupture.

○ **What other clinical entity can present in an identical fashion to a penile fracture?**

Rupture of the deep dorsal vein of the penis.

○ **True/False: It is important to rule out a ruptured dorsal vein of the penis since its management is different than a penile fracture.**

False. Treatment is essentially the same, as both entities need surgical exploration.

○ **True/False: Cavernosography can be used to confirm the diagnosis of penile fracture and localize the tear in difficult cases.**

True, although this is rarely necessary as the clinical presentation is usually sufficient.

○ **What are the potential complications of cavernosography in penile fractures?**

Contrast-reaction fibrosis from extravasated contrast, infection, and priapism.

○ **What imaging studies, if any, are recommended in suspected penile fractures?**

Sonography is the recommended study if any imaging at all is needed. A retrograde urethrogram is indicated in cases of suspected urethral injury. An MRI can also be done, but this modality is not always available. A clear clinical case should not be delayed while waiting for an MRI. Ultrasound in the ER has become the imaging modality of choice in most recent studies.

○ **How should penile fractures be treated?**

Immediate surgical exploration, evacuation of hematomas, and primary repair with buried, absorbable sutures through a circumferential subcoronal incision with degloving is the current recommended treatment. Complications of this approach include subcoronal skin necrosis, infections, abscess formation, transient distal edema, and penile curvature. A small, longitudinal skin incision has been suggested as an alternative surgical approach that would reduce some of the complications, but this limits the ability to fully inspect the entire tunica and urethra.

○ **How should a concomitant urethral injury be handled and what complications are possible?**

A diverting cystostomy may be sufficient treatment for a partially torn urethra although a direct repair gives equally good results. A complete transaction requires an end-to-end anastomosis and cystostomy. Urethral strictures and corporourethral fistulas are possible complications when a urethral injury is involved with a penile fracture.

○ **What is the expected outcome of conservative (nonsurgical) treatment of penile fractures?**

Significant complications are likely including development of a firm, fibrous plaque similar to Peyronie disease (which can occur in 30%–53% of patients treated conservatively), organized hematoma formation, cavernous fibrositis, penile angulation, ED, and delayed chordee.

Adult Urinary Tract Infections

David M. Albala, MD and
Udaya Kumar, MD, FRCS Urol, Dip Urol (Lon)

○ **How common are urinary tract infections (UTIs) in young women?**

UTIs occur in approximately 1% of schoolgirls (age 5–14). This proportion rises to 4% by young adulthood.

○ **Should patients with asymptomatic bacteriuria be treated?**

Pregnant women, children younger than 4 years, patients with severe diabetes, and patients with *Proteus* infections should be treated regardless of symptoms.

○ **Which bacteria are urea splitting?**

Majority are *Proteus* and *Providencia* species. *Pseudomonas, Klebsiella, Staph. epidermidis,* and mycoplasma are also capable of producing urease. *Escherichia coli* is not a urea-splitting organism.

○ **What is emphysematous pyelonephritis?**

It is a rare complication of pyelonephritis that can occur in diabetic patients. Nonresolving pyelonephritis despite therapy and the triad of fever, vomiting, and flank pain should be investigated. Presence of intraparenchymal gas on plain kidney, ureter, bladder (KUB) or computed tomography (CT) is diagnostic.

○ **What is significant bacteriuria?**

The number of bacteria that exceeds the number usually caused by contamination. 10^2 CFU/mL or more of a known pathogen in a patient with dysuria would be significant. Previously $\geq 10^5$ had been the cutoff limit. However, 20% to 40% of women with symptomatic UTIs had colony counts between 10^4 and 10^5.

○ **What are bacterial pili?**

Bacteria have surface structures called adhesins to mucosal surfaces. The most important adhesins are long filamentous appendages called pili fimbriae.

○ **What is phase variation?**

Changes in environmental growth conditions of bacteria can cause them to rapidly shift between piliated and nonpiliated phases.

○ **What patient genetic factors affect susceptibility to UTIs?**

Variation in bacterial adherence to vaginal, urethral, and buccal cell surfaces is genetically determined. Women with nonsecretor blood group phenotypes are more prone to UTIs.

○ **How common are *E. coli* infections?**

In the community setting, *E. coli* account for 85% of the UTIs. In the hospital setting, this proportion reduces to 50%.

○ **What tests are used to localize UTIs to the upper or lower tract?**

Fairley bladder washout and Stamey ureteral catheterization tests.

○ **How accurate are clinical signs in localizing UTIs to the upper or lower tract?**

Less than 50%. Fever and loin pain with significant bacteriuria, traditionally taught to be diagnostic of pyelonephritis, may occur with cystitis alone. Conversely, in patients with only bladder symptoms, the upper urinary tract is often involved.

○ **What is the recommended duration of therapy for uncomplicated UTIs?**

In a patient with a structurally normal urinary tract, a single dose or a 3-day course of antimicrobial treatment is adequate. Success rates are lower with single-dose therapy compared to multiday regimens. In men, all UTIs should be presumed complicated and treated for 7 days or more and an underlying cause sought.

○ **Is antibiotic prophylaxis necessary for TURP?**

No. If the preop urine shows no growth ($<10^2$ CFU/mL), prophylaxis is not necessary. In patients with significant growth, urethral catheters, risk of endocarditis, or whose bacterial status is unknown, prophylaxis is warranted. The risk of bacteremia is 50% if antimicrobials are not given when a UTI is present.

○ **What antibiotics are suitable as prophylaxis for transrectal biopsy of the prostate?**

Metronidazole with ampicillin or trimethoprim–sulfamethoxazole (TMP–SMX) is often used. A fluoroquinolone is a suitable alternative. Due to increasing resistance patterns, a rectal culture prior to the biopsy is now recommended by some experts.

○ **When are imaging studies needed in UTIs?**

Infections in males, febrile infections, failure to respond to appropriate therapy, bacterial persistence, and suspected urinary obstruction warrant imaging studies.

○ **What are the common causes of unresolved bacteriuria during therapy?**

- Bacterial resistance to drug (resistance may develop during the course of therapy).
- Mixed bacterial growth with varying drug susceptibilities.
- Rapid reinfection with a new organism.
- Renal insufficiency.
- Papillary necrosis.
- Bladder or Staghorn calculi.
- Self-inflicted infections or deception in taking medications.
- Urinary obstruction.
- Enterovesical fistulas.

○ **What is bacterial persistence?**

Despite clearance of bacteriuria with appropriate antimicrobial treatment, the same organism can reappear in the urinary tract from a site within the urinary tract that was excluded from the high concentrations of the antimicrobial agent, for example, a struvite stone.

○ **Which antibiotics are suitable for long-term, low-dose prophylaxis?**

Nitrofurantoin, TMP–SMX, TMP, and cephalexin. A low dose of the antibiotic is given, typically at bedtime for 6 to 12 months.

○ **Are there alternatives to long-term, low-dose prophylaxis?**

Intermittent 3-day, self-start therapy or post-intercourse therapy may be used instead.

○ **What does urinary microscopy show in patients with acute pyelonephritis?**

Numerous white cells and bacteria. WBCs exhibit Brownian motion of cytoplasm (glitter cells); granular and leukocyte casts; bacteria may be seen in casts.

○ **True/False: Nitrofurantoin and TMP–SMX are generally ineffective against Pseudomonas species.**

True. TMP alone or with SMX is effective against most uropathogens except enterococci and *Pseudomonas* sp. Nitrofurantoin is ineffective against *Proteus* and *Pseudomonas* sp.

○ **Why does an infection with *Proteus* cause more concern than *E. coli*?**

Patients who have a protracted infection with *Proteus* risk formation of struvite calculi due to the alkalinization caused by the urea-splitting bacteria. This leads to precipitation of Ca, Mg, NH_4, and PO_4 salts. *E. coli* does not produce urease.

○ **True/False: Prophylactic antibiotics should be given to catheterized patients to reduce risk of UTI.**

False. This does not reduce risk of infections. In fact, they give rise to infections with organisms resistant to several antibiotics.

○ **What are the radiologic features of xanthogranulomatous pyelonephritis?**

It is usually unilateral. Intravenous urogram (IVU) shows renal calculi in 38% to 70% of cases, a nonfunctioning kidney in 27% to 80%, a renal mass in 62%, and a calyceal deformity in 46%. On CT scan, a large renal mass with the renal pelvis tightly surrounding a central calcification is seen.

○ **What are the diagnostic features of malacoplakia histologically?**

Large histiocytes called von Hansemann cells and small basophilic calculospherules called Michaelis–Guttmann bodies, which may be intra- or extracytoplasmic.

○ **Why should a hydatid cyst not be aspirated?**

The contents of a hydatid cyst are highly antigenic and may cause anaphylaxis if it ruptures and spills during aspiration.

○ **What is the initiator of gram-negative septic shock?**

Endotoxin, a lipopolysaccharide component of bacterial cell wall, activates the macrophages and humoral pathways in septic shock. Most of the toxicity of endotoxin is contributed by lipid A, which is bound to the core oligosaccharide.

○ **Why do postmenopausal women have UTIs more frequently?**

Lack of estrogen causes changes in vaginal pH and microflora including loss of lactobacilli and colonization with *E. coli*. In addition, some women may have residual urine after voiding.

○ **When is screening for bacteriuria worthwhile?**

The first trimester of pregnancy. There appears to be little advantage in screening healthy women.

○ **True/False: In women with bacteriuria, acute pyelonephritis occurs more commonly in pregnant women than in nonpregnant women.**

True. Nonpregnant women with screening bacteriuria (SCBU) rarely develop pyelonephritis in contrast to 28% of pregnant women with SCBU.

○ **Which antimicrobials are suitable for use in pregnancy?**

Penicillins (including ampicillin and synthetic penicillins) and cephalosporins are safe throughout pregnancy. Short-acting sulfonamides and nitrofurantoin may be used in the first 2 trimesters. The former can cause neonatal hyperbilirubinemia and the latter hemolytic anemia in newborn if used near term.

○ **What is the incidence of bacteriuria in the elderly?**

Greater than 20% of women and >10% of men older than 65 years have bacteriuria. In contrast to young adults, in whom bacteriuria is 30 times more prevalent in women than in men, the ratio in women to men with bacteriuria progressively decreases to 2:1. Most elderly patients with bacteriuria are asymptomatic; estimates among women living in nursing homes range from 17% to 55%, as compared with 15% to 31% for their male cohorts.

○ **What is the treatment for elderly patients with bacteriuria?**

Prospective randomized comparative trials of antimicrobial or no therapy in elderly male and female nursing home residents with asymptomatic bacteriuria consistently document no benefit of antimicrobial therapy. There was no decrease in symptomatic episodes and no improvement in survival. In fact, treatment with antimicrobial therapy increases the occurrence of adverse drug effects and reinfection with resistant organisms and increases the cost of treatment. Therefore, asymptomatic bacteriuria in elderly residents of long-term care facilities should not be treated with antimicrobial agents.

If patients present with lower tract symptoms, 7 days of therapy is recommended. For individuals presenting with fever or more severe systemic infection 10 to 14 days of therapy is recommended.

○ **What is the difference between bacterial persistence and unresolved bacteriuria?**

Unresolved bacteriuria implies that the urinary tract is not sterilized during therapy. Bacterial persistence means recurrence of infection with the same organism after initial clearance.

○ **What is the significance of squamous cells in urine?**

Numerous squamous cells in the urine would indicate preputial, vaginal, or urethral contamination.

○ **Why is plasmid-mediated (R factor) resistance important?**

It is more common than selection of resistant clones. The resistance is transferable and produces multiple-resistant strains making therapy difficult.

○ **What problems do diabetic patients encounter with regard to urinary infections?**

Diabetic women appear to be more prone to UTIs. Diabetic patients often have glomerulopathy, with difficulty concentrating antimicrobials. They are also more prone to complications such as papillary necrosis and emphysematous pyelonephritis.

○ **What is the classic presentation of septic shock syndrome?**

Fever and chills followed by hypotension, but this occurs only in 30% of cases.

○ **What is the earliest metabolic abnormality in septic shock syndrome?**

Metabolic alkalosis as a consequence of hyperventilation. This occurs even before chills or fever.

○ **What are the x-ray findings of malacoplakia?**

On IVU, enlarged kidneys with multiple filling defects (best appreciated on U/S or CT). On CT, the foci are less dense than parenchyma. Unifocal lesions are indistinguishable from other inflammatory lesions and neoplasia.

○ **What is the added advantage in using low-dose TMP–SMX prophylaxis in renal transplant patients?**

In the immunosuppressed patient, TMP–SMX not only prevents UTIs but also provides protection against *Pneumocystis carinii* pneumonia, listeriosis, and nocardiosis.

○ **How do you treat candiduria in the renal transplant patient?**

As untreated candiduria can lead to the formation of obstructing candidal fungal balls, they should be treated promptly with fluconazole or with low-dose amphotericin plus rucytosine if it fails.

○ **True/False: Steroids increase the risk of UTI.**

True. The incidence of UTI increases approximately 3-fold in patients on prolonged steroid therapy.

○ **Why are fluoroquinolones contraindicated in children and pregnant women?**

They have the potential to damage developing cartilage.

○ **Why are trimethoprim and fluoroquinolones particularly suited for UTI prophylaxis?**

Both drugs are actively secreted in the vagina and bowel, thereby inhibiting growth of uropathogens at these sites.

○ **What is the most reliable form of urine collection?**

Suprapubic aspiration is the least prone to contamination.

○ **What is the most common form of recurrent UTI in women?**

Reinfection (new infection from bacteria outside the urinary tract) is the most common cause.

○ **What is the basis for leukocyte esterase test?**

Leukocyte esterase is produced by neutrophils and catalyzes the hydrolysis of an indoxyl carbonic acid ester to indoxyl. The latter oxidizes a diazonium salt on the dipstick to produce a color change.

○ **How sensitive and specific is the nitrite dipstick test for bacteriuria?**

Specificity is more than 90%, but sensitivity varies from 35% to 85%. The test is less reliable in detecting bacterial concentration $<10^5$. The most common cause of a false-positive test is contamination.

○ **Why is nitrofurantoin not suitable for the treatment of pyelonephritis?**

Nitrofurantoin is rapidly excreted in urine, but does not achieve therapeutic levels in most body tissues including the kidney.

○ **What constitutes significant bacteriuria in a catheterized patient?**

A count of $>10^2$ CFU/mL implies significant bacteriuria since these counts usually persist or increase in a catheterized patient within 48 hours.

○ **What measures are useful in reducing catheter-associated UTIs?**

Use of closed catheter drainage reduces catheter-related UTIs from 90% at 4 days to 30% to 40%. Periodic instillation of a chemical, for example, hydrogen peroxide into the collecting bag may delay the onset of infection.

○ **What is the most common organism associated with Fournier gangrene?**

Either staphylococcal or streptococcal infections may be solely responsible, although it is increasingly recognized that mixed infections, including gram-negative and anaerobic organisms, are the rule rather than the exception.

○ **How is Fournier gangrene treated and what is the mortality rate?**

Prompt treatment is critical as the mortality is 20% or more otherwise. Even with prompt therapy, the mortality rate is 5% to 6%. Intravenous hydration and multiple antibiotics with adequate surgical debridement are mainstays of treatment. Hyperbaric oxygen has been useful in some cases.

○ **How often is an orchiectomy necessary in Fournier gangrene?**

Orchiectomy is almost never needed. The testicles have a separate blood supply and can often be preserved by placement in a thigh pouch even if the scrotum is removed.

○ **Which antibiotics are suitable for the treatment of chronic prostatitis?**

Nonlipid-soluble drugs are unable to reach prostatic acini. Lipid-soluble drugs, weakly basic antibiotics that are concentrated in the prostate are most suitable. Fluoroquinolones are the drugs of first choice. Trimethoprim–sulfamethoxazole, clindamycin, erythromycin, and doxycycline are also appropriate choices.

○ **Which bacteria are usually resistant to the carbapenems?**

Carbapenems (ertapenem, imipenem, and meropenem) are active against gram-positive pathogens, gram-negative pathogens, and anaerobic bacteria and maintain efficacy against most β-lactamase-producing bacteria. They are not effective against *P. aeruginosa*, methicillin-resistant *Staphylococcus aureus*, and enterococci including vancomycin-resistant enterococci. Doripenem, the new carbapenem, and meropenem have activity against some strains of *Pseudomonas*.

○ **What issues complicate UTIs in patients with chronic renal insufficiency?**

Uremia impairs the immune system making it difficult to clear infections. The delivery of antibiotics to the urinary tract, including the kidneys, is compromised because of the reduced blood flow to the kidneys, low urine volume, and reduced renal drug-concentrating ability. Patients on dialysis are also more prone to acquiring secondary UTIs from elsewhere in the body.

○ **True/False: Circumcision is protective for HIV infection.**

True. It provides approximately 60% protection.

CHAPTER 26

Interstitial Cystitis and Other Inflammatory Conditions of the Lower Urinary Tract

Kelly C. Johnson, MD,
J. Nathaniel Hamilton, MD,
and Eric S. Rovner, MD

○ **How common is interstitial cystitis (IC) in the United States?**

Two large studies have estimated the prevalence of IC. The National Health Interview Study (NHIS) reports the overall prevalence at 500 per 100,000 population and 865 per 100,000 women. The third National Health and Nutrition Examination Survey (NHANES III) reports a prevalence of 470 per 100,000 population and 850 per 100,000 women. This equates to 83,000 men and 1.2 million US women with IC.

○ **What is the term preferred by the International Continence Society (ICS) for IC?**

ICS prefers the term Painful Bladder Syndrome (PBS) defined as "the complaint of suprapubic pain related to bladder filling, accompanied by other symptoms such as increased daytime and night-time frequency, in the absence of proven urinary infection or other obvious pathology."

○ **Are there racial differences in the prevalence of IC?**

Yes. 94% of patients are Caucasian.

○ **What percentage of patients with IC are female?**

90%.

○ **Is the incidence of childhood bladder problems increased in patients with IC?**

Yes. The incidence is 10 times higher in patients with IC than controls.

○ **What is the natural history of IC?**

Median presentation is at age 40. Spontaneous remission occurs in up to 50% of patients at a mean of 8 months. Patients may have complete and spontaneous relief from the symptoms, have a waxing and waning course, may be completely asymptomatic with intermittent "flares," or have a chronically progressive course of increasing symptoms over several years.

○ **What is the etiology of IC?**

Unknown. The most commonly cited hypotheses include (1) a pathogenic role of mast cells in the detrusor and/or mucosal layers of the bladder as a primary or secondary process, (2) a deficiency in the glycosaminoglycan layer (GAG) on the luminal surface of the bladder resulting in increased permeability of the surface layer and thus exposure of the underlying submucosal tissues to toxic substances in the urine, (3) an infection with a poorly characterized agent such as a slow growing virus or extremely fastidious bacterium which is unable to be cultured, (4) the production of a "toxic" substance in the urine, (5) neurogenic hypersensitivity or neurogenic inflammation mediated locally within the bladder or at the level of the spinal cord, (6) a manifestation of pelvic floor muscle dysfunction or dysfunctional voiding, and (7) autoimmune disorder.

○ **What other diseases or conditions have been associated with IC?**

Allergies (41%), irritable bowel (30%), inflammatory bowel disease (7%), Sjögren syndrome, vulvar vestibulitis syndrome, systemic lupus erythematosus, fibromyalgia, and sensitive skin.

○ **What are the characteristic voiding symptoms of patients with IC?**

Irritative voiding symptoms including urinary urgency, urinary frequency (>8 times per day by national institute of diabetes & digestive & kidney diseases (NIDDK) criteria) with nocturia, and pain with negative urine cultures. Obstructive symptoms including a sensation of incomplete bladder emptying and double voiding may be present. Absence of nocturnal symptoms suggests an alternative diagnosis.

○ **What are the 2 subgroups of IC?**

IC is often divided into 2 distinct subgroups based on intraoperative findings at cystoscopy and bladder overdistension. These categories are the ulcerative (ie, classic) and nonulcerative (ie, Messing–Stamey) types.

○ **Which of the following excludes a diagnosis of IC: endometriosis, pyuria, hematuria, bladder overactivity on urodynamics, or ureteral calculus?**

None. All of these conditions may coexist in patients with IC. Each of these may be related to a cause of lower urinary tract symptoms and should be properly investigated and treated prior to making a diagnosis of IC.

○ **What percentage of female patients with IC experience dyspareunia?**

Approximately 50% to 75%; such symptoms may be related to IC or associated conditions such as endometriosis or vulvodynia.

○ **What imaging studies are specific for IC?**

No known radiographic, ultrasonographic, or other imaging findings are specific for IC. Unless indicated to help exclude alternative diagnoses, radiographic studies have only a limited role in the evaluation of IC. Cross-sectional imaging including MRI, CT scan, and pelvic sonography may be performed when clinically indicated to evaluate for a suggestive pelvic mass that is causing compression of the bladder or for an adjacent inflammatory process (eg, diverticulitis). Cystography and voiding cystourethrography may be used to evaluate the bladder for other causes of irritative lower urinary tract symptoms, including intravesical masses, stones, bladder diverticula, urethral diverticula, urethral stricture, meatal stenosis, or findings suggestive of a neurogenic or nonneurogenic voiding dysfunction.

○ **Which urodynamic findings are common in IC?**

There is no urodynamic pattern that is pathognomonic for IC. On filling cystometry, most patients have a hypersensitive bladder with small volume at first sensation to void and at capacity. Filling may be limited by an intense urge to void or pain. Bladder compliance, flow, and postvoid residual are usually normal.

○ **What is the significance of finding detrusor overactivity on urodynamics?**

Involuntary bladder contractions may be found in 14% of IC patients. This is not different from the general population. Other than excluding the patient from clinical trials adhering to the NIDDK criteria, there is no other significance.

○ **What are the common findings at cystoscopy in patients with IC?**

Prior to hydrodistention—normal appearing bladder and urethral lumen, and rarely a Hunner ulcer (found in <10% of patients).

Following hydrodistention under anesthesia—glomerulations (petechial hemorrhages), submucosal hemorrhages, mucosal cracking, and bloody effluent upon drainage (terminal pinking).

○ **What are the findings during cystoscopy in a patient with "classic" IC as compared to the nonulcerative form of the disease?**

Classic IC (10% of IC patients)—reduced capacity under anesthesia (<400 mL during hydrodistention), ulcers, scars.

Nonulcerative disease (90% patients)—capacity >400 mL, no ulcers, scars, or mucosal cracking.

○ **What is the diagnostic utility of a bladder biopsy in IC?**

Although a higher proportion of IC patients may have detrusor mastocytosis as compared to normals, there are no-specific histologic findings on bladder biopsy which are pathognomonic of IC. Bladder biopsy is performed in patients being investigated for IC in order to eliminate carcinoma in situ or occult malignancy as a cause for their lower urinary tract symptoms.

○ **What is the significance of the NIDDK criteria for a diagnosis of IC?**

These criteria were developed at a national institutes of health (NIH) sponsored consensus conference to ensure a relatively homogenous and uniform population of patients for accrual and inclusion into IC research studies. Fulfillment of these criteria is not necessary for the diagnosis of IC in clinical practice.

○ **What is the potassium chloride (KCl) test?**

This is an in-office test used by some physicians in patients suspected of having a diagnosis of IC. After the intravesical instillation of 45 mL KCl (400 mEq/L), 70% of patients with a diagnosis of IC will experience pain versus only 4% of normals. This is felt to be due to a defect in the GAG layer of the bladder in patients with IC. Other conditions such as UTI may give a false-positive result.

○ **What is the role of hydrodistention in patients with IC?**

Hydrodistention is utilized both diagnostically and therapeutically in patients being evaluated for IC. A significant number of patients have transient relief of their symptoms following hydrodistention.

○ **Apart from IC, which conditions may manifest glomerulations following hydrodistention?**

Neoplasia, infectious cystitis, radiation cystitis, chemical cystitis, and a defunctionalized bladder (patients on dialysis or after urinary diversion).

○ **Are there any proven beneficial dietary restrictions for IC?**

No. However, many patients report improvement after altering their diet (changes in caffeine, alcohol, carbonated beverages, and juices). In the only prospective randomized trial performed, there was no benefit to diet modification and no association with a certain diet.

○ **Name at least 5 oral agents that have been utilized clinically in the treatment of IC?**

In uncontrolled trials, tricyclic antidepressants, sodium pentosan polyphosphate (Elmiron), hydroxyzine (antihistamines), L-arginine, nalmephene, anticholinergic agents (oxybutinin, hyoscyamine, etc), corticosteroids, cimetidine, antispasmodics, immunosuppressants, anti-inflammatories, and calcium channel blockers demonstrated some favorable effects in IC. To date, only sodium pentosanpolyphosphate (Elmiron) has shown some benefit (and only modestly) in a randomized placebo controlled trial.

○ **What is the only FDA-approved therapy for IC?**

Elmiron is the first and only oral medication approved by the Food and Drug Administration for the relief of bladder pain or discomfort associated with IC.

○ **What is the proposed mechanism of activity of Elmiron?**

Although its mechanism of action is not fully understood, Elmiron is thought to resemble glycosaminoglycans and adheres to the bladder epithelium in preclinical models. In this way, Elmiron may act as a buffer to control cell permeability, preventing irritating solutes in the urine from reaching epithelial cells.

○ **How effective is bladder hydrodistention in the management of IC?**

Temporary symptomatic improvement can be expected in up to 30% to 60% of patients.

○ **Which types of individuals are likely to respond to hydrodistention and how long does it last?**

There are no factors that are predictive of who will respond. Symptom improvement is usually transient (less than 6 months).

○ **What are the risks of hydrodistention?**

There have been reports of bladder necrosis and bladder perforation after hydrodistention. For this reason, any biopsies should be done after therapeutic hydrodistention.

○ **What is dimethylsulfoxide (DMSO) and how is it utilized to treat IC?**

DMSO is a product derived from the wood pulp industry. It has a number of pharmacologic properties, which may have some theoretical benefit in patients with IC including anti-inflammatory, analgesic, muscle relaxant properties, and mast cell histamine release. It is used as an intravesical lavage instilled on a weekly basis. It is sometimes administered in combination with steroids, alkalinizing agents, and heparin.

○ **When is urinary diversion indicated in IC/PBS?**

In the absence of a satisfactory response to other less invasive therapy, urinary diversion with or without cystectomy can be considered. However, in such cases, though the urinary frequency may be improved, pelvic pain may remain and even be aggravated following surgery. Thorough and complete patient counseling is necessary when urinary diversion is being considered for these nonmalignant, nonneurogenic cases.

○ **Per American urological association (AUA) guidelines, what is the role of the following interventions: long-term oral antibiotic administration, intravesical bacillus calmette-guérin (BCG), intravesical instillation of resiniferatoxin, high pressure/long duration hydrodistention, and systemic (oral) long-term glucocorticoid administration?**

All of these therapies are NOT recommended for PBS/IC.

○ **What is urethral syndrome?**

Urethral syndrome is a very nonspecific constellation of symptoms including urinary frequency, urgency, dysuria, and suprapubic discomfort without any objective findings of a urologic abnormality to account for the symptoms. The concept of urethral syndrome, chronic or acute, is now essentially historic, as this terminology is no longer used.

○ **What is the percentage of patients who develop radiation cystitis after external beam therapy?**

Early radiation cystitis usually occurs at 3 to 6 weeks after therapy in approximately 20% of patients. Late hemorrhagic cystitis will occur in 3% to 12% of patients. The risk of radiation cystitis varies with the dose and mode of delivery of the radiation. Radiation changes, including fibrosis and compliance changes, may occur years following the radiation treatments.

○ **What is the risk of transitional cell carcinoma of the bladder after pelvic radiation?**

Two- to four-fold increased risk. When found, the tumors tend to be high-grade and locally extensive.

○ **What is the approximate maximum radiation dose tolerated by the bladder?**

Approximately 65 to 70 Gy. Above 80 Gy, mucosal and/or full-thickness changes occur.

○ **What 3 factors of radiation delivery affect the occurrence of radiation cystitis?**

1. Volume and area of bladder treated (the trigone is especially sensitive).
2. Rate of delivery. Dose >2 Gy/Fraction increases risk.
3. Total dose.

○ **Which histopathologic changes lead to hematuria after pelvic radiation?**

Progressive obliterative endarteritis resulting in mucosal ischemia, telangiectasias, submucosal hemorrhage, and ulceration. Chronically, interstitial fibrosis ensues.

○ **How effective is hyperbaric oxygen therapy for control of radiation cystitis induced hematuria and how does it work?**

In uncontrolled studies, resolution of hematuria occurs in >90% of patients. Such therapy promotes neovascularization and generalized vasoconstriction.

○   **How many hyperbaric treatments are usually necessary for control of symptoms related to radiation cystitis?**

Thirty treatments at 2 atmospheres for 2 hours per individual treatment.

○   **What percentage of patients receiving cyclophosphamide will develop hemorrhagic cystitis in the absence of prophylactic measures?**

Up to 40% will develop hemorrhagic cystitis in low-dose chemotherapy protocols. This increased further in patients receiving high doses of cyclophosphamide in preparation for bone marrow transplantation.

○   **When is the usual onset of hemorrhagic cystitis in patients treated with cyclophosphamide?**

Cyclophosphamide can cause microscopic and gross hematuria. The onset of hematuria usually occurs within 48 hours of treatment.

○   **Which metabolite of cyclophosphamide is thought to be responsible for hemorrhagic cystitis?**

Acrolein.

○   **Which agents or therapies can be used to reduce the development of cyclophosphamide-induced hemorrhagic cystitis?**

Mesna—specifically binds acrolein. 20 mg/kg IM given at 0, 4, 8, and 12 hours after cyclophosphamide dosing.

N-acetylcysteine (Mucomyst)—oral, parenteral, or intravesical. Systemically reduces the antineoplastic effect of cyclophosphamide.

Hydration—hemorrhagic cystitis secondary to cyclophosphamide therapy is most prevalent in patients who are dehydrated.

Foley catheter—often placed to ensure immediate drainage of the bladder to minimize exposure.

CBI—continuous bladder irrigation is sometimes recommended to hasten acrolein clearance from the bladder.

○   **What is the risk of bladder cancer after cyclophosphamide therapy?**

Substantial. There is a 9-fold increased risk of bladder cancer with a short latency period (6-12 years). Most are muscle invasive at the time of diagnosis.

○   **What is the mechanism of action of epsilon aminocaproic acid (EACA) in treating hemorrhagic cystitis?**

Inhibits clot lysis by blocking plasminogen activation and fibrinolysis thereby promoting clot formation over bleeding surfaces.

○   **What is Alum and what is its mechanism of action in treating hemorrhagic cystitis?**

Potassium or ammonium aluminum sulfate (Alum) forms a salt–protein precipitate over the bleeding surface of the bladder.

○   **How is Alum administered?**

It is administered as a 1% intravesical lavage at 5 mL/min.

○ **What are the first steps for treatment if a patient on Alum bladder irrigation becomes confused or has an arrhythmia?**

Stop infusion and check serum aluminum as well as potassium or ammonia levels depending on the solution used. Once in the blood stream, aluminum can accumulate in the bone (leading to bone mass loss), liver, kidney and in very large doses, can cause cardiac arrest. Aluminum-citrate and aluminum-transferrin complexes can cross the blood–brain barrier and accumulate in brain cells, manifesting as memory loss, inability to concentrate, or dementia.

○ **What are the drawbacks of intravesical formalin for intractable hemorrhagic cystitis?**

Intravesical administration is quite painful requiring regional or general anesthesia. Reflux of formalin into the upper urinary tract may result in ureteral fibrosis, obstruction, and papillary necrosis.

○ **What is the mechanism of action of intravesical formalin?**

Formalin is used as a preservative and disinfectant in industry. Locally in the bladder, it precipitates cellular proteins of the bladder mucosa. Formalin has occluding and fixative actions on telangiectatic tissue and capillaries.

○ **What concentration of intravesical formalin should be used?**

Low formalin concentrations (1%-2%) should be used initially. This may be increased to a high concentration of formalin (10%) depending on the patient's clinical response, but the 10% concentration carries a greater risk of permanent bladder damage and loss of bladder function.

○ **What x-ray study should be performed prior to the initiation of intravesical formalin for hemorrhagic cystitis?**

A cystogram should be performed to exclude vesicoureteral reflux, as reflux of formalin into the upper tracts can have potentially devastating consequences.

○ **What is the mechanism of action of DDAVP (desmopressin) for intractable hemorrhagic cystitis?**

Increases factor VIII and von Willebrand factor levels.

○ **Which parasites have been associated with hemorrhagic cystitis?**

Echinococcus and schistosomiasis.

○ **Which viruses have been associated with hemorrhagic cystitis?**

Adenovirus types 11, 21, 35; papovarirus; influenza A; cytomegalovirus in immunodeficient states.

○ **What virus is associated with hemorrhagic cystitis following a bone marrow transplant?**

BK virus. This is a human polyomavirus that is present in approximately 60% of healthy adults and is usually acquired in childhood by the respiratory route.

○ **What percentage of bone marrow transplant recipients excrete BK virus in their urine?**

Up to 47%. The infection usually represents reactivation of latent virus.

○ **What is the first-line treatment for BK cystitis?**

Supportive measures and hyperhydration. Catheter placement should be avoided if possible because of the immunocompromised state of the patient.

○ **What is the antiviral medication given to patients with refractory BK cystitis?**

Cidofovir (3-5 mg/kg in 4-6 doses).

○ **A 68-year-old female is referred with *de novo* urinary retention. Physical examination reveals a vesicular eruption over the mons pubis and right buttocks. What is the most likely diagnosis?**

Herpes zoster may result in detrusor underactivity secondary to sacral root involvement. Characteristically, it involves a vesicular rash along sacral dermatomes. Intravesical vesicles may be seen. The urinary retention usually resolves spontaneously over 1 to 2 months.

○ **What is eosinophilic cystitis and how does it present?**

This is a pathologic diagnosis made on bladder biopsy in the setting of an eosinophilic infiltrate of the bladder lamina propria and detrusor. It has a nonspecific presentation: urgency, frequency, and hematuria. A history of allergies and peripheral eosinophilia may be present. Occasionally, a mass may be palpable, mimicking sarcoma in children.

○ **What are the endoscopic findings in eosinophilic cystitis?**

Yellow raised plaques, necrotic ulcerated lesions, edema, and erythema.

○ **Which radiologic findings are associated with eosinophilic cystitis?**

Vesicoureteral reflux is seen in one-third of patients. Bladder wall thickening may be seen on bladder sonography or other cross-sectional imaging.

○ **How is eosinophilic cystitis treated?**

Treatment is generally nonspecific with steroids and antihistamines. It often has a self-limiting course.

○ **What type of bladder cancer is associated with schistosomiasis?**

Bladder cancer in the setting of *S. hematobium* has an early onset (40-50 years) with a higher frequency of squamous cell carcinomas (60%-90%), and adenocarcinomas (5%-15%).

○ **What is malacoplakia?**

Malacoplakia means "soft plaque" in Greek. It is a rare inflammatory condition associated with abnormal microtubule assembly. This impairs the function of monocyte lysosomes, leading to inefficient killing and degradation of bacteria, resulting in incomplete eradication of bacterial infections.

○ **How do patients with malacoplakia present?**

Chronic urinary tract infections; 40% have associated systemic diseases such as immunodeficiency, malignancies, or autoimmune disease. Urine culture is positive in 90% of patients. Malacoplakia also commonly presents as a solid mass.

○ **What is the most common bacteria found in patients with malacoplakia?**

E. coli.

○ **What are the characteristic pathologic findings of genitourinary malacoplakia?**

Microscopically, infiltrates of bacteria-laden histiocytes (Michaelis–Gutmann bodies), lymphocytes, and plasma cells. Grossly, the lesions consist of raised yellow-brown plaques with hyperemic borders.

○ **What systemic diseases are associated with malacoplakia?**

Immunodeficiency states (especially organ transplantation patients on immunosuppressants), carcinoma, and autoimmune diseases. Mortality of malacoplakia is 50% when multifocal disease is present. Mortality approaches 100% when both kidneys are involved.

○ **What is emphysematous cystitis?**

This is a bladder infection characterized by gas within the bladder wall, which can spread to surrounding tissue or the upper urinary tracts in severe cases. Symptoms include abdominal pain, hematuria, and fever. This should be differentiated from air in the lumen of the bladder, which is very common and usually due to recent instrumentation or a recent UTI with a gas forming organism.

○ **Which factors predispose patients to develop emphysematous cystitis?**

Diabetes mellitus (50%), neurogenic bladder, chronic cystitis, bladder outlet obstruction, and immunodeficiencies.

○ **What are the most common pathogens in emphysematous cystitis?**

In decreasing frequency, *E. coli, Enterobacter, Klebsiella, Clostridia,* and *Candida.*

○ **How is emphysematous cystitis treated?**

Generally, in mild forms, patients may be treated with IV antibiotics, diabetic management, hydration and importantly, foley catheterization. Surgical intervention (debridement or cystectomy) can be used in extreme cases, which fail conservative management.

Prostatitis

Durwood E. Neal, Jr, MD, FACS

○ **How prevalent is prostatitis in the general population?**

Two to ten percent of men are currently experiencing prostatitis. It represents anywhere from 3% to 12% of urology office visits for men, and is the most common presenting diagnosis for men younger than 50 years. Prostatitis affects men of all ages, with the highest incidence between the ages of 20 and 49 years, but there is a second increase in incidence after the age of 65 years.

○ **What is the histologic definition of prostatitis?**

An increased number of inflammatory cells within the prostatic parenchyma.

○ **What is the most common histologic pattern of inflammation seen in prostatitis specimens?**

Lymphocytic infiltrate of prostatic stroma located immediately adjacent to the acini. Presence of polymorphonuclear cells in the prostatic acini may also be seen.

○ **Describe the 4 categories of the NIH prostatitis classification.**

1. Category I describes acute bacterial prostatitis seen in patients with acute febrile illness, a new onset of significant lower urinary tract symptoms, and possibly other systemic symptoms (chills, malaise, etc).

2. Category II represents chronic bacterial prostatitis. Patients may have constant, long-term symptoms or have recurrent episodes of acute episodes of prostatitis with asymptomatic periods. The most important finding in category II prostatitis is recurrent documented UTIs.

3. Category III denotes chronic nonbacterial prostatitis, more recently termed chronic pelvic pain syndrome (CPPS). It is divided into IIIA (inflammatory CPPS) and IIIB (noninflammatory CPPS). IIIB has historically been referred to as prostatdynia.

4. Category IV refers to asymptomatic inflammatory prostatitis. It is a histologic diagnosis only, typically made after evaluation of semen, prostate chips, or prostate biopsy specimens.

○ **What is the most common category of prostatitis?**

Type III (chronic prostatitis [CP]/chronic pelvic pain syndrome [CPPS]), which accounts for 90% to 95% of cases of prostatitis.

○ **What family of bacteria is the most common cause of category I and category II prostatitis?**

The enterobacteriaceae family of rod-shaped, gram-negative organisms is the most common bacteria implicated in both acute and chronic prostatitis. It is usually a normal part of gastrointestinal flora. *Escherichia coli* is the most common specific pathogen in bacterial prostatitis. Other genera are *Proteus, Serratia, Klebsiella,* and *Enterobacter.*

○ **What other pathogens have been implicated in bacterial prostatitis?**

Pseudomonas (gram-negative) and enterococci (gram-positive) have been found to be the causes of bacterial prostatitis. Various other organisms that are commonly found in the urethra of unaffected males have been theorized as possible causative pathogens, including *Staphylococcus* species, *Corynebacterium, Mycoplasma,* and *Ureaplasma.* Other postulated organisms include *Chlamydia, Candida* species, and nonculturable microorganisms. Fungal prostatitis may occur in patients who are immunosuppressed. *Mucorsp, Blastomyces, Cryptococcus,* and *Histoplasma* have been described.

○ **What role do prostatic calculi play in bacterial prostatitis?**

Although prostatic calculi do not lead to symptomatic bacterial prostatitis in every patient, it has been demonstrated that they can lead to persistent bacterial prostatitis that is recalcitrant to antibiotics. This is most likely related to bacterial aggregation and biofilm production along the surface and in the interstices of the stone. They also may cause blockage of prostatic ducts, preventing drainage of the secretions.

○ **Intraprostatic ductal reflux has been implicated as an important mechanism in the development of which categories of prostatitis? Which anatomic portion of the prostate is most susceptible to ductal reflux and why?**

All categories of prostatitis are either initiated by or at least affected by ductal reflux of urine into the prostate. Reflux of bacteria into the prostate can lead to infectious prostatitis, and it has been postulated that even sterile urine leads to prostatic inflammation secondary to immunologic response, or the presence of chemical irritants in the urine itself. The ducts to the peripheral zone are more horizontally oriented and seem to reflux more easily than other regions of the prostate.

○ **What happens to the levels of fructose, citrate, and acid phosphatase in prostatic secretions during acute bacterial prostatitis?**

The levels of these entities are reduced during infection of the prostate. Protein synthesis is dramatically reduced, and the cells are unable to acquire citrate during episodes of bacterial prostatitis.

○ **What happens to the levels of zinc and calcium in prostatic secretions during acute bacterial prostatitis?**

These divalent cations are normally sequestered in the prostate cells by an active transport mechanism. These processes are reduced during active infection, and secretory levels drop.

○ **How is the pH of prostatic secretions affected during acute bacterial prostatitis?**

The secretions become more basic during an acute infection. Some studies have proposed that this increase in pH reduces the diffusion and/or efficacy of antibiotics in the prostate tissue.

○ **What happens to prostatic blood flow during acute bacterial prostatitis?**

Prostatic blood flow increases in acute infections of the prostate, much like any other organ. There is most likely vascular redistribution to the periphery as a result of edema in the central portion of the gland.

○ **What is the most widely used index for research and clinical evaluation of prostatitis?**

The NIH Chronic Prostatitis Symptom Index is a valid and reproducible instrument to evaluate the symptoms and quality of life in individuals with prostatitis. The NIH-CPSI has become the primary instrument used for the quantification of CP/CPPS and has already been used in multiple placebo-controlled clinical trials.

○ **In what clinical scenario should a DRE never be performed while evaluating prostatitis?**

None. Most experts agree that a DRE can be done during the evaluation of any category of prostatitis, even category I (acute bacterial prostatitis). However, category I patients should have a single, gentle DRE, since a vigorous examination or prostatic massage can exacerbate the illness, or even result in bacteremia.

○ **Describe the Meares-Stamey test for evaluation of men with prostatitis.**

This test involves the collection of urine and prostatic fluid specimens before, during, and after prostatic massage. The first collected sample is the initial 10 mL of voided urine (voided bladder 1 or VB1) that represents urethral flora, followed by a midstream urine sample collected after 200 mL has been voided (VB2) that represents bladder flora. At this point, prostatic massage is performed and the expressed prostatic secretions (EPS) are collected, followed by the final voided urine sample (VB3). These samples are then sent for culture and microscopic analysis. The test is almost never performed by practicing urologists today, presumably due to the labor-intensive nature of the test. It has been shown that modifications of the test can be of benefit without being so onerous to perform.

○ **In what clinical scenario is the Meares-Stamey test contraindicated in the evaluation of a patient with suspected prostatitis?**

Patients with suspected category I (acute) prostatitis should not undergo the Meares-Stamey test, since the required prostatic massage could lead to bacteremia and acute worsening of symptoms.

○ **How can the Meares-Stamey test differentiate between category IIIA and IIIB prostatitis?**

Category IIIA is diagnosed when no pathogenic bacteria are cultured, but greater than 5 WBCs per HPF are seen on EPS or VB3 or both. Category IIIB is diagnosed when no pathogenic bacteria are cultured, and there are no significant levels of WBCs in the EPS and VB3.

○ **Describe the preprostatic massage and postprostatic massage test (two-glass test) and how it compares to the Meares-Stamey test.**

The patient gives a midstream urine sample prior to undergoing prostatic massage, then a urine sample (the initial 10 mL) following massage. It has been found to be 96% to 98% as accurate as the Meares-Stamey test. This is used more commonly today, when differentiation is indicated.

○ **In a patient with acute bacterial prostatitis being treated with appropriate intravenous broad-spectrum antibiotics, what diagnosis should be entertained if he continues to be febrile and highly symptomatic (chills, malaise) after 48 hours of therapy?**

Prostatic abscess should always be considered in patients with category I prostatitis who fail to respond to appropriate antimicrobial therapy. Urinary retention might also explain a failure of appropriate antibiotic therapy.

○   **What medical conditions place a patient at increased risk of developing a prostatic abscess?**

Immunocompromised patients (notably HIV-infected) are at a much greater risk of developing prostatic abscesses compared to the general population. Other important risk factors include urethral strictures, alcoholism, and chronic steroid use. Severely immunocompromised hosts are at an increased risk for prostatic abscesses caused by fungi.

○   **What are the best imaging modalities and what is the optimal treatment in a patient with a suspected prostatic abscess?**

CT scan is an acceptable imaging study to identify a prostatic abscess, but the gold standard is transrectal ultrasound. Transurethral unroofing of the abscess is considered the optimal treatment. Transperineal percutaneous drainage and transrectal drainage are other options.

○   **What is the appropriate antimicrobial management of a patient with category I prostatitis who presents with fevers, chills, and an elevated white blood cell count?**

Initial management with broad-spectrum parenteral antibiotics is considered the standard of care in acutely ill patients with category I prostatitis. Typically, a penicillin or penicillin derivative is coupled with an aminoglycoside. Once the patient has shown a good response to parenteral therapy, they can be switched to oral antibiotics, usually a fluoroquinolone, for 4 weeks.

○   **What other symptoms/complications should be addressed in patients with category I prostatitis?**

Many patients diagnosed with acute bacterial prostatitis experience varying degrees of urinary retention. α-Blockers might be needed for elevated postvoid residuals and acute LUTS, while suprapubic drainage might be required in those patients with more significant urinary retention during acute infection of the prostate. Avoidance of a urethral catheter is considered ideal when possible. Most authors recommend stool softeners, laxatives, warm sitz baths, and non-narcotic analgesics.

○   **What antibiotic class is usually recommended for category II prostatitis and why?**

Fluoroquinolones have been recommended as first-line therapy for chronic bacterial prostatitis. They show the best penetration into the prostate and seminal fluid (because of high lipid solubility), with the highest concentration by levofloxacin. The usual course is 4 to 6 weeks. Macrolides, sulfa/trimethoprim, and doxycycline are usually considered second-line therapies.

○   **What role, if any, does antibiotic therapy play in category III prostatitis?**

Patients with CP/CPPS with relatively new onset of symptoms (median of 4 weeks) might benefit from a course of antibiotics, but patients with longstanding symptoms almost never see benefit from prolonged courses of antibiotics.

○   **How long should patients with CP/CPPS be on α-blockers before they can expect to see a reduction in symptoms?**

A number of studies have shown that it takes a minimum of 6 weeks of α-blockade therapy before symptom amelioration begins to occur. Many men might need up to 3 months or more before they begin to see a significant improvement is symptoms.

○ **What anti-inflammatory agents have been found to reduce symptoms in men with CP/CPPS?**

Nonsteroidal anti-inflammatory drugs (NSAIDs) and corticosteroids have been shown to have a modest effect on symptoms related to CP. Pentosan polysulfate has also shown promise. Newer cyclooxygenase-2 inhibitors have also been studied and appear to be promising treatment options.

○ **What other pharmacologic agents have been shown to be potential treatment options for men with CP/CPPS?**

Quercetin, a bioflavinoid OTC supplement, has been shown to offer significant symptom relief in a few small trials. Tricyclic antidepressants have also been studied and showed modest improvement in symptoms. Recently the agents such as pregabalin or gabapentin have been used with fair efficacy. Many patients may benefit from the use of pentosan polysulfonate. The reasoning is that this condition may be the same as interstitial cystitis and thus treated accordingly.

○ **What role does surgical treatment play in CP/CPPS?**

Most experts recommend against TURP for the management of CP/CPPS unless a specific indication is found. TUMT has been studied with promising but inconsistent results.

○ **What other nonpharmacologic therapy options have been suggested for CP/CPPS?**

Prostatic massage, once the mainstay of prostatitis treatment, is still a controversial treatment option. There is no clear consensus regarding its use in prostatitis, while others recommend frequent ejaculation as a treatment option. Biofeedback, pelvic floor physical therapy, and myofascial release have each been supported by small clinical trials.

○ **Which antibiotic used in prostatitis has the most significant effect on male fertility?**

Doxycycline has been found to reduce both sperm production and semen quality secondary to toxic metabolites.

○ **How many tubuloalveolar glands are typically found in the prostate?**

Approximately 20.

○ **What are spermine and spermidine?**

These are natural host defenses found in prostatic fluid, as well as prostatic antibacterial factor, a zinc-containing protein. They are more effective against gram-positive organisms.

○ **Category I prostatitis is a recognized complication of what rectal surgical procedure?**

Sclerotherapy for rectal prolapse.

○ **Prostatic inflammation is found most commonly in which zone of the prostate?**

In both human and nonhuman primates, the peripheral zone is most commonly involved with the inflammatory process. This is most likely the result of the horizontal orientation of the ducts.

○   **What happens to PSA during acute prostatitis?**

PSA is elevated in the serum, sometimes markedly, during episodes of category I prostatitis, as well during acute exacerbations of category II prostatitis. This is usually due to cell disruption and loss of cell membrane integrity. It can also be elevated during other categories of prostatitis, but the degree of elevation is not clear.

○   **Patients originally misdiagnosed as prostatitis may actually have what other disorder?**

Interstitial cystitis.

○   **What are the risk factors for Type I and Type II prostatitis?**

Dysfunctional voiding, BPH (with LUTS), urethral catheterization, urethral stricture, and STDs.

CHAPTER 28 Genitourinary Tuberculosis

Thomas Chi, MD and Emil Tanagho, MD

○ **What is tuberculosis?**

Tuberculosis is a bacterial infection caused by *Mycobacterium tuberculosis*. It spreads from person to person by a pulmonary route followed by hematogenous seeding to the genitourinary (GU) tract.

○ **When was the first case of tuberculosis described?**

Tuberculosis is a disease that has been prevalent for many centuries. Dating back to 7000 BC, human skeletal remains have revealed pathologic findings consistent with tuberculosis (TB) infections.

○ **What are other historical names used for TB?**

Scrofula, consumption, phthisis, and Kings-Evil.

○ **Who first described *M. tuberculosis* and when?**

Robert Koch first identified *M. tuberculosis* as the causative organism in 1882.

○ **What is the incidence of TB worldwide?**

The WHO estimated a worldwide incidence of TB at 8.8 million cases per year in 2010 with 3 million deaths per year.

○ **What is the estimated number of people a TB-infected person could subsequently infect?**

30.

○ **How often does GU TB occur?**

Extrapulmonary TB is seen in 10% of all TB cases and of these, 30% to 40% are in the GU tract.

○ **What are the 2 main mechanisms for eradication of TB?**

Case identification and treatment, and Bacillus Calmette-Guerin (BCG) vaccination.

○ **What are the problems associated with BCG vaccination?**

The duration of response is only 15 years. It has little effect on the incidence of infection and is ineffective in patients with prior TB infections. BCG also carries many potential side effects.

○ **What are the unique microbiologic characteristics of *M. tuberculosis*?**

M. tuberculosis is an aerobic nonmotile bacterium with a high propensity to develop drug resistance. Its doubling time is slow at 24 hours. It can survive following phagocytosis in the lysosome of the macrophage.

○ **What type of immune response is seen in TB infection?**

A cell-mediated immune response from macrophages, T and B lymphocytes, and fibroblasts. Antibodies are not protective and viable bacilli within a tubercle consisting of Langhans giant cells can result in latent infection and reactivation.

○ **What are risk factors for TB reactivation?**

Diabetes mellitus, HIV infection, malignancies, chronic steroid use, chemotherapy, and immunosuppression.

○ **Describe the typical histologic findings associated with GU TB.**

Lymphocytes, macrophages, and fibroblasts aggregate to form a pathognomonic TB granuloma.

○ **What is the typical gross appearance of TB-infected renal tissue?**

Tissue demonstrates central caseating necrosis, sloughed renal papilla, and calyceal ulceration. Late-stage renal involvement demonstrates infundibular narrowing, ureteropelvic junction (UPJ) scarring, and segmental or generalized hydronephrosis.

○ **What are the typical pathologic changes of the ureter in TB infection?**

After tubercle formation, the ureteral mucosa undergoes ulceration, then fibrosis and scarring that ultimately cause stricture and obstruction, then fibrotic encasement of the ureter.

○ **What is the typical pathologic appearance of the bladder in GU TB?**

Mucosal caseation with an undermining tuberculous ulcer creates a "worm-eaten" appearance of the ulcer with ragged edges.

○ **What are the gross appearance of the epididymis, vas deferens, and testis in GU TB?**

Chronic inflammation causes obliteration of the epididymal lumen and nodular epididymitis. This can ulcerate to the skin, creating a tubercular sinus on the posterior scrotum. In a similar fashion, the vas deferens can take on a beaded appearance from segmental dense fibrosis. With chronic testicular infection, replacement of normal tissue with caseous material occurs.

○ **Do nontuberculosis mycobacteria cause pathogenic changes in the GU tract?**

This is very rare. Only a handful of cases have been reported. The mycobacteria involved include *M. kansasii*, *M. avium-intracellulare*, *M. xenopi*, and *M. fortuitum*.

○   **What test can be used to differentiate *M. tuberculosis* from nontuberculosis mycobacteria?**

p-Nitro-α-acetylamino-β-hydroxypropriophenone, the NAP test.

○   **What populations are at highest risk for developing TB?**

People living in underdeveloped countries, alcoholics, HIV patients, IV drug abusers, the homeless, and the elderly.

○   **What is the most common age group and gender to develop GU TB?**

GU TB is most commonly seen in the 20- to 40-year-old age group with a 2:1 male-to-female predominance.

○   **What is the classic triad of TB infections?**

Fatigue, weight loss, and anorexia.

○   **How does TB spread to the GU tract?**

GU TB is the result of metastatic spread of the mycobacterium via the blood stream. It usually results from a primary pulmonary focus. Only 25% of patients have a known history of TB.

○   **What is the mechanism that leads to TB of the lower urinary tract?**

Urinary excretion of the mycobacterium from the kidney causes seeding and infection of the lower urinary tract. Epididymal and prostatic TB are spread hematogenously.

○   **What are some of the clinical findings associated with GU TB?**

Sterile pyuria is the hallmark of GU TB. Other less specific signs are painless urinary frequency, nocturia, hematuria, hematospermia, suprapubic pain, and flank pain.

○   **How often is microscopic hematuria found in cases of GU TB?**

Microscopic hematuria is present in approximately 50% of cases.

○   **How should one culture the urine of a patient suspected of having GU TB?**

Five consecutive early morning urine specimens should be obtained and cultured on 2 separate media. Lowenstein–Jensen medium will isolate *M. tuberculosis*, BCG, and nontuberculosis mycobacterium. Radiometric media such as BACTEC 460 is much faster and takes only 2 to 3 days for results.

○   **What is the quickest way to diagnose TB?**

Polymerase chain reaction (PCR) testing is highly sensitive, specific, and quick. Results are available in 6 hours.

○   **A 41-year-old woman native of India is referred to her urologist with irritative voiding and sterile pyuria. What is the differential diagnosis?**

Carcinoma in situ of the bladder, GU TB, and interstitial cystitis.

○ **What are the most common sites of GU TB?**

The most common hematogenous sites of GU TB spread are the kidney, epididymis, and fallopian tubes. The prostate can be infected hematogenously, though its involvement is more often from a urinary source.

○ **What GU organs are spared from TB infections?**

None. All organs of the GU tract are targets for TB infections. However, TB of the penis, adrenal gland, and urethra are rare.

○ **What are typical signs of GU TB on plain radiographs?**

Thirty percent to fifty percent of involved kidneys have calcifications of the kidney. After autonephrectomy, a lobar calcified cast of the kidney can be seen. With late bladder contraction, bladder wall calcifications can be seen.

○ **What are the common radiographic findings of TB in the ureter?**

Ureteral strictures, beading of the ureter, hydroureterosis from distal stenosis, ureterovesical obstruction, and vesicoureteral reflux.

○ **What are the common intravenous pyelogram (IVP) findings of GU TB?**

The 3 most common findings are hydrocalycosis, hydronephrosis, and hydroureter. Additional findings include calcification, parenchymal loss, distorted calyces, calyceal loss, and poorly functioning or nonfunctioning kidneys. A moth-eaten appearance from calyceal erosion and papillary irregularity is typical during the excretory phase. Severe angulation of the UPJ can also be seen, called "Kerr kink." The ureter can have a rigid, straight, "pipe-stem" appearance.

○ **What are common CT findings in GU TB?**

Renal parenchymal scarring and masses (from coalescence of caseating granulomas) are common, as are thickened ureteral and bladder walls. In the prostate and seminal vesicles, necrosis can lead to cavity formation and resultant areas of hypoattenuation.

○ **What are typical endoscopic findings in GU TB?**

While there are no pathognomonic findings, the ureteral orifice may have a "golf-hole" appearance. Ulcers may be present and can mimic malignancy. The bladder lesions usually arise at the ureteral orifices. The lesions can be velvety, red, inflamed, and edematous with granulations as a later finding. More advanced disease can affect the entire bladder, leading to a small volume, contracted bladder.

○ **When is a bladder biopsy indicated in GU TB?**

Only to rule out malignancy if there is uncertainty. Isolated tubercles away from the ureteral orifices should be biopsied for this purpose. Positive urine cultures negate the need for biopsy, as biopsies are diagnostic in only 18% to 45% of cases. If the urine cultures are negative, the bladder biopsies will also be negative.

○ **What are the primary medications currently used to treat GU TB?**

Rifampin, isoniazid, pyrazinamide, streptomycin, and ethambutol.

○ **What is the current recommendation for the medical treatment of uncomplicated GU TB?**

At this time, a 6-month treatment regimen is the standard of care. Isoniazid, rifampin, pyrazinamide, and/or ethambutol (if isoniazid resistance is suspected) for 2 months and then isoniazid and rifampin for 4 additional months.

○ **What lab tests should be checked before initiating medical therapy and during a course of therapy?**

Baseline liver function tests, creatinine, complete blood cell (CBC), and platelet count should be checked. Periodic liver function tests should be performed to rule out rifampin hepatotoxicity. Uric acid levels should be monitored if pyrazinamide is used. Visual acuity and red-green color perception should be monitored if ethambutol is administered.

○ **A 45-year-old woman has just completed her course of medical therapy for renal TB. She is asymptomatic and feels well. How should she be followed?**

She should be seen at 3, 6, and 12 months following completed treatment. At each visit, she should have 3 consecutive morning urine specimens sent for TB cultures. Radiographic examination of her upper urinary tract would also be indicated. She should also return if symptoms recur.

○ **How long should one treat a patient with medical therapy for GU TB prior to embarking on a surgical intervention?**

At least 3 to 6 weeks to allow stabilization of lesions and decrease in the initial intense inflammation.

○ **What is a nonspecific test that can be used to monitor the effectiveness of treatment for TB?**

Erythrocyte sedimentation rate (ESR), if elevated prior to therapy, can be used to monitor the effectiveness of a specific treatment.

○ **Of the 5 most commonly used antituberculosis medications (rifampin, isoniazid, pyrazinamide, ethambutol, and streptomycin), which drugs are bactericidal?**

Rifampin, isoniazid, pyrazinamide, and streptomycin.

○ **Following institution of isoniazid, rifampin, and pyrazinamide for GU TB, the patient notices the development of a pruritic macular rash. This is followed by generalized myalgias and conjunctivitis. Which drug is most commonly associated with this hypersensitivity reaction?**

Rifampin and streptomycin are most commonly associated with hypersensitivity reactions.

○ **Which anti-TB drugs are to be avoided in the presence of renal failure?**

Ethambutol and streptomycin are primarily renally excreted and should be avoided in this situation.

○ **A 62-year-old man receiving isoniazid, rifampin, pyrazinamide, and ethambutol for GU TB has developed visual changes since the initiation of medical therapy. What is the most likely cause of his new symptoms?**

Ethambutol can lead to optic neuritis. It is recommended that all patients receiving the drug undergo monthly visual examinations.

○ **Three weeks following initiation of medical treatment for GU TB, the patient is noted to have a rise in the liver enzyme panel. Jaundice is not present. How should this be managed?**

Most patients will have a transient elevation in the liver enzyme panel for the first few weeks of therapy. If jaundice develops, the medications should be withdrawn until the jaundice resolves. Medical therapy can then be reinstituted.

○ **Which of the antituberculosis drugs is ototoxic?**

Streptomycin.

○ **A 34-year-old woman on oral contraceptive medications becomes pregnant following the initiation of an antituberculosis regimen. What is the likely cause for the failure of her contraceptive?**

Rifampin can affect the metabolism of estrogen in oral contraceptive preparations. This can lead to an increased failure rate of these contraceptives. Women of childbearing age should use an alternative means of contraception while taking antituberculosis drugs.

○ **A 40-year-old man with the new diagnosis of GU TB has severe cystitis secondary to bladder involvement. Anticholinergic medications did not improve his symptoms. What can be added to the usual drug regimen in order to improve his symptoms?**

Prednisone can reduce the symptoms of acute TB cystitis. Prednisone may also be of benefit if a distal ureteral stricture is present; however, this issue remains controversial. Rifampin will significantly decrease the bioavailability of prednisone.

○ **A 32-year-old man is being evaluated for left flank pain and sterile pyuria. What is the appropriate workup?**

This individual should have a repeat urinalysis, urine cytology, urine culture for TB, cystoscopy, and an IVP or CT scan. IVPs are preferred. If a CT scan is done, it should be with intravenous contrast.

○ **On a plain film of the abdomen, the patient is noted to have a large left upper pole calcification. The IVP reveals that he has minimal function of this kidney and blunting of his calyces. His urine cultures reveal TB. What would be the indications for nephrectomy in this individual?**

A nonfunctioning kidney, associated renal cell carcinoma, uncontrolled hypertension, persistent severe flank pain, and patient noncompliance with the appropriate medical treatments are all indications for nephrectomy in the described setting.

○ **What is the likelihood of finding hypertension in a patient with renal TB compared to the general population without TB?**

Patients with renal TB are approximately twice as likely to have hypertension as the general population.

○ **If the kidney is entirely destroyed with caseous decay, how should it be managed?**

These kidneys are best managed by nephrectomy.

○ **What are the indications for nephrectomy?**

As medical therapy is now first-line treatment for renal tuberculosis infection, nonfunctioning kidneys should be removed only if they fail adequate drainage and medical treatment. Extensive parenchymal destruction involving the whole kidney associated with hypertension is also an indication for nephrectomy.

○ **When is the appropriate time to perform the nephrectomy?**

3 to 6 weeks after the initiation of medical therapy.

○ **A 27-year-old woman with hypertension is found to have an atrophic right kidney from chronic renal TB. What is the likelihood that she will have an improvement in her hypertension with a nephrectomy?**

Approximately 65% of patients with significant unilateral renal involvement will have improvement in their hypertension.

○ **A 21-year-old man with renal TB has a small renal calcification resulting from the infectious process. He has been adequately treated for his TB. How should this calcification be managed?**

Calcification is associated with the normal tissue response from the destructive process and subsequent mineralization of the fibrous scar tissue. Small calcifications can be observed while larger ones should be removed in a parenchyma sparing fashion if there is adequate global kidney function in the remaining parenchyma.

○ **What is the most common portion of the ureter to be affected by TB?**

The ureterovesical junction.

○ **How does TB lead to vesicoureteral reflux?**

Scarring in the bladder at the level of the ureteral orifice can cause contraction of the surrounding tissue leading to a contracted rigid golf hole type ureteral orifice. This same process can also lead to stenosis of the ureteral orifice.

○ **A 50-year-old man was diagnosed with a distal ureteral stricture secondary to GU TB. He is placed on the standard medical regimen for GU TB. After 3 weeks of medical therapy he has no improvement in his ureteral obstruction. What is the next appropriate step in management?**

The addition of prednisone to his regimen would be indicated and should improve his ureteral stenosis.

○ **Following 3 more weeks of medical management, his obstruction persists. What are the remaining options for the treatment of his distal ureteral stricture?**

Accusize balloon dilation/incision, psoas hitch reimplantation, Boari flap reimplantation, and ileal interposition.

○ **A 55-year-old man was treated for severe GU cystitis with isoniazid, rifampin, pyrazinamide, and prednisone for 6 months. Following treatment, he remains disease free. However, he has severe persistent urgency, frequency, and nocturia. His bladder capacity is 120 mL. What would be the next appropriate therapy?**

Augmentation cystoplasty.

○ **A 20-year-old man presents with a superficial ulcer of his glans penis. Biopsy of the lesion rules out a malignancy, but reveals TB. How could he have contracted this disease?**

Hematogenous spread from a primary pulmonary source or direct inoculation from the female genital tract.

○ **How does TB orchitis develop?**

TB orchitis is almost always a direct extension of TB of the epididymis. TB is spread to the epididymis via the blood stream.

○   **A 22-year-old HIV-positive man presents with scrotal swelling and a tender right testicle and epididymis. Upon palpation, he has beading of his associated vas deferens. He has a poorly defined fullness to the globus major of the epididymis that is directly associated with the testis. What would be the next step in the management of this patient?**

A scrotal ultrasound should be obtained to further delineate the fullness.

○   **The ultrasound reveals a solid mass involving the testis and epididymis as well as a small associated loculated hydrocele. What is the next step in the management?**

The patient should have tumor markers drawn and undergo a radical orchiectomy. This lesion may represent a testicular malignancy.

○   **A 40-year-old man with prior pulmonary TB has epididymal fullness that on ultrasound is consistent with TB. The testis is uninvolved. What technique could be used to evaluate for active TB in his scrotum?**

Fine needle aspiration can frequently yield active TB within the epididymis.

○   **What complication can arise from epididymal TB?**

Obstructive azoospermia can occur and with more advanced disease, nodular epididymitis can lead to fistulization of sinus tracts to the skin.

○   **How should isolated epididymal infections be treated?**

Isolated epididymal involvement can be treated with epididymectomy. Meticulous sparing of the testicular blood supply is important. If testicular involvement is seen, then a scrotal orchiectomy can be performed.

○   **A young couple wish to have children. Female factor infertility has been ruled out. The potential father was treated for pulmonary TB. His workup has revealed findings consistent with epididymo-orchitis related to his history of TB. He is found to be profoundly azospermic. How should they proceed?**

Natural conception in unlikely is this setting. Most patients will require epididymal or testicular sperm aspiration followed by in vitro fertilization.

○   **Antituberculosis antibiotics should be used for how long in HIV-positive patients?**

Nine months is usually recommended.

○   **Patients with HIV account for what percent of the total TB population?**

Ten percent worldwide. TB testing is recommended in all HIV patients.

Medical Aspects of Urolithiasis

Elizabeth A. Phillips, MD and
David S. Wang, MD

○ **How common is nephrolithiasis?**

The overall prevalence of stone disease is approximately 8%.

○ **How many Americans experience a bout of renal colic caused by nephrolithiasis annually?**

Approximately 1,200,000.

○ **How does region affect the incidence of nephrolithiasis?**

More common in the southeast United States and less common in the northwest.

○ **Is the worldwide incidence of kidney stones increasing, decreasing, or about the same and why?**

The rate of kidney stone disease is increasing worldwide. This is thought to be the result of more cultures adopting a Western diet as well as global warming contributing to increased dehydration.

○ **Is nephrolithiasis more common in men or women and by what ratio?**

The male:female ratio is shifting, in the last few years it has been closer to 3:1, but is currently 1.7:1. Roughly 7% of women and 13% of men will develop at least one stone at some point in their lifetimes.

○ **What type of calculus is equally common in men and women?**

Cystine and uric acid stones.

○ **What type of calculus is more common in women than men?**

Struvite stones are twice as likely to occur in women because of the higher incidence of urinary tract infections in females.

○ **What is the most common age at presentation with nephrolithiasis?**

A peak incidence for nephrolithiasis occurs from 30 to 60 years old with 35 to 45 being the peak decade.

○ **What are the most common associated (non-chemistry) reasons for formation of stones in children, women, and men, respectively?**

- Children:
  ◦ Voiding dysfunction
  ◦ Anatomic abnormalities (ie, valves)
- Women:
  ◦ Prolapse
  ◦ Neurogenic bladder
  ◦ Foreign bodies
  ◦ Urinary tract infection
- Men:
  ◦ BPH, urethral stricture, bladder diverticulae
  ◦ Neurogenic bladder

○ **Bladder stones make up what percentage of all urinary calculi?**

5%.

○ **What is the current estimated yearly cost of kidney stone disease in the United States?**

More than 2 billion dollars a year and rising.

○ **Does family history of stones increase patient's risk of stone formation?**

Yes, 3-fold increased risk.

○ **What is the risk for stone recurrence after an initial symptomatic episode of urolithiasis? How does risk of stone formation change over time?**

- Increasing risk each year:
  ◦ Year 1: 10% to 15% risk of additional stone formation
  ◦ Year 5: 50% to 60%
  ◦ Year 10: 70% to 80%

○ **What are some risk factors for stone formation?**

- Dehydration
- Increased weight (obesity)
- Family history
- High sodium diet
- High animal protein diet
- Previous history of stones

○ **What populations of patients necessitate treatment of asymptomatic renal calculi?**

- Pediatric
- Woman planning pregnancy
- Solitary kidney or transplant
- Occupational hazard—military, pilot, etc

○ **What is the recommended antibiotic prophylaxis for stone manipulation?**

- Single systemic quinolone
- Cephalosporin

○ **What effect, if any, does obesity have on kidney stone formation?**

Obesity is a strong predictor of stone recurrence especially in first-time stone formers. Obesity causes changes in urine chemistry reflecting increased calcium, uric acid, sodium, and decreased citrate in the urine. Urine of obese patients has also been found to have a lower pH. Obesity is associated with a higher risk for both uric acid and calcium oxalate stones.

○ **How does obesity affect nephrolithiasis?**

Through purine gluttony, dietary excesses, diabetes, and insulin resistance.

○ **How might insulin resistance contribute to stone forming?**

Insulin resistance at the cellular level results in hyperinsulinemia, which in turn causes defects in renal production of ammonia, lowering the pH of the urine.

○ **What medications can be used to facilitate ureteral stone passage in urolithiasis?**

α_1-Adrenergic antagonists facilitate stone passage. Tamsulosin and other α-blockers, used often in BPH, facilitate passage of stones less than 10 mm. The rate of stone passage increases approximately 30% with the use of α-blockers, and the need for narcotics and surgical intervention decreases. Steroids may be used to reduce ureteral edema for easier stone passage. In addition, calcium channel blockers such as nifedipine have been shown to cause ureteral dilatation and relaxation resulting in increased spontaneous stone passage rates.

○ **What percentage of patients requires intervention for passage of a stone?**

It is 20% overall; 50% of patients with stones ≥ 5 mm. A proximal ureteral stone will have a lower chance of spontaneous stone passage (50%) than a distal ureteral stone (85%). In general, a stone 4 mm or less in size has a 90% chance of eventual passage.

○ **In a patient presenting with a ureteral stone, is antibiotic therapy indicated?**

Patients with bacteriuria and a ureteral stone should be treated with antibiotics given the increased risk of infectious complications and urosepsis (according to American urologic association (AUA) guidelines). Patients with planned interventions should be treated with antibiotics prior to the intervention.

○ **In patients presenting with a ureteral stone, with well-controlled symptoms, what are the recommendations for medical expulsion therapy?**

- Patients should be comfortable with this treatment and have good renal reserve.
- Patients should be informed that α-blocker therapy is used "off label."
- Patients should have radiologic follow-up to assess for progression.

○ **What is the average time to spontaneous stone passage?**

The time to spontaneous passage correlates with stone size. The average time to stone passage is 1 week for <2 mm, 2 weeks for 2 to 4 mm, and 3 weeks for >4 mm.

○ **How long should one wait for an asymptomatic stone to pass or move before considering doing a surgical procedure?**

For stones <10 mm approximately 95% will pass spontaneously within 4 to 6 weeks, following that time, if the stone has not passed spontaneously, one should consider intervention. After that time, the risk of possible long-term complications, such as strictures, increases.

○ **What are the indications for hospitalization in the acute setting of renal colic?**

Severe pain requiring continuing parenteral pain medication, fever and infection, intractable vomiting, renal insufficiency or rising creatinine, and a solitary kidney. Urinary tract infection with an obstructed system is an indication for emergent decompression of the collecting system with ureteral stenting or placement of a percutaneous nephrostomy tube.

○ **What medication decreases the need for narcotics to control renal colic?**

Ketorolac (Toradol) IV has been demonstrated to decrease the need for narcotics in acute renal colic. IV Acetaminophen has also been used.

○ **Can stone disease be ruled out in the absence of hematuria?**

No, approximately 15% of patients with ureteral stones have no RBC/HPF on microscopic urinalysis.

○ **What diagnostic imaging should be used if there is clinical suspicion of urolithiasis?**

Noncontrast spiral/helical CT. Patients with BMI <30 may have low-dose noncontrast CT as this will reduce the amount of exposure to radiation in these patients. Obese patients should have standard noncontrast CT as their body habitus precludes a low-dose study. CT can also assist in diagnosing other nonrenal causes of flank pain.

○ **Should a kidneys, ureter, bladder (KUB) be performed when the CT scan has already identified a stone? Why or why not?**

Yes, a KUB should be immediately performed when the CT scan has demonstrated a stone for several reasons. First, it provides a baseline study to easily track progress of the stone. Next, it quickly separates radiopaque from radiolucent stones. Finally, it provides a clear idea of the shape and size of the stone as well as its surgical orientation.

○ **What is the recommended imaging for follow-up of ureteral stones for patients that are being managed expectantly?**

For radio-opaque stones, ultrasound and KUB should be the preferred method of imaging. If stones are not radio-opaque, low-dose noncontrast CT should be employed.

○ **Compare modalities of imaging as diagnostic tests for urolithiasis.**

- Ultrasound detects 50% to 60% of stones.
- KUB detects 60% to 70%.
- Intravenous urogram (IVU) detects 70% to 90%.
- Noncontrast CT scan detects 90% to 100%.

○ **What differential diagnoses with urolithiasis may be evaluated using noncontrast CT?**

Pyelonephritis	Tumor with urinary retention	Pancreatitis
Diverticulitis	Renal mass or tumor	Ileus
Appendicitis	Duodenal ulcer with perforation	Benign stenosis of the ureter
Aortic aneurysm	Renal pelvis tumor	Pancreatic tumor

○ **What are some of the limitations of CT imaging of renal stones?**

CT cannot identify pure indinavir stones. It also cannot differentiate between radiolucent and radiopaque stones, and it does not always give an accurate rendering of the exact size or shape of some stones. It is also expensive and has significant radiation exposure so it cannot be used in pregnancy.

○ **How accurate is CT in diagnosing urolithiasis?**

98% sensitivity, 95% specificity, 98% positive predictive value, and 95% negative predictive value.

○ **Is MRI a useful imaging study in urolithiasis?**

MRI does not visualize stones and should not be used to make the diagnosis of urolithiasis. MR urography may have a role in the evaluation of flank pain in pregnancy, although ultrasound is the first choice in imaging.

○ **What is first- and second-line imaging modality for stones in pregnancy?**

- US
- IVP
- MRI can also be used, it is not very effective in visualizing stones, but may pick up filling defects

○ **What risk factors contribute to stones in pregnancy?**

- Multiparity
- Caucasian
- Prior stone episode
- Renal disease
- Hypertension

○ **During what trimester is a pregnant woman most likely to have a symptomatic stone?**

Second and third.

○ **What is the recommended treatment for a symptomatic ureteral stone in a pregnant woman?**

Ureteroscopy is acceptable treatment in the second and third trimester.

○ **According to AUA guidelines, what is the first-line treatment for pediatric stones?**

While both ureteroscopy and extracorporeal shock wave lithotripsy (ESWL) can be used, some literature favors ESWL for first-line treatment of pediatric renal/ureteral stones.

○ **Are forced fluids helpful in the management of acute renal colic?**

A recent randomized trial demonstrated that fluid bolus in the emergency department did not impact pain or stone passage. As such, forceful hydration may not help with stone expulsion although many patients with acute renal colic will be dehydrated and may need IV fluid replenishment for other reasons.

○ **What fluids and drinks should generally be avoided in stone formers?**

Phosphoric acid in soda drinks will acidify the urine and increase the risk of kidney stones. Performance drinks are often high in sodium content and will increase the risk of stones.

○ **How does dietary sodium impact the risk of stone formation?**

Every teaspoon of salt increases urinary calcium by 23 mg. It leads to higher rates of bone resorption and fluid retention while decreasing urinary citrate levels by 20%.

○ **Is significant oral calcium restriction recommended for calcium stone formers?**

Aggressive calcium restriction increases the risk of stone formation. Calcium is important for bone homeostasis and to bind oxalate in the bowel. A moderate limitation of calcium intake is reasonable.

○ **What complementary approaches are available for patients with hypercalciuria?**

Fish oil supplementation (Eicosapentaenoic acid, *n*-3 fatty acid) competes with arachidonic acid (*n*-6) resulting in a decrease in prostaglandin E2. This leads to a decrease in renal calcium excretion, increase of renal calcium reabsorption, and decreased bone resorption. It has been demonstrated to decrease urinary supersaturations for both calcium phosphate and calcium oxalate.

○ **What dietary changes can influence calcium excretion in the urine?**

Increased sodium intake results in increased urinary calcium. An increase of 100 mEq of dietary sodium will increase urinary excretion by 50 mg/day.

○ **What oral medication can effect hypercalciuric stone formation?**

Thiazides are used to blunt the increased calcium excretion in the urine. High sodium diet can block this effect.

○ **How does low calcium diet effect stone formation?**

Low calcium diets increase urinary oxalate, therefore encouraging stone formation. Low calcium diet is NOT recommended.

○ **How does dietary oxalate affect stone formation?**

Urinary calcium and oxalate are excreted in a bound state, thereby staying in solution. If there is less calcium excreted, oxalate is not bound and is free to facilitate oxalate stone formation.

○ **What food products contain high levels of oxalate?**

Chocolate, green leafy vegetables (spinach), and nuts.

○ **What effect does a high animal protein diet have on calcium, uric acid, pH, and citrate?**

- Increase in calcium and uric acid in the serum.
- Decrease in urinary pH and urinary citrate.

○ **Which patients should undergo a full metabolic evaluation for nephrolithiasis?**

1. Pediatric stone formers
2. Stone composition: cystine, uric acid, and struvite
3. Nephrocalcinosis
4. Renal failure and transplant patients

5. Strong family history

6. High stone recurrence (>1 per year)

7. Strongly motivated to follow through on long-term treatment

○ **What else is included in a full metabolic evaluation for nephrolithiasis?**

1. History and physical—including diet history, fluid intake, medications, history of recurrent urinary tract infections, personal and family history of stone events

2. Stone analysis—chemical analysis of stones or fragments recovered

3. Urinalysis

4. Serum electrolyte/ metabolic panel—serum sodium, potassium, chloride, bicarbonate, creatinine, uric acid, phosphate, magnesium, calcium, and alkaline phosphatase

5. Parathyroid hormone level (intact) and 25 (OH) vitamin D depending on calcium level

6. 24-hour urine collection on normal diet

7. 24-hour urine collection with dietary changes and increased fluid. (Some literature suggests that a single 24-hour urine may be sufficient for metabolic analysis of most patients, and some practitioners use 2 random 24-hour urine collections.)

○ **What are the components of a complete 24-hour urine evaluation?**

1. Total urine volume

2. pH urine

3. Calcium urine

4. Oxalate urine

5. Uric acid urine

6. Citrate urine

7. Sodium urine

8. Sulfate phosphorus urine

9. Magnesium urine

10. Ammonium urine

11. Potassium urine

12. Creatinine urine

13. Calcium oxalate

14. Brushite

15. Sodium urate

16. Struvite

17. Uric acid

○ **What is the most common reason for an inaccurate 24-hour urine evaluation?**

Inadequate collection, not collecting for full 24 hours.

○ **In what percentage of patients can at least one metabolic abnormality predisposing to urolithiasis be identified?**

A probable metabolic etiology for nephrolithiasis is found in 97% of patients who are properly evaluated.

○   **What is the most common type of stone formed?**

Calcium oxalate stones make up approximately 70% of all renal calculi.

○   **What types of crystal are depicted in this urine sample?**

Figure A.   **Figure B.**

Cystine: hexagonal shape.   Calcium oxalate: star-box shape.

Figure C.

Calcium phosphate: coffin shape.

○ **What are the 5 most important urinary chemical abnormalities found in stone formers?**

Hypercalciuria, hypocitraturia, hyperuricosuria, hyperoxaluria, and low urinary volume.

○ **What are some promotors of urinary stone formation?**

1. Calcium
2. Sodium
3. Oxalate
4. Urate
5. Cystine
6. Low urine pH
7. Tamm-Horsfall proteins
8. Low urine flow/volume

○ **What are some inhibitors of stone formation?**

1. Citrate
2. Magnesium
3. Pyrophosphate
4. Tamm-Horsfall protein
5. Urinary prothrombin fragment 1
6. Protease inhibitor
7. Glycosaminoglycans
8. Osteopontin (uropontin)
9. Renal lithostathine
10. Bikunin
11. Calgranulin
12. High urine flow/volume

○ **How does potassium citrate aid in prevention of stone formation?**

Potassium citrate corrects acidosis and increases urinary citrate levels. Citrate is a potent inhibitor of stone formation, inhibiting calcium stone crystallization and lowering the saturation of calcium in urine.

○ **Citrate is an important inhibitor of stone formation. What drink is highest in citrate content?**

Grapefruit juice (14,500 mg/L of citrate). However, grapefruit juice is also moderately high in oxalate content. The most effective means to obtain dietary citrate is 4 oz of concentrated lemon juice per day, usually as lemonade.

○ **How does citrate supplementation affect citrate levels in the urine?**

Citrate absorbed from the intestines is converted to bicarbonate in the liver. This increased alkali load stimulates renal excretion of citrate, raises the urinary pH, and increases urinary citrate levels.

○ **What role does citrate play in urinary stone formation?**

Citrate is an stone inhibitor for calcium oxalate stones.

○ **What physical states result in hypocitraturia?**
- Metabolic acidosis
  - Distal RTA (Type 1)
  - Chronic diarrhea
  - Physical exercise (lactic acidosis)
  - High protein diet
  - Hydrochlorothyazide (HCTZ) use, potassium wasting
- Urinary tract infection
  - Citrate is degraded by organism

○ **How does acidosis effect stone formation?**

Acidosis increases calcium resorption in the GU tract and from the bone, therefore there is more circulating calcium, and decreased renal resorption of calcium in the kidney. Calcium is then excreted in the urine.

○ **In what ways does citrate inhibit calcium stone formation?**

Citrate binds calcium, forming a soluble complex in urine and competing with its binding with oxalate or phosphate. Citrate will also alkalinize the urine, thereby inhibiting the formation of both calcium oxalate and uric acid crystals.

○ **What is the optimal level of oral citrate supplementation and how can this be determined clinically?**

An optimal concentration of 320 to 340 mg of citrate/L of urine and 24-hour urine levels $\geq$600 to 650 mg of citrate have been suggested as long as the urinary pH remains at or below 7. While a 24-hour urine test for citrate would be optimal, it is impractical to perform this test too often. Another method is to maximize the potassium citrate supplementation until the patient reaches maximum tolerance or the pH exceeds 7. FDA-approved urinary dipsticks to specifically monitor urinary pH are now available commercially (www.uridynamics.com).

○ **What is the most important chemical mediator of intestinal absorption of calcium?**

The most important chemical mediator of calcium absorption is calcitriol (1,25-dihydroxyvitamin D_3), which increases calcium transport across the intestinal lumen. The conversion of precursors to calcitriol is initiated by hypophosphatemia and parathyroid hormone (PTH).

○ **What additional effects does PTH have on calcium homeostasis?**

PTH is a polypeptide that stimulates the osteoclasts to resorb bone, releasing calcium and phosphate into the bloodstream. PTH also acts upon the kidney to resorb calcium from the urine into the blood.

○ **PTH increases calcium resorption in the kidney, so explain why we find hypercalciuria in patients with hyperparathyroidism.**

The calcium resorption effect of PTH is overcome in hyperparathyroidism by the extremely high serum calcium levels.

○ **True/False: The incidence of stone formation in hyperparathyroid patients is unrelated to the degree of serum calcium or PTH elevations.**

True.

○ **What percentage of hyperparathyroid patients will have nephrolithiasis as their presenting or initial symptom?**

22%.

○ **In what ways are hyperparathyroid stone formers different from hyperparathyroid patients without nephrolithiasis?**

Hyperparathyroid stone formers are more likely to be younger and have hypercalciuria. Their hyperparathyroidism is almost always caused by parathyroid adenomas as opposed to hyperplasia.

○ **How much dietary calcium is absorbed on a daily basis?**

Approximately 33% of the total dietary calcium (600-1200 mg or 15 mg/kg) is absorbed and 100 to 200 mg is secreted into the intestinal tract for a net absorption of approximately 100 to 300 mg. Calcium ions that are complexed in the gastrointestinal (GI) tract to phosphate, oxalate, citrate, and sulfate are not absorbed.

○ **How is hypercalciuria defined? (Give at least 3 definitions.)**

(1) The excretion of greater than 200 mg/24 h on a diet of 400 mg calcium and 100 mEq sodium for a week. (2) On an unrestricted diet, hypercalciuria can be defined as >275 mg calcium/day for men, >250 mg/day for women. (3) Another definition is more than 4 mg of calcium/kg body weight/day.

○ **What is the estimated percentage of patients with calcium oxalate stones who will demonstrate hypercalciuria?**

Approximately 35%.

○ **What are the 3 basic types of hypercalciuria?**

1. Absorptive hypercalciuria caused by increased intestinal absorption of calcium.

2. Renal leak hypercalciuria caused by an abnormality in renal absorption of calcium.

3. Resorptive hypercalciuria caused by augmented bone demineralization.

Hypercalciuria types:

- *Absorptive hypercalciuria*
  - Increased calcium absorption in the GI tract leading to increased plasma calcium, decreased PTH, and increased urinary calcium.
- *Renal leak hypercalciuria*
  - Increased calcium excretion into the urine, decreased calcium in plasma, increased PTH and increased GI calcium absorption, and increased bone absorption.
- *Resorptive hypercalciuria (primary hyperparathyroidism)*
  - Increased PTH → increased bone resorption and increased GI Ca absorption, increased plasma calcium, and increased urinary calcium

Using the below table, test your knowledge of hypercalciuric states. Options are "Normal", "Increased", or "Decreased."

	Absorptive	Renal	Resorption
Serum Ca			
Parathyroid hormone			
GI calcium absorption			
Fasting urinary Ca			

	Absorptive	Renal	Resorption
Serum Ca	Normal	Normal	Increased
Parathyroid hormone	Decreased	Increased	Increased
GI calcium absorption	Increased	Increased	Increased
Fasting urinary Ca	Normal	Increased	Increased

○ **How important is the differentiation of the type of hypercalciuria in clinical practice?**

Not very, except for research purposes and for the identification of hyperparathyroidism. What is more important is the patient's response and compliance with therapy.

○ **What is the "simplified" approach to a metabolic workup for hypercalciuria?**

First, exclude hyperparathyroidism by checking a serum calcium and parathyroid hormone level. Dietary measures, such as limitations on oral calcium intake, can be used initially. If these measures fail and the hypercalciuria persists, then a thiazide diuretic should be used.

○ **When should a calcium-loading test be performed?**

There is virtually no current role for a calcium-loading test outside of a research or investigative protocol.

○ **Describe the pathophysiology, diagnosis, and treatment of type 3 absorptive hypercalciuria?**

Type 3 absorptive hypercalciuria or renal phosphate leak hypercalciuria is caused by a defect in renal phosphate reabsorption. This leads to high urinary phosphate levels and hypophosphatemia that stimulates vitamin D activation to increase intestinal phosphate absorption to correct the low serum phosphate. The increased vitamin D levels will also inadvertently increase intestinal calcium absorption, where the excess calcium is eventually excreted in the urine as hypercalciuria. The diagnosis is made by the concurrent finding of hypercalciuria, relative hypophosphatemia, high urinary phosphate, and increased serum vitamin D levels. Treatment is by oral phosphate that suppresses the vitamin D activation. Thiazides are relatively ineffective in this particular form of hypercalciuria.

○ **Is an elevated serum calcium an effective screening test for absorptive hypercalciuria?**

No. The increased absorption of calcium secondarily increases the filtered calcium presented to the kidneys, thereby suppressing parathyroid function and subsequently decreasing renal resorption of calcium. The hypercalciuria offsets the increased intestinal absorption, thereby keeping serum calcium in the normal range.

○ **Is an elevated serum calcium an effective screening test for renal hypercalciuria?**

No. Renal leak of calcium results in lowering of serum calcium that stimulates PTH and 1,25-dihydroxy-vitamin D_3. This results in an increase in intestinal absorption of calcium, which normalizes the serum calcium levels.

○ **What is the medication of choice for renal hypercalciuria?**

Thiazides specifically correct the renal leak of calcium by augmenting calcium reabsorption in the distal and proximal tubules.

○ **How does thiazide help in prevention of recurrence of stones in some stone-formers?**

It lowers urinary calcium excretion by reabsorbing calcium in the proximal and distal tubules and inhibiting sodium reabsorption.

○ **How effective is thiazide in reducing hypercalciuria and preventing kidney stone recurrences in these patients?**

Thiazides reduce urinary calcium excretion by approximately 30% and can reduce stone recurrences by up to 80%.

○ **What other medication besides thiazide can also reduce renal excretion of calcium?**

Indapamide (Lozol) acts similarly but is technically not a thiazide.

○ **What should one consider if thiazide is not effective in preventing stone recurrences or controlling hypercalciuria?**

Look for an increase in dietary sodium or calcium as well as a decrease in potassium leading to intracellular acidosis and hypocitraturia. Also consider optimizing other aspects of metabolic stone disease such as uric acid, urinary oxalate, and total volume.

○ **Thiazides are contraindicated or ineffective in a subset of hypercalciuric patients. What other treatment modalities can be used to help control hypercalciuria?**

Amiloride, sodium cellulose phosphate, and orthophosphates as well as reasonable dietary calcium limitations.

○ **Is an elevated PTH diagnostic of resorptive hypercalciuria?**

No. PTH is secondarily increased in renal hypercalciuria. An oral calcium load will suppress the hypersecretion of PTH in renal hypercalciuria. This can help differentiate this entity from primary hyperparathyroidism.

○ **How does sodium cellulose phosphate work to inhibit stone formation and what are the potential side effects?**

Sodium cellulose phosphate is a nonabsorbable ion exchange resin that binds calcium and inhibits calcium absorption in the intestine. Side effects include hypomagnesemia via binding of intestinal magnesium. Patients also get secondary hyperoxaluria since more divalent cations are bound in the gut leaving more oxalate available for absorption. Lastly, there can be a negative calcium balance with consequent stimulation of PTH. Supplementation of magnesium and limitation of dietary oxalate are important adjuncts with the use of this agent.

○ **How do orthophosphates work and what are their side effects?**

Orthophosphates exert their hypocalciuric effect by inhibiting $1,25\text{-}OH_2\text{-}D_3$ synthesis. Side effects include secondary PTH stimulation and soft tissue calcification. Orthophosphates are indicated in vitamin D-dependent absorptive hypercalciuria and in cases of hypophosphatemia. They are also the drugs of choice for renal phosphate leak hypercalciuria (absorptive hypercalciuria type 3).

○ **What is the drug of choice for absorptive hypercalciuria type 1 in patients at risk for osteoporosis?**

Thiazides. They act by causing diuresis and increasing renal absorption of calcium. The main side effects include hypokalemia and hypocitraturia. These can be overcome by the addition of potassium citrate supplements.

○ **Why is it important to limit sodium intake when taking thiazides for stone disease?**

Thiazides inhibit sodium reabsorption in the ascending limb of the Loop of Henle, causing contraction of the extracellular volume. This leads to increased sodium and calcium reabsorption in the proximal convoluted tubule. Excess sodium intake would inhibit the ability of thiazides to contract the extracellular volume and limit their hypocalciuric response.

○ **Is the hypocalciuric response to thiazides routinely permanent?**

No. If the response to thiazides is lost, a 6-month "drug holiday," during which time sodium cellulose phosphate therapy or orthophosphates can be utilized, will often reinstate responsiveness to thiazides.

○ **When are thiazides contraindicated with hypercalciuria?**

Hyperparathyroidism and patients with severe sulfa allergies.

○ **Why are thiazides contraindicated in these patients?**

Resorption of calcium from bone and from the kidney in hyperparathyroidism causes hypercalcemia, which would be further increased after thiazide therapy. Thiazides contain sulfa molecules and so should be used cautiously in those with a documented sulfa allergy.

○ **What is the most common cause of hypercalcemia in the outpatient setting?**

Hyperparathyroidism. It should be suspected in all patients with high or high-normal serum calcium and calcium urinary lithiasis.

○ **How does one diagnose hyperparathyroidism?**

Assays that measure the intact molecule or the carboxy-terminal portion of PTH are approximately 90% sensitive in detecting elevations in blood levels of PTH. PTH also causes an increase in cAMP, which can be measured in the urine.

○ **What is "subtle" or "subclinical" hyperparathyroidism and how is it diagnosed?**

"Subtle" or "subclinical" hyperparathyroidism is defined as a condition where the serum calcium and PTH levels are both elevated or high normal but are not diagnostic of overt hyperparathyroidism. A temporary course of thiazides with increased oral calcium intake (a thiazide challenge test) should decrease serum PTH levels except in cases of true hyperparathyroidism. Even if negative, repeat testing should be done periodically to rule out true or clinical hyperparathyroidism that might develop later.

○ **What are alternative treatments for primary hyperparathyroidism if the patient cannot undergo parathyroidectomy?**

Orthophosphates, bisphosphonates, and potassium citrate can be used if surgery is contraindicated. Estrogen supplements can be tried in postmenopausal women.

○ **What is the most common cause of hypercalcemia in the inpatient setting?**

Malignancy. Less than 1% of patients with urinary lithiasis have a malignancy. The most common tumors in descending order of occurrence are lung, breast, renal cell, head and neck, and hematologic.

○ **Why does malignancy cause hypercalcemia?**

The mechanism for most hypercalcemia-related malignancy is osteoclastic bone resorption stimulated by cytokines and other substances released by the tumor, such as PTH-related polypeptide, prostaglandins, tumor necrosis factors, and transforming growth factors.

○ **What are other causes of hypercalcemia?**

Hyperthyroidism, glucocorticoid excess, pheochromocytoma, prolonged immobilization, familial hypocalciuric hypercalcemia, thiazides, lithium, milk-alkali syndrome, vitamin A toxicity, and granulomatous diseases such as sarcoidosis, histoplasmosis, tuberculosis, leprosy, silicosis, and coccidiomycosis. Sarcoid granulomas may produce calcitriol.

○ **How is hypercalcemia treated?**

Hypercalcemia is treated by addressing the underlying cause, hydration, bisphosphonates, calcitonin, and mithramycin.

○ **How does allopurinol help to prevent stone formation, and what stones will it prevent?**

Allopurinol lowers urinary uric acid by inhibiting the conversion of xanthine to uric acid, which is effective for patients with uric acid stones and hyperuricosuria.

○ **Which calculi are radiolucent?**

Uric acid, sodium urate, ammonium urate, xanthine, silica, protease medication, and 2,8-dihydroxyadenine calculi.

○ **What type of stones do patients form if they are hyperuricosuric?**

Calcium or uric acid stones.

○ **What is the pH of patient's urine with hyperuricemia (gouty diathesis)?**

Urine pH <5.5

○ **How does hyperuricosuria lead to stone formation?**

Stones secondary to hyperuricosuria are a result of the precipitation of sodium-urate crystals in the urine. These crystals can initiate both urate and calcium oxalate stones. They also remove certain inhibitors of stone formation and lower urinary pH.

○ **Would a person on a high-protein, low-carbohydrate diet (such as the Atkins diet) be more likely to form renal stones and, if so, why?**

High purine content of meat may lead to the formation of uric acid stones and hyperuricosuria. Patients on the Atkins diet have been shown to have more acidic urine, higher urinary calcium and uric acid, and low urinary citrate levels.

○ **What evidence supports the causal relationship between increased animal protein intake and nephrolithiasis?**

Population studies show that the increase in societal consumption of protein is associated with increased incidence of stone disease. Protein intake increases urinary calcium, uric acid, and oxalate. Protein moderation is recommended—aggressive protein restriction can increase the risk of stones. Patients should target a dietary protein intake of 0.8 to 1 g/kg/day.

○ **Why are humans and dalmatians the only mammals prone to uric acid urolithiasis?**

We both lack uricase, a hepatic enzyme that converts uric acid to soluble allantoin.

○ **What causes hyperuricosuria?**

Hypersecretion of urate can be caused by increased dietary purines, gout, or states of overproduction of purines such as malignancy, myeloproliferative diseases, and glycogen storage diseases. Urate stones may also be found in states of chronic diarrhea such as Crohn disease, ulcerative colitis, or jejunoileal bypass, which produce a state of acidosis via bicarbonate loss and dehydration.

○ **What is another effect of systemic acidosis that promotes stone formation?**

Systemic acidosis is the most important etiologic factor for the development of hypocitraturia.

○ **What foods are highest in purine content?**

Beef, poultry, pork, peanuts, and fish.

○ **What is the strongest urinary chemical promoter of kidney stone production?**

Oxalate is the strongest chemical promoter, approximately 15 times stronger than calcium.

○ **Does urinary oxalate come primarily from dietary sources?**

No. Approximately half of the enteric oxalate is degraded by luminal bacteria. Most (80%) of the urinary oxalate comes from hepatic conversion.

○ **Name 2 common GI bacteria that degrade intestinal oxalate?**

Oxalobacter formigenes and *Pseudomonas oxaliticus.*

○ **What are the characteristics of Oxalobacter formigenes?**

It is a gram-negative rod and obligate anaerobe that has a nutritional requirement for oxalate, degrading 70 to 100 mg of oxalate daily in a normal person with normal anatomy, bowel function, and diet. It usually prevents excessive absorption of oxalate, which may impact hyperoxaluria and stone formation.

○ **In what conditions would one see decreased colonization of *Oxalobacter formigenes* in the gut?**

Oxalobacter colony counts have been demonstrated to be decreased in stone formers. There is evidence that patients who have undergone bariatric surgery have fewer colonies of oxalobacter present in the GI tract; however, studies are ongoing to evaluate the effects of modern day bariatric surgery. Oxalobacter is sensitive to antibiotic therapy and may be decreased or absent in those receiving antibiotics.

○ **Besides hyperoxaluria, what other disorder is found in patients after bariatric surgery that would increase their overall risk of kidney stones?**

Hypocitraturia.

○ **In what conditions does dietary oxalate contribute significantly to urinary oxalate?**

Secondary hyperoxaluria (enteric hyperoxaluria) occurs in patients with short bowel syndrome, inflammatory bowel disease, jejunoileal bypass, or intestinal malabsorption. Intestinal fat malabsorption characteristic of ileal disease results in saponification of calcium and magnesium. This decreases the amount of calcium available to complex with oxalate in the intestinal lumen, raising the free oxalate pool available for intestinal absorption.

○ **What are the specific organ and enzymatic defects associated with hyperoxaluria?**

- Hyperoxaluria is associated with an enzyme deficiency in the liver.
  - Type 1: Alanine-glyoxalate aminotransferase.
  - Type 2: D-glycerate dehydrogenase.

○ **What is the main treatment for primary hyperoxaluria?**

Combined liver/kidney transplant.

○ **What other conditions can lead to hyperoxaluria?**

Pyridoxine deficiency, excess ascorbic acid ingestion, ethylene glycol ingestion, and methoxyflurane anesthesia.

○ **What is type 1 primary hyperoxaluria and what causes it?**

Primary hyperoxaluria type 1 is an extremely rare autosomal recessive disorder resulting in increased hepatic production of oxalate. It typically presents in childhood. It is caused by a deficiency of the enzyme alanine-glyoxylate aminotransferase that converts glyoxylate to glycine. Without this enzyme, oxalate levels increase substantially; 50% of patients develop end-stage renal disease by age 15 and 80% by age 30.

○ **How is type 1 primary hyperoxaluria treated?**

Pyridoxine (vitamin B_6) supplementation is a cofactor in the glyoxylate pathway and may be helpful. Early liver transplantation can avoid renal failure and other problems if the disease can be diagnosed early. If not, then a combined liver–kidney transplant is the only curative treatment available.

○ **What dietary restrictions would you recommend for hyperoxaluria?**

Leafy green vegetables, rhubarb, spinach, cocoa, okra, potatoes, peanuts, turnips, chocolate, pecans, carrots, berries, tea, powdered coffee, nuts, and broccoli are known to be generally high in oxalate content.

○ **What are some medical therapies for hyperoxaluria?**

High doses of oral calcium 0.25 to 1.00 g/day or more are recommended especially in cases of enteric hyperoxaluria. This complexes with the free oxalate in the intestinal tract. Large doses of pyridoxine 100 to 200 mg/day are beneficial in primary hyperoxaluria. Side effects of pyridoxine include hypomagnesuria. Doses higher than 200 mg/day can be associated with peripheral neuropathy. Cholestyramine helps in enteric hyperoxaluria by binding free intestinal oxalate where calcium cannot be used. Iron supplements can also do this and may be helpful in controlling hyperoxaluria.

○ **What other stone disease is characterized by autosomal recessive inheritance?**

Cystinuria is a rare autosomal recessive disorder characterized by >250 mg/day urinary excretion of cystine and flat hexagonal crystals in the urinary sediment, which increase in solubility with the increase in pH (especially pH >7.5).

○ **Can cystinuria be ruled out on the basis of patient age at presentation?**

No. Some patients do not present until the 5th or 6th decade.

○ **Cystinuria is defined by a defect in the breakdown of which 4 amino acids?**

Cystine, **O**rnithine, **L**ysine, and **A**rginine. COLA is a useful mnemonic. These amino acids are more soluble than cystine, so that they do not form calculi.

○ **What specific gene is responsible for cystinuria?**

The dibasic amino acid transporter gene SLC3A1.

○ **What is a characteristic radiographic appearance of cystine stones?**

Ground glass appearance. Less opaque than calcium stones.

○ **What are the treatment goals for patients with cystinuria?**

- Decrease cystine concentration in urine and increase cysteine solubility.
  - Decrease dietary cystine and increase fluid intake/urine output.
  - Chelating agents to make cystine more soluble.

○ **What 2 medications are most frequently used to treat cystinuria?**

- D-penicillamine
- Thiola (α-mercaptopropionylglycine)

○ **What is the first line of medical therapy for cystine stones?**

Aggressive hydration (aiming for 3-4 L of urine per day) and alkalinization to a pH of 7 to 7.5.

○ **What is a potential side effect of alkalinization beyond a pH of 7.5?**

Calcium phosphate crystallization.

○ **What are the advantages of potassium citrate over sodium bicarbonate as an alkalinizing agent?**

Limits sodium intake, which is of special importance in patients with congestive heart failure and hypertension. It does not promote calcium oxalate crystallization to the same degree and it tends to last longer.

○ **What other medications may be used to treat cystine stones?**

Drugs that contain a disulfide structure can reduce cystine to form soluble cysteine. These include D-penicillamine, α-mercaptopropionylglycine, and captopril. Penicillamine has been associated with frequent side effects including nephrotic syndrome, exfoliative dermatitis, and pancytopenia. α-mercaptopropionylglycine has a more favorable safety profile, making it the drug of choice. Dietary restriction of methionine should be instituted, but is usually of limited benefit due to tolerance and lack of compliance.

○ **What vitamin should be supplemented if D-penicillamine is utilized?**

Pyridoxine (vitamin B_6). Deficiency of vitamin B_6 leads to gastrointestinal upset, glossitis, dermatitis, and seizures.

○ **What is the sodium nitroprusside test?**

Examination of a spot urine sample for cystine can be performed by the nitroprusside test. The cyanide-nitroprusside colorimeter test gives a magenta ring at urinary cystine levels of greater than 75 mg/L.

○ **What is the chemical composition of struvite stones (infection stones)?**

Calcium carbonate apatite or magnesium ammonium phosphate (struvite).

○ **What types of bacteria are associated with struvite stones?**

Urinary tract infection caused by urease-producing organisms leads to the formation of struvite stones. The most common culprits include *Proteus, Pseudomonas, Klebsiella,* and *Staphylococcus. Escherichia coli* does not produce urease.

○ **Why is urease important?**

Urease splits urea in the urine to ammonia (contributes to ammonium in struvite stones) and bicarbonate. Bicarbonate creates alkaline urine, promoting the crystallization of struvite stones. Struvite does not precipitate unless the pH is >7.

○ **What is a staghorn calculus?**

Staghorn calculus describes the appearance of a calculus that has formed on a matrix cast of the pyelocalyceal system of the kidney. It is most commonly a struvite calculus, however, cystine and uric acid calculi may form staghorn configurations.

○ **In an asymptomatic patient with a staghorn calculus, what are the indications for intervention?**

Staghorn calculi should be treated after initial diagnosis. These stones have been shown to affect renal function over time and have a high incidence of infectious complications. Unless a patient is too ill to undergo treatment, treatment should be offered to all patients with staghorn calculi.

○ **What is the goal of medical therapy for struvite stones?**

Antibiotics are used to maintain sterile urine. Antibiotic suppression after clearance of the offending organism is useful, but complete elimination of the stone is the ultimate goal of therapy. Urine culture results should direct the selection of the most appropriate antibiotic.

○ **What adjunctive medications are useful for treatment of struvite stones?**

Urease inhibitors such as acetohydroxamic acid are useful. Acetohydroxamic acid reduces the urinary saturation of struvite and retards calculus formation. The recommended dosage is 250 mg 3 times per day. Limiting side effects include gastrointestinal upset, headaches, anxiety, and hallucination.

○ **How does acetohydroxamic acid help with treatment of struvite stones?**

Acetohydroxamic acid (Lithostat) inhibits urease formed by urea-splitting bacteria, thereby decreasing the ammonia content and lowering the pH of the urine.

○ **What potentially serious complication is associated with the use of acetohydroxamic acid?**

Deep venous thrombosis is a rare but potentially serious complication associated with this medication.

○ **Increased stone formation is seen in renal tubular acidosis. Does this defect affect the proximal or distal tubule?**

Distal.

○ **Which renal tubular acidosis type is associated with nephrolithiasis?**

Renal tubular acidosis (RTA) describes several conditions (types 1, 2, and 4), where defects in renal/urinary acidification lead to metabolic acidosis. Only type 1 RTA is characterized by nephrolithiasis, hypokalemia, hyperchloremia, and nonanion gap metabolic acidosis. Approximately 70% of adults with distal RTA (type 1) have renal calculi.

○ **What is the metabolic defect in RTA type 1 and what urinary abnormalities does it produce?**

Defective excretion of hydrogen ions by the distal tubule results in a high urinary pH. The urine remains relatively alkaline (pH >6.0) despite systemic acidosis caused by the inability of the distal tubule to maintain a proton gradient. Systemic acidosis results in hypercalciuria due to decreased renal reabsorption, increased bone resorption, and hypocitraturia.

○ **What is the pathophysiology of RTA type 1?**

There is impaired tubular excretion of hydrogen ion; therefore, the urine cannot be acidified. pH is generally >6.5. Patients excrete alkaline urine with LOW citrate content. Urinary calcium is increased.

○ **What type of stones are seen in RTA type 1?**

Calcium phosphate.

○ **What metabolic derangements are seen in patients with RTA type 1?**

Hyperchloremic hypokalemic metabolic acidosis.

○ **What type of stones are seen in patients with multiple myeloma?**

Uric acid stones.

○ **When should you suspect RTA type 1?**

Clinical suspicion is raised by hypocitraturia, hypokalemia, systemic acidosis (serum bicarbonate <23 mEq/L), nephrocalcinosis on radiographs, recurrent calcium phosphate stones (>30% of total stone burden), and urine pH >6.

○ **How do you diagnose RTA type 1 and how is it treated?**

Ammonium chloride load test. Diagnostic if urine pH >5.5 after taking 100 mg NH_4Cl/kg body weight the day prior. However, since the therapy for RTA type 1 and severe hypocitraturia is essentially the same (potassium citrate supplementation), there is little need for this particular test in clinical practice.

○ **What medications may promote stone formation and should be elicited in the medication history? (Identify at least 5 by name.)**

Indinavir and other protease inhibitors used for HIV as well as triamterene can form stones from the medication. Carbonic anhydrase inhibitors such as acetazolamide can cause overly alkaline urine and calcium phosphate stones. Excess vitamin C can be metabolized to oxalate. Excess vitamin D can cause absorptive hypercalciuria. Uricosuric agents such as probenecid lead to hyperuricosuria. Topiramate (Topamax), a migraine prevention medication, can cause metabolic acidosis that can lead to stones. Other agents that can promote stone formation include antacids, calcium supplements, chemotherapeutics, theophylline, and furosemide.

○ **When is allopurinol used and how does it work?**

Allopurinol (300 mg/day) is used for hyperuricosuric calcium oxalate nephrolithiasis and uric acid nephrolithiasis. It decreases urate synthesis by inhibiting hepatic xanthine oxidase and lowers blood and urinary urate. Allopurinol should be given with a moderate sodium restriction. Allopurinol dosage should be adjusted in hyperuricemic (gout) patients to maintain a serum uric acid level at or below 6.

○ **What type of stone may form as a result of allopurinol therapy?**

Xanthine, although this is quite uncommon.

○ **What new drug may be used as a nonpurine analogue inhibitor of xanthine oxidase?**

Febuxostat is a newer, orally administered drug. Dosing is 80 to 120 mg/day. It is metabolized by the liver. It has not been studied specifically in stone disease at this time.

○ **What medications are associated with the formation of ammonium urate calculi?**

Laxatives, acetazolamide, allopurinol, triamterene, and sulfonamides. Of these, laxative abuse is by far the most common.

○ **How is urine pH helpful in predicting the stone chemical composition?**

Low urine pH ($<$5.5) suggests the presence of uric acid or cystine calculi while an alkaline pH ($>$7.5) suggests the presence of struvite or calcium phosphate stones.

○ **What is gouty diathesis and how is it treated?**

Gouty diathesis is defined as calcium nephrolithiasis associated with hyperuricemia or gout. Patients typically are aggressive stone formers. The mainstay of treatment is to alkalinize the urinary pH to approximately 6.5. Potassium citrate has been demonstrated to provide adequate alkalinization with minimal side effects. Potassium citrate 30 to 60 mg/day is given in 2 or more divided doses. Sodium bicarbonate is a less expensive option; however, it should be used with caution in patients with hypertension or congestive heart failure. Elevation of the urinary pH above 7 should be avoided to prevent precipitation of calcium phosphate.

○ **When should allopurinol be used in the prophylaxis of kidney stones and what is the dosage?**

Allopurinol is recommended in all active stone patients with gout or hyperuricemia, especially if they also have uric acid stones or hyperuricosuria. Uric acid stones that are not adequately controlled with alkalinization therapy alone and patients who cannot take sufficient alkalinizing medication to obtain an optimal pH may also be candidates for allopurinol therapy. While the standard dose is 300 mg/day, the dosage should be titrated in hyperuricemic patients to obtain a serum uric acid level of 6 or less. No more than 300 mg should be taken at one time. Initial dosing should begin at 100 mg/day to avoid stimulating a gout attack and then increased weekly. Maximum dosage is 800 mg/day.

○ **Allopurinol has been associated with skin rashes and peripheral neuropathy. What treatments are used as prophylaxis for these complications?**

Allopurinol should be stopped for a skin rash as it represents a potentially serious allergic response. No prophylaxis is available. However, vitamin B_6 can be helpful in minimizing the potential neuropathy from allopurinol use.

○ **What is an intravenous alternative for alkalinization?**

Sodium lactate (1/6 M). Infuse 500 mL every 8 hours. Sodium lactate is completely converted to bicarbonate within 1 to 2 hours.

○ **When should the liquid version of potassium citrate be used instead of tablets?**

In any case where there is more rapid intestinal transit time, patients have difficulty swallowing the tablets, or urinary citrate levels fail to increase on tablet therapy alone.

○ **How should potassium citrate therapy be titrated?**

Adjust the dosage based on keeping the pH at or below 7.0 while maximizing the 24-hour urine citrate level. A bedtime dose helps supplement the normal nocturnal "alkaline tide."

○ **What diseases are calcium phosphate stones associated with?**

Primary hyperparathyroidism, renal tubular acidosis, and sodium alkali therapy.

○ **Who should be offered prophylactic testing with a 24-hour urine study?**

All kidney stone patients who are children should definitely be tested as well as those with kidney transplants, solitary kidneys ureteral reimplantations, and renal failure. Patients with multiple stones or frequent recurrences should be encouraged to have the testing. Ultimately, any kidney stone patient who is motivated to follow long-term preventive treatment suggestions is potentially a candidate for 24-hour urine testing. Patients need to understand that kidney stones are a lifelong problem and even the best preventive treatment plan may occasionally fail.

○ **What are the critical elements of a successful kidney stone preventive testing program?**

Correct urine collection procedures are very important. But even more important is making sure that interested patients understand that stone preventive therapy is ongoing and lifelong. Those without the motivation and discipline to follow a reasonable treatment plan indefinitely should not receive the testing. The most critical elements of 24-hour urine testing are total volume, calcium, uric acid, sodium, oxalate, and citrate. Phosphate, magnesium, and sulfate are also recommended as well as blood testing for uric acid, calcium, and CO_2.

○ **What general advice should be given to kidney stone formers who do not elect to perform 24-hour urine testing?**

Increase water intake. Moderate your diet, particularly purines and high-oxalate foods. Limit salt intake. For calcium oxalate stone formers, ask them to consider at least a nightly potassium citrate supplement.

○ **What is the recommended daily water intake for kidney stone formers?**

While 8 separate 8 oz glasses of water daily is often quoted, the better answer is whatever is necessary for that patient to generate 2000 mL or more of urine per day. This is roughly just a little more than half gallon.

○ **Is it necessary or recommended to have patients wake up during the night to drink extra water?**

This is almost never necessary, with the possible exception of cystine stone formers where a 3000 mL daily urinary volume is sometimes necessary.

○ **What are the statistical odds for other family members of stone formers to eventually develop stones?**

Approximately 25% for male children of stone formers. Female children approximately 8%. The highest risk ratio would be between brothers where the lifetime risk is approximately 50% if one brother is a stone former.

○ **Medullary sponge kidney is associated with what 3 urinary abnormalities associated with kidney stones?**

Medullary sponge kidney is associated with an increased risk of urinary tract infections, renal leak hypercalciuria, and hypocitraturia.

○ **What tests should be obtained prior to percutaneous chemolysis of calculi?**

Stone composition should be known. Urinary tract infection should be excluded by urine culture. Urinary extravasation should be excluded by antegrade contrast study.

○ **What is the solution of choice for chemolysis of uric acid calculi?**

Sodium bicarbonate (50 mEq in 1 L of 0.45% NaCl, pH 8).

○ **What is the solution of choice for chemolysis of cystine calculi?**

Acetylcysteine (0.3 M) in tromethamine E (Tham E, pH 10).

○ **What are the main ingredients in Suby G solution and hemiacidrin solution, utilized for struvite calculi dissolution?**

Citric acid and magnesium citrate. Both these solutions maintain a pH of 4.

○ **What was a potentially lethal complication of irrigation with hemiacidrin?**

Hypermagnesemia. Magnesium is added to the solution to decrease uroepithelial irritability. With high intrapelvic pressures (>25 cm H_2O), hypermagnesemia can occur, leading to respiratory depression.

○ **What laboratory studies should be monitored during hemiacidrin irrigation?**

Daily magnesium levels, creatinine and phosphorus levels. Urine culture every 3 days.

○ **What is a finding on physical examination suggestive of a high magnesium level?**

Depressed deep tendon reflexes.

○ **How would hypermagnesemia be treated?**

Intravenous calcium, furosemide, and saline.

○ **What are some changes during pregnancy that could alter stone formation?**

Placental production of 1,25-$(OH)_2$ vitamin D can stimulate hypercalciuria through increased intestinal absorption. This may be offset by increased renal excretion of citrate and nephrocalcin.

○ **True/False: Pentosan polysulfate (Elmiron) can be used to treat otherwise intractable recurrent stone disease.**

True. Reports indicate that Elmiron coats urinary crystals with a synthetic GAG layer reducing crystal aggregation and subsequent stone formation.

○ **What are the 2 most common metabolic problems in pediatric stone formers?**

Hypocitraturia and hypercalciuria are the most common.

○ **Pyridoxine (vitamin B₆) may decrease hepatic oxalate production by facilitating what chemical reaction?**

Pyridoxine helps convert glyoxalate to glycine.

○ **Randall plaques are always of what chemical composition?**

Calcium phosphate (hydroxyapatite).

○ **Hypermagnesemia is a potential complication of irrigation with Renacidin (magnesium carbonate) or Suby solution. What are the symptoms and treatment for hypermagnesemia?**

• Hypermagnesemia is characterized by confusion, lethargy, paralysis, and possibly coma.
• Treatment involves saline infusion with Lasix diuresis. In severe cases, IV calcium gluconate can be used.
• Hemodialysis is the preferred treatment in patients with renal failure.

○ **What percentage of bladder stones are 100% uric acid?**

Approximately 50%.

○ **What 4 medical problems are associated with abnormally elevated vitamin D levels?**

Hyperparathyroidism, sarcoidosis, malignant tumors, and granulomatous disease.

○ **When should orthophosphate therapy for calcium nephrolithiasis not be used?**

In renal failure with a GFR of 30 mL/s or less.

○ **Do obese patients actually have more kidney stones, or does it just seem that way?**

Obese patients actually do make more stones.

○ **True/False: Oxadrop, a freeze-dried product containing 5 different lactic acid bacteria, has been shown to significantly reduce urinary oxalate excretion in idiopathic hyperoxaluria.**

False. A randomized, placebo-controlled trial by Goldfarb et al. (2007) failed to show any benefit.

○ **Should patients with struvite (infection) stones have 24-hour urine metabolic testing?**

Yes, just like other stone formers.

○ **What is the most common urinary metabolic problem found in struvite stone formers other than infection?**

Hypercalciuria.

○ **At what 24-hour urine excretion of cystine should specific therapy be initiated?**

Usually at 250 mg of cystine per 24 hours.

○   **What is the optimal pH for most cystine stone formers and for calcium stone formers?**

Usually a pH of 7.5 is suggested even though this may increase the risk of calcium phosphate stones. The feeling is that the increased solubility of cystine at this pH level justifies the risk. Calcium stone formers are generally optimized at a pH of approximately 6.5.

○   **What is the formula for estimating the total 24-hour urinary creatinine excretion in men and women and why is it important?**

Women: 17 × body weight (kg).

Men: 22 × body weight (kg).

This is useful in determining the reliability of a 24-hour urine collection.

○   **What diagnosis is suggested by urolithiasis with hypercalciuria, hypercalcemia, and hyperuricemia together with parathyroid suppression and azotemia? What specifically causes the calcium abnormalities?**

Sarcoidosis. Overproduction of 1,25-$(OH)_2$ vitamin D by pulmonary macrophages causes the calcium metabolism abnormalities.

○   **What additional study is recommended in calcium stone forming hypercalciuric children besides blood and 24-hour urine testing?**

Bone mineral density testing for osteoporosis and osteopenia.

○   **What are the 3 acceptable surgical treatments for symptomatic ureteral stones in pregnancy?**

Percutaneous nephrostomy, double J stents, and ureteroscopic stone extraction.

CHAPTER 30 Genitourinary Trauma

James M. Cummings, MD

○ **What percentage of all hospital trauma admissions involve renal trauma?**

Approximately 3%.

○ **What percentage of all abdominal trauma involves the kidneys?**

Approximately 10%.

○ **True/False: The presence or absence of hematuria is not a good indicator of traumatic injury.**

True. In one study, 13% of proven renal gunshot victims had no hematuria.

○ **What are the indications for imaging of the kidneys following blunt trauma?**

Gross hematuria or microhematuria combined with shock defined as systolic BP <90 at any time following the injury are absolute indications for genitourinary (GU) tract imaging.

○ **In children, what are the indications for imaging of the kidneys following blunt trauma?**

All children who sustain blunt trauma and have greater than 5 RBC per high-power field on a microscopic urinalysis or a positive dipstick should undergo radiographic assessment of the kidneys. Also, children with significant deceleration injuries (ie, falls from heights) may need renal imaging even in the absence of hematuria.

○ **Staging of renal trauma is best accomplished with what radiographic test?**

CT scanning of the kidneys provides detailed images of the kidneys that allow for a clear delineation of most renal injuries and their severity.

○ **What are the advantages, if any, of an IVP over CT scans in the evaluation of GU trauma?**

An IVP can be done in the operating room (OR) when needed during emergent exploration. However, CT gives a better assessment of the renal anatomy and permits diagnosis of concurrent injuries. Therefore, CT scans are the standard for trauma imaging of the kidneys.

○ **The kidney is rich in tissue factor. What does this do and why is this important?**

Tissue factor activates the extrinsic coagulation cascade that promotes hemostasis after an injury.

○ **A small cortical laceration in the kidney with a small perirenal hematoma would be classified as what grade injury?**

Grade II.

○ **A renal injury extends through the parenchyma into the collecting system. What grade injury is this?**

Grade IV.

○ **What are the absolute indications for renal exploration following blunt trauma and how is it done?**

An expanding or pulsatile retroperitoneal hematoma must be explored. Initial control of the involved renal pedicle prior to opening of the hematoma must be achieved by means of a retroperitoneal incision medial to the inferior mesenteric vein and anterior to the aorta. The dissection is carried cephalad until the involved renal pedicle is encountered. Vascular control is achieved and the hematoma can now be entered.

○ **An attempt to repair a traumatic injury to the main renal artery should be pursued under what circumstances?**

Repair of the main renal artery should be attempted only in a hemodynamically stable patient who has no other associated major organ system injuries, an ischemia time of less than 8 to 10 hours, bilateral renal injuries, or injury to a solitary kidney.

○ **A patient has severe hematuria after a renal needle biopsy. What is the most likely diagnosis and treatment?**

The most likely diagnosis is arteriovenous fistula. Angiographic arterial embolization is the preferred therapy.

○ **The parents of a 12-year-old child with a solitary kidney want to know the risk of the child losing the remaining kidney in contact sports. What are the risk statistics you should tell them?**

It has been estimated that 6 kidneys per 1 million children will be injured per year with only one kidney lost per 2.67 million children per year.

○ **Hypertension following renal trauma can result from what 2 mechanisms?**

1. Renal vascular injury leading to stenosis or occlusion of the renal artery or one of its branches.
2. Compression of the renal parenchyma from extravasated blood and urine (Page kidney).

○ **A 1-cm segment of the left ureter is damaged during an elective left colectomy. The injury is recognized intraoperatively. The best choice for management at that time is?**

Debridement of any devitalized tissue, mobilization of the 2 ends of the ureter, and a spatulated ureteroureterostomy over a stent. The area must be adequately drained postoperatively.

○ **You are called to the OR to consult on a patient with a massive gunshot injury to the left abdomen. The trauma team has identified a 5-cm defect in the middle left ureter. The patient has become unstable and the trauma team wants to close and move the patient to the ICU for further resuscitation. What is your best option?**

Ligate the proximal ureter and have a percutaneous nephrostomy placed when the patient has stabilized. Perform operative reconstruction at a later date when the patient is better prepared.

○ **Does a ureteral injury sustained during an aortobifemoral grafting procedure require a nephrectomy?**

No. In the past it was felt that with a 50% risk of mortality from graft infection, a nephrectomy was a safer option than reconstruction. However, with better stenting and diversion techniques, newer antibiotics, and improved graft materials, ureteral reconstruction can be performed as long as adequate diversion and drainage is done. The risk is also lowered if omentum or some other tissue barrier is placed between the graft and the ureter.

○ **Which portion of the ureter is most likely to be injured during a hysterectomy?**

The ureter is most likely to be injured at the level of the broad ligament where the ureter passes beneath the uterine vascular pedicle in close proximity to the cervix.

○ **Following a ureteral reimplant with a psoas hitch, a patient complains of anterior thigh numbness. What is the most likely etiology for this complaint?**

The genitofemoral nerve lies on the anterior aspect of the iliopsoas muscle. Injury to this nerve can occur during suturing of the bladder to the tendon of the psoas minor muscle resulting in numbness of the anterior ipsilateral thigh.

○ **What are the options for closing a large gap between the proximal end of a damaged ureter and the bladder when a psoas hitch will not reach?**

Initially, the bladder should be mobilized on the contralateral side to the injury. This often involves division of vascular structures (superior vesical artery, obliterated umbilical artery, etc). A Boari bladder flap can gain considerable length. Another option is to do a caudal nephropexy that can gain additional length to allow for closure of the defect. When these maneuvers are unsuccessful, a transureteroureterostomy can be performed in the patient with unprepared bowel, otherwise an ileal interposition graft may need to be employed.

○ **Where should you anastomose the distal end of the ileal interposition graft?**

Directly to the bladder. This allows freer passage of mucus than an anastomosis to the distal ureter.

○ **Contraindications to the use of an ileal ureter for ureteral repair include?**

Impaired renal function (Cr >2 mg/dL), untreated bladder outlet obstruction, or poor bladder emptying for other reasons.

○ **The arterial vascular supply of the ureter comes most commonly from what sources?**

- Upper ureter—renal artery.
- Middle ureter—iliac artery.
- Lower ureter—superior vesical artery.

○ **A retrograde pyelogram done at the end of a difficult ureteroscopic stone extraction shows moderate extravasation at the previous location of the stone. Visual inspection reveals a perforation of the ureter and a wire placed initially is still in place in the renal pelvis. Appropriate management at this time is?**

Placement of a ureteral stent along with a Foley catheter to maximally drain the system and allow for healing of the ureter. A follow-up retrograde pyelogram should be performed at approximately 6 weeks postoperatively to assess healing of the involved area.

○ **Avulsion of the ureter during ureteroscopy occurs under what circumstances?**

The most common cause is a basket engaging a stone and trapping ureteral mucosa simultaneously. A basket can also cut directly into the ureter and trap the mucosa. Engaging a stone that is too large, especially in the proximal ureter. Finally, the ureteroscope alone can cause avulsion if it fits tightly in the ureter and intussuscepts when withdrawn.

○ **A woman presents with continuous urinary leakage 2 weeks following an abdominal hysterectomy. On physical examination, urine is identified in the vaginal vault. A cystogram is normal. What is the diagnosis and what test should be done next?**

The diagnosis is ureterovaginal fistula. CT scanning with coronal and sagittal reconstructions will effectively demonstrate the anatomy.

○ **In an adult suspected of having bladder trauma, what volume of contrast should be instilled into the bladder and how many films are required?**

The bladder should be filled under gravity pressure with up to 400 mL of contrast, or until a bladder contraction occurs. Following adequate anterior-posterior (AP) filling views, oblique views need to be obtained as well as drainage views of the anatomic pelvis.

○ **What is the major pitfall of CT cystography in the evaluation of a bladder injury?**

If done with IV contrast only, the bladder may not be sufficiently distended to reveal the injury and thus gives a false-negative result.

○ **Extraperitoneal bladder ruptures may be managed nonoperatively under what circumstances?**

If adequate bladder drainage via a large Foley catheter or suprapubic catheter can be achieved, there is no perforating bony fragment in the bladder wall, and the injury does not involve the bladder neck, nonoperative management can be successful. Close clinical follow-up is mandatory in this situation.

○ **What is the correct management of an intraperitoneal bladder rupture?**

Most commonly intraperitoneal bladder ruptures should be managed with surgical exploration, a multilayered closure, adequate bladder drainage, and possible drainage of the space of Retzius.

○ **You are called to the OR during a cesarean section for a bladder injury. On inspection, there is a 2-cm laceration of the anterior bladder. Your next step should be?**

Open the bladder sufficiently to be able to inspect the entire bladder for other possible bladder injuries and to ensure that the ureteral orifices are intact. Only after ensuring the integrity of the bladder and ureters should a bladder closure be performed.

○ **In the United States, what is the most common event leading to a vesicovaginal fistula?**

Iatrogenic injury during gynecologic surgery (particularly hysterectomy) is the most common etiology of fistulas. Fistulas from childbirth are more common in underdeveloped countries.

○ **Vesicovaginal fistulas following hysterectomy are a result of what etiologic event?**

An unrecognized bladder injury during hysterectomy with subsequent urinary extravasation into the surgical field and drainage via the vaginal cuff suture line leads to formation of the fistula.

○ **What is the best time to repair a vesicovaginal fistula following an uncomplicated hysterectomy?**

Timing of the repair depends largely on the time interval to the diagnosis of the injury as well as the clinical condition of the patient. Although 3 to 6 months have been recommended in the past, early intervention can be successful if there is minimal inflammation in the tissues and there are no other complicating factors.

○ **Tissues commonly used for interposition grafts in surgical repair of vesicovaginal fistulas include?**

Labial fat pad (Martius graft), gracilis muscle, peritoneum, and omentum.

○ **When used for interposition for vesicovaginal fistula repair, the omentum is mobilized on which vessel?**

The omentum is mobilized off the greater curvature of the stomach and the right gastroepiploic arterial supply is preserved. This is usually the dominant vessel supplying the omentum, and mobilization in this manner often allows the omentum to reach the deep pelvis.

○ **What are the most common causes of spontaneous rupture of an augmented bladder?**

Mucus plugging, chronic distension, or poor patient compliance with catheterization schedules.

○ **What are the 2 major classifications of pelvic fractures?**

The Tile classification and the Young classification.

○ **Physical findings of a posterior urethral injury include?**

Blood at the meatus, a distended bladder, and a high-riding prostate gland on rectal examination are all consistent with a posterior urethral injury.

○ **How does one diagnose a posterior urethral injury?**

Retrograde urethrography with the patient in a semioblique position is an effective method of diagnosing this injury. Extravasation of contrast is diagnostic. Attempted catheterization is controversial and can convert a partial urethral disruption into a complete disruption.

○ **A 32-year-old male victim of a motor vehicle accident suffers a pelvic fracture. Retrograde urethrography shows extravasation at the level of the membranous urethra. He is otherwise stable and no other immediate management is planned by the trauma team or orthopedics. What is the best urological management at this point?**

Management of a posterior urethral injury is controversial. In an otherwise stable patient, options include immediate realignment and delayed repair. Primary realignment may be possible in patients with limited pelvic bleeding. In this scenario, every attempt is made to avoid the pelvic hematoma and a urethral Foley catheter as well as a suprapubic catheter is placed. In a delayed repair, a suprapubic catheter is placed and plans are made for a possible urethroplasty after convalescence from the other injuries.

○ **What steps can be taken to gain length for an end-to-end bulboprostatic urethral anastomosis for repair of a stricture from a membranous urethral injury?**

- Mobilization of the urethra up to the penoscrotal junction.
- Division of the intercavernosal septum.
- Inferior pubectomy.
- Routing of the urethra over one of the cavernosal crura.

○ **What are the causes of erectile dysfunction (ED) following a pelvic fracture?**

Arteriogenic problems may occur as a result of injury to the internal pudendal artery. Venogenic impotence may ensue if there is direct injury to the corpus cavernosum. Neurogenic impotence can result from injury to the cavernous nerves, pelvic plexus, or sacral nerve roots. Most believe that impotence after pelvic fracture is a result of the injury itself and not the subsequent urethroplasty needed to repair the urethra.

○ **The best candidates for penile revascularization for traumatic impotence have what characteristics?**

- Demonstration of a focal arterial obstruction without diffuse atherosclerosis.
- Young patients and otherwise healthy patients.
- Patients have strong sexual desire and are highly motivated.

○ **A man presents with priapism. He gives a history of falling on a ladder and straddling one of the rungs 2 months ago. What type of priapism does the patient have, what are the likely characteristics of the blood aspirated from the penis, and how should the patient be treated?**

Blood gas determinations will show high oxygen levels since the likely etiology is arteriovenous fistula from the straddle injury. Arteriography with selective embolization of the fistula is the recommended treatment.

○ **True/False: A Winter shunt is a useful adjunct to the management of traumatic (high-flow) priapism.**

False. Surgical drainage of the corpus cavernosum is usually not required with high-flow priapism.

○ **A 24-year-old male suffers a gunshot wound to the penis. On examination, there is an entrance wound in the lateral midshaft with an exit wound at the ventral penoscrotal angle. The next step should be?**

Performance of a urethrogram to check for urethral injury is mandatory prior to any planned surgical intervention.

○ **A urethrogram in a male with a gunshot wound to the penis demonstrates stretching and elongation of the urethra in the penile urethra, but no extravasation. The best management for this injury is?**

The best management for this patient is careful placement of a small urethral catheter. It should be left indwelling for 10 to 14 days, followed by a voiding cystourethrogram.

○ **A urethrogram in a male with a gunshot to the penis shows extravasation in the midpenile urethra. There is minimal swelling on physical examination. The patient is stable without other significant injuries. How should the injury be managed?**

Exploration, debridement, and primary repair if the defect is small.

○ **In penile amputation injuries, how should the amputated portion of the penis be optimally preserved for transport?**

Wrapped in saline-soaked gauze and placed within a plastic bag, which is then immersed in a cooler with ice slush surrounding the bag.

○ **What are the clinical signs reported by the patient with a penile fracture?**

A "cracking" sound or "pop" followed by pain, rapid detumescence, and pronounced swelling.

○ **What is the single diagnostic test recommended for patients presenting with an obvious penile fracture?**

Retrograde urethrogram.

○ **What percentage of penile fractures will also have a urethral injury?**

Approximately 10% of these patients will have an associated urethral injury.

○ **What is the best management of penile fractures?**

Surgical exploration, identification of the tunica injury, and primary closure of the defect.

○ **A male presents with the skin of the penis dark from ischemia from a constricting ring left on at the base of the penis for 24 hours. Management should be?**

Excision of the ischemic penile skin is the first step. Following resolution of the inflammatory process, split-thickness, unmeshed skin grafts can be applied to cover the penis.

○ **The flap of choice for penile or phallic reconstruction is?**

The free forearm flap based on the radial artery.

○ **How should testis ruptures from blunt trauma be managed?**

Exploration, debridement of nonviable tissue, and reconstruction of the tunica defect.

○ **Describe the recommended immediate management of the testes after a major scrotal skin loss.**

Place the testes in thigh pouches to preserve them for future reconstruction.

○   **How should major scrotal skin loss be repaired?**

Meshed split-thickness skin grafts covering the testes and sutured to the remaining skin at the groin and perineum gives a good cosmetic appearance.

○   **Emergency reversal of clopidrogel (Plavix) is required to control bleeding in a trauma patient. How is this done?**

Platelet transfusion.

○   **What is the incidence of ED following traumatic injuries to the posterior urethra and how is it best treated?**

The incidence is more than 90%. PDE5 inhibitors are relatively ineffective. Intracavernosal injection is the most effective and successful medical therapy in this group with an 82% success rate reported in previously potent patients.

○   **True/False: The best way to manage a paraphimosis that cannot be easily reduced manually is immediate surgery.**

False. Usually the problem is distal edema. This can often be managed with simple manual compression for 5 minutes. If this is not successful, a moist gauze pad and an elastic compression wrap can be applied. This will almost always reduce the swelling and edema of the distal penis and allows for manual reduction of the paraphimosis. Surgery is a last resort.

○   **Hematuria that is out of proportion to the degree and nature of the apparent injury suggests what?**

Pre-existing renal pathology is suggested.

○   **What is the false-negative rate for hematuria by dipsticks?**

Published reports suggest a false-negative rate of 2.5% to 10% for urinary dipsticks.

○   **Emergency reversal of clopidrogel (Plavix) is required to control bleeding in a trauma patient. How is this done?**

Platelet transfusion.

CHAPTER 31 Adrenal Physiology

Matthew J. Resnick, MD and
Daniel A. Barocas, MD, MPH

○ **What is the weight of a normal adult adrenal gland?**

5 g.

○ **Embryologically, does the adrenal arise from a single structure? Describe the process.**

No, the adrenal cortex and medulla are derived from embryologically distinct structures. The cortex develops from embryonic mesoderm and the medulla from embryonic neureoectoderm. The hormonal secretions of each have different actions. Regulation of cortical and medullary secretions are independent of each other.

○ **Describe the functional relationship between the adrenal cortex and medulla.**

Despite their anatomic proximity, there is virtually no functional relationship between the adrenal cortex and medulla.

○ **In patients with renal ectopia or agenesis, where does the ipsilateral adrenal gland lie?**

It lies in its normal orthotopic position. Since the adrenal gland and the kidney are of different embryologic origins, their migrations to their final anatomic positions take place independently.

○ **What percentage of the adrenal gland is made up of the adrenal cortex?**

The cortex constitutes 90% of the gland.

○ **What are the 3 zones of the adrenal cortex?**

Zona glomerulosa lies immediately beneath the capsule of the gland, the zona fasciculata is the middle zone and is the largest portion of the cortex, and the zona reticularis is the innermost zone.

○ **Is there a functional significance between the anatomic zonations of the adrenal gland?**

Yes, each anatomic zone is also a functional zone. Aldosterone is produced exclusively in the zona glomerulosa. Cortisol is produced in the two inner zones, zona fasciculata and the zona reticularis. Adrenal androgens are produced in the inner cortical zone, the zona reticularis.

○ **What are the building blocks of adrenal hormones?**

Adrenal cells are capable of synthesizing cholesterol de novo, but most of the adrenal cholesterol used for steroidogenesis is derived from circulating lipoproteins and in particular from low-density lipoproteins (LDL).

○ **What is the first step in the production of adrenal steroid hormones?**

The first step is the production of pregnenolone from cholesterol via 2 hydroxylations followed by cleavage of the cholesterol side chain. Pregnenolone has no known biologic activity, but it is an intermediate in the production of all the biologically active steroid hormones.

○ **How are adrenal hormones stored?**

Adrenal hormones are steroid hormones, and as all biologic steroid hormones, adrenal hormones are not stored but are secreted immediately upon synthesis. The rate of steroid hormone secretion can be controlled by regulation of synthesis.

○ **Are active forms of adrenal hormones free or bound in serum?**

Only the free hormone is biologically active; however, all steroid hormones are largely protein-bound when they circulate in plasma. Because of the limited solubility of steroid hormones in water, protein binding acts to increase the amount of hormone that can circulate in the blood. Since the protein-bound fraction of hormone is relatively resistant to metabolism, protein binding also increases the plasma half-life of steroid hormones.

○ **Adrenal androgen production is limited by what factors?**

Many steroid compounds can be synthesized by the adrenal cortex; however, the enzymes required for the production of testosterone and estrogen are found in low concentration in the cortical cells. Consequently, androgens are normally produced in only very small quantities.

○ **Does the androgen precursor dehydroepiandrosterone (DHEA) have any androgenic activity in males?**

Only minimal; DHEA is secreted in large quantities by the adrenal cortex in males. DHEA has much less activity than testosterone, and in males, the overall effect of DHEA as an androgen is negligible. In females, both DHEA and androstenedione may be converted to testosterone at extra-adrenal sites, thus it has more androgenic activity in females.

○ **What stimulates adrenal androgen production?**

Adrenocorticotropic hormone (ACTH) influences adrenal androgen production and seems to be the primary stimulus. However, it is clearly not the only factor, as evidenced by dissociation of ACTH and adrenal androgen production during events such as puberty and stress. Other regulators are not completely delineated, but it appears to be independent of gonadotropins.

○ **What are the principal androgens produced by the adrenal glands?**

Dehydroepiandrosterone (DHEA), dehydroepiandrosterone sulfate (DHEAS), and androstenedione are the principal androgens produced by the adrenals.

○ **How substantial is adrenal androgen production compared to total androgen production?**

The major androgen products of the adrenals are weak in their androgen effect. They are converted to more potent androgens, testosterone, and dihydrotestosterone in peripheral tissues. Even so, adrenal androgens contribute 5% to 10% of the production rate of testosterone in an adult male, making a negligible contribution compared to testicular production. The proportion of adrenal androgen production is substantially higher in females (40%-60%). However, overall adrenal androgen production is rarely physiologically important in the natural state and is only clinically apparent in disease states of overproduction, such as congenital adrenal hyperplasia.

○ **How does ketoconazole affect adrenal androgen production?**

It inhibits the cytochrome P-450–dependent enzymes (CYP) important for steroidogenesis. Therefore, the conversion of cholesterol to pregnenolone is shut down, inhibiting production of testicular and adrenal androgens, as well as cortisol.

○ **True/False: Ketoconazole is a specific CYP inhibitor.**

False. Ketoconazole is a nonspecific CYP inhibitor that only weakly inhibits relevant enzymes at high doses. The dose-escalation required for effective CYP inhibition limits the widespread use of ketoconazole secondary to considerable patient intolerance.

○ **Which CYP enzyme has been implicated in the promotion of hormone-resistance in advanced prostate cancer?**

CYP17. Intratumoral overexpression of CYP17 has been implicated in the development of resistance to castration.

○ **Describe the role of adrenal androgens in the promotion of castrate-resistant prostate cancer (CRPC).**

In castrate prostate tumor tissues, levels of DHEA, DHEAS, and 5-androstenediol far exceed the concentrations of testosterone and dihydrotestosterone. These precursor adrenal androgens have been shown to activate both the wild-type and mutant androgen receptors (ARs).

○ **What is the mechanism of action of abiraterone acetate?**

Abiraterone acetate is a potent, selective inhibitor of CYP17, 17α-hydroxylase, and C17, 20-lyase.

○ **What are the side effects of abiraterone acetate, and why do these side effects occur?**

Side effects of abiraterone acetate include hypokalemia, hypertension, and fluid overload. The disruption of 17α-hydroxylase results in increased in deoxycorticosterone (10-fold) and corticosterone (40-fold). These changes result in secondary mineralocorticoid excess and the aforementioned symptoms.

○ **How does one manage the side effects of abiraterone acetate?**

Coadministration with prednisone avoids development of side effects by reducing ACTH secretion and thereby reducing production of downstream mineralocorticoid production. Alternatively, the addition of eplerenone, a specific mineralocorticoid receptor antagonist, is effective in controlling secondary mineralocorticoid excess associated with the administration of abiraterone acetate.

○ **Describe the differences between traditional antiandrogens (flutamide, bicalutamide) and enzalutamide.**

Traditional antiandrogens have low binding affinity for the AR, and in many cases, exhibit partial agonism resulting clinically in PSA declines upon withdrawal of these medications. Enzalutamide has a higher affinity for the AR than does bicalutamide and prevents nuclear translocation, DNA binding, and coactivator recruitment. Finally, enzalutamide has no demonstrable agonist activity.

○ **There are 5 enzymes involved in the conversion of cholesterol to cortisol. What are the consequences of deficiencies of these enzymes and what disease state does this produce?**

This family of disorders is known as congenital adrenal hyperplasia. In general, steroidogenesis is shunted to increased production of androgens in favor of cortisol and mineralocorticoid. The characteristic manifestations depend upon the enzyme affected, but typically include virilization of females and can include life-threatening salt-wasting due to lack of mineralocorticoid.

○ **What tests are used to distinguish adrenal tumors in women with hirsutism?**

Serum testosterone and DHEA.

○ **What is the most important mineralocorticoid produced by the adrenal cortex?**

Aldosterone, although produced in small quantities, is the most physiologically important mineralocorticoid. Other mineralocorticoids such as 11-deoxycorticosterone (DOC) have both glucocorticoid and mineralocorticoid properties, but are secreted in such small quantities that they are physiologically unimportant.

○ **What is the half-life of plasma aldosterone?**

Twenty to thirty minutes.

○ **What is the most significant regulator of aldosterone secretion?**

Angiotensin II (AII) is the primary physiologic control of aldosterone secretion. AII directly stimulates production of aldosterone by the zona glomerulosa. A second less important stimulus is an elevated serum potassium level. Hypokalemia blunts the adrenal gland's ability to synthesize aldosterone thus causing a decrease in production and secretion.

○ **What is the basis of aldosterone production and its role in the renin–angiotensin–aldosterone system (RAAS)?**

In response to multiple stimuli, but primarily hypovolemia and decreased renal perfusion, renin is released from the juxtaglomerular apparatus (JGA) of the afferent arteriole. Renin cleaves angiotensin I (AI) from angiotensinogen. Angiotensin-converting enzyme converts AI to AII primarily in the pulmonary vasculature. Secretion of aldosterone results from direct stimulation of the adrenal gland by AII. The actions of aldosterone include (a) increased renal conservation of sodium, (b) increased glomerular filtration fraction by increasing efferent arteriole tone, (c) increased peripheral vasomotor tone, and (d) increased thirst. The overall effect is an increase in plasma volume and renal perfusion.

○ **What are the main physiologic functions of aldosterone?**

To regulate sodium resorption in the kidneys, gut, salivary gland, and sweat glands.

○ **What is the site of action of aldosterone within the kidney?**

The principle site of aldosterone action is the distal tubule of the nephron.

○ **What is the mechanism of action of aldosterone within the kidney?**

Aldosterone stimulates transcription of the gene that encodes for a sodium–potassium ATPase, leading to increased numbers of sodium–potassium exchange pumps in the basolateral membrane of distal tubule epithelial cells. This conserves sodium in the nephron and water follows the sodium. The same mechanism is at play in the gut, salivary glands, and sweat glands.

○ **What is Conn syndrome?**

Conn syndrome is primary hyperaldosteronism.

○ **What are the clinical features of Conn syndrome?**

The clinical features of Conn syndrome include hypertension, hypokalemia, hypernatremia, alkalosis, and periodic paralysis.

○ **What laboratory abnormalities are typical of Conn syndrome?**

The laboratory abnormalities of Conn syndrome include hypokalemia, hypernatremia, alkalosis, decreased plasma renin activity (PRA <2 ng/mL), and high urine and plasma aldosterone (>15 ng/dL). Aldosterone-to-PRA ratio is >20:1.

○ **What is the phenomenon of renal escape?**

In primary aldosteronism after a gain of 1.5 kg of extracellular fluid, there is a decrease in absorption of sodium at the proximal tubules. Escape is associated with an increase in renal artery pressure and an increase in atrial natriuretic factor (ANF). Renal escape limits the clinical hypertensive response in patients with primary hyperaldosteronism.

○ **What is the most common cause of primary hyperaldosteronism?**

The most common cause is an aldosterone-producing adenoma of the adrenal gland.

○ **List the surgically correctable subtypes of primary hyperaldosteronism.**

Aldosterone-producing adenoma, primary unilateral adrenal hyperplasia, ovarian aldosterone-secreting tumor, and aldosterone-producing carcinoma.

○ **List subtypes of primary hyperaldosteronism not amenable to surgical correction.**

Bilateral adrenal hyperplasia, familial hyperaldosteronism type 1, and familial hyperaldosteronism type 2.

○ **What are the indications to screen for primary hyperaldosteronism?**

Hypertension with hypokalemia, resistant hypertension (3 or more oral agents with poor control); adrenal incidentaloma with hypertension, early-onset hypertension (<20 years) or stroke (<50 years), severe hypertension (≥160/≥110), whenever considering secondary causes of hypertension, unexplained hypokalemia, and evidence of target-organ damage disproportionate to degree of hypertension.

○ **True/False: The presence of a unilateral adrenal mass >1 cm mandates adrenalectomy in patients with primary hyperaldosteronism?**

False. Because adrenal lesions are commonplace among patients over 40 years old, the presence of a unilateral adrenal mass in the context of primary hyperaldosteronism does not mandate adrenalectomy. Instead, these patients should undergo adrenal vein sampling to confirm lateralizing aldosterone secretion. Indeed, studies have demonstrated that, in the absence of adrenal vein sampling, 25% of patients would have been inappropriately recommended adrenalectomy.

○ **What measurement(s) are required to document lateralization on adrenal vein sampling?**

Lateralization of aldosterone secretion is determined by comparing the aldosterone to cortisol ratios of the dominant to nondominant sides. Specifically, if the ratio of $(A_{dominant}/C_{dominant})/(A_{nondominant}/C_{nondominant})$ is greater than 2 to 4:1 (depending on the use of ACTH stimulation), aldosterone secretion is considered lateralizing.

○ **What is the most common cause of secondary hyperaldosteronism?**

The most common cause is renal arterial disease or renal parenchymal disease. This disease is a disorder with oversecretion of aldosterone secondary to excess production of AII and the RAAS.

○ **In treatment of an aldosterone-producing adrenal adenoma, adrenalectomy should be preceded by what preoperative measure?**

Adequate clinical treatment of hypertension and correction of hyperkalemia or other metabolic abnormalities.

○ **What is the treatment of primary aldosteronism caused by bilateral hyperplasia?**

The treatment is medication with the drug spironolactone, which is a competitive antagonist of the aldosterone receptor.

○ **What are the 3 endocrine glands required for regulation of cortisol synthesis and release?**

The hypothalamus, pituitary, and adrenal glands.

○ **Where is corticotropin-releasing hormone (CRH) produced and what is its function?**

CRH is synthesized in the hypothalamus and is carried to the anterior pituitary via the portal blood. CRH stimulates ACTH release.

○ **What are secondary stimulants of ACTH?**

Vasopressin, oxytocin, epinephrine, AII, vasoactive intestinal peptide, gastrin-releasing peptide, ANF, and γ-aminobutyric acid are all secondary stimulants.

○ **What complex is ACTH derived from?**

ACTH is a 39-amino acid polypeptide produced from the protein proopiomelanocortin (POMC). Other POMC derivatives include β-lipotropin, α-melanocyte-stimulating hormone, β-melanocyte-stimulating hormone, β-endorphin, methionine, and enkephalin.

○ **Is ACTH produced relatively constantly throughout the day?**

No, ACTH secretion is characterized by an intermittent diurnal rhythm leading to parallel changes with cortisol and ACTH.

○ **With respect to the normal diurnal variation with circulating cortisol levels, is the level typically higher in the morning or evening?**

Healthy subjects have a peak of cortisol levels in the morning with a fall throughout the day and into the evening. Patients with Cushing syndrome lose the diurnal variation of circulating cortisol.

○ **What is the relationship between ACTH and circulating cortisol?**

ACTH and circulating cortisol are reciprocally related.

○ **What effects do glucocorticoids have on cellular metabolism?**

Glucocorticoids are essential for life and affect a wide spectrum of cellular metabolism including increased glycogen synthesis, increased gluconeogenesis, decreased peripheral glucose utilization, protein catabolism, and decreased immune-mediated inflammation. In disease states and stress, hypertension, muscle wasting, myopathy, osteopenia, and glucose dysregulation are seen.

○ **What is Cushing syndrome?**

A symptom complex caused by excess glucocorticoid production. Manifestations include obesity, hypertension, diabetes, weakness, muscle atrophy, hirsutism, skin striae, moon facies, easy bruising, acne, and psychologic changes.

○ **What is the primary laboratory test to identify Cushing syndrome if it is clinically suspected?**

The key to diagnosing Cushing syndrome is establishing the presence of excess glucocorticoid. Therefore, a 24-hour urine to measure cortisol and creatinine is the primary laboratory test. The 24-hour urine collection commences following the first morning void and continues throughout a 24-hour period until completion of the next morning void. The urine should remain refrigerated in an opaque container until transported to the laboratory. Creatinine helps to confirm a complete collection.

○ **How accurate is urinary free cortisol as a screening test for Cushing syndrome?**

Although 3.3% of individuals without Cushing syndrome will have elevated values, this test is 95% specific for Cushing syndrome.

○ **What test may be used if urinary free cortisol is equivocal?**

A low-dose dexamethasone test; 1 mg of dexamethasone is given at 11 PM and the cortisol is checked at 8 AM the following morning. A normal person's cortisol will be suppressed to <2 ng/mL by negative feedback on ACTH and CRH production. If plasma cortisol is not suppressed, Cushing syndrome is present.

○ **How is the dexamethasone suppression test performed?**

One milligram of oral dexamethasone is ingested at bedtime. Serum cortisol is measured the next morning. Serum cortisol should be less than 2 μg/dL in normal individuals.

○ **False-positives may occur in what conditions?**

Obesity, alcoholism, renal failure, anorexia, and bulimia. Exercise and acute illness will also raise serum cortisol levels. Phenobarbital, phenytoin, and rifampin increase dexamethasone metabolism and may also cause false-positive results.

○ **What steps can be taken to identify the etiology of excess glucocorticoids?**

After the excess of glucocorticoids has been established by urinary free cortisol and/or a low-dose dexamethasone suppression test, the next step is to determine whether the hypercortisolism is ACTH-dependent or ACTH-independent. This can be accomplished by measuring late-afternoon ACTH with concurrent serum cortisol. A high ACTH value (>50 pg/mL) suggests ACTH dependence, whereas a low value (<5 pg/mL) suggests ACTH-independent Cushing syndrome.

○ **What are the etiologies of ACTH-independent Cushing syndrome?**

ACTH-independent causes of Cushing syndrome account for approximately 18% of cases of Cushing syndrome. Specific etiologies include adrenal adenoma, adrenal carcinoma, and bilateral adrenal hyperplasia.

○ **What are the etiologies of ACTH-dependent Cushing syndrome?**

ACTH-dependent causes of Cushing syndrome account for the majority of cases of Cushing syndrome. Specific etiologies include pituitary hypersecretion and ectopic ACTH production.

○ **What is Cushing disease?**

Pituitary hypersecretion of ACTH, usually secondary to a pituitary adenoma, which results in increased production and secretion of glucocorticoids.

○ **What percentage of patients with Cushing syndrome actually have Cushing disease?**

Seventy-five to eighty-five percent of Cushing syndrome is due to Cushing disease. Other causes of Cushing syndrome include adrenal adenomas, adrenal carcinomas, and ectopic secretion of either CRH or ACTH.

○ **What are the treatments of Cushing disease?**

Treatments for Cushing disease include transsphenoidal hypophyseal microsurgery to remove the pituitary adenoma. This treatment is effective in 85% to 95% of patients. Other treatments include pituitary external beam radiation and heavy particle proton beam therapy.

○ **If Cushing syndrome is diagnosed during pregnancy, is immediate treatment warranted or should it wait until the postpartum period?**

Both maternal and fetal morbidity have been reduced with treatment of Cushing syndrome during pregnancy, either by surgical removal of an adrenal adenoma during the second trimester or by transphenoidal adenomectomy or with medications such as metyrapone.

○ **What is the most common cause of ectopic or exogenous glucocorticoid excess causing Cushing syndrome?**

Exogenous steroid administration.

○ **ACTH may be produced ectopically by which tumors?**

Oat cell, small cell lung tumors, and carcinoid tumors.

○ **What is Nelson syndrome?**

Ten to twenty percent of individuals undergoing bilateral adrenalectomy for severe Cushing syndrome will suffer from growth of a pituitary adenoma (usually a chromophobe adenoma). Growth of the space-occupying lesion is attributed to the lack of hypothalamic/pituitary feedback and high levels of ACTH. Increased production of ACTH and melanocyte-stimulating hormone (a derivative of POMC) cause typical signs and symptoms of muscle weakness and skin hyperpigmentation. Mass effect can cause headaches, visual disturbances, and cranial nerve compression. With the development of treatments for Cushing disease other than bilateral adrenalectomy, Nelson syndrome is rarely encountered today.

○ **What is Addison disease?**

Addison disease is an inadequate production of corticosteroids by the adrenal cortex caused by a defect within the adrenal cortex rendering them unable to synthesize normal amounts of steroid hormones. Radiation therapy involving the adrenals can also cause Addison disease.

○ **What is the most common cause of adrenal insufficiency?**

The most common cause of Addison disease is withdrawal of exogenous steroid therapy. Additional causes include adrenal tuberculosis or lymphocytic adenitis with adrenal fibrosis, malignant infiltration of the adrenal, sarcoidosis, histoplasmosis, blastomycosis, and coccidioidomycosis. Additionally, Addison disease may occur with administration of aminoglutethimide, ketoconazole, mitotane, or suramin.

○ **What is the most common *primary* cause of adrenal insufficiency in Western countries?**

In the Western world, the most common cause of primary adrenal insufficiency is autoimmune adrenalitis. Adrenal insufficiency may occur as an isolated finding or as part of a complex of abnormalities known as autoimmune polyendocrine syndrome (APS), which includes hypoparathyroidism, autoimmune thyroid disease, hypogonadism, diabetes, and various other autoimmune conditions.

○ **What is the classic triad of Addison disease?**

Hyponatremia, hyperkalemia, and azotemia are the classic triad; however, the entire triad is present in only 50% to 60% of cases. Other disorders associated with Addison disease may include hypercalcemia, hyperthyroidism, hypothyroidism, and diabetes.

○ **What symptoms are associated with Addison disease?**

Symptoms associated with Addison disease are weakness, prostration, dehydration, and coma.

○ **How does one diagnose adrenal insufficiency?**

The clinical test for Addison disease is failure to increase plasma or urinary corticosteroid levels in response to an ACTH infusion. The screening test involves administration of ACTH or cosyntropin 0.25 mg IV. Cortisol is checked 60 minutes after administration and should be at least 18 μg/dL if normal.

O   **What can cause acute adrenal insufficiency?**

Acute adrenal insufficiency can be caused by withdrawal of exogenous steroids, sepsis, bilateral adrenal hemorrhage, surgical bilateral adrenalectomy, or surgical removal of a functional adenoma in a patient with an atrophic contralateral adrenal.

O   **What is the treatment of acute adrenal insufficiency?**

The treatment is administration of glucocorticoids along with replacement of saline.

O   **What is the treatment of chronic Addison disease?**

Maintenance with chronic glucocorticoids and mineralocorticoids.

O   **True/False: Mineralocorticoid replacement is necessary in patients with BOTH primary and secondary adrenal insufficiency?**

False. Aldosterone secretion by the adrenals is not contingent on ACTH. Accordingly, the zona glomerulosa continues to function appropriately in patients with secondary adrenal insufficiency. Only patients with primary adrenal insufficiency require mineralocorticoid replacement.

O   **What are the major catecholamines secreted by the adrenal medulla?**

Epinephrine, norepinephrine, and dopamine.

O   **Why is epinephrine secretion localized to the adrenal medulla?**

The enzyme phenylethanolamine-N-methyltransferase (PNMT) is located exclusively in the adrenal medulla, and catalyzes the methylation of norepinephrine to epinephrine. This can be clinically significant in patients with extra-adrenal pheochromocytoma, in which case only norepinephrine is produced because of the absence of PNMT at the extra-adrenal site.

O   **Are glucocorticoid and epinephrine production related?**

Yes, high levels of glucocorticoids are necessary to maintain levels of PNMT and thus epinephrine production. This may explain the proximity of the adrenal medulla to the venous drainage system within the adrenal gland.

O   **What are the substrates of epinephrine and norepinephrine?**

Dietary tyrosine and phenylalanine.

O   **What is the major regulation of catecholamine biosynthesis?**

Activation of tyrosine hydroxylase activity, which combines phenylalanine and tyrosine to form dopa as a precursor to norepinephrine. Tyrosine hydroxylase activity may be regulated by the adrenal cortex.

O   **How are catecholamines stored?**

They are stored in separate vesicles within nerve terminals.

○ **What causes preganglionic sympathetic nerves to release catecholamines?**

In general, catecholamine release is stimulated by sympathetic stimulation. Stress, pain, cold, heat, asphyxia, hypotension, hypoglycemia, and sodium depletion, all cause catecholamine release.

○ **What is the serum half-life of catecholamines?**

Less than 20 seconds.

○ **How are catecholamines degraded?**

They are degraded by the action of catechol-O-methyltransferase (COMT) and monoamine oxidase (MAO), following reuptake by nerve terminals.

○ **How are catecholamine breakdown products measured?**

The primary metabolite of catecholamine breakdown is urinary vanillylmandelic acid (VMA) with metanephrine and normetanephrine being secondary breakdown products. These are best measured by means of a 24-hour urine collection.

○ **Tumors of catecholamine-producing cells are known as what?**

Pheochromocytomas and paragangliomas in adrenal and extra-adrenal sites, respectively.

○ **Describe the clinical signs and symptoms of pheochromocytoma/paraganglioma.**

Headache (60%-90%), palpitations (50%-70%), sweating (55%-75%), pallor (40%-45%), nausea (20%-40%), flushing (10%-20%), weight loss (20%-40%), tiredness (25%-40%), psychologic symptoms (20%-40%), sustained hypertension (50%-60%), paroxysmal hypertension (30%), orthostatic hypotension (10%-50%), and hyperglycemia (40%).

CHAPTER 32 Adrenal Tumors

Paul L. Crispen, MD and
Matthew T. Gettman, MD

○ **How often are adrenal masses incidentally detected on CT scans?**

5% of the time.

○ **What is the relationship between age and the incidence of adrenal incidentalomas?**

The incidence for adrenal incidentalomas increases with age, with 0.5% incidence during the 3rd decade of life and 7% incidence during the 8th decade of life.

○ **What percentage of adrenal incidentalomas will be deemed potential surgical lesions upon further evaluation?**

20%

○ **What are the 2 general questions one needs to answer when working up an adrenal mass?**

1. Whether it is functional or nonfunctional.
2. Whether it is benign or malignant.

○ **What is the differential diagnosis of a benign incidental adrenal mass?**

The more common adrenal lesions are adrenal adenomas, myelolipomas, and adrenal cysts. Less commonly one encounters ectopic tissue, oncocytomas, ganglioneuromas, pheochromocytomas, aldosteronomas, and adrenal hemorrhage.

○ **List 4 pathologic conditions associated with hypersecretion of adrenal products.**

Pheochromocytoma, Cushing syndrome, primary aldosteronism, and adrenal carcinoma.

○ **How does adrenal hemorrhage following birth occur and which side is affected more often?**

Adrenal hemorrhage can occur following difficult childbirth and more often affects the right side. This phenomenon has been attributed to an increase in intra-abdominal pressure that is transmitted through the short right adrenal vein and into the parenchyma resulting in hemorrhage.

○ **What are the 2 most common adrenal lesions detected incidentally?**

Adenomas (75%) and myelolipomas (6%).

○ **What is the differential diagnosis of a malignant adrenal mass?**

Adrenocortical carcinoma, pheochromocytoma, neuroblastoma, and metastatic disease.

○ **What percentage of patients with an incidental adrenal mass will be diagnosed with pheochromocytoma?**

Approximately 5%.

○ **What percentage of pheochromocytomas will arise outside of the adrenal gland?**

10% to 25% of pheochromocytomas will be extra-adrenal.

○ **List the symptoms of pheochromocytoma.**

Headache, palpitations, sweating, pallor, flushing, weight loss, fatigue, anxiety, hypertension, and hyperglycemia.

○ **What is the 10% rule regarding pheochromocytomas?**

10% of pheochromocytomas are malignant, 10% are bilateral, 10% are found in the pediatric age group, 10% will be extra-adrenal, and 10% are associated with multiple endocrine neoplasia (MEN) syndrome.

○ **How accurate is the 10% rule in contemporary series evaluating pheochromocytomas?**

The classic 10% rule for pheochromocytomas does not seem to reflect contemporary findings. In more recent series up to 25% will be extra-adrenal, up to 30% will be associated with a hereditary syndrome, and malignant disease will be seen in only 5% of cases.

○ **List the hereditary conditions associated with pheochromocytoma.**

Multiple endocrine neoplasia type 2a, multiple endocrine neoplasia 2b, von Hippel–Lindau syndrome, neurofibromatosis type 1, familial paraganglioma syndrome type 4, and familial paraganglioma syndrome type 1.

○ **When is a partial adrenalectomy indicated?**

In patients with bilateral and hereditary adrenal tumors.

○ **Is the pattern of hypertension with pheochromocytomas sustained or paroxysmal?**

Sustained hypertension is found in 50% to 60% of patients, and is a more common finding in children and patients with multiple endocrine adenoma type-2 (MEA-2). Paroxysmal hypertension affects approximately 30% of patients. Orthostatic hypotension can be noted in 10% to 50% of patients.

○ **Is it possible to have a pheochromocytoma in a normotensive patient?**

Yes. Approximately 10% of pheochromocytomas are found in normotensive patients. This is why it is important not to eliminate pheochromocytomas from your differential diagnosis in a normotensive patient with an adrenal mass.

○ **How do the manifestations of pheochromocytoma in children vary from those in adults?**

Children manifest a higher incidence of familial pheochromocytomas (10%) and bilaterality (25%). Additionally, there is a 15% to 30% incidence of multiple pheochromocytomas in children and a 15% to 30% incidence of extra-adrenal location as well.

○ **What are the most common locations for extra-adrenal pheochromocytomas?**

The organ of Zuckerkandl (close to the origin of the inferior mesenteric artery), bladder wall, heart, mediastinum, carotid, and glomus jugulare bodies.

○ **What symptom is classically associated with extra-adrenal pheochromocytoma involving the urinary bladder?**

Micturition syncope.

○ **What laboratory tests confirm the diagnosis of pheochromocytoma?**

Free-fractionated plasma metanephrines and 24-hour urinary-fractionated metanephrine tests are the recommended studies to screen for and diagnosis pheochromocytoma.

○ **What is the utility of CT scanning for detecting pheochromocytomas?**

CT scanning detects >90% of pheochromocytomas of adrenal origin, and approximately 75% of extra-adrenal pheochromocytomas. Computed tomography alone cannot differentiate between pheochromocytomas and other adrenal lesions nor can one delineate malignant potential based upon the CT scanning alone.

○ **What is the average Hounsfield units of pheochromocytoma on unenhanced CT scans?**

35 Hounsfield units.

○ **What clinical, biochemical, and histologic features distinguish malignant from benign pheochromocytomas?**

Malignancy can be suggested by large tumor size, DNA ploidy pattern, local invasion, but is defined by the presence of metastases.

○ **What are the most common sites of metastatic pheochromocytoma?**

Bone, lung, liver, and lymph nodes.

○ **What is the characteristic appearance of pheochromocytoma on MRI scanning?**

They appear as a characteristically bright image on T2-weighted studies, but the diagnosis cannot be based upon MRI alone.

○ **What is an MIBG scan, what does "MIBG" stand for, and how is it useful?**

The metaiodobenzylguanidine (MIBG) scan images adrenal medullary tissue and is particularly useful for identifying pheochromocytomas of extra-adrenal origin or multiple pheochromocytomas. The MIBG scan has an overall sensitivity and specificity of 87% and 99%, respectively. The false-negative rate is 10%.

○ **What is the preoperative medical preparation for patients with pheochromocytomas?**

All patients must be vigorously hydrated in preparation for surgery since elevated catecholamine levels lead to significant dehydration. Additionally, patients are started on an α-adrenergic blocker such as phenoxybenzamine, with an initial divided dose of 20 to 30 mg orally, increasing to 40 to 100 mg as needed. Secondly, β-adrenergic blockers can be added to the α-blockers to protect against arrhythmias and permit reduction in the α-blocker requirement. β-Blockers are usually only added when cardiac arrhythmias are identified. Labetalol (Normodyne) is a nonselective β-blocker and a selective α-adrenergic blocker that has been shown to control hypertension associated with pheochromocytoma. Calcium channel blockers may also be utilized for controlling hypertension associated with pheochromocytoma.

○ **What problem can arise if β-blockers are initiated prior to α-blockers?**

There can be a marked rise in the total peripheral vascular resistance secondary to unopposed α-adrenergic activity that can lead to circulatory collapse.

○ **What additional drug might be used in the preoperative preparation of patients with pheochromocytomas who have cardiomyopathies, multiple catecholamine-secreting paragangliomas, or resistance to α-blockers?**

α-Methylparatyrosine (metyrosine) decreases the rate of catecholamine synthesis (the conversion of tyrosine to dopa).

○ **How should the surgeon and anesthesiologist be prepared for fluctuations in blood pressure at the onset of anesthetic induction in surgery?**

The patient must be volume-expanded with several liters of intravenous crystalloid prior to induction of anesthesia. In addition, α- and β-adrenergic blocking agents should be readily available for IV use. Phentolamine, a short-acting α-blocker (50 mg per 500 mL of ringers lactate), or sodium nitroprusside (50 mg per 250 mL of 5% dextrose in H_2O) should be on hand. Esmolol or propranolol should be available for persistent tachycardias or arrhythmias.

○ **What are the indications, advantages, and disadvantages for using a modified posterior incision for adrenal tumors?**

A modified posterior lumbotomy may be utilized in patients with right-sided adrenal aldosterone-secreting tumors or benign adenomas <5 cm. The main advantage over a flank or transabdominal incision is the excellent exposure of the vena cava in the region of the short right adrenal vein. The disadvantages include a limited visual field and compression of the abdominal contents and thoracic cavity that may impair respirations in the jackknife position. This approach is not recommended for pheochromocytomas or malignant adrenal tumors.

○ **Following surgical exposure of a pheochromocytoma, what anatomic structure must be initially addressed?**

The adrenal vein should be divided initially to avoid systemic release of catecholamines during manipulation of the adrenal gland.

○ **What other therapy can be used in patients with hypertensive pheochromocytoma crisis that is refractory to sodium nitroprusside, α-blockers, and β-blockers?**

Magnesium sulfate. It lowers catecholamine release and acts as a very effective α-adrenergic antagonist and arterial dilator. It is also an excellent cardiac antiarrhythmic in the presence of high epinephrine levels. The use of magnesium sulfate has reportedly been lifesaving in a number of cases of refractory pheochromocytoma crisis.

○ **What medical problem needs to be carefully monitored postoperatively after pheochromocytoma surgery and how should it be treated?**

Hypotension due to lack of catecholamine vasoconstriction is the most common medical problem encountered postoperatively, although hypoglycemia may also appear. The hypotension is best treated with volume replacement. Vasoconstricting medications should be avoided if possible.

○ **What is the difference between Cushing disease and Cushing syndrome?**

Cushing syndrome refers to the group of signs and symptoms that result from excessive glucocorticoids. Cushing disease refers to Cushing syndrome caused by the hypersecretion of adrenocorticotropic hormone (ACTH) from the pituitary gland.

○ **What are the 3 main causes of Cushing syndrome?**

Exogenous, ACTH-dependent, and ACTH-independent.

○ **What is the most common cause of Cushing syndrome?**

Use of exogenous steroids.

○ **List other disorders/causes of hypercortisolism that can mimic Cushing syndrome.**

Pregnancy, depression, alcohol dependence, and morbid obesity.

○ **What percentage of patients with endogenous Cushing syndrome will have Cushing disease?**

Approximately 70%.

○ **What are the symptoms of Cushing syndrome?**

Obesity, decreased libido, purple striae, hirsutism, hypertension, muscle weakness, glucose intolerance, depression, osteoporosis, and body bruising.

○ **What is subclinical Cushing syndrome?**

Hypercortisolism without the cushingoid phenotype. Diagnosis is typically made during the evaluation of an adrenal incidentaloma.

○ **What percentage of patients with adrenal incidentalomas will be diagnosed with subclinical Cushing syndrome?**

Up to 10% of patients with adrenal incidentalomas will be diagnosed with subclinical Cushing syndrome upon functional evaluation.

○ **What 3 tests can be used for the initial assessment glucocorticoid function in patients with suspected Cushing syndrome?**

24-hour urinary excretion of cortisol, low dose dexamethasone suppression test, and the late night salivary cortisol test.

○ **In the low dexamethasone suppression test, what serum and endpoint should change?**

There should be a decrease of plasma cortisol. Failure for cortisol to be suppressed suggests hypercortisolism.

○ **How does one determine if a patient has ACTH-dependent or ACTH-independent hypercortisolism?**

The simultaneous measurement of both plasma ACTH (corticotropin) and cortisol.

○ **When using the metyrapone-stimulation test to differentiate between pituitary Cushing and ectopic ACTH secretion, what result does one look for?**

Metyrapone blocks the conversion of 11-desoxycortisol to cortisol. As plasma cortisol concentrations fall, the pituitary gland secretes more ACTH, thus increasing urinary 17-hydroxy corticosteroid levels. Patients with Cushing disease have a normal or supranormal increase in 17-hydroxy corticosteroid urinary excretion. Patients with ectopic ACTH-secreting tumors will have little or no increase in urinary 17-hydroxy corticosteroid levels, since ectopic ACTH production will not be influenced by plasma cortisol feedback on the pituitary gland.

○ **Name 3 agents used to reduce the secretion of functional steroids in patients with Cushing syndrome.**

1. Aminoglutethimide blocks the conversion of cholesterol to pregnenolone. Patients given aminoglutethimide must be observed for adrenocortical insufficiency, since aldosterone production is also impaired.

2. Metyrapone blocks the conversion of 11-desoxycortisol to cortisone.

3. Ketoconazole blocks cytochrome P-450–mediated side-chain cleavage and hydroxylation at both the early and late steps in steroid biosynthesis.

○ **What is Nelson syndrome and when has it been seen in the treatment of Cushing disease?**

Historically, patients with Cushing disease often were treated with bilateral adrenalectomy. Ten to twenty percent of these patients subsequently developed pituitary tumors, usually chromophobe adenomas, secondary to the lack of hypothalamic/pituitary feedback and high ACTH production. This could occur years after bilateral adrenalectomy and can be treated by prophylactic pituitary radiation.

○ **What is the currently accepted treatment of choice for Cushing disease and what are the cure rates?**

Presently, transsphenoidal hypophyseal microsurgery for the removal of pituitary adenomas results in cure rates of approximately 60% to 80%.

○ **What is the role of adrenalectomy in the treatment of Cushing syndrome.**

Adrenalectomy can be performed in cases of unilateral cortisol secreting adrenal tumors. Bilateral adrenalectomy may be performed in cases of refractory Cushing disease and ectopic ACTH syndromes. Lifelong cortisol replacement therapy will be required in patients undergoing bilateral adrenalectomy.

○ **What findings suggest the diagnosis of primary hyperaldosteronism?**

Hypokalemia with metabolic alkalosis suppressed peripheral renin activity together with elevated urinary and plasma aldosterone levels in hypertensive patients.

○ **What percentage of patients with primary hyperaldosteronism will have hypokalemia in contemporary series?**

Only 10% to 30%.

○ **What factors can limit the evaluation of serum potassium and urinary aldosterone levels in patients with hyperaldosteronism?**

Hyponatremia can limit the evaluation of serum potassium and hypokalemia can limit the evaluation of urinary aldosterone. Additional several medications can alter the evaluation for primary aldosteronism including spironolactone, β-blockers, and angiotensin-converting-enzyme (ACE) inhibitors.

○ **What is the recommended screening test for hyperaldosteronism?**

Plasma aldosterone-to-renin ratio should be used as the screening test for primary aldosteronism.

○ **What are the indications for screening for primary aldosteronism?**

Hypertension with hypokalemia, resistant hypertension (3 or more medications with poor control), adrenal adenoma with hypertension, early-onset hypertension, severe hypertension (>160/>110), whenever considering secondary cause of hypertension, and unexplained hypokalemia.

○ **List causes of hyperaldosteronism.**

Solitary adenoma, bilateral adrenal hyperplasia, adrenal carcinoma, unilateral adrenal hyperplasia, familial hyperaldosteronism, and ectopic aldosterone-producing tumor.

○ **What is the most common cause of primary hyperaldosteronism?**

Bilateral adrenal hyperplasia (60%).

○ **What plasma aldosterone-to-renin ratio is suggestive of primary aldosteronism?**

A plasma aldosterone-to-renin ratio >30 (aldosterone ng/dL to PRA ng/mL/h).

○ **Can the diagnosis of primary aldosteronism be made based on the aldosterone-to-renin ratio alone?**

No. Confirmatory testing must be performed.

○ **List the subtypes of primary aldosteronism that are best managed with medical therapy.**

Bilateral adrenal hyperplasia and familial hyperaldosteronism.

○ **List the subtypes of primary aldosteronism that can be managed with surgical therapy.**

Aldosterone-producing adenoma, primary unilateral adrenal hyperplasia, aldosterone-producing carcinoma, and ectopic aldosterone-producing tumors.

○ **What is the best test to lateralize functional aldosterone-producing adenomas?**

Adrenal vein sampling of aldosterone is very sensitive in lateralizing these lesions.

○ **At the time of renal vein sampling to measure aldosterone, what else should be measured and why?**

Cortisol, in order to confirm correct positioning of the catheter during sampling.

○ **What is the management of a solitary unilateral adrenal mass identified on CT scan with biochemical criteria consistent with primary aldosteronism?**

After confirming functional status of the lesion, surgical extirpation would be appropriate. Adrenal vein sampling is not essential to lateralize the tumor, but can be helpful.

○ **What measures should be taken prior to surgical removal of a solitary adenoma associated with hyperaldosteronism?**

Treatment of hypertension with an aldosterone receptor antagonist or a calcium channel blocker and correction of potassium depletion.

○ **In patients with primary aldosteronism secondary to bilateral adrenal hyperplasia, what is the medical management of choice and how does it work?**

Medical therapy consisting of spironolactone or eplerenone, which are competitive antagonists of the aldosterone receptor.

○ **What is the relationship between the size and incidence of adrenal carcinoma?**

2% in adrenal tumors ≤4 cm, 6% in adrenal tumors 4 to 6 cm, and 25% in tumors >6 cm.

○ **Why is the size cutoff for an adrenal carcinoma reported to be both 5 and 6 cm?**

Studies have shown that tumors <6 cm in size pathologically are unlikely to be adrenal carcinomas. However, CT scanning underestimates the size of the adrenal glands, so a 5-cm cutoff is used radiographically as the equivalent of the 6-cm pathologic size.

○ **What percentage of adrenal carcinomas are functional?**

50% to 79% are functional in adults. 90% are functional in children.

○ **What is the most common hormone secreted by adrenal carcinomas?**

Cortisol.

○ **How does the presentation of adrenal carcinoma in children differ from that in adults?**

The majority of these tumors are hormonally active, usually presenting with Cushing syndrome, virilization in the female, and isosexual precocious puberty in males.

○ **What syndromes can be associated with adrenal carcinoma in children?**

Beckwith–Wiedemann syndrome (exophthalmos, macroglossia, gigantism, and neonatal hypoglycemia), isolated hemihypertrophy, and Li–Fraumeni syndrome.

○ **What is the differential diagnosis in the pediatric age group?**

In children younger than 5 years, neuroblastoma and Wilm tumor are likely.

○ **How do functional adrenal carcinomas present?**

Functional adrenal lesions typically present as Cushing syndrome (40%), Cushing syndrome and virilization (24%), virilization alone (20%) (virilization in females with either increased DHEA-17 ketosteroid or increased testosterone, feminizing syndrome in the male), hyperaldosteronism (2.5%), or a combination of the above.

○ **When evaluating functional status of an adrenal tumor suspicious for carcinoma what should be considered.**

Excess of glucocorticoid, mineralocorticoid, catecholamine, sexual steroid, and steroid precursors should be evaluated.

○ **What is the average size of adrenal carcinomas on cross-sectional imaging?**

10 to 12 cm. Over 90% of adrenal carcinomas are over 5 cm at the time of diagnosis.

○ **List common radiographic characteristics of adrenal carcinomas.**

Irregular borders, irregular enhancement, calcifications, and necrotic areas. The average Hounsfield units of adrenal carcinomas on noncontrast CT scans are 39.

○ **What is the primary indication for biopsy of an adrenal tumor suspicious for adrenal carcinoma?**

Biopsy is indicated in cases of unresectable, locally advanced, or metastatic disease in order to confirm the diagnosis prior to systemic medical therapy. Biopsy is not recommended in cases of clinically localized disease.

○ **Virilization in the absence of elevated urinary 17-ketosteroids in a female patient should raise the suspicion of what other lesion?**

In addition to adrenocortical tumors that secrete testosterone, one should also consider testosterone-secreting ovarian tumors.

○ **A male patient with a functional adrenocortical tumor presents with gynecomastia, testicular atrophy, and impotence. What is the presumed diagnosis, likelihood of malignancy, and prognosis?**

This patient likely has an estrogen-secreting adrenocortical tumor that secretes androstenedione, which is converted peripherally to estrogens. Eighty percent of these lesions are malignant, with the 3-year survival being <20%.

○ **What is the 5-year survival of adrenal carcinoma?**

Approximately 45%.

○ **What pathologic criteria are utilized when classifying adrenocortical carcinomas?**

The Weiss criteria based upon mitotic rate, atypical mitoses, venous invasion, nuclear grade, presence of clear cytoplasm, growth pattern, necrosis, sinusoidal, and capsular invasion.

○ **Describe the staging criteria utilized for adrenocortical carcinomas?**

T1: tumor ≤5 cm, invasion absent.

T2: tumor >5 cm, invasion absent.

T3: tumor involves adrenal fat.

T4: tumor invades adjacent organs.

○ **What is the standard recommended management of adrenal carcinoma?**

Surgical removal of the primary tumor, with an attempt to remove the entire lesion with contiguous organs (spleen, kidney) en bloc if necessary, and a regional lymphadenectomy.

○ **What is the local recurrence rate of adrenal carcinoma following complete resection?**

Up to 60% to 80%.

○ **How often does adrenal carcinoma present with metastases and how often is the inferior vena cava (IVC) involved?**

Approximately 32% of the time; 19% will have IVC involvement.

○ **What drugs are available for the medical management of advanced adrenocortical carcinoma?**

Mitotane, a DDT-derivative, has been shown to induce a tumor response in 35% of patients. Ketoconazole has an adrenolytic effect. However, these compounds, in addition to metyrapone, have not been shown to improve long-term survival.

○ **What radiographic criterion is utilized when distinguishing benign from potentially malignant adrenal masses detected on noncontrast-enhanced CT scans?**

Radiographic density measured by Hounsfield units. Adrenal lesions <10 Hounsfield units are considered benign.

○ **How many adrenal adenomas will present with Hounsfield units greater than 10?**

30%.

○ **What is the contrast washout test and how is it used?**

This test can be helpful in determining the presence of adenoma. An intravenous contrast agent is given and a CT scan is done after an 80-second delay. Another scan is done 10 minutes later, and the 2 scans are compared. A washout or decrease in contrast enhancement of 50% or more is indicative of an adenoma.

○ **What is the sensitivity and specificity of the contrast washout test?**

Sensitivity, 98%; specificity, 100%.

○ **True/False: It is recommended that all adrenal adenomas greater than 1 cm undergo metabolic evaluation.**

True. The national institutes of health (NIH) consensus statement recommends that all adrenal adenomas larger than 1 cm undergo metabolic evaluation. Surgical resection of metabolically active adenomas is suggested in acceptable surgical candidates.

○ **After the diagnosis of a nonfunctional adenoma, what does the recommended follow-up include?**

According to the NIH consensus statement, follow-up cross-sectional imaging should be performed 6 to 12 months following the initial study to evaluate for growth. Additionally, metabolic function should be reassessed yearly for 3 to 4 years.

○ **What percentage of nonfunctional adrenal adenomas will become functional during future follow-ups?**

Up to 20% of initially nonfunctional adrenal adenomas will become functional during follow-ups. Hypercortisolism is the most common perturbation to develop and two-thirds of these cases will be subclinical.

○ **What are the radiographic characteristics of adrenal myelolipomas?**

Well-circumscribed adrenal lesion with attenuation levels consistent with adipose tissue (–20 HU).

○ **Do calcifications in adrenal cysts suggest that these are actually malignant?**

No. Fifteen percent of adrenal cysts contain calcifications and this does not imply malignancy.

○ **What does the NIH consensus statement recommend in regard to the metabolic evaluation of adrenal incidentalomas?**

The NIH consensus statement recommends testing for excess catecholamine and cortisol production in patients presenting with adrenal incidentalomas. Testing for aldosterone excess should be considered in patients with hypertension.

○ **In a healthy individual, what is the recommended size threshold for surgical resection of adrenal incidentalomas?**

Incidental adrenal tumors >4 cm should undergo surgical resection following metabolic evaluation in otherwise healthy patients.

○ **When, if ever, is a bilateral adrenalectomy indicated?**

In patients who are surgical candidates but fail medical therapy. Also, in bilateral adrenal disease such as macronodular adrenal hyperplasia.

○ **What diagnosis should always be excluded prior to biopsy of an adrenal mass?**

Pheochromocytoma must be excluded prior to biopsy.

○ **What is the reported complication rate for percutaneous needle biopsy of the adrenal gland and what complications are most likely?**

3%. Pneumothorax and hemorrhage are most common. Pancreatitis can develop following the biopsy of left-sided lesions, especially if an anterior approach is used.

○ **What primary cancers metastasize to the adrenal gland?**

The most common metastatic lesions to the adrenal gland include melanoma and carcinoma of the breast and lung. Additionally, carcinomas of the kidney, contralateral adrenal gland, bladder, colon, esophagus, gallbladder, liver, pancreas, prostate, stomach, and uterus can metastasize the adrenal gland.

○ **In patients with previously diagnosed malignancies, what percentage of newly diagnosed adrenal tumors are metastatic?**

50%.

CHAPTER 33 Renal Physiology

Mary Ann C. Lim, MD

○ **What are the 3 major functions of the kidneys?**

1. First, the kidneys control the composition and volume of body fluids and maintain acid–base balance.

2. Second, blood is filtered in the glomerulus, forming a protein-free ultrafiltrate.

3. Third, the kidneys act as endocrine organs, producing hormones such as renin and erythropoietin (EPO), and produce active vitamin D_3.

○ **What is the nephron and what are the different segments that comprise each one?**

The kidney is composed of more than 1 million functional units called nephrons. Each nephron consists of the glomerulus contained within Bowman capsule, the proximal tubule, the loop of Henle, and the distal tubule, which ultimately drain into the collecting duct.

○ **What are the cells that comprise the glomerulus?**

The glomerulus is composed of a capillary network lined by endothelial cells, a central region of smooth muscle-like mesangial cells, which provide structural support, and an outer layer of epithelial cells called podocytes.

○ **What are the components of the glomerular filtration barrier?**

Blood in the capillary lumen is filtered through the fenestrated endothelial cells, an intervening glomerular basement membrane, and the interdigitated foot processes of the podocytes separated by slit diaphragms, producing a cell- and protein-free ultrafiltrate within the lumen of Bowman capsule.

○ **What prevents albumin from normally appearing in the urine?**

Filtration of albumin is hindered by its size, which is restricted by the filtration barrier to molecules less than 42 Å, and by its negative charge, which is repelled by sialoglycoproteins on the glomerular basement membrane.

○ **What percentage of total body weight is comprised by water and how is it distributed into different compartments?**

Total body water (TBW) comprises 60% of total body weight, of which 40% is intracellular fluid and 20% is extracellular fluid (ECF, includes plasma and interstitial fluid).

○ **Which electrolyte in the body regulates the volume of ECF?**

Sodium is the major extracellular solute; hence the retention or excretion of Na^+ by the kidneys is critical for the regulation of ECF volume. Sodium retention or increased oral intake leads to ECF volume expansion and Na^+ loss leads to ECF volume depletion.

○ **How does the kidney handle Na^+ in the setting of congestive heart failure?**

Congestive heart failure is a volume-excess state characterized by pulmonary and interstitial edema. However, the effective circulating volume in the body is decreased due to poor cardiac output and leads to low renal perfusion. This activates the renin–angiotensin system and the sympathetic nervous system, causing sodium retention; thus, further perpetuating the edema. Urine sodium levels are less than 10 mEq/dL. Sodium avidity is also seen in edematous states due to cirrhosis and nephrotic syndrome.

○ **What is the kidney's response to an increase in salt intake?**

Increased Na^+ intake leads to an increase in **ECF** volume. The renin–angiotensin system is inhibited and sympathetic tone is diminished. Atrial natriuretic peptide levels are elevated. These lead to decreased Na^+ reabsorption and increased urinary Na^+ loss or natriuresis.

○ **What is the juxtaglomerular apparatus (JGA) and what are its functions?**

The thick ascending limb of Henle loop comes into contact with the vascular pole (afferent and efferent arterioles) of its own glomerulus, forming the JGA. The JGA is important in the autoregulation of renal blood flow (RBF) and of the glomerular filtration rate (GFR). It also controls renin secretion.

○ **What are the 3 cells types that make up the JGA and which ones control renin secretion?**

Granular cells (also called juxtaglomerular cells), extraglomerular mesangial cells, and the macula densa cells. The macula densa cells of the JGA secrete renin.

○ **How does the kidney maintain a relatively constant RBF and GFR?**

The 2 mechanisms of autoregulation are the myogenic reflex and tubuloglomerular feedback. An increase in RBF will lead to vasoconstriction of the afferent arteriole caused by vascular smooth muscle contraction; thus decreasing flow. An increase in RBF will also enhance delivery of Na and Cl to the distal tubule. This is sensed by the macula densa, which will activate mechanisms that constrict the afferent arteriole.

○ **What are the effects of activation of the renin–angiotensin–aldosterone system?**

Renin stimulates angiotensin I (AI) production in the liver from angiotensinogen. Angiotensin-converting enzyme (ACE) converts AI to angiotensin II (AII). AII binds to AT_1 and AT_2 receptors, leading to systemic and efferent arteriolar vasoconstriction, increased Na^+ reabsorption by the proximal tubule, and production of aldosterone by the zona glomerulosa cells of the adrenal cortex. Aldosterone leads to Na^+ retention and K^+ loss and metabolic alkalosis as a result of H^+ secretion.

○ **What are the effects of ACE inhibitors and angiotensin receptor blockers (ARBs)?**

These drugs will decrease the glomerular filtration rate, decrease proteinuria, and lower systemic blood pressure. Hyperkalemia may result from decreased K^+ loss caused by hypoaldosteronism.

○ **How do nonsteroidal anti-inflammatory drugs (NSAIDs) affect the kidney?**

NSAIDs inhibit cyclooxygenase, an enzyme important for the synthesis of vasodilatory prostaglandin E_2 and I_2 in the kidneys. Low prostaglandin levels will lead to vasoconstriction of the afferent arteriole, hence decreasing GFR, and to Na^+ retention.

○ **What are the effects of norepinephrine and dopamine on RBF?**

Both afferent and efferent arterioles are innervated by sympathetic neurons. Norepinephrine constricts both and decreases RBF. Dopamine at low doses (up to 5 μg/kg/min when delivered exogenously) leads to vasodilation and increases RBF. At higher doses, it vasoconstricts the arterioles.

○ **How good are serum urea and creatinine levels as surrogate measures of an individual's GFR?**

Urea is reabsorbed in the kidneys and creatinine is secreted by tubules. As a consequence, urea levels underestimate the GFR, whereas creatinine levels overestimate it. Tubular secretion of creatinine increases with worsening kidney function.

○ **What factors are important to consider when using the serum creatinine levels to calculate creatinine clearance?**

Two commonly used formulas are the Cockroft-Gault and modification of diet in renal disease (MDRD) equations. The Cockroft-Gault formula takes gender, weight, and age into account. The MDRD equation has race as an added variable.

$$\textbf{Cockcroft-Gault: } C_{Cr}(\text{mL/min}) = (140 - \text{age in years}) \times (\text{weight in kg}) \\ \times 72 \times \text{serum creatinine (mg/dL)}$$

Multiply by 0.85, if female.

$$\textbf{MDRD: } \text{eGFR (mL/min/1.73m}^2) = 186 \times (S_{Cr})^{-1.154} \times (\text{age})^{-0.203} \\ \times (0.742 \text{ if female}) \times (1.210 \text{ if African American})$$

○ **Calculate the serum osmolality of a patient whose [Na] = 142 mEq/L, glucose = 180 mg/dL, and urea nitrogen = 12 mg/dL.**

$$\text{Osmolality (mOsm/kgH}_2\text{O)} = 2[\text{Na}] + \frac{\text{glucose}}{18} + \frac{\text{BUN}}{2.8} = 2(142) + \frac{180}{18} + \frac{12}{2.8} \approx 303$$

This patient has a serum osmolality of 303 mOsm/kg H_2O. The normal serum osmolality ranges between 280 and 295 mOsm/kg H_2O; hence, this person has hyperosmolal serum due to hyperglycemia.

○ **Where are osmoreceptors located and what do they control?**

Thirst is controlled by osmoreceptor cells in the anterolateral hypothalamus. A second set of osmoreceptors located in the wall of the third ventricle, which controls the secretion of antidiuretic hormone (ADH) from the supraoptic and paraventricular nuclei of the hypothalamus.

○ **What stimuli lead to ADH release?**

ADH is secreted in response to an increase in plasma osmolality more than 295 mOsm/kg H_2O as well as to volume contraction and hypotension.

○ **What are the effects of ADH on the kidney?**

ADH binds to V_2 receptors in the collecting duct, activating a G-protein that increases cyclic AMP levels. This stimulates the insertion of aquaporin-2 water channels in the apical membrane, permitting water entry into the cell. Exit of water into the interstitium occurs via aquaporin-3 and aquaporin-4 water channels in the basolateral membrane.

○ **Distinguish central from nephrogenic diabetes insipidus (DI).**

DI is characterized by polyuria. Hypernatremia and volume contraction may develop if the patient is unable to keep up with water loss. Central DI results from the absence of ADH caused by damage to neurons in the hypothalamus or posterior pituitary. In nephrogenic DI, there is resistance to circulating ADH caused by genetic defects in aquaporin-2 or V_2 receptor or to acquired conditions, such as hypercalcemia, hypokalemia, or lithium therapy.

○ **What is Fanconi syndrome?**

Proximal tubular reabsorption of amino acids, glucose, urate, phosphate, K^+, and HCO_3^- is defective in the Fanconi syndrome, leading to excess urinary excretion. These patients develop hypokalemia, hypophosphatemia, and metabolic acidosis due to type 2 or proximal renal tubular acidosis.

○ **How is Fanconi syndrome treated?**

Treatment is with replacement of fluids and lost electrolytes, usually phosphates, sodium bicarbonate, and potassium.

○ **What are the 5 classes of diuretics and where do they act to increase Na^+ excretion?**

1. Osmotic diuretics (mannitol) inhibit tubular reabsorption of Na^+ and water by the proximal tubule.
2. Carbonic anhydrase inhibitors (acetazolamide) inhibit proximal HCO_3^- reabsorption in the proximal tubule.
3. Loop diuretics (furosemide, bumetanide) inhibit the Na–K–2Cl cotransporter in the thick ascending limb of Henle loop.
4. Thiazide diuretics (hydrochlorothiazide, metolazone) inhibit the Na–Cl cotransporter in the early distal tubule.
5. Potassium-sparing diuretics include spironolactone, a competitive inhibitor of aldosterone action in the cortical collecting duct, and amiloride and triamterene, which inhibit the Na^+ channel in the collecting duct.

○ **Why does hyponatremia develop with thiazide diuretics and not with loop diuretics?**

Volume contraction stimulates ADH to increase water reabsorption. In patients taking thiazides, this increase in body water dilutes the serum Na concentration. However, loop diuretics wipe out the hypertonicity in the renal medulla; hence, increased water reabsorption is not possible.

○ **How do thiazides and loop diuretics affect urinary calcium excretion?**

Thiazides increase Ca^{2+} reabsorption in the distal tubule; thus decreasing urinary calcium excretion and potentially leading to hypercalcemia. Loop diuretics increase urinary calcium loss. Hypocalcemia does not occur, since chronic use leads to increased proximal tubule Ca^{2+} reabsorption.

○ **How does one treat hyperkalemia?**

To increase K^+ uptake by cells, administer one ampule of $NaHCO_3$, 10 to 20 U of insulin and 50 g glucose, and nebulized albuterol. Intravenous 10% calcium gluconate is administered to counteract the membrane effects of hyperkalemia. Oral or rectal Kayexalate removes K^+ via the gut. If all else fails, hemodialysis is employed.

○ **What are the manifestations of hyperaldosteronism?**

Hyperaldosteronism leads to hypertension due to Na^+ retention, hypokalemia, and metabolic alkalosis.

○ **How does one calculate the anion gap and what is the usual normal range?**

Anion gap (AG) = $Na^+ - (Cl^- + HCO_3^-)$.

The normal anion gap ranges between 8 and 12.

○ **What are the causes of an anion gap metabolic acidosis?**

Methanol, uremia, diabetic ketoacidosis, paraldehyde, isoniazid, isopropyl alcohol, lactic acidosis, ethylene glycol, ethanol, salicylates, and starvation ketosis.

○ **What are the causes of a nonanion gap metabolic acidosis?**

Hyperalimentation, acetazolamide, renal tubular acidosis, diarrhea, ureteral diversion, posthypocapnia, and spironolactone.

○ **Which of the renal tubular acidoses (RTA) is associated with stone formation?**

Type 1 (distal) RTA is associated with hypercalciuria, hyperphosphaturia, and nephrolithiasis, usually with calcium phosphate stones (although struvite stones are also seen). Several mechanisms are responsible for this: (1) hypercalciuria and hyperphosphaturia, both from bone buffering of acidosis and decreased tubular reabsorption; (2) high urine pH, thus promoting formation of calcium phosphate stones (as opposed to calcium oxalate stones); and (3) low urinary citrate from increased citrate reabsorption as a result of acidosis (citrate is a potent inhibitor of stone formation).

○ **What is type 4 renal tubular acidosis?**

Type 4 RTA refers to metabolic acidosis caused by aldosterone deficiency or resistance. Hyperkalemia develops as a result of decreased K^+ secretion and the metabolic acidosis is often mild. It is commonly seen in patients with chronic kidney disease. Fludrocortisone (Florinef) may be used to treat it, but it leads to Na^+ retention and edema.

○ **What are the metabolic abnormalities seen after prolonged vomiting?**

Loss of gastric acid (HCl) leads to metabolic alkalosis. The resulting volume contraction and Cl^- depletion increases renal HCO_3^- reabsorption. In addition, hypokalemia ensues and this further enhances HCO_3^- reabsorption.

○ **What mechanisms lead to contraction alkalosis?**

Volume contraction leads to metabolic alkalosis (increase in serum HCO_3^-) and several mechanisms are involved. The compensatory increase in Na^+ reabsorption enhances HCO_3^- reabsorption, and the increase in aldosterone stimulates urinary H^+ loss. In patients taking diuretics, hypokalemia will stimulate HCO_3^- reabsorption.

○ **What other electrolyte abnormalities are frequently seen in patients with hypomagnesemia?**

Hypomagnesemia impairs the secretion of parathyroid hormone (PTH) and leads to skeletal resistance to the action of PTH. Thus, patients may manifest positive Chvostek and Trousseau signs due to hypocalcemia. For unclear reasons, hypomagnesemia also leads to increased urinary K^+ loss; hence, hypokalemia often ensues.

○ **What are the mechanisms by which PTH increases serum calcium?**

PTH increases serum calcium by

- stimulating bone resorption by activating osteoclasts;
- increasing the synthesis of active vitamin D_3 by enhancing 25-OH cholecalciferol-1α-hydroxylase activity, thereby increasing intestinal Ca^{2+} absorption; and
- by increasing Ca^{2+} reabsorption in the distal tubule.

○ **What mechanisms lead to secondary hyperparathyroidism in chronic kidney disease?**

- Phosphate retention due to decreased urinary excretion of phosphorus.
- Decreased renal production of active vitamin D_3.
- Hypocalcemia.

○ **Why do patients with chronic kidney disease develop anemia?**

Peritubular interstitial cells in the kidney produce EPO in response to hypoxia. EPO stimulates the formation of red blood cells. In chronic renal failure, EPO levels are decreased.

○ **How does the antibiotic trimethoprim–sulfamethoxazole cause hyperkalemia?**

Trimethoprim blocks sodium channels in the distal collecting tubules, impairing sodium reabsorption, thus preventing potassium secretion and causing hyperkalemia. Trimethoprim-induced hyperkalemia is dose-dependent, usually seen in AIDS patients taking high doses of the antibiotics; however, it can also occur when trimethoprim is given in normal doses, particularly when given in the elderly.

○ **What causes pseudohyperkalemia? What can be done to measure the appropriate potassium level during these instances?**

Potassium levels are usually measured from the serum rather than the plasma. During the coagulation process, a small amount of potassium usually moves out of the white cells and platelets, resulting in a mild and insignificant increase in the potassium level in the serum (as opposed to plasma) in normal patients. In patients with leukocytosis (white cells >100,000/mL) or thrombocytosis (400,000/mL), the rise in potassium may be as high as 9 mEq/L. In these cases, it is advisable to check a plasma potassium level instead.

○ **What is the minimum dose of metformin that can cause lactic acidosis?**

It is unclear what minimum dose of metformin can lead to toxicity. Lactic acidosis usually occurs with acute overdose, but can occur in patients taking conventional doses but with the following comorbidities resulting in decreased clearance of the drug: kidney disease (serum creatinine >1.4 mg/dL in women, and >1.5 mg/dL in men), liver disease, or hemodynamic instability.

○ **What clinical conditions cause urine that is heme-positive on dipstick but show no RBCs on urine microscopy?**

Myoglobinuria and hemoglobinuria.

○ **How does fasting lead to hyperkalemia in dialysis patients?**

Insulin promotes potassium entry into the cells. The ingestion of glucose leads to endogenous insulin secretion. Fasting can lead to decreased insulin secretion and thus to hyperkalemia. In dialysis patients, this can be more pronounced. For dialysis patients who are kept NPO before surgery, the administration of glucose and insulin, or glucose alone in nondiabetic patients can help minimize this problem.

CHAPTER 34
Renovascular Hypertension

Marcus W. Balters, MD and
Jay Laurence Bloch, MD*

○ **True/False: Renal artery occlusive disease is the most common form of surgically correctable hypertension.**

True. Systemic BP elevations in these patients follow reductions in renal perfusion with activation of the renin–angiotensin system. While this tends to restore renal circulation to normal, it does so in a pathological manner producing systemic hypertension (*Greenfield's Surgery: Scientific Principles and Practice*, 2nd ed.).

○ **Renovascular hypertension is caused by hypoperfusion leading to renin release, renin converts angiotensinogen to angiotensin I, which is subsequently converted to angiotensin II by angiotensin-converting enzyme (ACE). List at least 3 physiologic effects of angiotensin II.**

1. Direct systemic vasoconstriction.

2. Stimulation of aldosterone secretion resulting in extracellular volume expansion.

3. Preferential glomerular efferent arteriolar vasoconstriction, thus maintaining glomerular filtration despite renal artery hypoperfusion.

4. Recent studies have also revealed additional mechanisms including sympathetic nervous system activation and formation of reactive oxygen species (Garovic and Textor, 2005).

○ **How does the stimulation of aldosterone by the renin–angiotension system contribute to systemic hypertension?**

Increased aldosterone levels lead to increased retention of sodium and water. This increased water retention can be compensated for if the patient has unilateral renal artery stenosis (RAS) and a normal second kidney, but the patient will still be hypertensive due to the vasoconstrictive effects of angiotension II. In patients with bilateral RAS, or patients with single kidney and RAS, they are unable to achieve the pressure diuresis required to handle the aldosterone-induced sodium and water retention so they will have volume component to their hypertension.

○ **What percentage of renovascular disease is due to atherosclerosis?**

It is estimated that 70% to 90% of renal arterial lesions are due to atherosclerosis, making it the most common form or renovascular disease resulting in hypertension. These lesions more often affect the ostium and proximal third of the renal artery. The adjacent aorta is also affected. Fibromuscular dysplasia frequently involves the distal two-thirds of the main renal artery as well as its branches (Kim et al., 2007).

---

*Dr. Bloch was contributing author from the previous edition of the work.

○ **What is the second most common type of renal artery disease resulting in hypertension and how common is it?**

Arterial fibrodysplasia (AF) accounts for up to 25% of renovascular hypertension. AF can be secondary to intimal fibroplasia (which affects children and young adults more than the elderly and makes up 5% of fibrodysplasia cases). AF can be secondary to medial fibroplasias (almost all women and makes up 85% of AF cases). AF can be secondary to perimedial dysplasia (which is also most common in women and makes up 10% of AF cases).

○ **True/False: Pulmonary edema is not a clinical feature of atherosclerotic RAS.**

False. Clinical features most suggestive of renovascular hypertension include rapid onset of hypertension after age 50 or development of hypertension in childhood, malignant hypertension or hypertension difficult to manage with 3 or more medications, sudden worsening of mild-to-moderate essential hypertension, and initial diastolic BPs >115. Additional suggestive clinical findings include peripheral vascular disease, severe retinopathy, azotemia (particularly in patients utilizing an ACE inhibitor or angiotensin II receptor antagonist), hypokalemia, renal atrophy, systolic and diastolic upper abdominal bruits, and pulmonary edema.

○ **True/False: The absence of an abdominal bruit essentially rules out RAS.**

False. In patients with angiographically proven RAS, abdominal bruits were audible with a sensitivity range of 39% to 63% and a specificity range of 90% to 99%. Thus, the presence of an abdominal bruit is highly indicative of RAS, but the absence of an abdominal bruit should not rule it out (Kim et al., 2007).

○ **What percentage reduction in renal artery cross-sectional area induces a pressure gradient sufficient to cause increased renin release from the kidneys?**

80%. Renin production and release from the kidneys is a complex process wherein renal baroreceptors, acting as stretch receptors, affect the release of renin from juxtaglomerular cells.

○ **Which 2 classes of antihypertensive medications precisely manage renovascular hypertension?**

ACE inhibitors and angiotensin II receptor antagonists. Most renovascular hypertension can be managed with these and other antihypertensive medications introduced over the past 2 decades. Previously, less than half of the patients with renovascular hypertension were adequately controlled by medications available at that time. It is arguable whether individuals with well-controlled blood pressure benefit much from revascularization (Garovic and Textor, 2005).

○ **True/False: Renal failure is a side effect of ACE inhibitors.**

True. Insofar as ACE inhibitors cause dilation of the glomerular efferent arteriole, there may be a decrease in glomerular filtration rate (GFR). In unilateral RAS, the change in total GFR is usually minimal due to compensatory increase in GFR by the contralateral kidney. However, vascular stenoses that involve both kidneys or a solitary kidney are more likely to be affected by ACE inhibitors resulting in acute renal failure. In 1 study, this occurred in 8 of 136 patients (6%) within 1 month of therapy. Discontinuation of the ACE inhibitor resulted in reversal of the acute renal failure in all, but 1 patient (Garovic and Textor, 2005).

○ **True/False: Endovascular stent placement is more often utilized in the elderly with at least grade 3 chronic kidney disease (QFR 45.5 mL/min/1.73 m^2) versus younger patients or those with lesser degrees of chronic kidney disease.**

True. In 1 study of 258 patients undergoing endovascular stenting, the mean age was 71 years and 85% of these patients had at least grade 3 chronic renal disease. These patients typically have additional cardiovascular problems and require additional risk-intervention strategies (reduction of cholesterol, discontinuation of smoking, and intensive hypertension control with medications) both before and after revascularization (Garovic and Textor, 2005).

○ **True/False: Restenosis is common following endovascular stenting of the renal arteries when compared with renal artery angioplasty alone.**

False. Endovascular stents have greatly improved the patency rates compared with angioplasty alone. Current studies report restenosis following endovascular stent placement as occurring in the range of 12% to 14% (complication rate 7%–9%). Endovascular procedures to restore patency to the renal arteries have increased quite remarkably since the mid-1990s. One reason maybe the number of "drive-by" renal angiographies performed during another catheterization, especially coronary angiography (Garovic and Textor, 2005).

○ **True/False: Randomized controlled prospective studies have clearly demonstrated the benefit of endovascular stents over medication alone.**

False. Currently, there is a lack of consensus regarding intervention with endovascular stents. Many nephrologists advocate the use of medication only, whereas interventional subspecialties, especially cardiologists, argue the potential benefits of stent placement. The cardiovascular outcomes in renal atherosclerotic lesions (CORAL) trial is an ongoing NIH-multicenter clinical trial whose enrollment ended in 2010. This trial, like several others before it, including the DRASTIC and the STAR trials, looks at 2 major groups, one treated by medication only, the other with medications and an endovascular stent. Hopefully, through such prospective trials, the true value of endovascular stenting will be determined (Garovic and Textor, 2005).

○ **How often is a clear abdominal bruit heard in RAS?**

Forty-six percent of patients.

○ **When does renovascular disease secondary to atherosclerosis most commonly present?**

Sixth decade of life. Men are affected twice as often as women. The lesions tend to affect the proximal one-third of the vessel (concentric or eccentric stenosis). 80% of the time, these lesions occur as continuation of diffuse atherosclerosis of the aorta. These lesions are bilateral in 75% of patients in whom they occur. When the lesion is unilateral there is no predilection toward right or left side.

○ **Do nonsteroidal anti-inflammatory drugs (NSAIDs) have any effect on plasma renin levels?**

Yes, they cause a decrease.

○ **True/False: Renal accessory arteries are better visualized with Gadolinium-DTPA–enhanced magnetic resonance angiography compared to nonenhanced images.**

True. Contrast images allow better visualization of accessory renal arteries. Studies are highly accurate in detecting RAS >50%, with a sensitivity of 93% and specificity of 98%. MRA is particularly useful in patients with impaired renal function who are at increased risk for contrast-induced nephropathy though nephropathy can occur with MRA-associated contrast materials. Additionally, it is important to remember that gadolinium, in approximately 5% of patients with renal insufficiency, has been associated with rare but serious conditions known as nephrogenic systemic fibrosis (NSF) and nephrogenic fibrosing dermopathy (NFD).

○ **Given a group of hypertensive patients on at least 3 antihypertensive medications with a diastolic BP ≥95 mm Hg, what is the prevalence of RAS?**

It is 25%. This may be a simple but useful set of criteria to select patients for diagnostic studies. Renovascular hypertension accounts for approximately 5% of all hypertensive patients, yet it is the most common cause of secondary hypertension. Not only can RAS cause hypertension, but it may also lead to progressive renal failure. Modern, less invasive diagnostic techniques, combined with percutaneous transluminal angioplasty and renal stenting, have stimulated a renewed interest in this subject.

○ **True/False: Ischemic nephropathy accounts for >5% of patients with ESRD on dialysis.**

True. Seventeen percent of patients are dialysis-dependent because of ischemic nephropathy. Significant RAS has been demonstrated in >50% of patients with a creatinine clearance <50 mL/min. Particularly at risk are patients with DM, hypertension, and generalized atherosclerosis. Median survival of patients on dialysis due to ischemic nephropathy is 27 months versus 56 months for other etiologies.

○ **True/False: Fibromuscular dysplasia rarely progresses to occlusion in cases of renal artery involvement.**

True. Nonatheromatous causes of RAS do not commonly progress to occlusion; conversely, 15% of atherosclerotic RAS cases progress to occlusion. The time to occlusion is brief (13 months) in patients presenting with >75% occlusion.

○ **True/False: Atherosclerotic RAS progresses from less than 60% to greater than 60% within 1 year in 30% of patients.**

True. The lumen narrows most rapidly from <60% to >60%; 44% of patients progress by 2 years and 48% by 3 years. The progression occurs bilaterally in 20% to 50% of these patients.

○ **In patients undergoing cardiac catheterization, risk factors for RAS include each of the following except which one: extent of CAD, female sex, smoking, or hypertension?**

Hypertension. Both multivariate and univariate analysis of patients undergoing cardiac catheterization failed to identify hypertension as a risk factor for significant RAS. Other risk factors that were identified include increasing age, CHF, PVD, and creatinine >1.06 mg/dL.

○ **True/False: Renal angiography is the gold standard for diagnosing RAS.**

True. Although angiography remains the gold standard for identifying RAS, risks include nephrotoxicity and possible complications of arterial puncture (hematoma, cholesterol embolization). Digital subtraction angiography may preclude the need for arterial puncture, but in so doing, requires a larger dose of contrast. CO_2 angiography obviates the need for iodinated contrast but is not readily available and is more operator-dependent. Lastly, conventional angiography may miss stenoses en face, requiring oblique imaging to project stenoses (as opposed to CT or MRI).

○ **True/False: A decrease in renal length of >1 cm is seen in most patients with RAS >60%.**

False. Renal dimensional changes of this magnitude are seen in only 26% of such patients. More important is Doppler interrogation of the extrarenal and intrarenal (segmental, interlobar) arteries. Extrarenal Doppler parameters include peak systolic velocity >200 cm/s, renal aortic ratio >3.3 to 3.5, and end-diastolic velocity >150 cm/s. Intrarenal Doppler parameters include a resistive index <0.45 to 0.59, difference of resistive index with contralateral kidney >0.05 to 0.08, pulsatility index <0.93 (difference of PI with contralateral kidney >0.14), acceleration time >60 to 120 milliseconds, and acceleration >7.4 m/s^2.

○ **True/False: Doppler renal sonography is highly accurate in screening for RAS.**

True. Five independent studies evaluating 597 patients demonstrated a sensitivity of 89% to 93% and a specificity of 92% to 98%. Positive predictive values of 88% to 98% and negative predictive values of 92% to 98% were reported. The lumbar approach to evaluating the intraparenchymal arteries is unaffected by the number of accessory arteries, bowel gas, or obesity. DRS is operator-dependent and may not yield accurate results regarding multiple renal arteries or branch occlusions. A galactose microbubble-based agent may enhance the Doppler signal but is generally not necessary.

○ **True/False: Spiral CT angiography requires contrast because predictions regarding RAS cannot be made by evaluating renal arterial calcifications.**

True. Seventeen percent of patients with no calcification, 30% of patients with <3 mm calcification, and 44% of patients with >3 mm calcification had ≥75% RAS. However, the data do not preclude the use of contrast for accurate diagnostic information. Contrast-enhanced CT studies may visualize vessels as small as 1 mm.

○ **True/False: Captopril challenge tests and renal vein sampling are poor screening tools for ischemic nephropathy.**

True. These tests are most useful in differentiating renovascular hypertension from other etiologies. Ischemic nephropathy is often secondary to atherosclerotic RAS. The tests are less sensitive in the situation of bilateral disease and renal compromise.

○ **True/False: Surgical revascularization for ischemic nephropathy virtually always results in substantial improvement in serum creatinine.**

False. Fifty-five percent of patients improved (ie, 20% decrease in serum creatinine), 32% of patients revascularized remained stable,14% of patients worsened, and 6% died perioperatively (accumulated data from 8 studies involving 352 patients from 1983 to 1992).

○ **List 3 preoperative criteria indicative of renal improvement following revascularization for total occlusion of the renal artery.**

Any of the following—collateral vessels with nephrogram on angiography, swift preop deterioration of GFR, patent vessels distal-to-proximal occlusion (back bleeding during revascularization surgery), viable nephrons on biopsy, renal length >9 cm, lateralization of renin secretion, and differential urinary concentration on split-function tests. The criteria need to be used together as a guide as individual parameters lack predictive value.

○ **True/False: 30% of renovascular operations for hypertension and renal insufficiency eventually fail.**

False. The failure rate is closer to 10%. Postoperative management following revascularization should include routine evaluation of blood pressure, serum creatinine, and periodic noninvasive radiologic assessment of renal blood flow (eg, Doppler renal sonogram, nuclear renography, and MRA). Approximately 10% of patients following revascularization will demonstrate recurrent hypertension or a diminution of renal function. This may be caused by restenosis of the operated vessel, stenosis of the contralateral renal artery, or progressive nephrosclerosis.

○ **Is PTA more successful with atherosclerotic or fibromuscular disease?**

Results are better with fibromuscular disease.

○ **What is eplerenone?**

It is a selective aldosterone inhibitor used for an antihypertensive. ACE inhibitor medications are still the preferred agents for medical treatment of RAS hypertension.

○ **What about angiotensin receptor blockers?**

They appear to be equally effective as ACE inhibitors.

○ **Serum creatinine may increase after therapy with ACE inhibitors. How much of an increase is acceptable?**

Usually up to about 35% above baseline.

○   **List the options for open surgical revascularization in patients with renovascular hypertension.**

- Aortorenal bypass (infrarenal, end-to-side or end-to-end, using vein or graft)
- Aortorenal artery thromboembolectomy
- Renal artery reimplantation
- Splenorenal bypass
- Hepatorenal bypass
- Aortorenal (supraceliac)
- Iliorenal bypass

○   **True/False: Splenorenal bypass is an ideal operation following a failed left aortorenal bypass.**

True. Although this is dependent on the author one reads. The success of the operation depends on the celiac trunk, which is visualized on the lateral aortic film of conventional angiogram, or by less invasive means. It is important to recognize that up to 40% or 50% of patients will exhibit celiac axis stenosis in this patient population. The splenic artery is divided proximally to avoid distal splenic atherosclerosis, and anastomosed end-to-end to the left renal artery. The spleen will remain viable, as collateral blood flow is derived from the gastroepiploic and short gastric vessels.

○   **True/False: Hepatorenal bypass is an ideal operation following a failed right aortorenal bypass.**

True. Patency of the celiac axis needs to be ascertained preoperatively for the same reason noted previously. A saphenous vein graft is interpositioned between the common hepatic artery (where it divides into the main hepatic artery and gastroduodenal artery, thus forming a trifurcation) and the renal artery. The proximal anastomosis is performed end-to-side and the hepatic artery is not divided because of ischemic risk to the gallbladder (ischemic risk to the liver is minimal due to portal venous circulation). An end-to-end anastomosis is performed to the kidney to reduce turbulent flow.

○   **True/False: Iliorenal bypass or supraceliac aortorenal bypass are the operations of choice following a failed aortorenal bypass.**

False. If the celiac axis is involved by advanced disease or is inaccessible due to prior surgery, the operations above are indicated. Iliorenal bypass is limited by possible progressive disease involving the iliac vessel and requires a long graft (saphenous vein or synthetic) directed cephalad. Supraceliac aortorenal bypass often requires a thoracic as well as an abdominal incision and is much more difficult to tunnel to the right renal artery.

○   **True/False: Renovascular surgery patients are commonly hypertensive in the postoperative period.**

True. In the immediate postoperative period, these patients are hypertensive due to hypervolemia, hypothermic vasoconstriction, or pain despite a patent arterial anastomosis. Management is with nitroprusside infusion to maintain the diastolic BP at approximately 90 mm Hg to insure adequate renal perfusion (avoiding graft thrombosis) yet, not so high to prevent anastomotic hemorrhage.

○   **True/False: Risk of hemorrhage following reoperation for renovascular disease is no different than that following the primary operation.**

False. Because of dense retroperitoneal fibrosis from the primary operation, hemorrhage is more likely to occur, as embedded lumbar vessels are more difficult to secure and the anastomosis itself is more arduous. Other likely sources of hemorrhage include the ipsilateral adrenal and an untied branch of a saphenous vein graft. Extra-aortic techniques during secondary operations avoid the potential complication of aortic hemorrhage requiring aortic clamping.

○ **Renal artery thrombosis postoperatively following renovascular surgery occurs because of what problems? (List at least 2, try to get all 4.)**

Hypotension, hypovolemia, arteriolar nephrosclerosis, or a hypercoagulable state may result in thrombosis. Kidneys with severe nephrosclerosis are best managed by nephrectomy. Technical problems are the most likely cause of postoperative thrombosis (mishandling, kinking, distortion, or angulation of the bypass graft, or atheromatous emboli).

○ **True/False: Secondary revascularization results in cure or improvement in BP in 97% of patients.**

True. Approximately 70% of patients will have normalization of their BP following surgical revascularization. Approximately 25% more have reduced hypertension that can be normalized with medical management, leaving less than 5% refractory to surgical revascularization. The operative mortality in 1 series was 1.4% with the incidence of nephrectomy being approximately 40% at reoperation. Nephrectomy will control BP as well as revascularization, and is indicated for the nonsalvageable kidney producing renin.

○ **True/False: Renal arterial bypass grafting (RABG) is more likely to normalize serum creatinine in patients with renovascular hypertension versus percutaneous transluminal renal angioplasty (PTRA) or percutaneous transluminal stent placement (PTSP).**

False. Actually all 3 failed to substantially alter creatinine in a study involving 130 patients. In comparing these modalities, the results are as follows:

	PTRA	PTSP	RABG
Technical success	91%	98%	92%
Complications	13%	16%	38%
Decrease in mean arterial BP at: 12 months following procedure	21 mm Hg	20 mm Hg	20 mm Hg
Initial treatment costs	$1400	$2600	$15,000

○ **True/False: PTSP is highly successful in preventing further episodes of congestive heart failure and pulmonary edema in patients with bilateral RAS or stenosis in a solitary functioning kidney.**

True. In 1 study, 23 of 56 patients (41%) had a history of CHF with associated pulmonary edema prior to PTSP of one or both arteries. Following the procedure, 77% of these patients remained free of congestive heart failure and pulmonary edema (mean follow-up, 18.4 months). In contradistinction, only 4 of 34 subjects (12%) with unilateral stenosis and a normal contralateral kidney had a history of congestive heart failure or pulmonary edema, and only 1 of 3 (33%) subjects was free of CHF and pulmonary edema following PTSP.

○ **True/False: PTRA for ostial atherosclerotic RAS yields results similar to PTSP.**

False.

	PTRA (%)	PTSP (%)
Primary success rate (<50% residual stenosis)	57	88
Secondary patency rate at 6 months	29	75
Restenosis following initial success	48	14

Secondary stent placement following early or late failure of PTRA resulted in success rates similar to patients undergoing primary PTSP. Despite the potential cost savings in stents using PTRA, the need for reintervention is greater. Therefore, PTSP is currently a better approach for ostial atherosclerotic stenosis.

○ **True/False: Renovascular hypertension is rare in children.**

False. It is relatively common as a cause of pediatric hypertension. Hypertension in children is most often secondary hypertension (70%–80%). The other common surgically correctable cause of secondary hypertension in children is coarctation of the aorta.

○ **What is the "nutcracker syndrome," where does it occur, how does it cause gross hematuria, how is it treated, and what other medical problem is associated with it?**

Nutcracker syndrome describes the uncommon situation where the left renal vein is compressed between the aorta and the superior mesenteric artery. This results in left renal venous hypertension, which over time leads to the development of collateral veins and varices. If any of these thin-walled varices should rupture into the collecting system, left-sided hematuria results. Usual symptoms are hypertension that may be uncontrollable, left-sided hematuria, and sometimes flank pain. Standard testing for hematuria such as urinary red blood cell morphology, IVP, cystoscopy, and even ureteroscopy are usually unrewarding except for identification of left-sided hematuria. If suspected, magnetic resonance angiography or CT scans looking for compression of the left renal vein are useful. Treatment with angioplasty and stenting is usually successful. Other treatment options include vein graft interposition, nephropexy, and renal autotransplantation.

○ **What type of trauma patients are more likely to develop renovascular hypertension?**

Post-trauma hypertension is not unusual. Occult renal injuries are one of many possible mechanisms. Patients with renal pedicle injuries have higher rates of renovascular hypertension than those with parenchymal injuries. Trauma patients with operative management of their renal injuries have a lower rate of hypertension compared to those with nonoperative management (17%–38%) (*Cameron's Current Surgical Therapy*, 8th ed.).

CHAPTER 35 Renal Transplantation

Michael C. Morris, MD, FACS

○ **Describe kidney stones following renal transplantation.**

Kidney stones following a renal transplant are an unusual complication. Stones may originate in the transplanted kidney following transplant secondary to any of the primary etiologies of kidney stones formation. Stones may also be transplanted with the stones having formed in the donor. Primary risk factors in the recipient include tertiary hyperparathyroidism, hypercalciuria, recurrent urinary tract infections, and urinary tract obstruction. Clinical presentation includes obstructive uropathy, hematuria, urinary tract infection, and allograft dysfunction. Renal colic is an unusual symptom in this population. Treatment can include observation and spontaneous passage of the stone, percutaneous or open nephrolithotomy, lithotripsy, cystoscopy, and ureteroscopy.

○ **What is a panel reactive antibody (PRA) and how are they usually formed?**

PRA is a panel of common human leukocyte antigen (HLA) antigens against which potential kidney transplant recipients are tested. The degree of reactivity is a reflection of the presence of preformed antibodies in the recipient. Patients develop HLA antibodies through 3 primary processes: (1) exposure through previous transplant, (2) pregnancy, and (3) blood transfusions. A high degree of reactivity against the panel suggests that there will be difficulty in identifying a cross-match negative donor.

○ **How can HLA antibodies be removed or diminished?**

HLA antibodies can be removed or depleted by the process of plasmapheresis and intravenous immunoglobulin (IVIG) therapy and/or rituximab therapy. A combination appears to be most effective. The results are best with the blood group antibodies. The removal of HLA antibodies is more difficult and the results in this group suggest a higher risk of both cellular and antibody-mediated rejection and poorer long-term survival.

○ **Describe donor exchange programs.**

The demand for organs for kidney transplantation has resulted in various exchange scenarios among incompatible donor recipient pairs. One such adaption has been the development of donor exchange programs. This program allows recipients with incompatible donors to exchange kidneys with other recipient donor pairs with similar incompatibilities. This exchange, which is frequently based on the blood group or cross-match incompatibilities, has increased the rate of transplant among these individuals. As more programs and patients enter into these exchanges the probability of finding compatible pairs increases. Paired donor exchange opportunities are currently being nationalized in the hopes of optimizing both transplant rates and the advantages of living donation.

○ **What is the average waiting time for a deceased donor transplant and what is the single most significant factor in determining how quickly a kidney may be available?**

Depending on the geographical region and blood type, the average waiting time for cadaveric transplant can vary from 2 to 6 years. Blood type "O" recipients tend to wait the longest. Blood type "AB" recipients tend to have the shortest waiting time. Other issues such as antibodies, age, and obesity can further increase waiting. Living donation avoids many of these issues. Recipients of living donor transplants have the shortest waiting time.

○ **What are the leading causes of end-stage renal disease in the United States?**

Diabetes is the single most common cause of renal failure. Other etiologies include hypertension, chronic glomerulonephritis, polycystic kidney disease, systemic lupus, interstitial nephritis, and various autoimmune nephritis syndromes.

○ **What is acute rejection, how is it diagnosed, and what is the current incidence?**

Acute cellular rejection is a T-cell–mediated rejection process and can occur at any time post-transplant. The diagnosis of acute rejection is most often made based on the findings of a rising serum creatinine and confirmed by transplant biopsy. Biopsies done for other reasons may also demonstrate rejection as well. Current maintenance immunosuppression is directed at the cellular rejection process. The incidence of acute rejection is currently 10% to 15%.

○ **What is the Banff system?**

The Banff system is a histologic standardized grading system for transplant rejection.

○ **What are the indications for native kidney nephrectomy?**

The indications for native kidney nephrectomy prior to transplant or at the time of transplant are: (1) the presence of large symptomatic polycystic kidneys, (2) severe reflux associated with pyelonephritis, (3) severe uncontrollable hypertension, and (4) uncontrolled proteinuria.

○ **What causes hyperacute rejection and how can it be prevented?**

The presence of preformed antibodies at the time of transplant can result in an accelerated rapid antibody-mediated rejection. This process is B-cell mediated. Frequently, antibodies can be removed prior to transplantation via a process that involves plasmapheresis, IVIG, and rituximab either alone or in combination. Currently, antibody reduction among the ABO blood group discrepancies prior to transplant appears to be the most effective antidonor antibody group to treat. Acquired antibodies against the HLA antigen groups are much harder to reduce and tend to have lower graft survival rates.

○ **What is induction immunosuppression?**

Induction agents are medications administered in the early or immediate postoperative period. These agents are potent immunosuppressants and are used to maximally suppress the immune response at the time of initial antigen exposure. Their effects can be long-lasting. These agents include both polyclonal antithymocyte and monoclonal (anti-IL-2 and anti-CD 52) agents. Induction therapy can be used in all patients or selectively. Induction therapy has increasingly been used in patients considered for maintenance immunosuppressive minimization. The use of induction therapy can be associated with a higher incidence of post-transplant infection and malignancy. These concerns weigh into the decision of when and how best to use these agents.

○ **What is maintenance immunosuppression?**

Chronic maintenance immunosuppressive medication is used to prevent acute rejection. Various combinations are used, which most commonly include a calcineurin inhibitor, antimetabolites, and steroids. Other agents frequently used include m-TOR inhibitors and most recently the costimulator blocking agent. The use of these medications in various combinations allows minimization of potential side effects. The variety of combinations used reflects an overall dissatisfaction with the trade-off between immunosuppression and immunosuppressive complications.

○ **What medications are used to treat acute cellular rejection?**

Acute cellular rejection is most commonly treated with high-dose steroids or antilymphocytic agents. Diagnosis of acute cellular rejection is made by finding an elevated creatinine and/or a suggestive biopsy. Treatment is generally successful especially when therapy is initiated early in the process. The success of treatment may best be determined by the established postrejection creatinine. The ability to return to baseline portends a better prognosis than a failure to do so.

○ **What is the overall graft survival for deceased and living donor transplants?**

Many variables affect long-term graft survival. Better immunosuppression has improved early graft survival but has had minimal impact on long-term graft survival. Cadaveric kidney survival is also impacted by the type of organ utilized. A standard criteria donor (a donor between the ages of 10 and 50) versus donors at higher risk whose kidneys tend to show poorer long- and short-term graft function. These include expanded criteria donors (over the age of 50 years and other defined criteria), deceased cardiac donors, and prolonged ischemic times. Living donors tend to have much better results than cadaveric donors. Deceased donor kidneys have a 1-year graft survival of approximately 87%, a 3-year graft survival of approximately 76%, and a graft half-life of nearly 8 years. Living donors have a 1-year graft survival of 93%, a 3-year graft survival of approximately 86%, and a half-life of nearly 18 years.

○ **What is an expanded criteria donor (ECD) kidney?**

ECD kidneys refer to cadaveric kidney donors greater than 60 years of age or between the ages of 50 and 59 years and meet one of the following criteria: (1) hypertension, (2) creatinine greater than 1.5, or (3) death from a cerebral vascular accident. These kidneys are believed to have a higher risk of delayed function (acute tubular necrosis, ATN) and a higher risk of primary nonfunctioning. The half-life of these organs is believed to be shorter than standard criteria donor organs. Careful recipient selection is required and utilization of these organs in younger patients is generally avoided.

○ **What is a deceased cardiac donor (DCD)?**

A DCD organ donor is a donor who most frequently has experienced a devastating, irreversible neurologic injury, but fails to progress to brain death. The decision is made to withdraw life-support and after cardiac activity terminates the potential donor is pronounced dead. Donation can only proceed after pronouncement. Careful criteria for acceptability are applied as extensive ischemic injury can occur. There is a higher risk of delayed primary function and of primary nonfunction. As many of these donors are otherwise young and healthy, they are potential organs for younger carefully selected recipients. DCD organs have had a significant positive impact on the donor pool.

○ **What is a high-risk organ donor?**

The social and medical history, lifestyle choice, or social and medical risk factors of a donor increase the probability of disease transmission. Of particular concern is the transmission of hepatitis B, hepatitis C, and HIV. Potential donors are carefully screened for these diseases and all testing is negative, but there is a window period between exposure and conversion that must be considered. The degree of risk varies with the nature of the behavior. High-risk donors are defined using the same center for disease control (CDC) criteria as for blood donors. Risk of disease transmission must be taken into careful consideration. Full informed consent is required.

○ **What is a post-transplant lymphocele and how is it treated?**

A lymphocele is the most common perinephric fluid collection found in the post-transplant period. The etiology of lymphatic fluid can be either retroperitoneal recipient lymphatics or lymphatics associated with the transplant kidney itself. The incidence of post-transplant lymphocele is believed to be approximately 15%. The incidence has increased with modern immunosuppression. Most lymphoceles are asymptomatic and require no treatment. Symptoms when they occur typically are compressive in nature and are associated with allograft dysfunction and/or leg edema. The differential diagnosis includes urinoma and abscess. The diagnosis is made by ultrasound and percutaneous drainage and/or aspiration. Treatment with percutaneous drainage is successful approximately half the time. Intra-abdominal marsupialization, which can be performed either as an open or as a laparoscopic procedure, is successful more than 80% of the time.

○ **What is the significance of ATN in the transplant setting?**

Acute tubular necrosis (ATN) is an ischemic injury to the kidney. This injury is often associated with both warm and cold ischemic times, donor age, cause of death, and an unfavorable recipient environment. ATN of the living donor kidney is relatively uncommon and is usually associated with surgical factors. ATN occurs in 20% to 40% of cadaveric donors. Clinically, ATN is defined as the need for dialysis in the early postoperative period. The more severe the ATN, the greater the risk of compromised long-term allograft function. The differential diagnosis includes vascular compromise, perinephric collections, hydronephrosis, acute cellular and antibody-mediated rejection, and drug toxicities. Diagnosis is supported by ultrasound findings and confirmed by biopsy. Treatment is supportive.

○ **What is post-transplant lymphoproliferative disease (PTLD)**

PTLD is one of the most common post-transplant malignancies. Most cases of early PTLD are the result of infection with the Epstein–Barr virus (EBV). Newly acquired or reactivated EBV infection can induce B-cell proliferation in the immunocompromised host. EBV-induced PTLD ranges from a polyclonal B-cell proliferation to a full-blown malignant monoclonal transformation. Diagnosis is frequently suggested by the findings of clinically significant adenopathy in the face of new or rising EBV titers and confirmed by biopsy. The initial step in the treatment of PTLD is the reduction or termination of immunosuppression. More aggressive disease may require the use of chemotherapy as well as immunosuppression withdrawal. CNS and bone marrow involvement suggest a poor prognosis.

EBV naïve patients receiving EBV positive donor organs are at greatest risk, particularly if exposed to lytic immunosuppressive agents.

○ **Describe the management of pregnancy in the kidney transplant patient. Which immunosuppressive agents are preferred or particularly toxic during pregnancy?**

Uremic infertility is rapidly corrected by successful renal transplantation, and pregnancy becomes a significant possibility. Patients are advised to take precautions to avoid pregnancy until allograft function has stabilized and immunosuppressive medications can be adjusted and overall risk reduced. If pregnancy occurs, careful management by a high-risk obstetrician/perinatologist is advisable. Pregnancy post-renal transplant, if carefully planned and monitored, is often a successful and rewarding experience. Immunotherapy may need to be adjusted to avoid agents with significant teratogenic potential. Immunosuppressants such as Mycophenolate mofetil (MMF) and the m-TOR inhibitors have been shown to be particularly toxic to fetal development. Calcineurin inhibitor agents have been used with minimal risk. Azathioprine and steroids may in fact be the safest options.

○ **How do calcineurin inhibitors work?**

Cyclosporine and tacrolimus are calcineurin inhibitors frequently used in maintenance immunosuppression. These agents bind to a class of immunophilins in the cytosol of T helper cells. This complex binds to calcineurin. This immunophilins–calcineurin complex blocks the signaling pathway, which results in upregulation of IL-2 cell surface receptors. By blocking T-cell proliferation, these medications exert their primary immunosuppressive effect. Various formulations of these medications currently exist. Drug monitoring is critical to the safe and effective management of these medications. Toxicities of this class of medications include lowering of the seizure threshold, nephrotoxicity, hyperkalemia, hyperglycemia, and dermatologic changes. Multiple drug interactions are also possible.

○ **How does MMF work?**

MMF is the prodrug of mycophenolic acid. As an antimetabolite, the drug binds to inosine monophosphate dehydrogenase preventing proliferation of T and B cells. Drug level monitoring is possible, but appears to be of limited benefit. Primary side effects of this medication include gastrointestinal (GI) disturbances (nausea, vomiting, and diarrhea), myelosuppression, and leukopenia. Several birth defects have been associated with the use of MMF during pregnancy.

○ **How do m-TOR inhibitors work?**

Currently, there are 2 primary formulations of this medication: sirolimus and everolimus. This drug acts in the cytosol of T cells by binding with a specific class of immunophilins and inhibits cellular proliferation signals. These agents have less nephrotoxicity compared to the calcineurin inhibitors and may have antitumor properties. Toxicities are often significant and include hyperlipidemia, pneumonitis, proteinurea, peripheral edema, leukopenia, mouth ulcers, and poor wound healing. Drug level monitoring is helpful, and these medications are often used in conjunction with the calcineurin inhibitors. Fear of complications and a lack of superior long-term allograft outcomes have limited the general use of this class of medications. This medication class is most often used selectively. It is often recommended that m-TOR inhibitors be stopped prior to major surgical intervention because of their negative impact on wound healing.

○   **Describe the failed renal allograft.**

The best management of the failed renal allograft has not been defined. Concerns regarding the potential complications of a surgical procedure, the risk of ongoing immunosuppression, the risk of chronic ongoing inflammatory response, and the risk of developing HLA antibodies all weigh into the clinical decision-making process. Currently many centers use a selective approach with nephrectomy reserved for patients with symptomatic graft failure and graft loss due to early immunologic or technical graft issues. Decisions regarding withdrawal of immunosuppression in failed allografts that remain in place vary from center to center. Some choose to maintain a low level of reduced immunosuppressive medications. Some will taper all immunosuppressive medications. Following nephrectomy, immunosuppressive therapy can be stopped.

○   **What is the pretransplant management of hyperoxaluria and renal failure?**

Primary oxalosis (Type 1 and 2) results from a hepatic enzymatic defect, which causes increased serum oxalate levels and the deposition of calcium oxalate in the tissues. The enzymatic defect is transmitted as an autosomal recessive trait. Secondary oxalosis is the result of other disease processes and does not have a genetic component. In secondary oxalosis treatment of the underlying process is indicated. The deposition of calcium oxalate level occurs in all tissues and can lead to renal failure. The treatment of hyperoxaluria depends on the underlying etiology. In renal failure, intensive dialysis therapy can decrease a patient's oxalate load to a level at which tissue deposition does not occur—less than 50 mg/mL. Patients with primary oxalosis are best managed with early combined or staged liver–kidney transplant.

○   **What are the complications of bladder drainage of pancreatic exocrine secretions in kidney–pancreas transplantations?**

There are many technical variations for pancreas transplantation. The drainage of pancreatic exocrine secretions by the anastomosis of the duodenal segment of the allograft to the bladder was a major technical advancement in the clinical evolution of the procedure. Nowadays this anastomosis is most frequently replaced by an enteric one. This change was a result of the frequent complications associated with bladder drainage. These complications are: (1) metabolic acidosis secondary to the significant loss of sodium bicarbonate and fluid comprising pancreatic exocrine juices, (2) graft pancreatitis associated with a neurogenic bladder and reflux of bladder contents into the transplanted duodenal segment, (3) frequent urinary tract infections associated with an alkaline urine and a neurogenic bladder, and (4) cystitis/urethritis associated with mucosal exposure to the activated pancreatic enzymes. The severity of symptoms dictated the need for conversion to an enteric drainage and could be required in 15% to 20% of cases.

○   **Describe renal transplantation in the face of a dysfunctional bladder.**

A significant number of patients present for renal transplantation with a history of poor bladder emptying, frequent urinary tract infections (UTIs), incontinence, or other bladder abnormalities. In the face of such a history a thorough urologic evaluation is required. Preoperative definition and preparation for the management of these problems can have a significant impact on the success of the transplant.

○ **Describe the management of renal artery stenosis.**

Renal artery stenosis is one of the more common vascular complications of renal transplantation. Lesions may be asymptomatic or may present with hypertension, fluid retention, worsening renal function, or congestive heart failure. An abdominal bruit over the allograft may or may not be present. Pathogenic processes involved include immunologic, infectious, and/or progressive atherosclerotic disease. The diagnosis is frequently made by the findings of elevated systolic velocities on duplex renal ultrasound and can be confirmed by either MRA or angiography. The primary therapy for significant disease is percutaneous transluminal angioplasty (PTA). Surgical correction is complex and generally reserved for cases not amendable to PTA.

○ **10 days after transplant a patient develops drainage from the wound. An ultrasound demonstrates hydronephrosis and a perinephric collection. Drainage of the collection demonstrates sterile fluid with a fluid creatinine of 38 mg/dL. A nephrostomy is performed and demonstrates a leak at the ureteroneocystostomy. How should this be treated?**

Currently the instance of ureteral complications post-renal transplant is approximately 2%. Ureteral obstruction/stricture is the most common post-transplant ureteral complication and urine leak the least common. Most urine leaks occur at the ureteroneocystostomy and are technical in nature. Factors such as ischemia and urinary retention can play a significant role. Small urine leaks can often be managed by placement of a Foley catheter with or without nephrostomy and stenting. Large leaks may best be dealt with direct surgical repair, frequently involving revision of the ureteroneocystostomy, pyeloureterostomy, or pylocystostomy. Revisions and repairs are most commonly done over a stent. Routine stenting at the time of transplant remains a subject of debate. In the above case, a ureteral stent was positioned and a Foley catheter was placed. A nephrostogram 6 weeks later confirms no further leak or stricture.

○ **What are the indications for native nephrectomy?**

The indications for nephrectomy prior to renal transplant include (1) chronic infections, (2) heavy proteinuria, (3) intractable hypertension, and (4) symptomatic polycystic kidney disease. Native nephrectomy is infrequently required and can be performed prior to or at the time of transplant.

○ **Describe chronic allograft nephropathy (CAN).**

CAN is a histologic diagnosis of varying severity with findings of interstitial fibrosis and tubular atrophy. Patients may be asymptomatic or have evidence of progressive deterioration of allograft function. Multiple etiologies have been associated with CAN and include chronic ongoing immunologic injury either of a cellular or antibody-mediated process, evolving ischemic/traumatic injury, and chronic medication exposure particularly to calcineurin inhibitors.

○ **What is cellular rejection?**

Cellular rejection is a T-cell–mediated process. Antigen-presenting cells present antigen to the T-cell antigen receptor. This interaction in conjunction with various costimulators can activate a T-cell response characterized by clonal expansion and the upregulation of various cell surface proteins. This activation results in the infiltration of the allograft by activated T cells, an associated inflammatory response, cellular injury, and death. Current maintenance and induction immunosuppression is designed to block T-cell activation and interfere with the interaction between the donor antigen and recipient T-cell. The incidence of acute rejection under current immunosuppression protocols is 10% to 20%.

○   **Describe post-transplant cytomegalovirus infection (CMV).**

CMV can be transplanted from the donor or reactivated in the recipient following kidney transplant. CMV disease is associated with significant morbidity and mortality in the recipient. Antiviral agents are available for prophylaxis and treatment. Those at highest risk for CMV infection are recipients without previous CMV exposure who receive a kidney from a CMV positive donor. These patients frequently receive CMV antiviral prophylaxis in the first several months post-transplant. Those at the lowest risk for CMV infection are CMV naïve recipients who receive kidneys from CMV naïve donors. Prophylaxis is not usually given in this circumstance. Clinically CMV infection presents as an asymptomatic viremia or presents as a syndrome of fever, leukopenia, and allograft dysfunction. CMV gastritis and colitis are also common presentation. Active disease may require a reduction in immunosuppression.

Pediatric kidneys being separated from small bowel in combined kidney/donor small amount pediatric en bloc kidneys on profusion machine.

Duplex ultrasound of transplant kidney demonstrating arterial and venous flow transplant.

Transplant kidney.

Pediatric kidney on perfusion machine.

CHAPTER 36

Benign Renal Cystic Disease

John Chandler Williams, MD, MS

○ **Describe the radiographic characteristics of a simple renal cortical cyst on intravenous pyelography and CT scan images.**

On intravenous pyelography, a simple cyst is a well-circumscribed recent mass that may distort the contour of the kidney and may show a "beak sign" with normal parenchyma. Computed tomography demonstrates a mass with water density (−10 and +20 HU) with an imperceptible wall, sharp margins with the renal parenchyma, and no enhancement after intravenous contrast administration.

○ **Describe the radiographic characteristics of a simple renal cortical cyst on MRI scans and ultrasound.**

On T1-weighted MRI, the mass is homogenous with low signal intensity (less than liver or renal cortex), and on T2-weighted images the lesion is homogenously hyperdense. There is no enhancement following intravenous administration of gadolinium-DTPA. On ultrasound, cysts are well demarcated with no internal echoes. They are usually spherical in shape and demonstrate an increase in through transmission with acoustic enhancement within the cyst.

○ **Describe the radiographic characteristics of a complicated cyst.**

A complicated cyst has an unusual contour, internal septations, calcifications, and/or evidence of enhancement on a contrasted CT scan.

○ **What are the Bosniak criteria for cyst classification?**

Morton A. Bosniak, MD, originally described his classification in 1986 and has subsequently updated it many times. The classification delineates cysts into 5 categories of renal cysts. The categorizations have management implications associated with the potential risk of malignancy.

○ **What is Bosniak I?**

Bosniak I cysts are solitary and fit the sonographic and CT criteria for simple cysts. Cysts would be sharp, thin, smooth walled, spherical, or ovoid water density lesions (−10 to +20 HU), with no internal echoes and no enhancement after intravenous contrast administration on CT. There is less than a 2% chance of being associated with a malignancy.

○ **What is Bosniak II?**

Bosniak II cysts have thin central septations, thin peripheral calcifications, or they can be hyperdense nonenhancing lesions with 50 to 100 HU. They are less than 3 cm in size. There is a 10% to 13% chance of being associated with a malignancy.

○ **What is Bosniak IIF?**

These cysts can have several thin central septations, thickened peripheral calcifications, or they can be hyperdense minimally enhancing lesions. They are greater than or equal to 3 cm in size. They may be totally intrarenal. There is a 14% to 25% chance of being associated with a malignancy. "F" is for follow-up. These cysts need follow-up examinations to demonstrate stability. About 10% of IIF cysts will progress. Radiographic changes in the cyst warrant excision.

○ **What is Bosniak III?**

These are complicated cysts with extensive calcifications, thickened walls (greater than or equal to 1 mm thick), and irregular borders. They have irregularly enhancing walls. There should be a high level of suspicion for malignancy in these lesions. There is approximately a 50% to 54% chance of being associated with a malignancy. Bosniak III cysts warrant excision.

○ **What is Bosniak IV?**

Bosniak IV describes a complex renal cystic mass with thick septa and/or thick walls, thickened calcifications that can be central or peripheral, and/or an enhancing component on contrasted images. These lesions can be found in association with a solid tumor. There is a 90% to 92% chance of being associated with a malignancy. Bosniak IV cysts require excision.

○ **In the Bosniak renal cyst criteria, which is more ominous: tissue calcification or tissue enhancement with contrast?**

Tissue enhancement with contrast is more ominous and more likely to be associated with malignancy.

○ **What are other factors to consider in regard to renal cyst imaging and chance of malignancy?**

Bosniak IIF and III cysts have a higher malignancy rate in patients with a history of primary renal malignancy or either a coexisting Bosniak IV lesion and/or a solid renal neoplasm.

○ **Should a complex cystic renal mass be biopsied?**

Percutaneous needle biopsy plays a limited role in the evaluation of cystic renal masses. Differences of opinion can arise regarding which category a particular case should be placed (whether Bosniak category II, IIF, or III). Follow-up imaging is advocated in these situations to determine progression. Some centers advocate needle biopsy of Bosniak III lesions.

○ **What would be the expected positive biopsy rate of a Bosniak III lesion?**

Centers that advocate biopsy of Bosniak III lesions report 39% nonmalignancy rate in their biopsy experience, thus saving patients from unnecessary surgery. In addition, biopsy as part of a percutaneous ablation of the renal lesion has also been advocated. With current laparoscopic and robot-assisted laparoscopic techniques, excisional biopsy of the entire lesion or partial nephrectomy is possible with low morbidity to the patient.

○ **What findings would suggest an inflammatory etiology, what should be done to confirm this, and how should it be treated if inflammation is confirmed?**

If the urologist suspects the cystic mass is inflammatory (pyuria, etc) or there is radiological evidence suggesting inflammation (such as perinephric fat stranding), puncture is acceptable. When the outcome is infection, the lesion can be treated and followed.

○ **What are the risks of percutaneous needle biopsy of a cystic renal mass?**

Risks of percutaneous renal cyst biopsy include bleeding, infection, and possible tumor track spread. Although considered rare, Dr Bosniak considered needle track spread of tumor an underestimated and underreported risk of cyst biopsy. A core biopsy of the wall of a cystic lesion (benign or malignant) can cause it to rupture and spill its contents into the surrounding tissues. Furthermore, a negative biopsy result does not absolutely rule out malignancy, particularly in cystic lesions that have less bulk of tissue to sample.

○ **What are the clinical or historical correlates to a complicated renal cystic mass found on imaging study?**

Urologists are frequently consulted for complicated cysts found incidentally on abdominal imaging studies. Review of the patient's family history to determine if there are genetic diseases that may affect the kidney or any family history of renal malignancies should be done. A review of prior medical history should be performed to determine if there is a history of prior renal malignancy, masses, neoplasms, or cysts in the patient. Any prior renal imaging studies can be extremely helpful in diagnosis of the renal cystic disease. Laboratory studies demonstrating current and historical renal function tests and urinalysis should be reviewed. There is little on physical examination that may be helpful.

○ **What is the current classification of cysts based upon?**

Several classifications have been proposed upon microscopic findings, clinical presentation, or radiographic appearance. Most recent publications in the urologic literature followed in 1987 classification given by the Committee on Classification, Nomenclature and Terminology suggestions of the American Academy of Pediatrics, Section of Urology. The primary distinctions are genetic and nongenetic.

○ **What are genetic renal cystic diseases?**
- Autosomal dominant (adult) polycystic kidney disease.
- Autosomal recessive (infantile) polycystic kidney disease.
- Juvenile nephronophthisis–medullary cystic disease complex.
- Juvenile nephronophthisis (autosomal recessive).
- Autosomal dominant interstitial kidney disease (misnomer medullary cystic disease).
- Congenital nephrosis (familial nephrotic syndrome) autosomal recessive.
- Familial hypoplastic glomerulocystic disease (autosomal dominant).
- Rare multisystemic disorders (Von Hippel–Lindau disease, tuberous sclerosis, etc).

○ **What are the nongenetic renal cystic diseases?**
- Multicystic dysplastic.
- Benign multilocular cysts.
- Simple cysts.
- Medullary sponge kidney.
- Sporadic glomerulocystic kidney disease.
- Acquired renal cystic disease.
- Calyceal diverticulum.

○ **What is autosomal dominant polycystic kidney disease (ADPKD) and what percentage of dialysis patients have this disorder?**

Also known as adult polycystic kidney disease, this is an important cause of renal failure and accounts for almost 10% of all dialysis patients. The incidents are approximately 1 in 500 to 1 in 1000. While this condition typically presents in the 3rd to 5th decades of life, it has been identified in newborns. Large irregular cysts of varying size appear diffusely through the renal cortex and medulla. Renal function is impaired, and hypertension and microscopic hematuria are common.

○ **What is autosomal recessive polycystic kidney disease (ARPKD), when is it most likely to be diagnosed, and by what means?**

ARPKD is typically diagnosed during infancy and carries 50% mortality rate in the first few hours to days of life. This disease has a spectrum of severity with the most severe form being diagnosed at birth and the less severe forms are diagnosed later in infancy and childhood. The affected newborn has massively enlarged kidneys. They are hyperdense on sonography due to the presence of multiple subcapsular cysts. All patients have some degree of hepatic fibrosis with lesions in the periportal region of the liver. This pathologic entity can be readily diagnosed by the gross appearance of the kidneys.

○ **What is juvenile nephronophthisis?**

Both juvenile nephronophthisis and medullary cystic disease cause polydipsia and polyuria in more than 80% of cases. The cysts are medullary in position. This is severe renal tubular defect associated with the inability to conserve sodium. The polyuria is refractory to vasopressin and a large salt intake diet is required to maintain sodium balance. There is associated growth retardation in juvenile nephronophthisis.

○ **Describe the renal cysts associated with tuberous sclerosis and particularly what makes these cysts unique.**

The renal cysts of tubular sclerosis are unique in that they have a lining of hypertrophic, hyperplastic eosinophilic cells.

○ **Describe the renal cysts associated with Von Hippel–Lindau disease.**

The cysts usually resemble simple benign cysts with flattened epithelium that some investigators consider precancerous.

○ **What is the sonographic appearance of ARPKD in the newborn?**

Bilateral, symmetrically enlarged, homogenously hyperechoic kidneys, usually without evidence of large discrete cysts.

○ **In which polycystic kidney disease (autosomal dominant or recessive) would you suspect liver pathology?**

Both. **ADPKD** is associated with hepatic cysts that become evident in adulthood and increase in incidence with age. **ARPKD** is associated with congenital hepatic fibrosis in all affected individuals.

○ **What is the essential histopathologic finding to diagnose dysplasia?**

Primitive ducts.

○ **In what renal cystic disease is there a high incidence of renal cell carcinoma and what is that incidence?**

The highest incidence, 35%, is in Von Hippel–Lindau disease. Tuberous sclerosis has a 2% incidence of associated renal malignancy. All others carry the same incidences of renal cell carcinomas as in the general population.

○ **How do patients with medullary sponge kidney present?**

Renal colic, gross hematuria, nephrolithiasis, and urinary tract infections.

○ **Patients with medullary sponge kidney also have a higher than normal incidence of which 2 metabolic abnormalities that increase their kidney stone risk?**

They tend to have a higher incidence of low urinary citrate and renal leak type hypercalciuria.

○ **Can ureteropelvic junction obstruction (UPJ) obstruction be differentiated from multicystic kidney disease based only on sonographic findings?**

Yes, it is possible. In multicystic kidney disease, the cysts are arranged in a random fashion. In UPJ obstruction, the largest cyst-like structure is medial or central representing the renal pelvis and communications can be demonstrated between the central "cyst" or renal pelvis and the "peripheral cysts" which are actually the calyces.

○ **In unilateral multicystic kidney disease, what is the typical contralateral urologic finding?**

20% to 40% of patients have contralateral vesicoureteral reflux. 3% to 10% of patients will have a contralateral UPJ obstruction.

○ **What is acquired renal cystic disease (ARCD) and what other renal disorder is associated with it?**

ARCD is a feature of end-stage renal disease rather than a response to dialysis. The cysts are predominantly in the cortex, generally less than 1 cm in diameter, and are associated with a significantly increased risk of renal cell carcinoma.

○ **What is the most common presentation of ARCD?**

Loin pain, hematuria, or both.

○ **What is the incidence of renal cell carcinoma in ARCD?**

Renal cell carcinoma is 3 to 6 times higher in **ARCD** than in the general population.

○ **What is the incidence of ARPKD?**

Incidence is 1 in 40,000 births.

○ **What is the typical clinical presentation of ARPKD?**

Enlarge kidneys or a flank mass is the typical presentation. Other findings include oligohydramnios, oliguria, cysts of the renal tubules, and congenital hepatic fibrosis of varying degrees.

○ **What specific genetic abnormality is associated with ADPKD and what percentage of their offspring will be affected?**

In ADPKD, 95% are caused by a gene located on the short arm of chromosome 16; 50% of the patient's offspring will be affected; and 5% are caused by a defect of chromosome 4. Usually they will have symptoms later in life.

○ **What is the usual age and typical clinical presentation of ADPKD?**

ADPKD usually presents between the ages of 30 and 50 years. It occurs uncommonly in newborns. The clinical presentation is usually with hypertension, flank pain, hematuria, and urinary tract infections.

○ **What other systemic anomalies are associated with ADPKD?**

Other anomalies associated with ADPKD include aneurysm of the circle of Willis (10%-40%), cysts in the liver, spleen, pancreas, and lung, as well as diverticula of the colon and mitral valve prolapse.

○ **What is the differential diagnosis for a neonate with bilateral renal enlargement and homogenous hyperechoic kidneys?**

- Autosomal recessive polycystic kidney disease (ARPKD).
- Autosomal dominant polycystic kidney disease (ADPKD).
- Sporadic glomerulocystic kidney disease.
- Contrast nephropathy.
- Renal vein thrombosis.

○ **On which chromosome do we find the genetic defect for ARPKD?**

Chromosome 6.

○ **What is the histology of ARPKD and how much normal renal tissue is typically found?**

The kidney retains fetal lobulation, with small cysts and no normal renal parenchyma. The renal vessels and ureter appear normal. Collecting duct ectasia is present.

○ **In ARPKD, the cysts develop from which specific part of the nephron?**

The cysts are derived principally from the collecting duct.

○ **What is the histology of ADPKD?**

Cyst sizes range from a few millimeters to several centimeters. Focal tubular dilatation, epithelial hyperplasia, or adenomas of the cyst wall are typically found. The vessels show atherosclerosis and interstitial fibrosis in advanced stages.

○ **In ADPKD, the cysts develop from which specific part of the nephron?**

Microcysts and macrocysts are derived from the entire nephron.

○ **What percentage of renal failure in children is caused by juvenile nephronophthisis?**

10% to 20%.

○ **Which chromosome contains the genetic defect of juvenile nephronophthisis?**

Chromosome 2.

○ **What is the inheritance pattern of juvenile nephronophthisis and for adult dominant interstitial kidney disease (ADIKD)?**

Juvenile nephronophthisis is autosomal recessive on chromosome 2. ADIKD (medullary cystic disease) is autosomal dominant with an unidentified chromosomal abnormality.

○ **What are the clinical manifestations of Von Hippel–Lindau disease?**

Von Hippel–Lindau is an autosomal dominant condition manifested by cerebellar hemangioblastomas; retinal angiomas; cysts of the pancreas, kidney, and epididymis. It is also associated with pheochromocytomas in approximately 20% of the patients with renal cell carcinomas.

○ **What are the clinical manifestations of tuberous sclerosis?**

Tuberous sclerosis is part of a triad of epilepsy, mental retardation, and adenoma sebaceum. The hallmark lesion is a superficial cortical hamartoma of the cerebrum. Although renal cysts have been associated with tuberous sclerosis, angiomyolipomas are more common than cysts.

○ **What is a multicystic kidney and how common is it?**

Multicystic kidney (multicystic dysplastic kidney) is a severe form of dysplasia in which there is no functioning renal parenchyma. The kidney does not have a reniform shape and calyceal drainage is not present. A "bunch of grapes" has been used to describe the gross appearance of the kidney. Renal size is variable. Multicystic kidney is the most common type of renal cystic disease and one of the most common causes of an abdominal mass in infants.

○ **What are the characteristics of medullary sponge kidney?**

Medullary sponge kidney is characterized by the dilatation of the distal portion of the collecting ducts, which may be associated with cysts and diverticula. The dilated collecting tubules have a distinct appearance on pyelography and look as if they were brushed on with the "bristles of a paintbrush." One-third of patients have hypercalciuria that tends to be the "renal calcium leak type." Patients with medullary sponge kidneys also tend to have a relatively high incidence of renal calculi, urinary tract infections, and hypocitraturia.

CHAPTER 37 **Renal Tumors, Adults**

Paul L. Crispen, MD and
Matthew T. Gettman, MD

○ **How quickly is the incidence of renal cell cancer increasing?**

Two percent annually. Although renal cancer is more common in men, the incidence in women is rising faster (2.2% vs 1.7%). The greatest increase has been noted in tumors <4 cm in diameter.

○ **What is the incidence of renal cell carcinoma (RCC)?**

Renal cell cancer accounts for 3% of adult malignancies. Approximately 65,000 new cases of RCC are expected to be diagnosed in 2012, with approximately 14,000 RCC-related deaths. RCC accounts for up to 90% of all kidney tumors.

○ **What are the risk factors for RCC?**

Tobacco use, hypertension, obesity, male gender, and urban dwellers. The majority of RCC occur in the 5th to 7th decade of life; however, a recent trend suggests a higher incidence in younger females and adolescents.

○ **What is the typical clinical presentation for most RCC cases and how does it differ from the classic triad?**

Incidental in the modern era. Hematuria (gross or microscopic), mass, and flank pain are not uncommon. The classic triad of pain, hematuria, and flank mass occurs in only 10% to 15% of patients. Presenting symptoms can often be attributed to metastasis or paraneoplastic syndromes.

○ **What is responsible for the increased detection of incidental renal tumors?**

The routine use of cross-sectional imaging (CT scans) to evaluate abdominal symptomatology.

○ **What must be considered prior to the administration of IV contrast in the evaluation of renal mass?**

Renal function. Impaired renal function places patients at risk for complications following the administration of iodine and gadolinium-based contrast agents. Iodine-based contrast is associated with the risk of acute nephrotoxicity and worsening renal function. Gadolinium has been associated with nephrogenic systemic fibrosis.

○ **What are Hounsfield units and how do they help to differentiate renal tumors on computed tomography?**

Hounsfield units are a measure of radiodensity on CT scans. Enhancement of 15 or more Hounsfield units following the administration of contrast are suggestive of a malignancy; however, benign lesions such as oncocytoma will also enhance. Whereas, tumors containing areas with negative Hounsfield units, suggestive of fat, are likely angiomyolipomas (AMLs).

○ **Can information from a percutaneous needle biopsy of a renal mass be considered reliable?**

Analysis of biopsies on permanent section is significantly more reliable than frozen-section analysis. With experienced pathologists and radiologists, the expected sensitivity and specificity of a percutaneous needle biopsy is 97% and 100%, respectively. The primary limitation of renal mass biopsy in contemporary series is nondiagnostic biopsies, not false negatives.

○ **What are the indications for a biopsy of a renal mass?**

Percutaneous biopsy is advocated only when clinical or radiologic evidence suggests a diagnosis other than RCC (such as lymphoma or metastases from another primary tumor), or when a definite diagnosis is absolutely necessary. However with the improved accuracy of renal mass biopsy, its role may be expanding to help guide treatment decisions in patients with small renal tumors.

○ **How is renal cancer staged?**

By TNM staging system.

- T1a: confined to the kidney <4 cm.
- T1b: confined to the kidney >4 cm and <7 cm.
- T2a: confined to the kidney >7 cm and ≤10 cm.
- T2b: confined to the kidney and >10 cm.
- T3a: perinephric fat, ipsilateral adrenal gland involvement, and tumor extends into the renal vein or segmental branches.
- T3b: tumor extension into the vena cava, but not extending above the diaphragm.
- T3c: tumor extension into the renal vein extending above the diaphragm or invasion into the wall of the vena cava.
- T4: tumor extension beyond Gerota fascia, involvement of adjacent organs other than the ipsilateral adrenal gland.

○ **What is the standard of care in the treatment of renal tumors clinically localized to the kidney?**

Nephrectomy—partial or radical.

○ **What are additional treatment options for patients with T1a tumors?**

Observation, cryoablation, and radiofrequency ablation.

○ **Synchronous metastases occur in what percentage of RCC patients?**

Up to one-third of patients will have synchronous metastases. Metachronous metastases occur in 10% to 20% of patients at 5-year follow-up. The prognosis is much worse for patients with synchronous metastasis.

O **How frequently does RCC invade adjacent organs?**

RCC invades adjacent organs in approximately 10% of cases. Invasion of adjacent organs is associated with a very poor prognosis with reported 5-year survival rates of less than 5%. In many cases, surgical intervention can require partial resection of contiguous structures including colon, pancreas, liver, or spleen. Preoperative imaging often overstates the possibility of direct liver invasion.

O **A patient undergoes a partial nephrectomy for organ-confined RCC. What recurrence rates would be expected in the ipsilateral kidney and the contralateral kidney?**

Recurrence in the ipsilateral kidney would be 1% to 5% and 1% to 3% in the contralateral kidney.

O **What percentage of RCCs occur bilaterally?**

One to five percent of RCC patients have tumors present in both kidneys simultaneously.

O **What is the incidence of the different histologic types of RCC?**

Clear cell (80%) followed by papillary (15%), chromophobe (5%), collecting duct cancer (1%), and renal medullary carcinoma (<1%).

O **What is the prognosis for cystic clear cell RCC?**

Excellent. Cystic clear cell RCC is associated with a low rate of systemic progression following complete surgical excision.

O **True/False: At least 50% of RCCs are vimentin-positive on immunohistochemical analysis.**

True. In addition, high-grade tumors, clear cell cancers, and those with sarcomatoid differentiation are more commonly vimentin-positive. Almost all RCCs stain positively for keratin 8 and 18 and the majority stains positively for epithelial membrane antigen. This is useful in diagnosing metastases.

O **What cystic renal diseases are associated with an increased incidence of RCC?**

Acquired renal cystic disease is associated with a 4- to 6-fold increased risk of RCC over the general population. Von Hippel–Lindau (VHL) disease has a known incidence of bilateral renal cysts in 76% of affected individuals with a 35% to 38% incidence of RCC in affected individuals. Tuberous sclerosis is associated with a 2% increased risk of RCC over the general population.

O **Which types of RCC are more aggressive?**

Renal medullary carcinoma and collecting duct carcinoma are more aggressive subtypes. The behavior of clear cell, papillary, and chromophobe types are best predicted by stage and grade.

O **Which type of RCC is associated with multifocality?**

Papillary RCC is associated with a 15% incidence of multifocality within the affected kidney.

O **What is the predominant group of patients in whom the renal medullary type of RCC appears?**

Renal medullary carcinomas occur almost exclusively in association with sickle cell trait or hemoglobin SC disease. These are very aggressive tumors and tend to occur in younger patients.

○ **What is the renal cell type of origin of clear cell and papillary RCCs?**

Proximal convoluted tubule.

○ **What is the renal cell type of origin of Bellini tumors?**

The origin of the Bellini tumors is the collecting duct. Renal medullary carcinomas are thought to arise from the calyceal epithelium.

○ **List the hereditary forms of RCC?**

Von Hippel–Lindau (VHL) disease, Birt–Hogg–Dube (BHD), hereditary papillary RCC, and hereditary leiomyomatosis and RCC syndrome.

○ **What percentage of RCCs are familial?**

Only 2% to 3%, the majority are considered sporadic.

○ **What are the specific genetic abnormalities associated with each of the hereditary forms of RCC?**

- VHL: VHL gene on chromosome 3p.
- Birt–Hogg–Dube: BHD1 gene on chromosome 17p.
- Hereditary papillary RCC: c-met protooncogene on chromosome 7q.
- Hereditary leiomyomatosis and RCC: fumarate hydratase on chromosome 1q.

○ **What is Von Hippel–Lindau disease?**

A rare, autosomal dominant, multiorgan syndrome associated with a 50% incidence of RCC; 75% incidence of renal, epididymal, and pancreatic cysts; cerebellar hemangioblastomas; retinal angiomas; and pheochromocytoma. Typically, RCC in this instance tends to be multiple and bilateral (80%). Historically, one-third of patients die from RCC.

○ **What is the most common cause of hereditary pheochromocytoma?**

VHL syndrome.

○ **Can the size or appearance of renal lesions in VHL disease predict the presence of RCC?**

No. No correlation exists between the size of a lesion and the diagnosis of RCC. Twenty-five to thirty-five percent of RCC in VHL occur in cystic lesions.

○ **A patient with VHL has small bilateral renal tumors. At what point is surgical intervention indicated?**

The balance between oncologic control and preservation of renal function is crucial in patients with small renal tumors. In VHL patients, tumors less than 3 cm have been associated with a low rate of progression to metastatic disease. For this reason, close surveillance with surgical intervention when a tumor reaches 3 cm in size can be employed in this population.

○ **A patient with VHL has diffuse, high-volume, bilateral renal lesions. What treatment is best?**

The best treatment in this case would be bilateral nephrectomy with subsequent transplantation. Nephron-sparing surgery, while technically feasible in many cases, is best reserved for patients with cystic and low-volume, nondiffuse solid lesions.

○ **What is the function of the VHL gene?**

The VHL gene is a tumor suppressor gene. The VHL protein complex helps to maintain appropriate levels of HIF-1, depending on oxygen availability. When VHL is mutated, HIF-1 levels increase, leading to the activation of angiogenesis pathways.

○ **Do sporadic clear cell RCC have mutations of the VHL gene?**

Yes, 50% to 60% of clear cell RCC have mutations of the VHL gene. Another 15% to 20% have hypermethylation of the VHL gene.

○ **Describe Birt-Hogg-Dube syndrome (BHD).**

Autosomal dominant disorder characterized by cutaneous fibrofolliculomas, lung cysts, and renal tumors. Renal tumors are noted in approximately 30% of patients with BHD syndrome. The most common renal tumors are oncocytomas and chromophobe RCC; these tumors are often multifocal and bilateral.

○ **Describe hereditary papillary RCC syndrome (HPRCC).**

Autosomal dominant disorder characterized by bilateral multifocal type 1 papillary tumors.

○ **Describe hereditary leiomyomatosis and RCC syndrome (HLRCC).**

Autosomal dominant disorder characterized by type 2 papillary tumors and cutaneous and uterine leiomyomas. Although only 20% to 30% of patients with HLRCC syndrome develop renal tumors, the tumors have been noted to be very aggressive.

○ **What accounts for the yellowish gross appearance of many clear cell RCCs?**

The presence of cholesterol causes the gross yellow appearance of these tumors. The lipid substances tend to dissolve during histologic preparation, creating the microscopic appearance of clear cells.

○ **True/False: Nuclear grade is a predictor of survival that is independent of pathologic stage.**

True. Nuclear grade has a significant impact on survival for all stages of RCC.

○ **Differentiate between the Bosniak classification of renal cysts and their relationship to malignancy.**

- Category I: A simple cyst with through transmission on ultrasound and a clearly defined wall. There are no internal septa, echoes, or calcifications. This portends a remote chance for cancer.
- Category II: A septated, nonenhancing cyst that can have thin peripheral calcifications and minimally thickened wall. This lesion carries roughly a 15% chance of malignancy.
- Category III: A complex cyst with a thickened wall, a hyperdense cyst that shows no enhancement with contrast administration, can have thick calcifications, or thickened septa that carry roughly a 50% cancer.
- Category IV: An enhancing, thick-walled cyst with irregular borders, thick calcifications that may be central, and carries roughly a 95% chance of malignancy.

○ **What is the most common benign renal lesion?**

Renal cysts are the most common benign renal lesions, representing more than 70% of asymptomatic renal lesions.

○ **What is the recommended treatment for Bosniak class III and IV cysts?**

Definitive therapy, surgical excision, or thermal ablation due to the increased risk of malignancy.

○ **List treatment options for symptomatic simple renal cysts.**

Treatment options include aspiration, resection, decortications, and sclerotherapy.

○ **What is the most common benign solid renal tumor?**

Renal cortical adenoma. These lesions are less than 5 mm and are seen in up to 35% of autopsies.

○ **How are renal cortical adenomas differentiated from papillary renal cell carcinoma?**

Renal cortical adenomas and papillary renal cell carcinomas cannot be distinguished histologically. The only distinction beyond size is potential trisomies of chromosomes 12, 16, and 20 noted in papillary renal cell carcinomas.

○ **What are the indications for a partial nephrectomy?**

Solitary kidney, bilateral renal masses, renal insufficiency, or anticipated renal insufficiency secondary to a comorbid disease process are imperative indications. However, partial nephrectomy has been shown to offer equivalent oncologic efficacy in small renal tumors compared to radical nephrectomy in small renal tumors (≤4 cm). With the additional benefit of preserving renal function, the "elective" application of partial nephrectomy has greatly expanded and is now considered the gold standard for the treatment of small renal tumors.

○ **What percentage of renal tumors are clinical T1a?**

Nearly 70% of newly diagnosed renal tumors in contemporary series are less than 4 cm in diameter.

○ **True/False. Radical nephrectomy offers better oncologic outcomes compared to partial nephrectomy when treating T1a renal cell carcinomas.**

False. There is no difference in cancer-specific survival when treating T1a renal cell carcinoma comparing partial versus radical nephrectomy.

○ **When treating clinical T1a renal tumors does partial nephrectomy afford an overall survival advantage over radical nephrectomy?**

Several retrospective series have suggested an advantage in overall survival with partial nephrectomy versus radical nephrectomy. However, a randomized EORTC trial failed to demonstrate an overall survival advantage.

○ **When treating clinical T1a renal tumors does partial nephrectomy afford an advantage in preserving renal function?**

Partial nephrectomy has been shown to offer improved preservation of renal function compared to radical nephrectomy.

○ **According to the 2009 AUA Guidelines for the Management of a Stage 1 Renal Mass, when should nephron-sparing surgery be considered?**

The guidelines recommend nephron-sparing surgery be considered for all stage 1 renal masses presuming adequate oncologic control. Radical nephrectomy remains an option when nephron-sparing surgery is not technically feasible or advisable.

○ **According to the 2009 AUA Guidelines for the Management of a Stage 1 Renal Mass, when should active surveillance be considered?**

The guidelines recommend consideration of active surveillance for patients with decreased life expectancy or extensive comorbidities that make them high risk for other management strategies.

○ **What is the reported average growth rate of small, <4 cm, renal tumors during active surveillance?**

The growth rate of small, <4 cm, renal tumors during active surveillance is approximately 3 mm per year.

○ **What is the reported rate of metastatic progression during the active surveillance of small, <4 cm, renal tumor?**

The reported rate of metastatic progression is 1% to 2% during follow-up ranging from 3 to 5 years.

○ **True/False: Renal tumor biopsy should always be performed prior to thermal ablation.**

True. Renal tumor biopsy should always be performed to define histology.

○ **Intraoperatively, what maneuver is recommended prior to proceeding with a partial nephrectomy?**

Complete exposure of the kidney to exclude multifocality. Ipsilateral multifocal disease is noted in up to 5% of patients at the time of nephrectomy. Intraoperative ultrasound is a valuable adjunct in this regard.

○ **How commonly are paraneoplastic syndromes associated with RCC?**

Paraneoplastic syndromes are seen concurrently with or develop in 30% of patients with RCC and are more common in patients with advanced disease.

○ **Describe Stauffer syndrome.**

Reversible hepatic dysfunction in the absence of metastatic disease. Patients have abnormal liver function tests, fever, and hepatic necrosis, which typically resolve after nephrectomy. Persistence or recurrence of disease is a poor prognostic sign.

○ **What other disease is associated with Stauffer syndrome?**

Xanthogranulomatous pyelonephritis.

○ **Which type of RCC is frequently observed in patients with Stauffer syndrome?**

Clear cell type.

○   **What is the etiology of hypercalcemia in patients with RCC?**

Hypercalcemia has been noted in approximately 15% of patients with RCC. Osteolytic bone metastasis or paraneoplastic syndrome frequently cause hypercalcemia. Stromal cells of RCC are thought to produce a parathyroid hormone-like peptide responsible for the paraneoplastic syndrome.

○   **List the levels of tumor thrombus associated with RCC.**

- Level 0: limited to the renal vein.
- Level 1: extending into the inferior vena cava (IVC), <2 cm above the renal vein.
- Level 2: extending >2 cm above renal vein, but below the hepatic veins.
- Level 3: extending to the hepatic veins, but below the diaphragm.
- Level 4: extending above the diaphragm.

○   **What is the incidence of venous involvement by a tumor thrombus in RCC?**

Renal vein only, up to 25%; inferior vena cava, 5% to 10%; atrial, 1%.

○   **What clinical findings are suggestive of an increased risk for venous involvement by RCC?**

The presence of a varicocele, leg edema, deep vein thrombosis, recurrent pulmonary emboli, and caput medusae are reported manifestations but are found infrequently. A high index of suspicion for patients with larger, centrally located tumors is an important finding.

○   **What is the blood supply of the vena cava tumor associated with RCC?**

When vascularized, parasitized vessels from the renal artery typically feed the tumor thrombus.

○   **Describe the collateral venous circulation in cases where the IVC is occluded secondary to tumor thrombus.**

IVC occlusion at the level of renal veins leads to dilatation and increased venous return via the retroperitoneal (hemiazygous system, lumbar veins, and Batson plexus), gonadal, mesenteric, and pelvic plexus.

○   **What is the differential diagnosis and incidence of a vena cava tumor thrombus?**

Wilms tumor, transitional cell carcinoma, sarcoma, lymphomas, primitive neuroectodermal tumors, adrenal cortical carcinoma, testis tumors, and pheochromocytoma. Five percent of RCC cases have vena cava involvement.

○   **What is the role of routine lymph node dissection at the time of nephrectomy for suspected RCC?**

Results of a randomized trial did not demonstrate a benefit of routine lymphadenopathy at the time of nephrectomy. For this reason, lymphadenectomy is reserved for select cases with increased risk of lymph node involvement.

○   **What is the role of adrenalectomy at the time of nephrectomy for suspected RCC?**

Ipsilateral adrenalectomy at the time of nephrectomy is recommended only in cases with radiographic adrenal enlargement or in cases when the tumor located immediately adjacent to the adrenal gland.

○   **Where are the most common sites of metastasis from RCC?**

The most common sites are the lung, bone, lymph nodes, liver, adrenal glands, brain, heart, spleen, and skin.

○ **List the 6 predictors of decreased survival utilized in the Memorial Sloan-Kettering Cancer Risk Stratification System for metastatic renal cancer.**

Karnofsky performance status ≤70, high lactate dehydrogenase (>1.5 times upper limit of normal), low hemoglobin levels (less than lower limit of normal), high corrected serum calcium (>10 mg/dL), time from initial diagnosis to randomization <1 year, and >2 sites of organ metastasis. Number of risk factors are used to categorize risk (0 = low risk, 1-2 = intermediate risk, ≥3 = high risk).

○ **Describe general 5-year survival for RCC with tumor confined to the kidney, with perinephric fat involvement, with vena cava thrombus, with node-positive disease, or metastasis.**

The 5-year survival for organ-confined RCC is 85% to 90%, 70% to 75% for perinephric fat involvement, 40% to 60% for vena cava thrombus, 10% to 20% with node involvement, and 0% to 5% for metastatic disease.

○ **What is the role, if any, of cytoreductive nephrectomy for patients with metastatic RCC?**

Cytoreductive nephrectomy can be completed prior to the systemic therapy, for palliation, in conjunction with resection of select solitary metastasis and prior to the initiation of systemic therapy. In fact, randomized series have demonstrated a significant increase in survival in patients undergoing cytoreductive nephrectomy prior to cytokine therapy compared to patients not undergoing nephrectomy.

○ **What is the role of cytoreductive nephrectomy for patients who are to be treated with tyrosine kinase inhibitors?**

The role of cytoreductive nephrectomy prior to the use of tyrosine kinase inhibitors for metastatic renal cancer is unknown. The routine use of cytoreductive nephrectomy in this population is based on the data evaluating cytokine therapy and that the majority of patients enrolled in trials evaluating the efficacy of tyrosine kinase inhibitors having undergone nephrectomy prior to treatment.

○ **Should solitary metastases in RCC be surgically resected if possible?**

Yes. Metastasectomy has been associated with increased long-term survival. Nephrectomy in conjunction with resection of a solitary pulmonary metastasis has yielded 5-year survival rates of 30% to 35%. Patients with CNS metastasis represent a special case in which they are treated preferentially prior to cytoreductive nephrectomy.

○ **List the various forms of systemic therapy for metastatic RCC.**

Immunotherapy and targeted therapy. Since the introduction of targeted therapy, the use of immunotherapy has decreased significantly. However, immunotherapy is the only form of therapy for metastatic RCC that has been associated with the potential for a complete treatment response.

○ **List the various forms of immunotherapy for metastatic RCC.**

- *Active specific immunotherapy:* stimulation of T cell by immunization of patient with inactivated autologous tumor cells, limited proven benefit.
- *Adoptive immunotherapy:* typically involves either in vitro or in vivo interleukin stimulation (usually IL-2) of peripheral lymphocytes (lymphocyte-activated killer cells or LAK cells), reported response rates up to 20%.
- *Cytokines:* typically α-interferon or IL-2 therapy with direct or indirect cytotoxic effects on the tumor, response rates of 5% to 25%.
- Vaccines and stem cell transplantation techniques are being developed.

○ **List the various forms of targeted therapy for metastatic RCC.**

Tyrosine kinase inhibitors, mTOR inhibitors, and vascular endothelial growth factor (VEGF) monoclonal antibodies.

○ **List the benefits of targeted therapy compared to immunotherapy.**

Decreased toxicity, oral administration (tyrosine kinase and mTOR inhibitors), increased partial response rate, and disease stabilization compared to cytokine therapy.

○ **Which receptors are targeted by the tyrosine inhibitors approved for metastatic renal cancer?**

Multiple receptors are targeted by each agent; however, all inhibit the tyrosine kinase domains of VEGF and platelet-derived growth factor (PDGF) receptors.

○ **What is the proposed mechanism of action of tyrosine kinase inhibitors for treating metastatic renal cancer?**

Inhibition of angiogenesis and cellular proliferation of endothelial cells.

○ **What is the mechanism of action of bevacizumab?**

Monoclonal antibody which binds to circulating VEGF.

○ **True/False: Bevacizumab is approved as monotherapy for metastatic RCC.**

False. Bevacizumab is approved in combination with interferon-alpha for the treatment of metastatic RCC.

○ **What is the proposed mechanism of action of mTOR inhibitors?**

Decreased transcription of hypoxia-inducible factor, VEGF, and PDGF ligands.

○ **What are common side effects of mTOR inhibitors?**

Anemia, fatigue, stomatitis, hyperglycemia, dyspnea, pain, infection, rash, edema, and hyperlipidemia.

○ **What are common side effects of the oral tyrosine kinase inhibitors?**

Hand-and-foot syndrome, rash, mucositis/stomatitis, hypertension, neutropenia, hypophosphatemia, anemia, fatigue, hypothyroidism, and diarrhea.

○ **True/False: Tyrosine kinase inhibitors have been associated with hypothyroidism during the treatment of metastatic renal cancer.**

True. Hypothyroidism has been noted in 21% to 84% of patients treated with tyrosine kinase inhibitors. It should be treated with replacement therapy when noted.

○ **What is the most common renal sarcoma in adults?**

Leiomyosarcoma accounts for 60% of renal sarcomas and is best treated with surgical removal. Other less common tumors include osteogenic sarcoma, liposarcoma, carcinosarcoma, fibrosarcoma, rhabdomyosarcoma of adults, and malignant fibrous histiocytoma.

○ **What is the characteristic substance secreted by juxtaglomerular cell tumors?**

Renin. These are extremely rare, profusely vascular benign tumors that not uncommonly are difficult to locate because of the small size. They occur in young adults and adolescents. Patients typically present with severe hypertension, polydipsia, polyuria, myalgia, and headaches. A partial nephrectomy should be considered if the diagnosis is made preoperatively.

○ **True/False: Patients with juxtaglomerular cell tumors typically have hyperkalemia.**

False. The hyperreninemia causes a secondary hyperaldosteronism followed by hypokalemia.

○ **At autopsy, what percentage of hematologic malignancies will have renal involvement?**

Up to 50%. Usually hematologic malignancies appear in the kidney as part of the systemic disease process. Non-Hodgkin lymphoma is more common than Hodgkin disease. Multiple, bilateral renal masses are common. The treatment is systemic for the most part. Hematologic malignancies are the most common secondary tumors of the kidney.

○ **Besides hematologic malignancies, where are the sites of primary tumors that metastasize to the kidney?**

Virtually any solid neoplasm can metastasize to the kidney. Lung cancer (squamous cell) frequently metastasizes to the kidney as well as breast cancer and uterine cancer. Up to 20% of patients with lung cancer have occult renal metastases. Malignant melanoma is also frequently noted in the kidneys at autopsy.

○ **Which renal tumors contain fat?**

Angiomyolipomas are the most common. Less common tumors that contain fat include lipomas, liposarcoma, some Wilms tumors, an occasional oncocytoma, and very rarely RCC.

○ **What hereditary syndrome is associated with AML?**

Tuberous sclerosis. This is an autosomal dominant inherited disease associated typically with multiple and bilateral AML, mental retardation, and adenoma sebaceum. AML in these patients develop frequently in late childhood. Although AML occur in 50% of patients with tuberous sclerosis, less than 40% of patients with AML have features of tuberous sclerosis.

○ **What is another name for angiomyolipoma?**

Renal hamartoma. These tumors contain fat, smooth muscle, and blood vessels. The incidence is 0.3% to 2%. Isolated AML are commonly seen in middle-aged women. The majority of AML appear as single asymptomatic lesions and are not associated with tuberous sclerosis.

○ **Does AML occur in other locations besides the kidney?**

Angiomyolipoma (hamartoma) have been reported to occur in the bone, heart, lung, brain, and eye.

○ **What is the name of the pulmonary condition that can be seen concurrently with AML?**

Pulmonary lymphangiomyomatosis.

○ **Which renal tumor is most frequently associated with spontaneous hemorrhage?**

Angiomyolipoma.

○ **What is Wunderlich syndrome?**

Spontaneous retroperitoneal hemorrhage associated with an AML.

○ **Are any other renal tumors associated with tuberous sclerosis?**

Renal cell carcinoma has been observed concurrently with AML in patients with tuberous sclerosis.

○ **How do patients with AML typically present?**

Tumor size correlates well with symptoms. Most small lesions are asymptomatic. Lesions larger than 4 cm are at increased risk for hematuria, spontaneous rupture, retroperitoneal bleeding, pain, and possibly fever. At least 10% of patients with AML develop acute hemorrhage requiring intervention.

○ **What hormone receptors are associated with AML?**

AMLs have been noted to express androgen, estrogen (α and β subtypes), and progesterone receptors.

○ **What chromosomal abnormalities are associated with AML?**

Loss of heterozygosity at chromosome 16p13 has been observed in 50% of AML occurring in association with tuberous sclerosis and 10% of sporadic AML. Changes in chromosome 9q and 16p have also been linked to tuberous sclerosis.

○ **What are the treatment options for AML?**

Observation, angioinfarction, and partial nephrectomy. Asymptomatic patients with small tumors are often followed with serial imaging unless renal function decreases or tumor diameter increases. It has been suggested that asymptomatic tumors larger than 4 cm be treated. All symptomatic tumors should be treated.

○ **What is the most common solid enhancing benign renal tumor larger than 1 cm in diameter?**

Oncocytoma.

○ **What pathologic features are rarely seen with oncocytoma?**

Hemorrhage, cystic degeneration, and necrosis.

○ **What is the characteristic organelle seen in oncocytomas on electron microscopy?**

Mitochondria. The abundant mitochondria are responsible for the eosinophilic cytoplasm seen in the polygonal, uniform cells of oncocytomas. Mitotic figures are rare.

○ **What is the incidence of multifocal or bilateral oncocytomas?**

Oncocytomas are multifocal in 3% to 5% of cases. Bilateral oncocytomas can occur in approximately 3% to 5% of cases.

○ **True/False. The incidence of oncocytomas decrease with increasing age.**

False. The incidence of oncocytomas increases with increasing age.

○ **Do oncocytomas ever occur concurrently with RCC?**

Yes. Ten percent of oncocytomas occur concurrently with a **RCC** in either the ipsilateral or contralateral kidney.

○ **What chromosomal changes are associated with oncocytoma?**

Oncocytomas are characterized by loss of the Y chromosome and translocations involving the long arm of chromosome 1. Abnormalities of chromosomes 3, 7, and 17 are rare in oncocytomas.

○ **What are the classic radiographic signs associated with the appearance of oncocytomas?**

Oncocytomas can have a "spoke wheel" appearance on angiography created by the vessels, whereas on CT, the presence of a stellate scar has been reported. Oncocytomas are also sharply demarcated, with no calcification, and isodense with a homogeneous pattern of enhancement.

○ **Can oncocytomas be reliably differentiated from RCC on imaging alone?**

No.

○ **True/False: Oncocytomas occur exclusively in the kidney.**

False. Oncocytomas have also been reported in the parathyroid and thyroid glands, salivary glands, and the adrenal glands.

○ **How common are renal oncocytomas?**

They account for 10% of all renal tumors. They are more common in men with a peak incidence in the 6th to 8th decade. Paraneoplastic syndromes and spontaneous rupture are uncommon. The radiographic differentiation from RCC is difficult.

○ **What is the renal cell type of origin for oncocytomas?**

Intercalated cells of the renal collecting tubules.

○ **True/False: Wilms tumor in adults is typically associated with a better prognosis than presence of Wilms tumor in children.**

False. The prognosis is generally not as good in adults compared to children. Furthermore, adults typically present with a more advanced stage compared to children.

○ **What is the most common malignant tumor observed in a horseshoe kidney?**

RCC followed by Wilms tumor. The incidence of Wilms tumor in horseshoe kidneys, however, is much higher than normal kidneys.

○ **What are classic features for cystic nephroma?**

An uncommon multicystic tumor that is solitary, unilateral, and multilobular. Predilection for middle-aged women, frequently in the upper pole.

○ **Can a cystic nephroma and a cystic RCC be differentiated radiographically?**

No. For this reason, all complex cysts (Bosniak III-IV) should be surgically explored in appropriate surgical candidates.

○ **What is the best way to predict postoperative renal insufficiency in patients undergoing nephrectomy for RCC?**

Probably a combination of creatinine clearance and Technetium-99m-mercaptoacetyltriglycine (Tc-MAG3) renal scintigraphy. A preoperative Tc-MAG3 clearance rate of 130 mL/min/1.73 m^2 has been suggested as a cutoff point in predicting significant renal insufficiency postop.

○ **When is a bone scan clearly indicated in the metastatic workup of patients with RCC?**

In patients with unexplained bone pain or elevated serum alkaline phosphatase levels.

○ **How often are metastases found at the time of initial presentation of RCC?**

Approximately one-third will have metastatic disease when their cancer is first diagnosed. Ten to twenty percent will develop metastases over the subsequent 5 years.

○ **What is the incidence and significance of adrenal metastases in RCC and how does adrenalectomy affect the outcome?**

The incidence of adrenal metastases at the time of nephrectomy for renal cell cancer is just under 4%. Reports indicate that the prognosis for these cases is generally poor regardless of whether or not an adrenalectomy is done. This suggests that there may be little therapeutic benefit in performing a simultaneous adrenalectomy.

○ **During a laparoscopic nephrectomy, the patient develops sudden hypotension and a new "mill-wheel" cardiac murmer is detected. What is the diagnosis and recommended treatment of this condition?**

The patient has developed a gas embolism. The earliest sign of this entity is an extremely rapid and sudden decrease in end-tidal carbon dioxide, which literally happens in a matter of seconds. This is due to the gas embolism blocking the pulmonary outflow from the heart. This is why all laparoscopic cases should be appropriately monitored for carbon dioxide. Severe hypotension, development of the typical mill-wheel cardiac murmer, and a rapid decline in oxygen saturation occur somewhat later and are associated with a poorer prognosis. Treatment involves immediate removal of carbon dioxide gas from the abdomen and placing the patient in a steep left lateral decubitus/Trendelenburg position to minimize any right ventricular outlet obstruction. Central venous catheter aspiration of the gas embolism may be necessary.

○ **Following a partial nephrectomy, a patient develops increased output from their flank drain after their Foley catheter was removed. Analysis of the drain fluid is consistent with urine. How should the patient be managed?**

Urine leak following partial nephrectomy is best managed with Foley catheter drainage. Occasionally, a ureteral stent will also need to be placed to maximize drainage. However, the vast majority of urine leaks heal with these conservative measures. Repeat surgical exploration should not be performed and is associated with the risk of completion nephrectomy.

○ **If renal ischemia is required during a partial nephrectomy, what measure can be performed to decrease renal injury?**

Limit ischemic time, utilization of cold ischemia, adequate hydration, and IV administration of mannitol and furosemide prior to vascular clamping.

○ **Five days following a partial nephrectomy a patient develops gross hematuria, flank pain, and hypotension. What potential postoperative complication must be ruled out?**

Pseudoaneurysm. Vascular disruption and suturing during tumor resection can lead to fusion of arteries and veins creating an arteriovenous fistula. Most cases present with hematuria, pain, hypotension, flank mass, or ecchymosis. Selective angioembolization should be attempted prior to consideration of nephrectomy for treatment.

Renal Tumors, Children

Jessica C. Lloyd, MD and
Jonathan C. Routh, MD, MPH

○ **What is the incidence of Wilms tumor in children in North America?**

Roughly 500 cases of Wilms tumor occur in North America per year, giving an incidence of roughly 8 per 1,000,000. Wilms tumor is the most common malignant pediatric renal tumor, and accounts for 7% of all childhood cancers.

○ **How often are congenital anomalies associated with Wilms tumor?**

Fifteen percent of cases. Congenital anomalies are much more common in patients with bilateral or simultaneous multifocal tumors.

○ **What are the major Wilms tumor study groups?**

In North America, the renal committee of the Children's Oncology Group (COG) is the major cooperative Wilms tumor study group. In Europe, the International Society of Pediatric Oncology (SIOP) is the major cooperative Wilms tumor study group.

○ **What is the relationship of aniridia to Wilms tumor?**

Aniridia is caused by an abnormality of the PAX6 gene located adjacent to WT1, and is seen in 1% of patients with Wilms tumors. Of patients with aniridia, 40% of those having a chromosomal deletion that includes the locus for WT1 will develop Wilms tumor. Conversely, those with a normal WT1 do not develop Wilms tumor.

○ **What genitourinary abnormalities are associated with Wilms tumor?**

Horseshoe kidney and other renal fusion anomalies, renal ectopia, Mullerian duct anomalies, hypospadias, and cryptorchidism have been reported in 5% of cases.

○ **How frequently does hemihypertrophy occur with Wilms tumor?**

Three percent of cases. Hemihypertrophy can be complete, partial, unilateral, or crossed. It is more common in females than males. This is also associated with 11p abnormalities and may occur as isolated hemihypertrophy or in the context of Beckwith–Wiedemann syndrome (BWS).

○   **What skin lesions are associated with Wilms tumor?**

Hemangiomas, cafe au lait spots, neurofibromas, and nevi are seen in 3% of cases.

○   **What is Beckwith–Wiedemann syndrome?**

BWS is a rare congenital overgrowth syndrome defined by macroglossia, anterior abdominal wall defects (ranging from umbilical hernia to omphalocele), visceromegaly (particularly hepatomegaly and nephromegaly), posterior helical indentations (pits of the external ear), neonatal hypoglycemia, and hemihypertrophy. Most cases are sporadic; 15% have autosomal dominant inheritance. BWS is associated with WT2 abnormalities, and 10% of children with BWS will develop a pediatric tumor, usually Wilms tumor, adrenal carcinoma, hepatoblastoma, and/or rhabdomyosarcoma.

○   **What other syndromes are associated with an increased incidence of Wilms tumor?**

Microcephaly, Perlman, Sotos, and Simpson–Golabi–Behmel syndromes, developmental delay, spina bifida, intersex, trisomy 18, mixed gonadal dysgenesis, and nephrotic syndrome.

○   **What is the risk of Wilms tumor development in the following syndromes/conditions: WAGR, Denys–Drash, Perlman, Beckwith–Wiedemann, Simpson–Golabi–Behmel, Li–Fraumeni, Sotos, and neurofibromatosis?**

WAGR: 50%

Denys–Drash: 50%

Perlman: >20%

Beckwith–Wiedemann: 5% to 10%

Simpson–Golabi–Behmel: 10% (in males)

Li–Fraumeni: low

Sotos: low

Neurofibromatosis: low

○   **True/False: No study has recommended screening ultrasound for Wilms tumor.**

False. Screening with serial renal ultrasonography has been recommended for children suffering from conditions that confer a ≥5% chance of developing Wilms tumor. Serial ultrasounds are recommended from the age of diagnosis until 5 years of age, at 3 to 4 month intervals. In children with Beckwith–Wiedemann Syndrome, Simpson–Golabi–Behmel syndrome, and familial Wilms histories, screenings are recommended through age 7 years.

○   **Has a familial basis for Wilms tumor been described?**

Yes, approximately 1% of patients have a positive family history for Wilms tumor. This is thought to be inherited in an autosomal dominant manner, but with variable penetrance. Familial Wilms tumor often presents at an earlier age, with an increased frequency of bilateral disease.

○   **What chromosomal abnormalities have been associated with Wilms tumor?**

Deletions in chromosome 11p13 are most commonly reported. The gene at this locus has been cloned and designated the WT1 tumor suppressor gene. A second Wilms tumor locus, WT2, has been also identified on chromosome 11p15. 20% of Wilms tumor patients have loss of heterozygosity on chromosome 16q and 11% of Wilms tumor patients have loss of heterozygosity on chromosome 1p.

○ **What is the function of the WT1 gene?**

WT1 is important for normal kidney and gonadal development. It encodes a zinc-finger transcription factor that is expressed in the kidneys, gonads, spleen, and mesothelium. WT1 is necessary for ureteric bud outgrowth and is also important in nephrogenesis.

○ **What is WAGR syndrome?**

The WAGR syndrome is seen in children with **W**ilms tumor, **A**niridia, **G**enitourinary malformation, and mental **R**etardation. Most children with WAGR syndrome have a chromosomal deletion on chromosome 11p13. WAGR patients are at high risk of renal failure and of bilateral tumors.

○ **What is Denys–Drash syndrome?**

Denys–Drash is a rare syndrome which consists of the triad of ambiguous genitalia (disorders of sex development, most commonly pure gonadal dysgenesis), nephrotic syndrome (renal or diffuse mesangial sclerosis), and Wilms tumor. It is associated with mutations of the zinc-finger DNA-binding region of WT1 on chromosome 11p13. Children with Denys–Drash are at high risk of end-stage renal disease following treatment for their Wilms tumor.

○ **What is the incidence of bilateral Wilms tumors?**

Bilateral disease occurs in 5% of patients (4% synchronous, 1% metachronous).

○ **Do sporadic, heritable, and bilateral cases of Wilms tumor have varying mean ages of presentation?**

Yes. Bilateral and heritable cases of Wilms tumors present with a mean age of 2.5 years, whereas sporadic cases have a mean age of presentation of 3.5 years.

○ **How common is Wilms tumor in neonates?**

Wilms tumor is rare in the newborn. The more likely solid renal tumor in this age group is congenital mesoblastic nephroma, while the most common solid abdominal tumor is neuroblastoma.

○ **True/False: Wilms tumor occurs most commonly after the age of 6 years.**

False. Fifty percent of patients are 1 to 3 years old, 75% are younger than 5 years, and 98% are younger than 10 years at diagnosis. The peak incidence occurs between 1 and 3 years.

○ **What is the prognostic significance of Wilms tumors occurring in older children?**

Patients presenting at an older age typically have a more advanced tumor that is less responsive to treatment.

○ **What are the common presenting symptoms for patients with Wilms tumors?**

Abdominal mass is most common (90%), followed by hypertension (0%-60%), pain (20%-30%), nausea and vomiting (15%), fever (10%-20%), and gross hematuria (5%-10%).

○ **An acquired von Willebrand disease is observed in what percentage of newly diagnosed Wilms tumor patients?**

In 5% to 10% of patients. All newly diagnosed patients should undergo a coagulation screen with platelet count, bleeding time, prothrombin time, and activated partial thromboplastin time prior to surgery.

○ **What percentage of Wilms tumors have a tumor diameter greater than 5 cm?**

90%.

○ **How frequently does Wilms tumor display venous extension?**

Four percent of patients have a tumor thrombus extending to the renal vein, inferior vena cava, or right atrium.

○ **What are the common sites of metastasis for Wilms tumor?**

The most common site of distant metastasis is the lungs. Pulmonary metastases are present at diagnosis in 8% of patients. The other common site of metastasis is the liver.

○ **What histopathologic features are classically seen with Wilms tumor?**

The gross appearance of the tumor is a fleshy ("brain-like") tan tumor with a pseudocapsule. Hemorrhage or cysts may be present. Microscopically, one will typically see blastemal, stromal, and epithelial elements. Sixty percent of cases will have a predominant component.

○ **What is the most important prognostic indicator in Wilms tumor?**

Unfavorable or anaplastic histology. Unfavorable histology has the most significant prognostic impact when the tumor extends beyond the kidney, that is, in higher-stage tumors. Anaplasia is associated with resistance to chemotherapy.

○ **True/False: Unfavorable histology is most commonly seen in Wilms tumors of patients younger than 2 years of age.**

False. Unfavorable histology (anaplasia) is rare in Wilms tumors presenting in the first 2 years of life.

○ **What is the incidence of unfavorable histology among Wilms tumor patients?**

Unfavorable histology accounts for 5% to 10% of Wilms tumor cases, but is responsible for 50% of Wilms tumor deaths.

○ **What possible precursor lesions have been implicated in Wilms tumor?**

Nephrogenic rests. Precursors to Wilms tumor are found in 25% to 40% of cases. Presence of precursor lesions in one kidney is highly suggestive of precursor lesions in another kidney and, therefore, helps in identifying patients at risk for tumor in the contralateral kidney.

○ **What are nephrogenic rests?**

Clusters of abnormally persistent nephrogenic cells; microscopically, these are not easily distinguished from Wilms tumor. These are thought to be premalignant lesions, although most do not develop into Wilms tumor. They may be classified as perilobar or intralobar.

○ **What is nephroblastomatosis?**

Bilateral, symmetrical enlargement of kidneys characterized by diffuse proliferation of nephrogenic rests.

○ **True/False: A 3-year-old child's CT scan demonstrates a large Wilms tumor in the left kidney with a normal right kidney. Proper management includes left nephrectomy with right renal exploration to exclude occult metastasis or nephroblastomatosis.**

False. Under current guidelines, it is no longer necessary to explore the contralateral kidney if a preoperative fine-cut CT or MRI shows no abnormality.

○ **What clinical scenarios preclude primary surgical excision for Wilms tumor?**

Most patients with bilateral disease, extensive intravascular tumor extension, or tumors that require resection of adjacent organs to complete excision should undergo neoadjuvant chemotherapy, then surgery.

○ **How are bilateral Wilms tumors best treated?**

Give neoadjuvant chemotherapy, with the goal of tumor shrinkage and bilateral renal-sparing surgery.

○ **Is open biopsy necessary to confirm the diagnosis in patients with suspected bilateral Wilms tumor?**

No. In North America, ARENO534, the current Children's Oncology Group protocol, states that children with apparent bilateral Wilms tumor seen on imaging should be given 6 to 12 weeks of vincristine, actinomycin, and doxorubicin. Surgery (nephron-sparing if possible) should be performed no later than week 12. Similar protocols are used in Europe under the guidance of SIOP and various national Wilms tumor networks.

○ **What effect does tumor spillage at the time of surgery have on the local abdominal relapse rate?**

Tumor spillage results in a 6-fold increase in local abdominal relapses.

○ **What is the staging system used for Wilms tumors?**

Stage I—tumor completely confined to kidney and completely excised.

Stage II—tumor extends beyond kidney capsule but is completely removed without spillage.

Stage III—residual abdominal disease: nodes involved, diffuse spillage, peritoneal implants, positive margin, incomplete resection.

Stage IV—hematogenous metastasis.

Stage V—bilateral disease (each side should also be staged).

○ **True/False: In Wilms tumor, the treatment protocol for patients with unfavorable (focal anaplasia) stage I disease is the same as patients with favorable stage II disease.**

True. Both groups of patients should receive 18 weeks of adjuvant actinomycin D and vincristine, without radiotherapy.

○ **What is the preferred approach for radical nephrectomy in the setting of suspected Wilms tumor?**

Transperitoneal approach with selective sampling of lymph nodes. Formal retroperitoneal lymph node dissection is not recommended.

○ **Do primary Wilms tumors appear exclusively in the kidneys?**

No. Extrarenal Wilms tumors have been reported in the retroperitoneum, sacrococcyx, cervix, groin, and gonads. The prognosis of patients with extrarenal Wilms tumors is comparable to patients with intrarenal Wilms tumors. Extrarenal Wilms tumors are thought to arise from displaced metanephric elements or mesonephric remnants.

○ **What chemotherapeutic agents are currently used for Wilms tumor?**

For stage I and II favorable histology tumors, actinomycin and vincristine are used. For stage III and IV favorable histology tumors, doxorubicin is added, along with radiation. For high-stage unfavorable histology tumors, patients will usually receive 5 drugs and radiation: actinomycin, vincristine, doxorubicin, cyclophosphamide, and etoposide.

○ **Are any chemotherapy drugs used for Wilms tumor associated with the development of long-term side effects?**

Doxorubicin is associated with long-term risk of cardiotoxicity. This risk is directly proportional to the dose of doxorubicin used. Roughly 20% of children with Wilms tumor who receive doxorubicin will develop congestive heart failure.

○ **True/False: Second malignancies have not occurred in patients with Wilms tumor.**

False. Sarcomas, adenocarcinomas, lymphomas, and leukemias have all been reported. The incidence of second malignancies at 15 years post-treatment is 1.6% in the National Wilms Tumor Study Group.

○ **True/False: Selected patients with Wilms tumor can be treated with nephrectomy alone.**

True. Very low-risk disease (stage I tumor with favorable histology weighing <550 g, in patients <2 years of age) can be treated with nephrectomy alone.

○ **What factors place patients at an increased risk for second malignancy?**

Prior treatment for relapse, the amount of abdominal radiotherapy, and use of doxorubicin place patients at increased risk for a second malignancy.

○ **Do horseshoe or fused kidneys predispose patients for Wilms tumor?**

Wilms tumor is 2 to 8 times more common in patients with horseshoe or fused kidneys.

○ **True/False: All pediatric renal tumors have a better prognosis when diagnosed at a younger age.**

False. Although the predominant renal tumors of childhood, Wilms tumor, and neuroblastoma, do have a better prognosis when diagnosed at a younger age, this is not true of all tumors. Rhabdoid tumor of the kidney, for example, is associated with a much poorer prognosis when diagnosed in infants.

○ **What pediatric renal tumor is associated with polyhydramnios?**

Congenital mesoblastic nephroma is associated with a maternal history of polyhydramnios; 15% of patients will have other associated congenital abnormalities.

○ **An abdominal ultrasound in a 6-month-old female reveals a right kidney with multiple cysts, appearing like a bunch of grapes, and an atretic right ureter. The left kidney is normal. What is the likely diagnosis and what will a functional renal scan reveal about the right kidney?**

Multicystic dysplastic right kidney. Renal scan will likely reveal a nonfunctioning right kidney.

○ **What are the most common urologic abnormalities seen with multicystic dysplastic kidney (MCDK)? What test should be obtained for these patients?**

Contralateral vesicoureteral reflux (~30%) and ureteropelvic junction obstruction (~10%) can be seen in MCDK patients; voiding cystourethrogram (VCUG) should therefore be obtained.

○ **What are the most common cystic renal tumors in children?**

Multicystic dysplastic kidney, cystic Wilms tumor, and multilocular cystic nephroma.

○ **What cystic renal tumor commonly occurs in both young males and young adult women?**

Multilocular cystic nephroma. This benign renal tumor is cured by nephrectomy. Gross pathology reveals a well-encapsulated multilocular tumor composed of varying-sized cysts compressing the surrounding renal parenchyma. Only mature cell types are seen within the septa of the cyst walls.

○ **A 12-year-old boy presents with diastolic hypertension and hypokalemia. He has a 3.0-cm renal mass on CT scan. What laboratory tests should be obtained?**

Serum renin level. The suspected diagnosis is a juxtaglomerular tumor and serum renin levels would be elevated.

○ **True/False: By definition, patients with juxtaglomerular tumors have primary hyperaldosteronism.**

False. Juxtaglomerular tumors secrete renin, which causes profound hypertension and *secondary* hyperaldosteronism.

○ **A 16-year-old girl with Klippel–Trenaunay syndrome presents with hematuria. What diagnosis should especially be considered?**

Renal hemangioma. Renal hemangiomas have been reported in the cortex, medulla, or renal pelvis. Most are small, single lesions and 50% are below the limits of radiologic detection. Symptomatic lesions appear more commonly in adults often with hematuria, which may become massive.

○ **A 9-year-old girl has microscopic hematuria and a honeycombed peripelvic renal mass noted on abdominal CT. What is the most likely diagnosis?**

The appearance of a honeycombed mass in a peripelvic location is most consistent with a lymphangioma. About one-third of lymphangiomas have been reported to occur in children.

○ **What tumor is referred to as the bone-metastasizing renal tumor of childhood?**

Clear cell sarcomas. The other tumor to consider in the setting of a child with a bony metastasis and a primary renal tumor is renal cell carcinoma.

○ **What are the most common solid renal tumors at the following ages: 1 month, 3 years, 10 years, and 18 years?**

At 1 month, congenital mesoblastic nephroma; at 3 years, favorable histology Wilms tumor; at 10 years, Wilms tumor and renal cell carcinoma are equally likely; and at 18 years, renal cell carcinoma.

○ **How do clear cell sarcomas differ from Wilms tumors?**

These tumors have a significant component of clear cells, predilection for bone and brain involvement, and a poor prognosis. They represent 5% of all pediatric renal tumors and 50% present before 2 years of age.

○ **True/False: The majority of clear cell sarcomas have bone metastases.**

False. Despite its nickname, clear cell sarcoma has bone metastasis in only 15% to 20% of cases.

○ **Have rhabdoid tumors of the kidney been reported in conjunction with brain tumors?**

Yes, rhabdoid tumors have coexisted with medulloblastoma and other intracranial neoplasms and have been known to metastasize to the brain. The other renal tumor with propensity for brain metastasis is clear cell sarcoma. Patients with either diagnosis should have a brain MRI or CT performed in the early postoperative period.

○ **What are typical survival rates for patients with favorable and unfavorable Wilms tumor, clear cell sarcoma, and rhabdoid tumor of the kidney?**

Four-year survival rates for these tumors are 90%, 70%, 75%, and 25%, respectively.

○ **A 2-month-old boy has a unilateral renal mass. What renal tumor is most commonly the cause?**

Congenital mesoblastic nephroma. More common in boys, it is effectively treated with nephrectomy.

○ **Microscopically, congenital mesoblastic nephroma resembles what other types of tumors?**

Congenital mesoblastic nephroma demonstrates 3 histological subtypes: classical, cellular, and mixed. The classical subtype, with interlacing sheets of bland spindle cells, resembles infantile fibromatosis. The cellular variant, with a solid, sheet-like growth pattern and frequent mitoses, resembles congenital fibrosarcoma. On gross pathology, this lesion has the yellowish-gray appearance of leiomyoma.

○ **What are the typical characteristics of RCC in children?**

RCC accounts for only 3% to 5% of renal tumors in children. The tumors typically present above 10 years of age, most commonly with an abdominal mass. No sex predilection exists. Survival for RCC in children is worse than Wilms tumor survival.

○ **What is a translocation carcinoma?**

A solid renal mass found in preteen children, often following treatment for neuroblastoma or Wilms tumor. Histologically, this appears similar to papillary renal cell carcinoma, but has a distinct genetic abnormality: translocation of chromosome 17 to chromosome X. Lymph node involvement by translocation carcinoma appears to have a fair prognosis, although hematogenous metastasis remains prognostically grim.

○ **A 13-year-old boy with sickle cell trait is found to have a renal mass with multiple pulmonary nodules. What is the likely diagnosis?**

Medullary renal cell carcinoma is found in patients with sickle cell hemoglobinopathy and is highly lethal. Mean age at diagnosis is 13 years.

○ **True/False: All cases of angiomyolipoma reported in children have been associated with tuberous sclerosis.**

False. While angiomyolipoma is a very rare tumor in children, cases have been reported without features of tuberous sclerosis.

○ **What are the distinctive pathological features of Wilms tumor?**

Pathologically, Wilms tumor is characterized as a triphasic tumor with 3 distinct patterns. There is an epithelial component, a stromal element, and a blastemal component, although biphasic or monophasic tumors can occur.

○ **What is the significance of elevated urinary catecholamines in the evaluation of childhood neoplasms?**

Urinary homovanillic acid (HMA) or vanillylmandelic acid (VMA) is elevated in over 90% of patients with neuroblastoma. There is an inverse relationship between the VMA/HMA ratio and survival in disseminated disease.

○ **What is the most common extracranial solid tumor in children?**

Neuroblastoma, which accounts for 10% of all childhood cancers.

○ **What molecular and genetic markers are important in neuroblastoma?**

MYCN amplification is associated with a less favorable prognosis, as are elevated levels of neuron-specific enolase, ferritin, and chromosome 1p deletion. Tumor DNA aneuploidy is associated with a more favorable prognosis.

○ **At what age is Wilms tumor more common than neuroblastoma?**

Wilms tumor is more common than neuroblastoma in children older than 2 years of age. Younger children are more likely to have neuroblastoma or another primary renal tumor.

○ **Bright blue nodules are found subcutaneously in a newborn. What problem does this suggest?**

Possible disseminated neuroblastoma. Particularly in a newborn, this may represent Stage IV-S neuroblastoma, a distinct staging category, referring to infants with a small primary tumor and liver, skin, or bone marrow metastases without radiographic evidence of bone metastases. Stage IV-S neuroblastoma carries a good prognosis, with survival ranging upward of 80%.

○ **What is the significance of stippled calcifications noted in a solid retroperitoneal mass?**

Approximately 50% of neuroblastomas have such stippling. These can help distinguish neuroblastoma from Wilms tumor.

○ **True/False: When hypertension appears in the setting of neuroblastoma, mass effect on the renal vessels is the most common underlying etiology.**

True. Often, the tumor will compress the renal vessels, activating the renin–angiotensin–aldosterone axis, leading to hypertension. Rarely is hypertension related to the direct effect of catecholamines secreted by the tumor.

○ **A newborn presents with an abdominal mass and hematuria. What diagnosis does this suggest, what causes it, and how is it treated?**

Renal vein thrombosis. This is usually due to a hypercoagulable state or reduced intravascular volume such as from dehydration or infection. Renal vein thrombosis is usually unilateral and treatment generally involves only supportive measures. Thrombolytic therapy and/or anticoagulants are generally used only when there is vena caval or bilateral involvement.

○ **Are the kidneys usually palpable in normal neonates?**

Yes, both kidneys can usually be palpated.

○ **Turner syndrome is associated with what urologic abnormality?**

Horseshoe kidney is more common in patients with Turner syndrome (and, like all children with horseshoe kidney, children with Turner syndrome and horseshoe kidney are also at an increased risk of Wilms tumor).

CHAPTER 39

Renal/Ureteral Stone Surgery

Derek Prabharasuth, MD, Andrew I. Fishman, MD, and Michael Grasso III, MD

○ **What are the most common renal stones in North America and their percentages?**

Calcium stones (calcium oxalate, calcium phosphate, mixed) account for approximately 70% of stones in the United States, while infection stones account for 15% to 20%. Uric acid stones make up 5% to 10% and cystine stones 1% to 5% of stones diagnosed in this country.

○ **What are the ingredients of "triple phosphate" stones?**

Triple phosphate stones are composed of calcium, magnesium, and ammonium phosphate.

○ **Which stones are associated with laxative abuse?**

Ammonium acid urate stones.

○ **Which stones are most dense on plain radiograph?**

Calcium hydrogen phosphate stones (brushite), followed by calcium oxalate monohydrate.

○ **Which stones are radiolucent on plain radiography?**

Uric acid, sodium urate, ammonium acid urate, xanthine stones, 2,8-dihydroxyadenine (rare), matrix, and indinavir stones are all radiolucent on plain radiography.

○ **Which of these stones cannot be seen on CT scan without IV contrast?**

Indinavir (Crixivan) is a protease inhibitor used for treatment in HIV patients, which cause stone formation. Indinavir can obstruct the ureter as a precipitate or as a pasty sludge. This type of stone is most commonly diagnosed endoscopically. If there is suspicion of a kidney stone and the patient is taking protease inhibitor drugs such as indinavir, an intravenous pyelogram (IVP) would be a better choice for a confirmatory imaging study.

○ **Do all cystinuric patients produce kidney stones?**

No. Cystinuria is an inherited disorder of renal tubular reabsorption of cystine, ornithine, lysine, and arginine. These 4 amino acids can be remembered by the mnemonic COLA. Of these 4, only cystine is relatively insoluble in urine and will precipitate to form stones. Patients with 24-hour urine cystine levels less than 400 mg/day rarely produce stones, while those with elevated levels over 1000 mg/day will produce large stone fragments unless treated medically.

○ **What are the most common specific medications used as medical therapy for cystinuria and their most frequent complications?**

Thiola and D-penicillamine are the 2 agents that are commonly used to treat cystinuria. Both agents act on the disulfide bond creating a more soluble compound. Patients on these agents require 24-hour urine protein collections to rule out nephrotic syndrome, which is often reversible when the medications are stopped. Goal of therapy is to titrate the medications until 24-hour cystine excretion is 250 mg or less. Nephrotic syndrome, dermatitis, and pancytopenia are more common with D-penicillamine, while asthenia, gastrointestinal (GI) distress, rashes, joint aches, and mental status changes are more common with Thiola.

○ **What other treatments are available for cystinuria?**

Initial therapy includes a high fluid intake sufficient to generate 3000 mL of urine per day or more. Cystine solubility rises when the urine pH increases so alkalinization therapy with potassium citrate is recommended although substantial alkalinization is difficult to maintain and overalkalinization can lead to calcium phosphate. Sodium intake restrictions are also helpful.

○ **Which gas is produced by Holmium: YAG laser lithotripsy of cystine stones?**

A malodorous sulfur dioxide gas is given off during laser lithotripsy of cystine stones.

○ **What are the 4 common components of ESWL?**

Energy source to produce shockwave, focusing device, coupling medium, and stone localization system.

○ **Which geometric principle is the basis for most ESWL generators?**

The first ESWL generator employed clinically was the Dornier HM3. This device employs a sparking electrode (electrohydraulic generator) to generate spherically shaped shock waves at the origin site (termed F1). The firing of this electrode creates shock waves that are focused by an ellipsoid focusing device to the site of the kidney stone (F2 position). Newer types of shock wave generators such as the piezoelectric and electromagnetic generators utilize nonspherically shaped shock waves with different coupling mediums and shapes.

○ **What are the main clinical differences in newer generation lithotripters compared to the original nonmodified electrohydraulic lithotripter?**

Newer second and third generation lithotripters sometimes employ wider apertures to spread the delivering energy over a greater surface area of the body, thereby limiting cutaneous pain. However, this increased aperture also narrows the focal treatment field leading to a lower stone-free rate in some of the newer models.

○ **What are the factors that limit success with ESWL therapy?**

Large stone burdens (size and number), stone composition, stone location, and clinical features such as body habitus and obesity are all factors that limit the stone clearance rate. A slower ESWL rate (60-90 shocks/min), pretreatment with 250 to 300 low energy shockwaves, good coupling, and general anesthesia also help improve the efficiency of the shock wave therapy. Using a single, large dollop of gel has been shown to leave fewer air gaps than other methods and is now the preferred way to place the coupling gel.

○ **Which stones are most resistant to ESWL therapy?**

Cystine stones are most resistant, followed by brushite stones, and then calcium oxalate monohydrate stones. Calcium oxalate dyhydrate are the most brittle.

○ **Stones in which position are the most difficult to fragment with ESWL—proximal, mid, or distal ureteral stones?**

Midureteral calculi, especially those located between the level of the inferior and superior margin of the sacroiliac joint are hardest to approach with ESWL. The patient is positioned prone and the stone may be difficult to visualize/localize against the background of the pelvic bones with current imaging. Only a few ESWL machines allow the treatment head to be rotated 180° so the patient can remain prone even with stones over the sacrum.

○ **What are the 2 absolute contraindications to ESWL?**

Pregnancy and uncorrected coagulopathy.

○ **What is "steinstrasse"?**

Steinstrasse, meaning "stone street" in German, refers to a column of stone fragments that may line up in the ureter following ESWL. This may lead to symptoms of obstruction.

○ **How is steinstrasse treated?**

In mild cases, observation alone may be enough. Double pigtail catheters, ESWL, and ureteroscopy are other available options. In cases of sepsis secondary to steinstrasse, percutaneous nephrostomy should be considered first line therapy.

○ **What is the most common clinically significant acute complication of ESWL therapy?**

Subcapsular hematoma formation. Patients with uncontrolled hypertension (HTN) are believed to be at greatest risk.

○ **What is the most common, serious long-term complication associated with ESWL?**

Increased risk for HTN.

○ **Which medications have been shown to help facilitate stone passage rates?**

Tamsulosin (Flomax), nifedipine, and corticosteroids can improve stone passage from the distal ureter by approximately 30%. Other α-blockers also increase spontaneous passage. Such treatment is called "medical expulsive therapy."

○ **What is the most important factor in predicting spontaneous stone passage?**

Stone size. If 4 mm or less, 90% will pass spontaneously.

○ **A patient presents with flank pain. Laboratory work is normal. CT shows a 4-mm distal ureteral stone with hydronephrosis and forniceal extravasation. Is surgical intervention always indicated?**

No. Given the small size, a trial of spontaneous passage is warranted. Forniceal extravasation is noted to occur more frequently in small, obstructing stones, and is not always an indication for surgery by itself.

○ **What are the 3 areas of functional narrowing of the ureter?**

The ureteropelvic junction (UPJ) is the proximal site of narrowing, followed by the level at which the ureter traverses the iliac vessels, and finally the ureterovesical junction.

○ **Which of these areas is most often the narrowest point in the ureter?**

The intramural segment at the ureterovesical junction.

○ **What are the 2 major complications associated with ureteropyeloscopy and what is their frequency?**

The 2 major complications are acute, intraoperative ureteral wall perforation or avulsion and postoperative ureteral strictures. In the largest series, this complication rate occurred less than 0.5%.

○ **Which portion of the ureter is the most common location for ureteral avulsion during ureteroscopy?**

The proximal one-third of the ureter is the most common site for ureteral avulsion secondary to the thin muscularis layer.

○ **What is the next step in treatment if a ureteral avulsion is encountered?**

Prompt proximal drainage, most often performed with a percutaneous nephrostomy tube, with subsequent delayed repair.

○ **What are the indications for hospitalization in a patient with a ureteral calculus?**

The following are indications for hospitalization and/or treatment: intractable pain requiring continuing parenteral analgesics, severe colic and/or intractable nausea and vomiting with dehydration, fever, leukocytosis, or bacteriuria, a stone in a solitary kidney, simultaneous bilateral ureteral stones with obstruction, complete obstruction of the kidney which is not transient, and azotemia.

○ **What are the different types of endoscopic lithotripters?**

Electrohydraulic, ultrasonic, laser, and ballistic.

○ **What endoscopic instrument is required for retrograde treatment of a lower pole calculus?**

Actively deflectable, flexible ureteropyeloscopes are essential in treating intrarenal stones, particularly those in the lower pole. Active endoscopic tip deflection facilitates placement of laser fibers and extractors (eg, baskets and graspers). The application of a semirigid ureteroscope in treating intrarenal stones is limited.

○ **Laser lithotripsy of uric acid stones produces which toxic chemical?**

Cyanide.

○ **True/False: Blind basketing of ureteral calculi is an acceptable method of extracting ureteral stones.**

False. With the advent of ureteroscopic lithotripsy, blind basketing has been completely abandoned. Stone extraction with force using this method often results in severe tissue trauma, and a stone could occasionally be engaged within a basket that subsequently could not be safely extracted from the ureter resulting in an adverse situation.

○ **What is the potential consequence of a submucosal stone?**

A stone granuloma may form; this may lead to a ureteral stricture.

○ **What is the incidence of symptomatic urinary calculi in pregnancy?**

The incidence has been estimated at 1 in 1500 pregnancies.

○ **True/False: The incidence of urinary stone formation is higher among pregnant women.**

False. Elevated urinary citrate levels are a protective mechanism correcting for the significant hypercalciuria associated with pregnancy.

○ **Which imaging modality should be considered first line in the diagnosis of nephrolithiasis in the pregnant patient?**

Ultrasound, given that there is no associated risk of radiation to the fetus. Resistive indices >0.7, documentation of ureteral jets, and transvaginal ultrasound can help improve detection rates.

○ **What is physiologic hydronephrosis and on which side is it more commonly found?**

Physiologic hydronephrosis is a physiologic phenomenon that occurs during pregnancy secondary to compression of the ureter by the uterus. It is more common on the right, begins around 6 to 10 weeks of gestation, and may not resolve until 6 weeks after pregnancy.

○ **What happens to GFR and renal plasma flow during pregnancy?**

GFR and renal plasma flow increase during pregnancy leading to a decrease in serum BUN and creatinine.

○ **What are the indications for urologic intervention of symptomatic ureteral calculi in the pregnant woman?**

Severe intractable pain, urosepsis, and obstruction of a solitary kidney with azotemia are all well-established indications for intervention. Ureteral stenting and percutaneous nephrostomy may be placed for stones that are unlikely to pass spontaneously with definitive stone management deferred until after pregnancy. Percutaneous drainage is less favored due to patient discomfort and bacterial colonization. Ureteral stent changes should occur every 4 to 8 weeks to avoid encrustation.

○ **What factors affect the success of endoincision for ureteral strictures?**

Long stricture length >2 cm, periureteral fibrosis (eg, secondary to endometrioma, idiopathic retroperitoneal fibrosis, etc), and a history of prior abdominal radiation are all factors that negatively affect the success of endoincision of a ureteral stricture.

○ **What is Dietl crisis?**

Flank pain that occurs or is exacerbated by increased fluid intake or a diuretic effect from ingestion of fluids such as alcohol. This is often associated with UPJ obstruction.

○ **What is a struvite stone?**

A struvite stone is an infectious stone caused by urea-splitting bacteria (*Proteus*, *Pseudomonas*, and *Klebsiella* are common examples). A struvite stone comprises a mixture of magnesium ammonium phosphate and carbonate apatite.

○ **Which bacteria never forms a struvite stone?**

Escherichia coli never forms struvite stones since it is unable to manufacture urease to make the urine consistently alkaline.

○ **A patient has multiple recurrent urinary tract infections (UTIs), all showing *Proteus*. In addition to antibiotics, what additional work-up is warranted?**

Given the strong association between *Proteus* infections and struvite stones, a noncontrast CT should be obtained to rule out an offending staghorn calculus. A renal ultrasound and a KUB are reasonable alternatives to a CT for this purpose as they would be less expensive and have reduced radiation exposure.

○ **Can struvite stones form in acidic urine?**

No, they cannot. An alkaline urine of pH >7.0 is necessary.

○ **What is the consequence of an untreated staghorn struvite calculus?**

Over time, an untreated staghorn calculus has a significant chance of causing death (~28%) due to renal failure or sepsis. As such, the American Urological Association Nephrolithiasis Clinical Guidelines panel recommends that newly diagnosed struvite staghorn calculi be treated actively rather than be followed conservatively and observed.

○ **How are staghorn calculi removed?**

Anatrophic nephrolithotomy is effective but rarely performed today. Percutaneous nephrolithotomy (PCNL) is considered the standard of care as it is associated with lower transfusion rates, shorter hospital stays, and shorter procedure times. Other modalities, including shock wave lithotripsy, can be used adjunctively.

○ **What is "sandwich therapy?"**

Combination of SWL and PCNL.

○ **Does "sandwich therapy" lead to a greater stone-free rate compared to PCNL monotherapy?**

No, PCNL monotherapy has higher stone-free rates than combination therapy and also requires a total lower number of procedures performed compared to combination therapy. Additionally, if combination therapy is employed, PCNL should be the last interventional modality as it allows direct visualization of residual stone fragments and a higher chance for stone-free status.

○ **What is the indication for treating large intrarenal stones ureteroscopically?**

Metabolic noninfectious stones can be treated successfully using retrograde ureteroscopic techniques. When stone burdens exceed 2.5 cm, staged therapy is commonly necessary. In patients where PCNL is contraindicated such as certain ectopic kidneys, ureteroscopy offers an alternative treatment modality.

○ **True/False: Percutaneous nephrostomy tracts should always be placed through anterior calyces.**

False. The posterior approach is preferred except in special circumstances. The anterior approach has a higher risk of bowel injury.

○ **Why should one avoid placing a percutaneous nephrostomy tube directly into the renal pelvis?**

A direct approach to the renal pelvis may injure the renal hilar vessels. Entry into the collecting system should be through a posteriorly located fornix. Additionally, a pyelotomy tract closes slower than a nephrostomy tract, and is associated with greater urinary leakage postoperatively.

○ **What is the transfusion rate following percutaneous nephrostomy?**

Recent studies show transfusion rates <1%.

○ **What are the risk factors for pneumothorax with PCNL?**

Supracostal access has a higher risk of pneumothorax and hydrothorax. It is approximately 10% over the 12th rib, but can approach approximately 50% over the 11th rib. Treatment is based on thoracentesis and/or placement of a small caliber thoracostomy tube.

○ **What are the different methods available to dilate a nephrostomy tract?**

Balloon dilatation (employed with a hydronephrotic system), Amplatz dilators (employed commonly with a branching stone), and metal telescoping dilators (employed when there is significant retroperitoneal fibrosis from prior renal surgery) are the commonly used methods.

○ **What are the common causes of delayed bleeding following PCNL?**

This complication, which occurs in less than 1% of patients, is usually secondary to pseudoaneurysm formation or an arteriovenous fistula.

○ **What is the most common postoperative complication following PCNL for a staghorn calculus?**

Fever from urinary extravasation and/or atelectasis.

○ **During placement of a nephrostomy tube during PCNL, fluoroscopy confirms placement of the nephrostomy tube through the colon and into the collecting system. What is the next step?**

Urinary diversion with ureteral stent, withdrawal of the nephrostomy tube into the GI tract to allow fecal diversion, and closure of the nephrocolic fistula. If delayed imaging confirms closure of the fistula, the nephrostomy tube can be removed.

○ **What is tubeless PCNL?**

PCNL without percutaneous drainage after the procedure. In most cases, a ureteral stent is used for antegrade drainage and a pro-sealant is used for closure of the nephrostomy tract.

○ **What are contraindications for tubeless PCNL?**

Large volume disease, traumatic access, multiple access attempts, hemorrhage, perforation, and obstruction.

○ **Which calculi are the least amenable to chemolysis?**

Calcium oxalate stones, the most common of all renal calculi, are the least amenable to chemolysis.

○ **Which electrolyte must be monitored closely when using Renacidin chemolysis?**

Magnesium levels. Hypermagnesemia, although occurring mainly in those with severe renal impairment, may also occur in those with normal renal function. Mucosal erosions, UTIs, and elevated intrarenal irrigation pressures may contribute to elevated serum magnesium levels.

○ **Exactly how big is 3 French?**

3 French = 1 mm = 0.038 inch.

○ **How does one differentiate between a calyceal diverticulum and a hydrocalyx?**

Calyceal diverticula are considered to be congenital in origin and arise from a fornix of a minor calyx. A hydrocalyx is considered to be an acquired condition secondary to infundibular stenosis caused by various conditions (TB, stones, prior surgery, inflammation). Renal papillae are present within and diagnostic of a hydrocalyx. A calyceal diverticulum will not have a renal papilla inside it but will be lined only by transitional epithelium.

○ **What is the optimal recommended treatment for a severely septic patient with pyonephrosis?**

Prompt percutaneous nephrostomy drainage, which can usually be done with only a local anesthetic. Depending on the consistency of the infected fluid, a larger-caliber catheter may be required. A retrograde catheter can also be placed but usually requires anesthesia and is more difficult to irrigate if it becomes obstructed by thick inspissated material.

○ **What nonkinking flexible metal is the preferred component of guidewires and baskets?**

Nitinol (nickel–titanium alloy) is a strong but flexible metal, which is the preferred component for ureteroscopic access guidewires. The Terumo guidewire is the premier ureteral access wire. This lubricious and flexible guidewire is commonly employed with ureteral strictures and impacted stones.

For flexible ureteroscopic access, the Teflon-jacketed nitinol-based zebra wire is commonly employed by many urologists. Stainless steel Segura baskets have been largely replaced for renal stone extraction by tipless nitinol designs. In the ureter, a small net-like basket called the "Escape" is carved out of a single nitinol wire and is small enough that a laser fiber can also be used alongside it.

○ **What are the standard stone basket types along with their relative individual strengths and weaknesses?**

The Dormia basket is the standard, symmetrical, spiral wire design. It is effective but usually requires a twisting motion to encompass the stone. A double wire design is also available that increases the radial, spreading force while keeping the space between wires relatively open.

The Segura type basket uses 4 flat wires arranged in a symmetrical fashion. It cannot be twisted or safely turned, but has good radial spreading force that is useful in narrowed ureters or in tight quarters. Newer models have rounded edges on the flat wires.

The Leslie type baskets use an asymmetrical design that works something like a net. Two distal base pillars split into a 4- or 8-wire net. The open "front" allows for easy entry of stones while the "back" prevents distal migration of the stone. Essentially the basket works like a net. These designs work best when the proximal ureter is somewhat dilated so they can fully deploy. They also work well as a backstop when using intracorporeal lithotripsy to prevent proximal migration of larger stone fragments. To do this, the basket is opened above the stone before starting lithotripsy. The stainless steel "Parachute" and the popular nitinol "Escape" baskets are examples of this design.

○ **Which patients should undergo metabolic testing after passing a first stone?**

In general, patients who have their first episode of renal colic without significant underlying diseases do not require an extensive metabolic workup. A stone chemical analysis, urinalysis, and serum electrolytes including phosphate, calcium, uric acid, and alkaline phosphatase should be performed. Those considered high risk (patients with bowel disease, gout, renal tubular acidosis, staghorn stones, cystine stones, metabolic bone disease, or pediatric stone formers) or those who have had recurrent stone formation should have a more extensive workup including 24-hour urine studies. Some will recommend 24-hour urine testing in any stone patient who is strongly motivated to follow long-term treatments to prevent future stones.

○ **Is ureteral dilation always required for ureteroscopic access?**

No, with less than 8-French semirigid and flexible ureteroscopes, the need to dilate the intramural tunnel for access is low (<5%). As a general rule, dilators up to 12 French are preferred in this setting and cause the least ureteral trauma.

○ **When is open surgery indicated for intrarenal calculi?**

In cases with large intrarenal stones and/or multiple infundibular stenosis, where an excessive number of access tracts would be required, anatrophic nephrolithotomy is indicated. This open procedure also facilitates infundibuloplasty that is key to intrarenal drainage.

○ **What are the indications for laparoscopic pyelolithotomy or ureteral lithotomy?**

Patients who failed prior endoscopic treatments can be treated laparoscopically. In addition, those patients who have renal or ureteral stones and are going to undergo laparoscopic reconstruction such as pyeloplasty can have them both treated simultaneously.

○ **What is the indication for a laparoscopic or open nephrectomy in a patient with a large staghorn calculus?**

Xanthogranulomatous pyelonephritis (XGP) is characterized by a large, obstructing stone with resultant infection and destruction of the renal unit. Diagnosis is confirmed pathologically by the presence of foamy macrophages. Laparoscopic, robotic, or open nephrectomy is indicated in this setting although rare, anecdotal cases of percutaneous drainage have been reported in patients judged unfit for surgery.

○   **What is the most commonly used double-J stent length?**

26 cm is the most commonly used length.

○   **How can the ureteral length be measured?**

The ureteral length can be estimated from a retrograde pyelogram directly. Once a measurement is done, subtract 10% to offset the usual x-ray magnification effect.

If this is not possible, the length can be measured directly. An open-ended ureteral catheter can be placed over a guide wire with the tip at the UPJ and confirmed on fluoroscopy. The ureteral length can then be measured by identifying the centimeter markings on the catheter.

TCC of the Upper Urinary Tracts

Thomas W. Jarrett, MD

○ **What is the mean age of occurrence of transitional cell cancer of the upper urinary tracts?**

65 years.

○ **What is Balkan nephropathy?**

A degenerative interstitial nephropathy common to certain rural Balkan areas. Affected individuals are 100 to 200 times more susceptible to upper tract transitional cell carcinoma (TCC). Tumors tend to be low grade, multiple, and bilateral.

○ **What is the most common presenting sign of upper tract urothelial tumors?**

Hematuria is seen in 75% of cases followed by flank pain in 30% of cases. Rarely do upper tract tumors remain asymptomatic.

○ **What percentage of urothelial tumors are located in the upper urinary tract?**

Approximately 5% to 8% of all urothelial tumors are located in the ureter and/or renal collecting system.

○ **What percentage of primary renal tumors will be of urothelial origin?**

Five percent of primary renal tumors will be of urothelial origin.

○ **What histology is most commonly found with urothelial tumors of the upper urinary tract?**

TCC accounts for more than 90% of upper tract urothelial tumors. Squamous cell and adenocarcinoma make up the majority of the remaining tumors.

○ **What are some of the tumor markers reported for upper tract tumors?**

These include cyclooxygenase 2, EP4 receptors, oncoprotein p53, proliferation marker Ki67, and tissue inhibitor of metalloproteinase I. p53 over expression tends to correlate with tumor progression.

○ **What are acceptable ways of making the diagnosis of upper urinary tract TCC?**

Diagnosis was traditionally made by the characteristic radiolucent filling defect of the upper urinary tract as well as cytologic evaluation of the urine. In some cases, sonography or cross-sectional imaging may be necessary to rule out a radiolucent stone as the cause of a filling defect. With improvements in upper urinary tract endoscopy, ureteroscopy with biopsy should be strongly considered in all patients to confirm the diagnosis.

○ **Are there any limitations of ureteroscopic biopsy?**

Ureteroscopic biopsy has a high correlation with final tumor grade but does not accurately diagnose tumor stage.

○ **What other histologic patterns are found with upper tract tumors?**

Squamous cell carcinoma and adenocarcinoma are less commonly seen and are usually associated with chronic inflammation from kidney stones, obstruction, and/or infection.

○ **What is the most common risk factor contributing to the development of upper urinary tract TCC?**

Cigarette smoking is the risk factor most strongly associated with transitional cell carcinoma of the bladder and upper urinary tracts. The risk increases 3-fold in a patient with a history of significant tobacco abuse when compared to the general population.

○ **What are some other risk factors for upper tract TCC?**

Exposure to cyclophosphamide, phenacetin, arsenic, and various aromatic amines and amides.

○ **What is acrolein?**

A metabolic breakdown product of cyclophosphamide. It is thought to be the causative agent in the development of TCC.

○ **True/False: Tumors linked to chemotherapy use tend to be high grade.**

True.

○ **What is Lynch syndrome II?**

An autosomal dominant hereditary syndrome involving upper urinary tract tumors and early colon tumors.

○ **What is the incidence of a bilateral upper tract involvement (either synchronous or metachronous)?**

Approximately 2% to 5% of patients with upper tract TCC will have involvement of the contralateral system at some point in their lives. The percentage may be higher in patients with associated carcinoma in situ (CIS).

○ **How is bilateral disease treated?**

Renal-sparing surgeries are recommended when possible. These techniques include ureteroscopic, percutaneous, and segmental resections. Rarely, autotransplantation and pyleoneocystostomy may be necessary.

○ **What percentage of patients who initially present with TCC of the bladder will subsequently develop a tumor of the upper urinary tract?**

Upper urinary tract cancer occurs in 2% to 4% of patients with bladder cancer.

○ **What percentage of patients who initially present with TCC of the upper urinary tract will subsequently develop a bladder tumor?**

Approximately 50% of upper urinary tract TCC patients will develop bladder tumors at some point in their lives. This necessitates vigilant lifetime bladder surveillance in all patients with upper urinary tract tumors.

○ **What are the 2 most clinically important prognostic variables?**

Tumor grade and stage are the most important prognostic indicators. All studies have shown that the prognosis significantly worsens with higher grade and stage lesions.

○ **What is the incidence of multifocality with upper tract TCC?**

Multifocality is seen in approximately one-third of patients and is directly related to tumor grade.

○ **Are tumor grade and stage related?**

Tumor grade and stage are matched in the vast majority of cases. It is quite rare for a low-grade lesion to show potential for invasion and/or metastasis. The opposite is true for high-grade lesions.

○ **What percentage of upper tract TCC presents with metastatic disease?**

19% of patients present with metastatic disease. In general, upper tract TCC is associated with a poor prognosis.

○ **What is the pattern of spread for upper tract TCC?**

TCC of the upper urinary tract can spread by direct extension, lymphatic invasion, and/or vascular invasion.

○ **What is the traditional treatment of organ-confined TCC of the upper urinary tract?**

The propensity of upper tract TCC toward multifocality and ipsilateral recurrence has led to ipsilateral nephroureterectomy with a bladder cuff as the best treatment for reducing the risks of disease recurrence and progression.

○ **When can distal ureterectomy be considered?**

Distal ureterectomy with ureteroneocystostomy may be considered for solitary low-grade lesions of the distal ureter. Exceptions to this rule are patients who may be at risk for renal failure and hemodialysis following removal of a renal unit. Examples include patients with solitary kidneys, bilateral disease, chronic renal insufficiency, and/or other risk factors for renal failure. In such cases, the risks of long-term hemodialysis may be greater than the risks of the disease itself and an organ-sparing approach should be considered.

○ **What surgical approaches may be used for total nephroureterectomy?**

Nephroureterectomy requires surgical exposure of the kidney and bladder. This requires either a single midline or thoraco-abdominal incision or a 2-incision approach: flank and lower abdomen. Laparoscopic techniques have recently been incorporated to reduce the morbidity of the procedure.

○ **What are the advantages of a laparoscopic approach for total nephroureterectomy?**

Total laparoscopic, robotic-assisted laparoscopic, and laparoscopic-assisted procedures have been reported. Advantages include decreased blood loss, decreased postoperative pain, fewer convalescent days, and shorter hospital stays.

○ **Are there differences in oncologic outcomes between laparoscopic and traditional open approaches?**

No, both demonstrate equivalent cancer outcomes.

○ **What is the role of lymphadenectomy?**

Lymphadenectomy should be considered in all patients with high-grade and/or invasive lesions. It traditionally was performed for staging purposes, although there may be some therapeutic value based on studies with bladder TCC.

○ **What organ-sparing alternatives to nephroureterectomy are available in the treatment of localized TCC of the upper urinary tract?**

Open local excision and endoscopic resection are established alternatives to nephroureterectomy.

○ **What endoscopic techniques are acceptable for the treatment of upper urinary tract TCC?**

Endoscopic therapy can be performed in a retrograde ureteroscopic fashion or an antegrade percutaneous fashion. Rarely, a combined approach is necessary.

○ **Are patients with a normal contralateral kidney candidates for organ-sparing therapy?**

This is a controversial area of urologic oncology; however, it is generally accepted that patients with low-grade and low-stage TCC are at low risk for disease progression. A careful clinical correlation of cytology, pathology, imaging, and endoscopic findings is needed for decision making. Organ-sparing therapy is acceptable provided that the patient is compliant and committed to lifelong follow-up of the ipsilateral collecting system with ureteroscopy.

○ **When patients treated with organ-sparing therapy, is there any evidence that ipsilateral recurrence compromises patient survival?**

Especially when dealing with low-grade disease, there is little evidence to suggest that survival is compromised by ipsilateral recurrences. Recurrences can be addressed with repeat endoscopic treatment, surgical excision, or nephroureterectomy.

○ **What are the benefits of the retrograde ureteroscopic approach over the antegrade percutaneous method?**

The retrograde ureteroscopic approach has 2 distinct advantages: (1) ureteroscopy can generally be performed on an outpatient basis with minimal risk of complications, (2) ureteroscopic techniques maintain a closed system and thus have a lower theoretical risk of tumor seeding of nonurinary tract surfaces. The ureteroscopic approach works well for low-volume and low-grade tumors.

○ **What are the limitations of the ureteroscopic approach?**

Limitations of this approach include (1) inability to treat a large volume of tumor, (2) limitations of ureteroscopes to reach all portions of the kidney (ie, lower pole system), and (3) limitations of biopsy specimens. Specimens obtained ureteroscopically are generally sufficient to establish tumor grade but are of inadequate depth to establish stage by assessing depth of invasion.

○ **When is the percutaneous approach generally favored?**

The percutaneous approach is generally indicated for larger tumors and/or those that are not easily accessible through the ureteroscopic approach (ie, lower pole lesions). Unlike ureteroscopy, larger caliber instruments can be used for removal of larger tumor burdens. In addition, deep tissue specimens can be obtained for staging purposes.

○ **What is the best follow-up study for transitional cell carcinoma of the upper urinary tract treated with conservative management?**

Ureteroscopic evaluation is the most effective way of screening for ipsilateral tumor recurrences. Simple radiographic evaluation is not sufficient, as it has been shown that up to 75% of early tumor recurrences were visible endoscopically and not radiographically.

○ **With endoscopic management, what are the risks of tumor seeding of noninvolved urothelial surfaces or the nephrostomy tract?**

A significant concern of endoscopic therapy has been the theoretical possibility of tumor seeding of the normal urothelial surfaces and/or nephrostomy tract. Although there are individual case reports describing such problems, the majority of the literature has not supported this concern.

○ **Topical immuno- or chemotherapy has been effective adjuvant therapy for bladder TCC. Have any studies shown significant improvement with regard to tumor recurrence or prevention of disease progression when this therapy is used for the upper urinary tract?**

Adjuvant topical therapy via nephrostomy tubes and ureteral catheters has been described. To date, no study has shown a statistically significant benefit with regard to recurrence and disease progression. This may be due to low patient numbers or possibly due to inadequate contact time with the urothelial surfaces of the upper urinary tract.

○ **What systemic chemotherapy regimens are available for the treatment of metastatic upper tract TCC?**

Available chemotherapeutic protocols for TCC of the upper urinary tract are identical to their bladder counterparts. Because of the rarity of the disease, no large studies have been performed that show significant benefit. However, these tumors are similar to their bladder counterparts and should respond in the same fashion.

○ **Is there a role for radiation therapy in the treatment of TCC of the upper tracts?**

Limited. It can be used for hemostasis in patients where other therapies cannot be used. Radiation may also be helpful as an adjunct to chemotherapy in patients with advanced disease.

○ **True/False: Patients with upper tract TCC tend to have a worse prognosis if they had a previous history of bladder cancer?**

True.

○   **How often will TCC of the upper tracts develop in patients with CIS of the bladder?**

Approximately 25% of the time.

○   **Does endoscopic resection of upper tract TCC offer equivalent overall survival to standard definitive surgical extirpation?**

In appropriate patients, yes. Patients with clinically localized upper tract TCC can be offered an endoscopic approach initially while allowing for more aggressive surgery at a later date if necessary. Also, there is a higher rate of recurrence with endourological treatment.

○   **What is *Aristolochia fangchi* and why is it important urologically?**

It's a Chinese herb used for weight loss. Its use has been associated with TCC of the upper tracts.

Bladder Cancer

Emily Blum, MD and
Howard J. Korman, MD, FACS

○ **What is the most common kind of bladder cancer?**

Transitional cell carcinoma (TCC) accounts for more than 90% of all bladder cancers.

○ **What is the next most common kind of bladder cancer?**

Squamous cell carcinoma accounts for 3% to 7%, with adenocarcinoma and metastatic carcinomas uncommon.

○ **What specific agents in cigarette smoke are thought to be the most carcinogenic?**

Nitrosamine, 2-naphthylamine, and 4-aminobiphenyl.

○ **Other than smoking, what are other risk factors for bladder cancer?**

Analgesic abuse (phenacetin), exposure to chemicals in the workplace such as aniline dye, 2-naphthylamine, paints, oils, gasoline, zinc, and chromium as well as pelvic irradiation, chronic cystitis, and treatment with cyclophosphamide.

○ **Does coffee consumption increase the risk of bladder cancer?**

No.

○ **Does the risk of bladder cancer return to baseline after smoking cessation?**

Yes, the risk of bladder cancer returns to baseline 20 to 30 years after smoking cessation.

○ **What chromosomal abnormalities are associated with TCC?**

Loss segments of chromosome 9, aneuploidy of chromosome 3, 5, 7, 17, defects in p53, p16, p21, p27, Rb, and H-ras.

○ **On which chromosome is the tumor suppressor gene p53 found?**

Chromosome 17.

○ **What is the most common presentation of bladder cancer?**

Gross, painless hematuria is typical for bladder cancer.

○ **Frequency, urgency, and dysuria are associated with what type of bladder cancer?**

Frequency, urgency, and dysuria can be linked to carcinoma in situ (CIS).

○ **What urine markers are available for the evaluation of TCC besides urine cytology?**

Protein-based markers include NMP22 and BTA stat/TRAK. NMP22 is a nuclear matrix protein that is elevated in bladder cancer patient and BTA stat/TRAK (qualitative/quantitative) detects complement factor H. Cellular-based markers include ImmunoCyt and UroVysion FISH.

○ **Which method of urinary cytology has the best diagnostic yield: voided or bladder wash?**

It has been estimated that the sensitivity of a single barbotage (bladder wash) specimen is equivalent to that of 3 voided specimens (Matzkin et al., 1992).

○ **What is the UroVysion FISH detecting and on which chromosomes?**

UroVysion Fluorescence **In S**itu **H**ybridization (FISH) detects aneuploidy of chromosomes 3, 7, and 17, as well as the loss of the 9p21 locus.

○ **What is the effect of barbotage (bladder washing) on UroVysion FISH testing?**

Bladder washing samples may result in false-positive results on a UroVysion FISH test.

○ **Of patients who have a positive UroVysion FISH with a negative cystoscopy and imaging, how often does this occur and how many will eventually develop a urothelial tumor?**

"Anticipatory positive" results (when FISH is positive with negative cystoscopy) occur in up to 30% of screened patients. Approximately two-third of these cases will progress to disease recurrence. The likely explanation is that FISH detects precancerous DNA mutations that promote tumor development in the future (Yoder, 2007).

○ **What percentage of bladder cancer is noninvasive at presentation?**

75% of bladder cancer is nonmuscle invasive at presentation, 20% is muscle invasive, and 5% is metastatic.

○ **How often do synchronous upper tract urothelial tumors coexist when a bladder tumor is diagnosed?**

2.4% of the time.

○ **If a person has a known upper tract disease, what is the risk of developing a bladder tumor?**

30% to 75%.

○ **What are the most predictive factors of disease progression for superficial TCC of the bladder?**

Tumor grade, stage, and the presence of CIS are the most significant prognostic factors. Other risk factors include lymphovascular invasion, tumor size, architecture, multifocality, and frequency of prior tumor recurrences.

○ **What tumor parameters are the most predictive factors for lymph node metastasis in invasive TCC of the bladder?**

Tumor grade and depth of tumor invasion.

○ **What is the current TNM staging system for cancer of the urinary bladder?**

- Ta: Noninvasive papillary carcinoma.
- Tis: Carcinoma in situ.
- T1: Tumor invades lamina propria.
- T2: Tumor invades muscle.
  ○ T2a: Superficial muscle (inner half).
  ○ T2b: Deep muscle (outer half).
- T3: Tumor invades perivesical fat.
  ○ T3a: Microscopic invasion.
  ○ T3b: Macroscopic invasion.
- T4: Tumor invades adjacent organs.
  ○ T4a: prostate, rectum, uterus, or vagina.
  ○ T4b: pelvic or abdominal wall.

○ **What are the main indications for intravesical therapy?**

High-grade tumor, low-grade tumor with high risk of recurrence, multiplicity, CIS, and unresectable tumor.

○ **What are the risk factors for systemic side effects from intravesical chemotherapy?**

In general, anything that increases drug absorption may lead to systemic toxicity. These factors include low molecular weight of the intravesical agent (thiotepa), extensive area of resection, bladder perforation, persistent gross hematuria, urinary tract infections, and instillation close to the time of resection.

○ **What side effects are common to most forms of intravesical chemotherapy?**

Hematuria, cystitis, and irritative voiding symptoms.

○ **Which intravesical agent is most commonly associated with the side effect of myelosuppression?**

Thiotepa, because of its low molecular weight, is easily absorbed and can be associated with myelosuppression.

○ **Which intravesical agent is most often associated with the side effect of contact dermatitis?**

Mitomycin C is caustic to the skin when direct contact is made.

○ **What are common side effects associated with bacillus Calmette–Guerin (BCG)?**

Cystitis, hematuria, fever, sepsis, granulomatous prostatitis, pneumonitis, or hepatitis. Deaths have also been reported from systemic BCGosis.

○ **What is the mechanism of action of BCG?**

The BCG organism binds to the cell surface through fibronectin-binding sites, which activates the Th-1–mediated immune response.

○ **What is the effect of anticoagulants on BCG therapy?**

Anticlotting drugs inhibit the binding of BCG to fibronectin, thus patients should be off anticoagulants when receiving BCG if at all possible.

○ **What drugs are used to treat BCG infection or overtreatment?**

Isoniazid (INH), rifampin, and ethambutol are the primary therapies. Streptomycin may also be used.

○ **What is the treatment for systemic BCG sepsis?**

Patients with severe voiding symptoms/hematuria and a fever >38.5 °C should be hospitalized and started on oral isoniazid 300 mg and rifampin 600 mg a day until symptoms resolve. Patients with hemodynamic changes and persistent high-grade temperature should also receive ethambutol 15 mg/kg/day and possibly prednisone 40 mg/day in addition to isoniazid and rifampin. Isoniazid, rifampin, and ethambutol should be continued for 3 to 6 months. Cycloserine inhibits growth of the bacillus within 24 hours. It is usually used in combination with isoniazid, rifampin, and ethambutol. The major side effect of cycloserine is a lowering of the seizure threshold.

○ **How can the risk of BCG complications be diminished?**

BCG therapy should not be initiated until 2 to 4 weeks after transurethral resection of the bladder tumor (TURBT). If gross hematuria is present or catheterization is traumatic, BCG should be withheld. BCG should not be administered to immunocompromised patients or those with an active UTI.

○ **What are other immunotherapeutic agents that have been used?**

Keyhole limpet hemocyanin (KLH), oral bropirimine, and interferon have also been studied but are not currently first-line therapies.

○ **What is the reported response rate to valrubicin in patients who do not respond to BCG?**

21%.

○ **What is the optimal course of intravesical therapy?**

The optimal duration, dosage, and timing of intravesical therapy have yet to be determined and remain under investigation.

○ **What is the most commonly used induction and maintenance protocol for BCG therapy?**

Patients usually receive a 6-week induction course. Maintenance doses after induction are commonly 3 weekly instillations at 3 months, 6 months, and every 6 months thereafter.

○ **What are possible indications for partial cystectomy?**

Tumor in a diverticulum or a small (<2 cm) isolated invasive tumor away from the trigone. Total radical cystectomy remains the treatment of choice for most invasive bladder cancers due to high recurrence rates reported following partial cystectomy in patients with muscle invasive disease.

○ **What are the indications for radical cystectomy for superficial disease?**

Recurrent or persistent high-grade disease, diffuse CIS, failure of intravesical therapy, refractory hematuria from a large volume tumor, unresectable tumor, or a strong clinical suspicion of understaging (ie, lymphovascular invasion, unfavorable variant histology).

○ **What is the obturator reflex and why is it important to urologists?**

The obturator nerve runs in close proximity to the inferolateral wall of the bladder. Stimulation from electrocautery current during TURBT may cause sudden and unexpected external rotation and adduction of the thigh. Care must be taken during TURBT as stimulation of the obturator nerve may increase the risk of bladder perforation.

○ **What degree of clinical understaging is associated with T1 disease?**

Understaging as high as 33% has been reported.

○ **Is cytology or other urine markers indicated for evaluation of asymptomatic microscopic hematuria?**

No, recent AUA guidelines recommend that no urine markers or urine cytology are necessary for the evaluation of an initial episode of asymptomatic microscopic hematuria. Cytology may be utilized if patient is at high risk for bladder Ca (ie, smoking history or chemical exposure) or if irritative voiding symptoms are present. The recommendations do not include the use of other urine markers in these instances.

○ **What is the most accepted treatment for muscle invasive bladder cancer?**

Radical cystectomy. Bladder preservation with radiation and chemotherapy can be used for select patients but has not been shown to be better than surgical extirpation.

○ **What are local recurrence rates after radical cystectomy for invasive bladder cancer?**

Approximately 6% of patients have a local recurrence after radical cystectomy (Cornu et al., 2012).

○ **What are the expected 5-year survival rates for T2, T3, T4, and N1 disease after radical cystectomy without neoadjuvant therapy?**

Estimated 5-year survival is 74% to 89%, 57% to 62%, 50% to 62%, and 28% to 48%, respectively.

○ **What is the urethral recurrence rate following cystoprostatectomy if tumor was present in the prostatic urethra on final pathology? (Stein et al., 2005)**

Urethral recurrence following radical cystoprostatectomy is 5% (urothelium), 12% (ducts), and 18% (stroma) if urethrectomy is not performed.

○ **What is the risk of a urethral recurrence after cystectomy and when does it typically appear?**

The risk of a urethral recurrence is approximately 10% typically occurring within 2 years of cystectomy.

○ **In what percentage of patients is incidental adenocarcinoma of the prostate found at the time of radical cystoprostatectomy?**

Approximately 30% to 40% of patients undergoing radical cystoprostatectomy have incidental adenocarcinomas found in the pathological specimen.

○ **List the common complications associated with ileal conduit urinary diversions.**

Pyelonephritis, stomal stenosis, parastomal hernias, ureterointestinal anastomotic strictures, anastomotic leaks, hyperchloremic metabolic acidosis, and stone formation.

○ **List the common complications associated with orthotopic urinary diversions.**

Pyelonephritis, stomal stenosis, ureterointestinal anastomotic strictures, metabolic abnormalities, reservoir and renal stones, mucous retention, and nocturnal incontinence.

○ **What is the cut-off for renal function (maximum serum creatinine) for performing orthotopic diversions and why?**

Patients with a serum creatinine greater than 2.5 mg/dL are usually excluded due to the high likelihood of metabolic complications (Korman et al., 1996a, b).

○ **What percentage of patients undergoing continent urinary diversion develop metabolic acidosis and how is this treated?**

Metabolic acidosis can occur in up to 50% of patients, often requiring lifelong oral alkalinization therapy.

○ **Why is the distal 15 to 20 cm of the ileum commonly spared with the various diversion techniques?**

Vitamin B_{12} (cobalamin) is absorbed in the distal ileum. A B_{12} deficiency can lead to megaloblastic anemia with a mean red blood cell volume (MCV) >100 fL and hypersegmented neutrophils. This type of a deficiency usually takes about 5 years to develop from the time of surgery and results in demyelination injury to the dorsal and lateral columns of the spinal cord.

○ **What is the traditional systemic chemotherapy regimen for metastatic bladder cancer and what is the survival rate?**

Methotrexate, vinblastine, Adriamycin, and cisplatin (MVAC) traditionally was the most commonly used chemotherapeutic regimen for metastatic bladder cancer if the patient is healthy enough to tolerate the side effects of treatment with 50% to 70% response rates reported in the literature. Two-year survival is only 15% to 20%.

○ **How has the standard of care changed for the use of systemic chemotherapy for metastatic bladder cancer?**

The combination of gemcitabine (Gemzar) and cisplatin has been shown to have a similar survival outcome with lower toxicity compared to MVAC (Von der Masse et al., 2000). Although the newer treatment regimen is not without side effects (50% neutropenia/thrombocytopenia), its lower toxicity profile has made it the treatment of choice for most centers (Aparicio et al., 2005).

○ **Is a patient with diffuse CIS a candidate for radiation therapy?**

No, CIS is resistant to radiation.

○ **What is the most common hematogenous site of bladder cancer metastasis?**

Liver (38%), lung (36%), bone (27%), adrenal (21%), and bowel (13%).

○ **What is the most common site of metastasis overall for bladder cancer?**

Lymph node metastases are the most common (78%), and most frequently involve the obturator lymph nodes (64%).

○ **What is the reported response rate and the most common side effect associated with high-dose interferon used as intravesical treatment for refractory superficial TCC?**

A flu-like syndrome occurs in up to 20% of patients. Local symptoms are rare. The expense of high dose intravesical interferon has limited its use as a primary therapy. Complete response rates of 25% to 43% have been reported.

○ **What is the reported 5-year survival rate after treatment with external beam radiation therapy in stage T2-T3 disease?**

20% to 40%.

○ **Carcinoma in situ frequently has alterations of what molecular markers?**

P53 and RB.

○ **What is the 3-year mortality rate of untreated muscle invasive TCC of the bladder?**

Eighty to ninety percent by 3 years.

○ **True/False: The presence of hemorrhagic cystitis correlates with the later development of bladder cancer.**

False. No such correlation exists.

○ **What is MESNA and what is it used for?**

MESNA stands for 2-mercaptoethane sulfonate. It is a chemoprotective agent that is administered during cyclophosphamide or ifosfamide therapy to help reduce the incidence of hemorrhagic cystitis.

○ **What is acrolein?**

Acrolein is the most significant carcinogenic metabolite of cyclophosphamide with a latency period of 6 to 13 years.

○ **What are the differences between Brunn nests, cystitis cystica, and cystitis glandularis?**

Brunn nests are essentially benign urothelial growths in the submucosal layer of the bladder. They are caused by an invagination or invasive growth of the basal layer and are usually considered a normal urothelial variant. Cystitis cystica and cystitis glandularis are variations of von Brunn nests. Cystitis cystica has a cyst-like appearance with a liquid filling the center of the lesion. Cystitis glandularis occurs when additional glandular metaplasia has occurred and the cells become more columnar.

○ **Is cystitis glandularis considered benign or malignant and what other entities is it associated with?**

It is generally considered benign but may be associated with pelvic lipomatosis and can develop into adenocarcinoma.

○ **What is the most effective intravesical chemotherapy agent for TCC of the bladder?**

Mitomycin C is the most active intravesical chemotherapy agent. (BCG is technically considered immunotherapy.)

○ **What is the effect of a single intravesical application of chemotherapy after transurethral resection (TUR) of a Ta T1 bladder tumor?**

With solitary tumors, the reduction in recurrence rate was 39% compared to similar patients who did not get the instillation. Patients with multiple tumors did not see as much benefit.

○ **What is the preferred management of an inadvertent bladder perforation during TUR of a bladder tumor?**

Open repair is associated with a very high rate of extravesical tumor recurrence and should be avoided. Catheterization and/or percutaneous drainage should be employed when possible. Animal studies have suggested that a single immediate low dose (>0.3125 mg/m^2) intraperitoneal instillation of mitomycin C can be helpful.

○ **How is a Hautmann ileal neobladder created and why is the shape important?**

The Hautmann neobladder is created from a "W" of ileum with each limb approximately 15 cm in length and a 5-cm tail. The bowel is opened on its antimesenteric border and the edges sewn together to create a sphere. The shape is important because a sphere has the largest possible volume with the lowest luminal pressure. For a given vesicle radius and internal pressure, a spherical vessel will have half of the wall pressure of a cylinder (law of Laplace).

○ **What is the purpose of the tail on a Studer neobladder?**

The Studer neobladder has a 15- to 20-cm isoperistaltic limb that acts to carry urine toward the reservoir and theoretically prevent reflux.

○ **What are the risks and benefits of a nonrefluxing anastomosis?**

A nonrefluxing anastomosis is designed to prevent reflux of urine that could lead to high upper tract pressures and pyelonephritis (neither of which is actually prevented). A nonrefluxing type of anastomosis takes more surgery time to perform and is prone to stricture.

○ **What is fluorescent cystoscopy and how much can it improve standard cystoscopy?**

A photoactive porphyrin such as 5-aminolevulinic acid (5-ALA) or hexaminolevulinate (HAL) is instilled into the bladder. The porphyrins accumulate preferentially in neoplastic tissues. A blue light illuminates the areas of high porphyrin concentrations, emitting a red fluorescence. Preliminary studies have shown that 25% to 35% more cases of small papillary tumors and CIS are identified as compared to standard cystoscopy. Prospective studies suggest a decrease in recurrence rate of 16% with the use of fluorescent cystoscopy (Stenzl, 2010).

○ **At least how many lymph nodes should you remove during a cystoprostatectomy with pelvic lymph node dissection and which specific nodes should be included?**

Minimum of 12 lymph nodes. With lymph node-positive disease, patients who had more than 15 lymph nodes removed during dissection had 11% 10-year recurrence-free survival advantage compared to patients who had fewer than 15 nodes resected. At a minimum, pelvic lymph node dissection should include bilateral external iliac, hypogastric, and obturator nodes.

○ **What is the significance of the number of positive lymph nodes on recurrence rate? (Stein et al., 2005)**

<8 positive nodes: 40% 10-year recurrence-free survival versus 10% if less than 8 nodes were positive.

○ **What survival advantage can be gained by the administration of neoadjuvant chemotherapy?**

Fourteen percent survival advantage at 5 years. The South West Oncology Group compared cystectomy alone versus neoadjuvant MVAC and cystectomy, and found a 14% survival advantage at 5 years (Grossman et al., 2003).

○ **Do childhood cancer survivors (non-Hodgkin lymphoma, retinoblastoma, leukemia, and soft tissue sarcomas) have an increased risk of bladder cancer as adults?**

Yes. Their risk is 5 times greater than the general population.

CHAPTER 42

Squamous Cell Carcinoma and Adenocarcinoma of the Bladder

A. Ari Hakimi, MD and Reza Ghavamian, MD

○ **Non-transitional cell carcinoma (non-TCC) makes up what percentage of bladder cancers in developed nations?**

Less than 10% of all bladder cancers in developed nations are non-TCC.

○ **Are non-TCCs considered more aggressive or less aggressive than TCC of the bladder and by how much?**

Non-TCCs of the bladder typically present at a more advanced stage and setting than TCC and are almost always invasive. The 5-year relative survival of squamous cell carcinoma (SCC) patients is less than half the figure for TCC, while the survival for adenocarcinoma is roughly 25% lower than TCC.

○ **Why is SCC of the bladder an important public health problem in Egypt?**

In Egypt, where schistosomiasis is endemic, about 80% of SCCs of the bladder are caused by *Schistosoma haematobium*.

○ **Is schistosomiasis only associated with SCC?**

No, schistosomiasis also increases the incidence of TCC of the bladder.

○ **Can SCC coexist with TCC?**

Yes, transitional epithelium has tremendous metaplastic potential and therefore SCC elements are also frequently seen with invasive TCC.

○ **What is the difference between SCC and TCC with squamous differentiation?**

The diagnosis of SCC should be reserved for tumors with exclusive or predominant squamous differentiation.

○ **How does SCC of the bladder typically present?**

Most patients have irritative voiding symptoms with or without gross hematuria.

○ **What are the cystoscopic and histological characteristics of SCC of the bladder?**

SCCs of the bladder are almost always solitary lesions and tend to be sessile and ulcerated. They are well differentiated and have a low incidence of lymph node and distant metastases. Bilharzial lesions are less likely to be stage T4 and are usually bulky, nodular, and located in the upper hemisphere of the bladder.

○ **What are the proposed risk factors nonbilharzial squamous cell cancers?**

Reported risk factors include African American race, cigarettes smoking, chronic irritation of the bladder mucosa from bladder calculi or long-term indwelling Foley catheters, chronic urinary infectious, bladder diverticula, cyclophosphamide exposure, and intravesical bacillus Calmette–Guerin (BCG).

○ **What is the proposed carcinogenic mechanism?**

This is not completely understood, but could be the result of formation of nitrite and *N*-nitroso compounds that result from parasitic and bacterial metabolism.

○ **What other patients are found to have squamous epithelium in their bladder?**

Vaginal type nonkeratinizing stratified squamous epithelium is commonly found in the trigone of many women and in men receiving estrogen for prostate cancer. These patients should not be diagnosed with squamous metaplasia.

○ **What patient populations are at greatest risk for the development of squamous metaplasia?**

Eighty percent of paraplegic patients are found to have squamous metaplasia of the bladder.

○ **In squamous metaplasia, is keratinization considered a good or bad prognostic sign?**

Keratinization is somewhat ominous because it is more closely associated with carcinoma; 21% progress to malignancy.

○ **What is the name of the above condition?**

Leukoplakia.

○ **How should these patients be followed?**

Patients with biopsy-proven keratinizing squamous metaplasia of the bladder should have periodic (at least yearly) cystoscopy and urine cytology examinations.

○ **What percentage of paraplegic patients with squamous metaplasia will go on to develop SCC?**

Approximately 5% of paraplegics with squamous metaplasia will go on to develop SCC and 21% if keratinization is present.

○ **What other patient populations are at risk for SCC of the bladder?**

These tumors account for approximately 20% of bladder cancers arising within bladder diverticula, 50% occur in patients with nonfunctioning bladders and also account for 15% of bladder cancers in patients who have had renal transplants.

○ **How does nonbilharzial SCC differ from bilharzial SCC of the bladder?**

In bilharzial SCC, the tumors are usually well differentiated with a low incidence of lymph node or distant metastases. In nonbilharzial SCC of the bladder seen in the United States, the tumors tend to be poorly differentiated and advanced at diagnosis so the patients tend to have a poorer prognosis.

○ **What is the role of chemotherapy and radiation in the treatment of SCC of the bladder?**

Chemotherapy has not been very effective in the treatment of SCC of the bladder. In addition, transurethral resection, partial cystectomy, and radiation therapy alone have not been effective.

○ **What has been shown to be the most effective treatment against SCC of the bladder?**

The most effective treatment at this time is radical cystectomy with pelvic lymph node dissection. The role of preoperative radiation is not well defined and there are currently no large studies to prove its survival advantage.

○ **What percentage of patients with SCC of the bladder are found to have involvement of their urethra?**

Approximately 50% of patients are found to have urethral involvement; therefore, it has been suggested that urethrectomy should be routinely performed in all patients undergoing a cystectomy.

○ **What is the prognosis of SCC of the bladder? How does it compare to the prognosis for transitional cell bladder carcinoma?**

Stage for stage, the prognosis of squamous cell bladder cancer is equivalent to TCC of the bladder. A recent study from Egypt placed the 5-year survival at 50% for bilharzial cancers compared to 39% for nonbilharzial tumors. Another study from Turkey showed no difference in 5-year disease-specific survival between SCC and TCC when controlling for other disease-related factors.

○ **What percent of primary bladder cancers are adenocarcinomas?**

Adenocarcinoma of the bladder accounts for less than 2% of primary bladder cancers in Western countries, but up to 10% of bladder cancers in nations with endemic schistosomiasis.

○ **What are the different classifications of bladder adenocarcinoma?**

Bladder adenocarcinomas can be classified as primary vesical, urachal, and metastatic. Urachal carcinomas represent approximately one-third of primary bladder adenocarcinomas.

○ **What are the different cell types of primary vesical adenocarcinoma?**

In 1 large series, vesical adenocarcinomas were mucinous (23.6%), enteric (19.4%), signet-ring cell (16.7%), mixed (12.5%), or not otherwise specified (27.8%).

○ **What is a critical component of the workup of a patient with vesical adenocarcinoma?**

Ruling out other causes of malignancy. Routine workup should include sigmoid or colonoscopy, and assessment of the prostate in males and endometrium in females to rule out direct extension from adjacent organs.

○ **What are the histologic features?**

There is a predominantly glandular pattern, but in poorly differentiated tumors, areas of solid growth are evident. The glands resemble intestinal adenocarcinoma of typical or colloid type. The epithelial lining can have a mucinous character. Eight percent of the tumors can have papillary features.

○ **What is linitis plastica of the bladder?**

This is primary vesical adenocarcinoma of the signet-ring cell type. It accounts for 3% to 5% of primary adenocarcinomas of the bladder. It can present with a diffusely thickened bladder wall on imaging studies, especially computed tomography or ultrasonography. Sheets of tumor cells, fibrosis, and mural thickening typical of linitis plastica of the stomach is characteristic of these tumors and they are generally associated with a worse prognosis.

○ **Which patient populations are at increased risk for bladder adenocarcinomas?**

Patients with intestinal urinary conduits, augmentations, pouches, and ureterosigmoidostomies are at increased risk. Adenocarcinoma is also the most common type of cancer in bladder exstrophy (90%). Schistosomiasis is another risk factor.

○ **With what premalignant lesion in the bladder is adenocarcinoma associated?**

Adenocarcinomas of the bladder are most often associated with cystitis glandularis.

○ **What treatment offers the best chance for cure in patients with primary adenocarcinoma of the bladder?**

Radical cystectomy with a bilateral pelvic lymph node dissection offers the best chance of cure for localized adenocarcinoma of the bladder. Retrospective analysis of bilharzial adenocarcinoma indicates that adjuvant radiation may improve survival, but no such data exist in the nonbilharzial setting.

○ **What is the prognosis for bladder adenocarcinomas?**

There is no concrete evidence to suggest that adenocarcinoma of the bladder carries a worse prognosis stage than TCC. However, they are generally thought to be associated with a poor prognosis because 60% to 65% are stage T3-4 at diagnosis. Of the different cell types, signet-ring cell carcinoma is more undifferentiated and hence carries the worst prognosis.

○ **How common are urachal remnants and where are they located?**

They are found in up to 35% of autopsies, usually in the dome of the bladder.

○ **What is the incidence of urachal carcinoma?**

0.35% to 0.7%, with predilection for males (72%-80% of the cases).

○ **The majority of urachal tumors are of which cell type?**

Urachal tumors are usually adenocarcinomas; however, primary SCC, TCC, and even rarely sarcomas of the urachus have been described.

○ **How do urachal tumors present?**

Urachal tumors may present with a bloody or mucoid discharge from the umbilicus. Urachal tumors may also produce a mucocele, which occurs as a midline infraumbilical palpable abdominal mass. Fifteen percent of urachal tumors do not produce mucin.

○ **What are the other presenting symptoms?**

Tumors invading the bladder lumen can produce mucus in the urine. This happens in only 15% to 33% of cases. Tumors that complicate exstrophy are remarkable primarily for their presence on the anterior abdominal wall. Other symptoms include dysuria and frequency, and lower abdominal pain.

○ **What is the most common finding on radiography?**

Sixty percent of urachal tumors have areas of low attenuation on CT, which is reflective of the tumor's high mucin content.

○ **What is essential in the diagnosis of urachal carcinomas?**

Cystoscopy and transurethral biopsy is essential for tumor location assessment and tissue diagnosis. Usually cystitis, cystica/glandularis, and dysplasia are absent.

○ **What other neoplastic processes can mimic urachal carcinoma?**

Metastatic prostate, colonic, ovarian, and endometrial carcinoma all have the potential to locally invade the bladder. Therefore, tissue diagnosis is important.

○ **What is the prognosis of primary urachal adenocarcinomas?**

These tumors usually portend a worse prognosis than primary vesical adenocarcinomas. Patients with predominantly mucin histology have a 79% 5-year survival. Patients with papillary, tubular, or signet-ring cells had a 33% 5-year survival based on 1 study.

○ **What is the overall 5-year survival?**

43% to 50%.

○ **How should urachal tumors be treated?**

Radical cystectomy with an en bloc excision of the urachus is the treatment of choice in patients with large tumors as histologically these tumors exhibit wider and deeper infiltration of the bladder wall. However, for small localized tumors at the bladder dome, partial cystectomy with complete removal of the urachal ligament and umbilicus is acceptable. Extended partial cystectomy has been shown to be the treatment of choice as survival is related to the stage at presentation rather than extent of surgical resection.

○ **Are urachal tumors sensitive to radiation or chemotherapy therapy?**

Urachal tumors are usually unresponsive to chemotherapy, and radiation therapy is also ineffective. However, the MD Anderson group reported a 33% response rate using 5-fluorouracil, leucovorin, and cisplatin, with or without gemcitabine.

○   **Where are the common metastatic sites for urachal adenocarcinomas?**

Urachal tumors can metastasize to the iliac and inguinal nodes as well as the omentum, liver, lung, and bones.

○   **What are the more common primary sites for adenocarcinomas metastatic to the bladder?**

Rectum, stomach, endometrium, breast, prostate, and ovary.

○   **Are any additional investigations necessary once a diagnosis of adenocarcinoma of the bladder is established?**

Patients should be evaluated for a possible source of a primary adenocarcinoma site. This includes computed tomography of the abdomen and pelvis, barium enema, and colonoscopy when the index of suspicion is high and in patients in whom linitis plastica of the bladder is diagnosed, upper endoscopy to rule out a stomach primary is indicated.

CHAPTER 43 Urethral Lesions

Benjamin N. Breyer, MD, MAS and Badrinath R. Konety, MD, MBA

○ **From distal to proximal, what are the anatomic names of the urethral segments?**

- Fossa navicularis
- Penile–pendulous urethra
- Bulbous urethra
- Membranous urethra
- Prostatic urethra

○ **Describe the different types of epithelia lining the male urethra.**

- Prostatic and membranous urethra: transitional epithelium.
- Bulbar urethra: squamous epithelium distally and gradually changes to transitional epithelium.
- Penile urethra: simple squamous epithelium.
- Fossa navicularis: stratified squamous epithelium.

○ **What is the average length of the male urethra?**

The average length of the urethra from an anatomically normal male is 22 cm (range, 15-29 cm)

○ **What is the lacuna magna?**

The dorsal expansion of the fossa navicularis in the glans penis is called the lacuna magna.

○ **What portion of the urethra do Cowper glands and the glands of Littre open into?**

Cowper glands open into the membranous urethra, while the glands of Littre open into the dorsal urethra.

○ **What is the specific feature of the male urethral blood supply which is advantageous in planning urethral reconstructive surgery?**

The male urethra has a dual blood supply—proximally from the bulbar artery, a branch of the internal pudendal artery, and distally from the dorsal artery of the penis, which is a terminal branch of the pudendal artery. This fact allows for complete excision of diseased segments of the urethra during urethral reconstruction.

○ **What is the name of the deep penile fascia and its attachments?**

Buck fascia surrounds the corpus spongiosum and corpora cavernosa. Distally, Buck fascia is connected to the undersurface of the glans at the corona. Proximally, Buck fascia encloses each crus of the corpora cavernosa and the bulb of the corpus spongiosum.

○ **When Buck fascia remains intact after injury to the anterior urethra, what is the expected appearance?**

Typically, if Buck fascia remains intact, bruising, hematoma, and swelling will be confined to the penis.

○ **What is the name of the superficial penile fascia and its attachments?**

Colles fascia of the perineum attaches laterally to the fascia lata of the thigh, the ischia, and the inferior rami of the pubis. Anteriorly, Colles fascia is continuous with the Dartos layer of the scrotum and Scarpa fascia on the anterior abdominal wall.

○ **How do injuries that violate Buck fascia and leave Colles fascia intact appear?**

A butterfly or saddle perineal appearance of a hematoma may be present. In addition, a scrotal hematoma and bruising on the anterior abdominal wall to the level of the clavicles is possible.

○ **What are the most common sites of iatrogenic urethral injury?**

The penoscrotal junction and the external urethral meatus are the most common sites of iatrogenic urethral injury.

○ **What is the incidence of urethral injury following pelvic fractures?**

Approximately 10% of pelvic fractures are accompanied by urethral injury, whereas a majority of patients with urethral injury will have pelvic fractures. Approximately 10% of patients with posterior urethral injury will also have an accompanying bladder rupture.

○ **What is the most common cause of external urethral meatal stenosis requiring surgical repair?**

Lichen sclerosis is the most common cause of meatal stenosis requiring surgical repair.

○ **What is the proper technique for obtaining a retrograde urethrogram (RUG)?**

A RUG is obtained by positioning the patient obliquely at 45°, with the bottom leg flexed 90° at the knee and the top leg kept straight. A 12-F Foley catheter is introduced into the fossa navicularis, the balloon inflated with 2 mL saline to prevent dislodgement, the penis placed on gentle traction, and 20 to 30 mL of undiluted water-soluble contrast material is injected with the film exposed while injecting.

○ **How do blunt injuries to the urethra occur?**

Blunt urethral injuries typically result from straddle-type trauma incurred after forceful contact of the perineum with a blunt object. Any focused external force, as encountered in falls and vehicular accidents, can crush the immobile bulbous urethra against the inferior pubic symphysis.

○ **A 40-year-old male presents after a motorcycle crash with blood at his meatus. What is the next step in his urinary tract evaluation?**

Blood at the meatus is seen in at least 75% of patients after external anterior urethral trauma. No urethral instrumentation should be undertaken until a proper RUG is obtained if meatal blood is present or suspicion of urethral injury exists. If the urethra is in continuity or only partially disrupted, an attempt at placing a well-lubricated Foley catheter should be made.

○ **What other radiologic methods other than a RUG can be employed in evaluating urethral injuries?**

Urethral strictures resulting from urethral trauma can also be evaluated by a sonographic urethrogram at the time of delayed repair, but are not typically used in the acute trauma setting. A sonographic urethrogram allows determination of the extent of periurethral fibrosis, spongiofibrosis, and luminal size. This is important because in the case of most urethral strictures, subepithelial spongiofibrosis extends well beyond the grossly identifiable stricture area. MRI can be useful in the evaluation of posterior urethral disruptions.

○ **What is the main continence mechanism in men with complete urethral disruption?**

The bladder neck constitutes the main continence mechanism in men with complete urethral disruption.

○ **What are the 2 main principles to be kept in mind during the excision and reanastomosis of urethral strictures?**

Excision and reanastomosis should be avoided in pendulous urethral strictures because it can result in shortening of the penile urethra and chordee. A similar situation can result if >2 cm of bulbar urethra is excised and the urethra is not properly mobilized.

○ **What are the most common indications for 2-stage urethral reconstruction?**

The most common indications prompting a 2-stage urethral reconstruction are: pan-urethral stricture with a poor and narrowed urethral plate, multiple strictures, presence of urethrocutaneous fistula, periurethral inflammation, lichen sclerosis, or extensive local scarring.

○ **What are the principal advantages and disadvantages of immediate primary urethral reanastomosis versus delayed primary reanastomosis?**

This is a controversial topic in reconstructive urology. With improvements in endoscopic equipment endoscopic primary realignment is less traumatic than open primary realignment. Rates of stricture, while high, do not reach the nearly 100% seen in delayed repair. Those advocating delayed repair contend that endoscopic realignment may increase rates of erectile dysfunction and make the future reconstruction more challenging. Primary endoscopic alignment should only be attempted in the stable trauma patient. If significant difficulties in realignment are noted or prolonged time is needed, attempts should be stopped and a suprapubic tube left in place.

○ **A 38-year-old male accidentally discharges his handgun while carrying it under his belt. He has a large gash in his penile urethra. How should this be managed?**

Immediate repair is indicated. A tension-free, watertight closure with absorbable sutures should be employed over a Foley catheter. Careful inspection and repair of any corporotomies should be made.

○ **Which is the only genitourinary malignancy more common in women?**

Urethral carcinoma is the only genitourinary malignancy more common in women. Squamous cell carcinoma is the most common histologic type in both sexes, followed by transitional cell carcinoma.

○ **What are the most common risk factors for urethral carcinoma in men and women?**

Risk factors include urethral strictures, venereal disease, transitional cell carcinoma of the bladder, human papilloma virus (HPV) subtypes 16 and 18 infections. In women, urethral diverticula can also constitute a risk factor for urethral carcinoma. Biopsies should be done on all unusual appearing strictures and spontaneous fistulas.

○ **What are some common symptoms of urethral carcinoma?**

Frequently similar to those of benign voiding dysfunction. The onset is typically insidious. General storage symptoms such as frequency, hesitancy, and nocturia, obstructive voiding symptoms such as straining, weak stream, incontinence secondary to retention and urinary overflow, hematuria, purulent, necrotic watery discharge, urethral or perineal pain, and swelling.

○ **What are some common physical examination findings of urethral carcinoma?**

Palpable mass on the ventral surface of penis or the perineum, periurethral abscess, urethral diverticula, and urethral-cutaneous and urethral-vaginal fistulas.

○ **What is the key pathologic feature that determines the need for a urethrectomy along with a radical cystoprostatectomy in patients with transitional cell carcinoma of the bladder?**

Presence of transitional cell carcinoma invading the prostatic stroma on urethral biopsy necessitates a urethrectomy along with cystoprostatectomy in cases of transitional cell carcinoma of the bladder. Urethrectomy is not considered mandatory in cases with carcinoma in situ of the urethra or tumor invasion into the prostatic ducts and acini without stromal encroachment. In cases where urethrectomy is not deemed necessary, involvement of the prostatic urethral margin dictates the need for urethrectomy which can be performed simultaneously with the cystectomy or within the next 2 months following the cystoprostatectomy. ●

○ **How is male urethral cancer treated?**

Surgery is the main treatment. Low-stage urethral carcinoma, especially if located in the anterior urethra, is treated with local resection or Nd:YAG laser fulguration. More extensive disease requires wider resection with partial penectomy, total penectomy, or en bloc resection. There is no demonstrated benefit to prophylactic lymphadenectomy in these patients. Radiation and chemotherapy can be useful additions in advanced cases for palliation.

○ **What is the most common site of malignant melanoma in the genitourinary tract?**

The urethra is the most common site of malignant melanoma in the urinary tract. It is most often located at the fossa navicularis in men. It most often occurs in individuals in their sixties to eighties, survival is poor and dissemination can occur by direct extension, lymphatic, or hematogenous spread.

○ **What is commonly believed to be the site of origin of urethral adenocarcinoma in men?**

Cowper glands are commonly believed to be the site of origin of urethral adenocarcinoma in men.

○ **What is the most common histologic type of cancer occurring in a urethral diverticulum in women?**

Adenocarcinomas are the most common histologic type of tumor, which occur in urethral diverticula in women.

○ **What is the Grabstald classification of urethral tumors in women?**

According to the Grabstald classification, female urethral tumors are classified as involving the anterior (external meatus and distal one-third) or entire (posterior two-thirds may extend to anterior) urethra. However, survival from urethral carcinoma is only dependent upon stage at diagnosis and tumor size with location having no impact.

○ **What is the American Joint Committee on Cancer Tumor Node Metastasis (TMN) staging system for urethral cancer?**

- *Primary tumor (T) (men and women):*
  Tx: Primary tumor cannot be assessed.
  T0: No evidence of primary tumor.
  Ta: Noninvasive papillary, polypoid, or verrucous carcinoma.
  Tis: Carcinoma in situ.
  T1: Tumor invading subepithelial connective tissue.
  T2: Tumor invading any of the following: corpus spongiosum, prostate, periurethral muscle.
  T3: Tumor invading any of the following: corpus cavernosum, beyond prostate capsule, anterior vagina, bladder neck.
  T4: Tumor invades other adjacent organs.
- *Regional lymph nodes (N):*
  Nx: Regional nodes cannot be assessed.
  N0: No regional lymph node metastasis.
  N1: Metastasis in a single lymph node, 2 cm or less in greatest dimension.
  N2: Metastasis in a single lymph node, larger than 2 cm in greatest dimension, or in multiple lymph nodes.
- *Distant metastases (M):*
  Mx: Distant metastasis cannot be assessed.
  M0: No distant metastasis.
  M1: Distant metastasis.

○ **What is the prognosis for urethral cancer?**

Anterior lesions have a better prognosis, probably because penectomy offers a better opportunity for a wide surgical margin and because of symptoms they present earlier. Five-year survival for anterior urethral cancer is approximately 50%, while posterior cancers have only a 10% to 15% 5-year survival rate.

○ **What are the principles of management of female urethral carcinoma?**

Early-stage female urethral carcinoma can be managed with laser fulguration or radiation. Invasive tumors require local resection with or without neoadjuvant radiation therapy. Combined external beam and interstitial radiation therapy have been used for palliation.

○ **How many female patients with urethral cancer present with metastases at presentation?**

Approximately 14%.

○ **What are the demographic patterns of gonococcal and non-gonococcal urethritis (NGU)?**

Gonococcal urethritis caused by the gram-negative diplococcus *Neisseria gonorrhoeae* occurs more commonly in adolescent inner city males with a large incidence in African Americans. NGU, one of the major causes of which is *Chlamydia trachomatis*, is commonly found in educated Caucasians of higher socioeconomic class including students.

○ **Who are the carriers of *N. gonorrhoeae*?**

Both sexes can be asymptomatic carriers of *N. gonorrhoeae* and symptomatic infections can also occur in both sexes. Humans are the sole host for this organism.

○ **What are the criteria for diagnosing NGU?**

The presence of inflammatory cells on a urethral smear in the absence of *N. gonorrhoeae* suggests a diagnosis of NGU. Presence of significant inflammation is indicated by the presence of >4 neutrophils/oil immersion field (400×).

○ **What is the optimal means of documenting infection by *C. trachomatis*?**

C. trachomatis infection is best confirmed by culturing the organism from urethral swabs or staining with fluorescein conjugated antichlamydial monoclonal antibodies.

○ **What associations between gonococcal urethritis and NGU should be considered when evaluating patients with gonococcal urethritis?**

Forty-five percent of patients with gonococcal urethritis will have concomitant infection with *C. trachomatis*. Hence, all such patients should be treated for both infections simultaneously.

○ **What are the standard therapeutic antibiotic regimens used to treat gonococcal urethritis and NGU?**

- Gonococcal urethritis—single dose ofloxacin (400 mg po), ciprofloxacin (500 mg po), cefixime (400 mg po), or ceftriaxone (250 mg IM). Spectinomycin 2 g IM can also be used.
- NGU—recommended: azithromycin single dose (1 g po), doxycycline 7 days (100 mg po bid).

Alternative: erythromycin or tetracycline 7 days (500 mg po qid), ofloxacin 7 days (300 mg po bid). Ciprofloxacin is not effective in treating *C. trachomatis* infections. Partners though asymptomatic should be treated since 33% of them will be carriers.

○ **What are other organisms commonly implicated in NGU?**

Ureaplasma urealyticum, *Trichomonas vaginalis*, herpes simplex virus (HSV) types 1 and 2, and human papilloma virus (HPV).

○ **What are the best methods to establish infection with HSV and HPV?**

HSV infection can be established by viral culture, while HPV infection can best be established by testing for the presence of viral DNA.

○ **What are the standard therapeutic regimens used in the management of NGU caused by organisms other than *C. trachomatis*?**

Ureaplasma urealyticum responds to treatment with erythromycin and tetracycline (500 mg po qid for 7 days). *Trichomonas* is treated with metronidazole (250 mg po tid for 7 days). Partners though asymptomatic should also be treated since they could be carriers. HSV infections can respond to topical or oral acyclovir (for primary or recurrent episodes). HPV infections are treated with topical podophyllin, 5-Fluorouracil, cryotherapy, laser fulguration, electrocautery, or surgical excision.

○ **What are the common complications ensuing from urethritis?**

Epididymitis—*C. trachomatis* is the most common organism responsible for epididymitis in younger men. Urethral strictures can occur as a consequence of both gonococcal urethritis and NGU. Disseminated gonococcal infections with septic arthritis and tenosynovitis occur more commonly in pregnant women. NGU is associated with Reiter syndrome of uveitis and arthritis. It is the most common cause of peripheral arthritis in young men.

○ **What is the incidence of gonococcal resistance to tetracycline?**

Five to fifteen percent and increasing.

○ **Can probenecid and penicillin still be used for gonorrhea?**

Currently, resistance to this combination therapy from the past is too high, so other regimens are preferred.

○ **What is the recommended therapy for recurrent chlamydial urethritis?**

Prolonged 14- to 28-day course of erythromycin.

○ **Urethral prolapse most frequently occurs in which patient population?**

Urethral prolapse occurs almost exclusively in African American girls between ages 1 and 9 years.

○ **What is believed to be the pathophysiology of urethral prolapse?**

Urethral prolapse is thought to occur during episodes of increased abdominal pressure in a urethra, where there is poor attachment of the smooth muscle layers. The cleavage plane is usually between the inner circular and outer longitudinal muscle layers.

○ **What is the standard therapeutic management of urethral prolapse?**

Standard therapy for urethral prolapse entails topical application of estrogen cream and sitz baths. Formal surgical excision may be required if the prolapse is persistent.

○ **What is the pathophysiologic mechanism resulting in acquired urethral diverticula?**

Acquired urethral diverticula result from infected and obstructed periurethral glands that rupture into the urethral lumen.

○ **What are the tumors that have been found in urethral diverticula?**

Urethral adenocarcinoma, transitional cell carcinoma, squamous cell carcinoma, and nephrogenic adenoma are the tumors that have been found in urethral diverticula. Of these, adenocarcinoma is the most common.

○ **What are the 3Ds of symptoms that are characteristic of urethral diverticula?**

Dysuria, postvoid **D**ribbling, and **D**yspareunia.

○ **What is the diagnostic study to demonstrate the presence of a urethral diverticulum?**

Many believe MRI is the imaging modality of choice. While 100% sensitive, an MRI is expensive. A RUG with a double balloon catheter or voiding cystourethrogram can also be employed.

○ **What are the surgical principles employed to treat a urethral diverticulum?**

In the setting of small distal diverticulum, some may be simply marsupialized. For more proximal or larger lesions, complete excision is required. The urethral defect should be closed without tension with multiple layers utilizing the periurethral fascia and vaginal wall flaps. A Martius flap of labial fat maybe interspersed between suture lines to help prevent fistula formation.

○ **What is circinate balanitis?**

Circinate balanitis manifests as a shallow ulcer on the glans penis. It is painless, has gray borders, and is typically associated with Reiter syndrome.

○ **What is the difference between senile urethritis and a urethral caruncle?**

Both are benign conditions occurring in postmenopausal women, with the former being more common. Senile urethritis results in eversion of the external urethral meatus due to shortening of the vagina. It can be mistaken for a urethral caruncle and responds to estrogen replacement therapy. Urethral caruncle is a red, friable mass located on the posterior lip of the external urethral meatus. It is composed of connective tissue, blood vessels, and inflammatory cells. It may require local excision.

CHAPTER 44

Diagnosis and Staging of Prostate Cancer

George P. Hemstreet III, MD, PhD and
Sudhir Isharwal, MD

○ **What is the US Preventive Services Task Force (USPSTF) recommendation for prostate specific antigen (PSA) screening in 2012 and describe its significance?**

They recommend against prostate-specific antigen-based screening and gave it a "D" recommendation. USPSTF concludes that there is moderate or high certainity that prostate screening harms outweigh the benefits.

○ **Discuss the studies used as the basis for the USPSTF level D recommendation including the associated morbidities.**

- The USPSTF recommendation for not screening is the fact that there is no reduction in all-cause mortality in the PLCO (Prostate, Lung, Colon and Ovary) trial and the European Randomized Study of Screening for Prostate Cancer (ERSPC) study showed only a modest overall survival benefit.
- You have to screen 1000 people and diagnose 37 individuals with prostate cancer in order to prevent one death from prostate cancer.
- The USPSTF sees that risk versus benefit from screening leads to erectile dysfunction and urinary incontinence, which is as high as 20% to 30% in men who undergo therapy with no reduction in all-cause mortality.

○ **The basis for the American Urologic Association for continued screening are based on what scientific data?**

- Since widespread screening was initiated in 1992, there has been a 44% reduction in prostate cancer-specific deaths, of which 50% to 75% are attributed to prostate cancer screening. In addition, there has been 75% reduction in the number of men presenting initially with metastatic prostate cancer. There are also a number of trials such as those done in Tyrol—Austria and Goteborg—Sweden that suggest a 50% or better cancer-specific survival benefit in screened populations.
- The PLCO and ERSPC trials were highly flawed with over 50% of men in the control group getting PSA testing either before or during the trial. The test period for these studies was less than 10 years (7 and 9 years) when initially reported, and there were significant protocol violations where up to 70% of the men in the screened group who had an elevated PSA did not get the required biopsies.

○ **The identification and molecular analysis of prostate circulating tumor cells (CTC) has potential in the following areas:**
- Early prostate cancer detection
- Selection of cancer therapy
- Monitoring chemotherapy
- Determining surgical intervention
- All of the above

○ **True/False: Quantification of circulating prostate tumor cells for monitoring chemotherapy of hormone refractory prostate cancer is FDA approved.**

True.

○ **What does the Prolaris test for in prostate cancer, and what is its significance?**
- It tests for quantitative measures of RNA expression levels of multiple genes that are related to tumor cell division and progression.
- The significance of this test is that it can assess an individual's relative risk of mortality from prostate cancer within 10 years with a hazard ratio (HR) value of 1.67 in a multivariate analysis.

○ **Discuss the clinical utility of the PCA3 test in the management of a patient with a PSA positive and negative biopsy.**

The PCA3 test has a sensitivity of 62% and a specificity of approximately 90%. Thus, this test is useful in combination with PSA when deciding regarding repeat biopsy or initial biopsy of patients at risk for prostate cancer. In the receiver operating characteristic (ROC), the area under the curve increases 0.2 to 0.7 compared to PSA 0.5. Thus the accuracy of this test is improved when compared to the PSA test.

○ **Discuss the current role of CTC.**

CTC may be used to predict survival outcome in prostate cancer and can provide insight into patients with metastatic disease. CTCs may be more useful in monitoring patients with bone metastasis because they are more frequently elevated than in patients with visceral disease.

○ **What PCA3 values are useful for the clinical management of patients with prostate cancer?**

PCA3 score threshold of 20 may have the highest utility for selecting men with clinically insignificant prostate cancer while a PCA3 score of 50 may be used to identify men who are at significant risk for prostate cancer and are candidates for a radical prostatectomy.

○ **What is pro-PSA?**

[−2] pro-PSA, a truncated form of pro-PSA is the most specific cancer form, and is most preferentially expressed in cancer epithelium. There is evidence to suggest that percentage of pro-PSA over free PSA improves the specificity of both tPSA and fPSA.

○ **What is prostate health index (PHI)?**

Phi is defined as ($[−2]$ pro-PSA/fPSA) $\times \sqrt{tPSA}$.

○ **Laparoscopic pelvic lymphadenectomy prior to treatment is typically reserved for patients with what criteria?**

Gleason score greater than 8, extraprostatic extension on digital rectal examination (DRE), PSA greater than 20 ng/mL, or suspicion of enlarged lymph nodes on radiologic evaluation.

○ **In what groups of prostate cancer patients is a bone scan recommended?**

In patients with PSA greater than 20 ng/mL, a Gleason score of 8 to 10, clinical stage T3 or T4, or clinical symptoms of bone metastasis.

○ **What is the D'Amico stratification of prostate cancer?**

- Low-risk patients are those with clinical stage T1 to T2a, PSA 10 ng/mL or less, and Gleason score of 6 or less.
- Intermediate stage patients are those with stage T2b, PSA greater than 10 ng/mL but less than 20 ng/mL, or Gleason score of 7.
- High-risk patients include those with T2c, PSA greater than 20 ng/mL, or Gleason score 8 to 10.

○ **What other factors other than Gleason score determinations on prostate biopsies are used for risk prediction?**

The number of positive cores, the percentage of tumor involvement of those positive cores, the presence or absence of bilateral involvement, and the presence of perineural invasion all have some predictive value. Even worse prognosis is associated with seminal vesicle invasion. A new biomarker EN2 may be useful for defining tumor volume (Pandha et al., 2012). PCA3 has been shown in preliminary studies to correlate with tumor volume as well as capsular invasion and penetration.

○ **What information should be related to a patient prior to PSA screening?**

PSA screening should be limited to those individuals with a life expectancy of greater than 10 years. Patients should be informed that even though their PSA is elevated, this may not indicate that they have cancer and the chance of finding cancer based on PSA alone in an unscreened population is less than 25%. In addition, the patient should be informed that a positive biopsy based on an elevated PSA or clinical findings does not necessarily indicate the patient will be recommended for surgery or definitive radiation, but may be considered a good candidate for active surveillance. Information regarding the future management should be a joint decision between the patient and physician considering the risk versus benefit for each individual patient at each decision point.

○ **Describe the PIVOT trial and how its conclusions affect PSA screenings since it does not appear to show any benefit from surgical intervention in localized prostate cancer.**

The Prostate Intervention versus Observation Trial followed 2 groups of men with localized prostate cancer and good performance status. One group received radical prostatectomies, the other just observation. After 10 years, there was no significant difference in overall survival between the 2 groups. The study has been criticized for several reasons. The median age was 67 where, according to the Actuary Office of the Social Security Administration, the current average life expectancy would be slightly more than 17 years while in this study of mostly VA patients, the median life expectancy was only 10 years. A careful review of the data also shows that there was a trend beginning to show a cancer-specific benefit to treatment beginning at 10 years, but only a longer follow-up will be able to show this.

○   **What are the current recommendations for screening for prostate cancer in American men?**

To date, there is no consensus on screening for prostate cancer in American men. The American Urological Association currently recommends initiating screening at age 50 for white men with no family history of prostate cancer and age 45 for black men with no family history of the disease. In men with a first-degree relative with the disease, initiation of screening should begin at age 45 for whites and at age 40 for blacks. AUA recommends checking baseline PSA at age 40 for all men.

○   **What is considered a "normal" PSA?**

Normal PSA ranges have been determined to be 0 to 4 ng/mL. Age-specific normal reference ranges and acceptable rates of change in the PSA value over time (PSA velocity) have been delineated and may enhance the identification of individuals at risk for the disease.

○   **What are the age-specific normal reference ranges for PSA?**

- For men aged 40 to 49 years, the normal reference range is 0 to 2.5 ng/mL.
- For men aged 50 to 59 years, the normal reference range is 0 to 3.5 ng/mL.
- For men aged 60 to 69 years, the normal reference range is 0 to 4.5 ng/mL.
- For men aged 70 to 79 years, the normal reference range is 0 to 6.5 ng/mL.

○   **So which is better, the normal range or the age-specific range?**

It isn't yet clear exactly what the optimal range should be. If the criteria are too strict, curable cancers will not be detected. If too liberal, too many unnecessary biopsies will be done. While the 0 to 4.0 range has proved very effective, age-related adjustments seem reasonable. For age 65 and above, a PSA range of 0 to 4.0 can be used, and for age 64 and younger, a PSA range of 0 to 2.5 has been suggested.

○   **What is the current suggested PSA cut-off level for men aging 65 years and younger being screened for prostate cancer?**

2.5 is the current threshold level for men 65 years of age and younger.

○   **What percentage of the cancers detected in prostate screenings are estimated to be clinically insignificant?**

Less than 7%.

○   **At what point should routine prostate cancer screenings (DREs and PSA determinations) be stopped?**

The consensus opinion is that there is a declining benefit of treatment of screening detected prostate cancer with advancing age and that men with less than a 10-year life expectancy, usually age 75, should probably not undergo routine prostate cancer or PSA screenings.

○   **What is the normal function of PSA?**

PSA is a protease whose normal function is to help liquify the semen. It also liquify cervical mucus to help passage of sperm.

○   **When was PSA approved for prostate cancer screening by the FDA?**

1994.

○ **What percentage of prostate cancers are found in men with "normal" PSA levels?**

Approximately 20%.

○ **What is PSA velocity?**

PSA velocity is the rate of change of serum PSA over time. Studies have indicated that the acceptable rate of change in PSA over 12 months is <0.75 ng/mL for PSA levels between 4 and 10 ng/mL. Changes that exceed this rate are considered abnormal and should be carefully considered by the interpreting physician. An individual should have several PSA determinations over time intervals to provide for correct interpretation.

○ **What types of events can adversely affect PSA results?**

A number of factors will affect the accuracy of PSA results. A vigorous DRE, urinary retention, passage of a Foley catheter, acute prostatitis, recent prostate biopsy, and any maneuver that "manipulates" the gland will falsely elevate the PSA. Interpretation of serum PSA results following any of these events should be delayed for 21 days to allow sufficient time for resolution of the false elevation of the PSA.

○ **What is the serum half-life of PSA?**

Published reports have documented the serum half-life of PSA to be 2.2 ± 0.8 days and 3.3 ± 0.1 days depending upon the testing method used. Based on these data, one should wait at least 21 days following manipulation of the gland to allow for a sufficient number of half-lives to yield a reliable result before drawing a serum PSA.

○ **What is free PSA and what is the significance of free PSA?**

PSA is a glycoprotein produced by the prostatic epithelial cells and once in the serum approximately 40% is bound to α_2-macroglobulin and is unmeasurable. The remaining fraction of PSA is bound to α_1-antichymotrypsin or circulates free in the serum and both are measurable by commercial techniques. Conclusive studies have indicated that individuals with prostate cancer tend to have a lower percent free PSA, and cut-off limits have been assigned to this value. A free PSA less than 25% is considered to be a prognostic factor for prostate cancer. Levels of 10% or less are associated with a 50% incidence of prostate cancer.

○ **Can free PSA be used to assess the relative risk for carcinoma of the prostate in all men?**

No. The utility of free PSA is restricted to men with a total PSA between 4 and 10 ng/mL. There have been no definitive studies that indicate an application of free PSA to individuals with a total PSA less than 4 ng/mL. If the total PSA is less than 4.0 ng/mL, one may employ the age-specific reference ranges for PSA and PSA velocity to better assess an individual's risk for disease.

○ **Can the serum PSA level reliably predict pathological stage?**

No. The serum PSA level alone cannot be used to reliably predict the pathological stage of disease. Approximately 70% to 80% of patients with locally advanced prostate cancer have a serum PSA levels >10 ng/mL. The Gleason biopsy score may have more predictive value in predicting the extent of disease.

○ **You are sent an individual with an elevated PSA for evaluation. He has no symptoms or clinical findings suggesting BPH, LUTS, or prostatitis. What should be your next step?**

Rather than rush directly into a prostate biopsy, consider the patients age, general state of health, medications, and state of mind. If he is anxious about prostate cancer and demands a biopsy, it may be best to do so for his anxiety. For most patients, it is often best to repeat the PSA level after a 30-day course of antibiotics. A decision about a possible biopsy can be made at that time. In many cases, the PSA returns to baseline avoiding a potentially painful biopsy.

○ **A 54-year-old man with an enlarged prostate on rectal examination has a serum PSA of 3.6 ng/mL and a free PSA of 45%. There is no family history of prostate cancer. How would you counsel him about his risk for prostate cancer?**

Autopsy studies from 1954 indicate that the overall risk for prostate cancer in 50-year-old men is 30%. This individual has BPH by examination and although his free PSA is over 25%, which is consistent with the diagnosis of BPH, his total PSA is less than 4.0 ng/mL and therefore the free PSA may not have much bearing. This patient's current risk for indolent disease should parallel the age-matched general population. A reasonable course of follow-up may consist of serial PSA measurements to track his PSA velocity.

○ **What is the role for DRE in assessing patients at risk for prostate cancer?**

Data reported in the literature indicate that DRE alone detects less than 1.7% of all diagnosed prostate cancers even when there is a high index of suspicion of glandular abnormalities. However, DRE does provide useful information about the size and potential resectability of the prostate in individuals with prostate pathology. It may also detect asymmetry that could suggest a tumor.

○ **What is the accuracy of clinical staging based on DRE?**

The accuracy of DRE alone in men with palpable lesions approximates 50% and of those individuals diagnosed by this modality alone more than 70% will be upstaged at the time of pathological examination.

○ **What is the best role for DRE in assessing patients at risk for prostate cancer?**

DRE is utilized best in combination with PSA determination and transrectal ultrasound-guided biopsies. This combination provides for the most efficient means of evaluating men at risk for prostate cancer.

○ **Can ultrasound reliably diagnose prostate cancer?**

No. Numerous published studies have indicated the absence of a pathognomonic appearance of prostate cancer on ultrasound. Although a higher percentage of cancers are hypoechoic, prostate cancer can also be hyperechoic or isoechoic on transrectal ultrasound imaging.

○ **What is the role for ultrasound in diagnosing prostate cancer?**

Ultrasound is a very useful adjunct in diagnosing prostate cancer and has its greatest utility in directing the biopsy needle to particular areas of the prostate gland.

○ **When performing transrectal needle biopsy of the prostate, how many biopsies should be done?**

Historically, 6 cores were thought to represent a reasonable sampling of the gland with the cores including left- and right-sided biopsies from the base, mid, and apical portions of the gland. Reports in the literature over the years have indicated that 6 cores may be insufficient and performing 12 biopsies has now become the norm with the biopsies being more laterally located and adding medial apical biopsies in lieu of transitional zone biopsies. Recent publications indicate the lack of sufficient benefit and efficacy of saturation biopsy at the initial biopsy setting although this may be useful as a secondary measure in select cases.

○ **Is the biopsy result indicative of overall disease burden?**

Yes. There have been a number of studies that indicate that the biopsy result has prognostic information about overall disease burden. The Gleason score of the biopsy specimen is the most important prognostic factor for capsular extension of disease. Additionally, the percent of core involved and the number of cores involved can give predictive information for capsular extension and lymph node involvement.

○ **What is the strongest prognostic factor for prostate cancer-related death?**

The biopsy Gleason score has consistently been shown to be a significant prognostic factor for cancer-related death in individuals diagnosed with the disease. To date, there have been no reliable prognostic data reported for preoperative PSA results or free PSA results.

○ **What agents are being studied for their potential use in the prevention of prostate cancer and their proposed mechanisms?**

- Dutasteride (Avodart) inhibits both type 1 and type 2 forms of 5-alpha-reductase.
- Vitamin D induces cell-cycle arrest and has an antiproliferative effect on prostate cancer cells.
- Cox-2 inhibitors selectively block prostaglandin production and may reduce expression of several androgen-inducible genes.
- Lycopenes are antioxidants that may inhibit prostate cancer cell growth.
- Green tea-derived polyphenols induce apoptosis, inhibit cell growth, and dysregulate the cell cycle.
- Selenium inhibits cell proliferation and induces apoptosis. Vitamin E has shown direct antiandrogen activity.

○ **A 64-year-old man with a normal DRE undergoes a transrectal needle biopsy of the prostate for a PSA of 4.9 ng/mL. One out of 8 cores, the left base, is positive for Gleason 3 + 3 adenocarcinoma. What is his clinical stage?**

One of the more commonly used staging systems is that outlined by the American Joint Commission on Cancer (AJCC). Based on this staging system, this individual would be classified as having T1c disease, that is, tumor identified by needle biopsy.

○ **The patient in the previous question underwent a radical retropubic prostatectomy. The pathology report revealed disease involving the entire left side of the gland with no capsular penetration. The lymph nodes were negative. What is his pathologic stage?**

Using AJCC criteria, disease confined by the capsule and involving more than one-half of the lobe but not more than one lobe with negative lymph nodes is classified as pT2b, N0, M0 disease.

○ **A 58-year-old man underwent a radical perineal prostatectomy for unilateral Gleason 3 + 4 in 1 out of 8 core biopsies. His PSA was 4.3 ng/mL. The pathology specimen showed disease involving both sides of the gland with capsular penetration at the left apex. What is his stage?**

AJCC criteria support a diagnosis of pT3a, Nx, M0 in this individual. A pelvic lymph node dissection was not done and therefore one cannot assess the status of the lymph nodes.

○ **A 69-year-old man underwent a radical retropubic prostatectomy and the pathology report revealed disease on both sides of the gland with extension through the capsule bilaterally and 0 out of 13 lymph nodes involved. What is his pathologic stage?**

Based on the AJCC criteria, the correct diagnosis is pT3a, N0, M0 disease.

○ **A 63-year-old man whose father had prostate cancer has a total PSA of 11.8 ng/mL and a free PSA of 11%. A transrectal ultrasound-guided needle biopsy of his prostate revealed no evidence of cancer in 12 cores. What is a reasonable approach to his management?**

This individual certainly is at high risk for having prostate cancer and probably warrants a repeat biopsy. One could consider doing more extensive biopsies including biopsies of the transitional zone and far lateral peripheral zone biopsies. Mapping saturation biopsies done under anesthesia and often numbering as high as 24 or more cores in which the gland is more thoroughly sampled may be helpful.

○ **A 78-year-old healthy asymptomatic man presents with a PSA of 8 ng/mL and a free PSA of 20%. He has no voiding symptoms, minimal nocturia, and no history of past genitourinary (GU) problems. On physical examination, his prostate is enlarged, asymmetric but not clinically suspicious. What is the next best course of action?**

This individual has a minimally elevated PSA when one considers the age-specific reference ranges. He is asymptomatic from a GU standpoint. A conservative approach with serial PSA determinations is not unreasonable in this situation. In a younger man, a biopsy would be recommended.

○ **A 54-year-old man with no comorbid disease underwent a transrectal needle biopsy of the prostate for a PSA of 18 ng/mL and a free PSA of 8%. The pathology showed Gleason 4 + 5 in all cores and there was evidence of perineural invasion. What is your next course of action?**

This individual has a very poor chance of being cured of his disease. The overwhelming majority (approximately 80%) of patients with this Gleason pattern will suffer a biochemical failure within 5 years of monotherapeutic intervention. Furthermore, the likelihood of his having positive lymph nodes based on his biopsy results must be considered. Brachytherapy alone would be a poor choice, since it does not effectively treat disease in the extracapsular space. Radical prostatectomy for maximal local control of the disease with an option for early adjuvant radiation therapy to sterilize the field may be an option depending upon the lymph node status, but this will likely only extend his time period of biochemical freedom of disease rather than result in cure. A multimodality approach in this young individual with no comorbid disease will be required to maximize his outcome. A ProstaScint scan would be useful to see if he has localized or disseminated disease. If localized, cryotherapy would be another option.

○ **A 57-year-old healthy man presents with a PSA of 3.2 ng/mL. His previous PSA 6 months ago was 2.3 ng/mL and 6 months prior to that his PSA was 1.5 ng/mL. What is your next course of action?**

Although this man has a PSA within the age-specific reference range (0-3.5 ng/mL), his PSA velocity is out of the accepted range of normal. He has a sufficient PSA history to make this determination and his most recent findings warrant further investigation. A TRUS-guided biopsy of the prostate would not be unreasonable. Alternatively, a 30-day course of antibiotics can be given and then the PSA level repeated. Further therapy would depend on the second PSA level.

○ **A 69-year-old, obese, insulin-dependent diabetic man with a history of hypertension, coronary artery disease, s/p CABG, and a 70 pack per year smoking history presents with a PSA of 5.4 ng/mL. What is the next best course of action?**

This individual has significant comorbid disease and his PSA is minimally elevated. He is asymptomatic from a GU standpoint. A careful assessment of his overall condition reveals that he is not a good candidate for anesthesia. One must determine how aggressive they should be in evaluating patients at risk for disease, and whether the risk–benefit ratio warrants further evaluation/intervention. Close observation with repeat PSA measurements may not be unreasonable for this individual. If a biopsy is done and is positive for prostate cancer, watchful waiting, external beam radiation, and hormonal therapy are all possible treatments.

○ **Is there a role for MRI in the routine evaluation for prostate cancer?**

The role of MRI in diagnosing and staging prostate cancer has been studied extensively. Endorectal coil and newer body surface coil MRI of the prostate have shown utility in staging select patients with prostate cancer. However, the lack of sensitivity and specificity of MRI in differentiating benign from malignant prostate tissue preclude the use of MRI as a reliable means to diagnose the disease. Extracapsular extension and seminal vesicle involvement have been identified with MRI and correlated with pathologic findings, but the associated costs and the availability of the equipment are factors that preclude the use of MRI as a first-line imaging modality for patients with prostate cancer. MRI is used by a number of institutions for assessment of metastatic disease and confirmation of bony involvement as well as for Prostascint determinations.

○ **A 64-year-old man presents with a PSA of 52 ng/mL and a free PSA of 8%. He complains of back pain and left hip pain. What is the next best course of action?**

This individual likely has bony metastases from his disease. He requires prompt diagnosis with a prostate biopsy as well as a serum alkaline phosphatase level and a radiologic evaluation of his bones. If he has metastatic disease, initiation of hormonal deprivation therapy is reasonable. Radiation therapy to the bones should be considered.

○ **What are the risks of starting LHRH therapy alone in a patient with metastatic prostate cancer?**

Initiation of LHRH therapy is associated with a testosterone flare that usually lasts about 14 days, after which castrate levels of testosterone are achieved. During the flare period, individuals can suffer from exacerbation of obstructive voiding symptoms and increased bone pain, and if there is vertebral involvement with bony metastases, they can develop spinal cord compromise or even paralysis. Additionally, compression fractures of the spine or any other involved bone may occur during the flare period depending upon the degree of bony involvement. Therefore, it is wise to begin antiandrogen therapy at the time of initiation of LHRH therapy in an effort to minimize potential morbidity in these select patients. The duration of antiandrogen administration should be a minimum of 2 weeks. Orchiectomy avoids this flare phenomenon, as does LHRH antagonists.

○ **A thin, 52-year-old man is referred by his internist with complaints of obstructive voiding symptoms, pelvic pain and bilateral lower extremity weakness, and swelling. On physical examination, he has palpable nontender periaortic masses and his prostate is consistent with TIIIc disease. He also has 2+ pitting edema of the lower extremities. A phone call to the internist reveals a PSA was drawn and the result is 914 ng/mL. How would you proceed?**

This patient requires urgent intervention. A computed tomography (CT) scan of the abdomen and pelvis reveals massive retroperitoneal adenopathy with compression of the vena cava. There are large iliac lymph nodes identified on the CT scan. There is no evidence of vertebral bony involvement with disease or cord compression. His findings are consistent with advanced prostate cancer as well as vascular compromise from metastatic disease. An urgent orchiectomy is preferred since initiation of LHRH therapy will not result in castrate levels of testosterone for approximately 14 days. Additionally, one should consider CT-guided needle biopsy of the retroperitoneal lymph nodes to confirm the absence of a second primary such as lymphoma. If LHRH therapy is used, antiandrogens should also be used.

○ **Should all patients with prostate cancer have a bone scan as part of the staging evaluation?**

No. Bone scans are often employed to evaluate patients at risk for metastatic prostate cancer. Studies have indicated that the likelihood of a positive bone scan in an individual with a PSA less than 10 ng/mL in the absence of symptoms of bone pain is less than 1%. However, poorly differentiated cancers are known to have diminished PSA production, and therefore, PSA can be misleading in patients with poorly differentiated prostate cancer. If an individual has symptoms of bone pain and/or an elevated alkaline phosphatase, a bone scan is a reasonable staging examination.

○ **Which is more sensitive for the detection of bone metastases, bone scans or plain radiographs?**

Bone scintigraphy is much more sensitive than plain radiography for detection of bony metastases. Plain radiography generally requires a 50% change in the cortical bone density to diagnose a bony metastasis, whereas bone scintigraphy can detect disease with as little as 10% change in the cortical bone density. Ninety-five percent of bone lesions due to prostate cancer are osteoblastic, whereas 5% are osteolytic.

○ **A 73-year-old man presents with a PSA of 23 ng/mL 10 years following 64-Gy external beam radiation therapy for prostate cancer. He has significant bladder outlet obstructive symptoms and a clinical TIIIb prostate. There are no other pertinent findings on history and physical. What is your next course of action?**

This individual should be evaluated with a TRUS biopsy of the prostate to establish the diagnosis of recurrent disease. If the diagnosis of locally recurrent disease is made, LHRH therapy can be initiated cognizant of the fact that he may develop urinary retention due to the testosterone flare. This can usually be presented by using anti-androgen therapy such as Casodex or Flutamide. To address his bladder outlet obstruction, one might consider a "channel" TUR of the prostate, but the associated risk of incontinence in a previously radiated patient is as high as 30% in some series. LHRH therapy will not have impact on his voiding function for several months, and α-blockers are not always effective with a high tumor burden in the prostate. Finally, a metastatic evaluation would be predicated upon abnormal findings on physical examination or blood work. Generally, a PSA of 20 or more is necessary to justify a bone scan.

○ **Is there a role for CT scan in the routine staging of prostate cancer?**

No. CT scanning lacks sufficient sensitivity and specificity to reliably increase the accuracy of clinical staging for patients with prostate cancer. Numerous published studies have reported accuracy rates ranging between 15% and 65% for staging individuals with disease. In the absence of bulky disease, CT lacks the resolution necessary to delineate extracapsular extension, and CT cannot differentiate benign from pathologic tissue within the prostate.

○ **Is there a role for CT scanning in assessing the status of the pelvic lymph nodes?**

CT scanning cannot differentiate a suspicious (>1 cm) from an abnormal lymph node (>1.5 cm) with regard to a benign inflammatory condition versus a pathologic process. However, in select individuals with prognostic factors suggestive of lymph node involvement, that is, significantly elevated PSA, high Gleason score (>7), or bulky clinical disease CT scanning may have a role in staging the patient.

○ **Is there a role for Prostascint in staging patients with prostate cancer?**

Yes. Prostascint uses indium in III capromab pendetide, a radiolabeled monoclonal antibody to prostate-specific membrane antigen (PSMA) to identify soft tissue sites of prostate cancer metastasis. PSMA is selectively expressed in epithelial cells of prostate origin both normal and malignant. Expression is increased in prostate cancer compared to normal epithelium. The scan is best used when correlated with other modalities such as MRI and SPECT.

○ **How is Prostascint most effectively used?**

It is best used in patients with rising PSA to determine if they may still benefit from localized therapy. Purely anatomical tests such as CT and MRI cannot demonstrate low volume metastatic disease. It can also be used in higher-risk individuals to help detect extraprostatic disease. This would spare the individuals the complications of local definitive therapy in favor of systemic treatment.

○ **What is the impact of obesity on prostate cancer incidence and aggressiveness?**

Analysis of data from the CaPSURE database of over 10,000 men with prostate cancer showed no correlation between Gleason score and obesity. However, obese patients were more likely to be younger at the time of diagnosis and have more comorbidities. This is thought to be due to more frequent interactions of this group with the medical community, which would lead to earlier detection.

○ **What is the risk of fracture in prostate cancer patients receiving androgen ablation therapy?**

According to the SEER database of 50,613 men with prostate cancer, of those surviving at least 5 years after diagnosis, the risk of a fracture was 19.4%.

○ **What is the average amount of bone mass lost in the first 12 months after androgen deprivation therapy is started?**

From 2% to 8%.

○ **What treatments are recommended to reduce osteoporosis in men receiving androgen deprivation therapy?**

Vitamin D and calcium supplementation should be started. Decreasing excessive alcohol intake, stopping smoking, and increasing weight-bearing exercise have been shown to be helpful. If hypercalciuric, a thiazide diuretic may help reduce urinary calcium loss. Oral bisphosphonates have not been shown to increase bone mineral density, but they may reduce the rate of bone loss. Only zoledronic acid (Zometa) has been shown to actually increase bone in men receiving androgen ablation therapy for prostate cancer.

○ **What percentage of men on androgen deprivation therapy for prostate cancer typically receive osteoporosis testing or preventive therapy?**

Less than 15%, with only about 5% receiving bisphosphonate therapy.

○ **What is the most accurate way of measuring bone mineral density?**

Dual-energy x-ray absorptiometry (DEXA) is considered the best and most accurate way to measure bone mineral density. Ultrasound is less expensive and more convenient although it is less accurate.

○ **Is a higher free testosterone level associated with an increased risk of prostate cancer?**

Yes, particularly in older men. This suggests that caution should be used in hypogonadal seniors who are considering testosterone replacement therapy, which increases free testosterone levels.

○ **Does the presence of hematospermia increase the risk of prostate cancer?**

Yes. Although hematospermia is generally thought of as a benign and self-limiting problem, when it appears in the prostate cancer screening population, it is associated with a significantly higher risk of prostate cancer. This risk is roughly double the risk of the general screened population.

○ **Does a Gleason sum of 4 + 3 = 7 carry a worse prognosis than a Gleason sum of 3 + 4 = 7?**

It isn't clear. We tend to give more weight to the primary Gleason score, but in this case with Gleason 7, the studies are conflicting.

○ **True/False: Bicalutamide (Casodex) 150 mg should no longer be used as monotherapy for prostate cancer?**

True. While there is no problem with the standard approved 50 mg dose, the higher 150 mg daily dose was found to be associated with a higher death rate at 5 years in a large European study.

○ **Over 90% of prostate cancers are adenocarcinomas. What are the other types of prostate cancer that may be found?**

Transitional cell carcinoma and sarcoma are the most common after adenocarcinoma.

○ **What are the histological variations in adenocarcinoma of the prostate?**

Neuroendocrine, endometrioid, small cell, and mucinous are some of the histological variations of prostate cancer.

○ **What are the best nomograms for predicting prostate cancer outcomes and prognosis?**

There are a number of nomograms available but most have not been updated, validated, or had their predictions compared to actual results. Possibly the best and certainly the most well known are the Partin tables. The websites for a few of the most useful nomograms currently available are listed below. They are the Partin tables from Johns Hopkins, nomograms from Dr. Kevin Slawin of Baylor, and the Memorial Sloan Kettering tables.

- Partin Tables: http://urology.jhu.edu/prostate/partintables.php
- Dr. Kevin Slawin: www.drslawin.com/nomogram.html#
- Memorial Sloan Kettering: www.mskcc.org/mskcc/html/10088.cfm

○ **A 57-year-old man with 2-years status postexternal beam radiation therapy for localized prostate cancer presents with a rising PSA. His PSA at the time of diagnosis was 6.07 ng/mL. The PSA has increased from a nadir of 1.02 ng/mL to 2.02 ng/mL to 4.2 ng/mL over the past 12 months. History and physical examination are only revealing a firm radiated prostate. The best course of action is?**

This patient has radiation failure prostate cancer based upon the Phoenix criteria of a PSA nadir + 2 ng/mL. The next best course of action is to obtain pathologic confirmation of recurrent disease. A bone scan would be revealing in a minority of patients in this situation, but may be prudent if salvage therapy is entertained. Imaging to assess extraprostatic disease burden and spread is appropriate after a prostate biopsy has been performed. LHRH therapy is an option, but if the patient proves to have localized recurrent disease curative therapy with salvage radical prostatectomy or cryotherapy may be more appropriate and potentially lifesaving.

○ **A 67-year-old man presents 3-year status postexternal beam radiation therapy with concomitant LHRH analog therapy for localized prostate cancer. His PSA at the time of diagnosis was 13 ng/mL and the Gleason score was 4 + 3 in 8/14 biopsies. The PSA has increased from a nadir of 0.1 ng/mL to 0.75 ng/mL to 2.24 ng/mL over the past 9 months. Serum testosterone levels are consistently less than 50 ng/dL. What is the next best course of action?**

This patient has hormone-independent radiation failure prostate cancer. His PSA doubling time is less than 9 months, which is a very poor prognostic factor for long-term disease-specific survival. A metastatic evaluation is the best first course of action. Even in the setting of a negative metastatic evaluation, a salvage procedure would be of limited benefit given the following factors: his high primary Gleason score, the rapid doubling time of his PSA, and the hormone-independent progression of his disease. Systemic chemotherapy would usually be reserved until evidence of bony metastases.

○ **A 63-year-old man presents with a PSA of 2.78 ng/mL 6-years status postbrachytherapy for localized Gleason 3 + 3 prostate cancer. He has biopsy proven localized recurrent disease. A comprehensive history and physical examination reveal no significant findings. The next best course of action is?**

This patient is young with no comorbid factors and salvage therapy is a very reasonable option. Pathologic evidence of recurrent disease and a negative metastatic evaluation allow for options of salvage therapy. CyberKnife radiotherapy is not an option given his history of prior brachytherapy. Salvage prostatectomy is an option but is associated with higher procedure-related morbidity than salvage cryotherapy.

○ **A 64-year-old tile contractor presents with a PSA of 5.17 ng/mL. He has no LUTS and physical examination is revealing only for a mildly enlarged prostate that is asymmetric. The next best course of action is?**

This patient has a single elevated age-specific reference range PSA. Before offering a prostate biopsy it might be prudent to repeat the value to rule out an erratic abnormal result. Cognizant of the greater than 30% risk of indolent disease in this age population, confirmation of an abnormal PSA result is the best choice before proceeding with a biopsy. A 15 to 30 day course of antibiotics and a free/total PSA may be helpful in deciding whether or not a biopsy is necessary.

○ **Prior to the implementation of PSA into the physician's armamentarium, what percent of men had nonorgan-confined disease at the time of diagnosis of prostate cancer?**

Prior to widespread use of PSA, 50% to 60% of men had extracapsular extension at the time of surgical extirpation. With the utilization of widespread PSA screening, the incidence of organ-confined disease has increased to 75% to 85% of all prostatectomy specimens.

○ **In 2008, what is the likelihood of a man having metastatic prostate cancer at the time of diagnosis?**

With widespread use of PSA screening, the likelihood of a man having metastatic disease at the time of diagnosis is less than 5%. Additionally, the Partin tables have been revised due to the increased incidence of T1c disease. In the revised nomograms, approximately 77% of all men who underwent surgical extirpation had nonpalpable lesions at the time of diagnosis.

○ **What is uPM3?**

uPM3 was the first urine-based genetic test available to assess an individual's risk for carcinoma of the prostate. This test proved to be highly specific for detection of prostate cancer. uPM3 preliminarily proved to be an independent and specific biomarker that detects prostate cancer. This marker performed similarly to other conventional means of identifying patients at risk for disease. uPM3 is not able to distinguish large or aggressive cancers from more indolent disease.

○ **A 47-year-old man presents with an elevated PSA of 3.7 ng/mL and a nodule on the left base of the prostate gland. Detailed history and physical examination are negative. A TRUS-guided needle biopsy of the prostate is positive for 9/14 cores Gleason 3 + 3 disease. Based upon risk stratification criteria what is this patient's category?**

Favorable factors included in risk stratification include PSA less than 10 ng/mL, Gleason score 6 or less, and clinical T2a disease or less. Therefore, this patient is in the favorable-risk group for 10-year biochemical disease-free survival. A patient without one of the 3 risk factor criteria would be in the moderate-risk group and the lack of 2 or more factors place an individual in the high-risk group for 10-year biochemical disease-free survival.

○ **True/False: Black men tend to have higher serum testosterone levels than white men, which might explain their increased risk of prostate cancer.**

False. It's unproven that blacks have higher serum testosterone levels than whites.

○ **True/False: Serum testosterone levels do not affect prostate cancer risk.**

True. In a large collaborative review of 18 studies comprising nearly 4000 prostate cancer patients and 6500 controls, no relationship could be found between the risk of prostate cancer and serum concentrations of any sex hormones including testosterone, dihydrotestosterone, or estradiol. (Endogenous Hormones and Prostate Cancer Collaborative Group, 2008.)

○ **What is the median age for prostate cancer diagnosis?**

Approximately 70.5 years.

○ **What percentage of patients newly diagnosed with prostate cancer are 65 years of age or younger?**

Approximately 20%.

○ **True/False: A negative PSA velocity after a course of antibiotics reasonably eliminates the presence of prostate cancer.**

False. The PSA following the course of antibiotics must still fall below the biopsy threshold level.

○ **What is the significance of "atypical small acinar proliferation" (ASAP) on prostate needle biopsy specimens and how often, if ever, is it associated with prostate cancer?**

ASAP is generally considered suspicious for prostate cancer. Approximately 30% of subsequent biopsies demonstrate prostate cancer.

○ **Patients with large prostates (>80 g) are more, less or equally likely to have less aggressive prostate cancers than patients with smaller glands?**

More likely.

○ **In patients with increased PSA levels, a positive rectal examination increases the risk of high-grade prostate cancer by what amount?**

The risk is 2.5 times greater.

○ **What effect does vitamin D have on the development of prostate cancer?**

Vitamin D appears to be protective. Increased sun exposure and growing up in geographic locations with high solar radiation levels can reduce lifetime prostate cancer risk by 50%.

○ **True/False: Studies on docetaxel-based regimens have shown a survival benefit in all hormone refractory prostate cancer patient groups, including those with asymptomatic disease.**

True.

○ **True/False: Nonfat (skim) milk consumption has been linked to advanced prostate cancer.**

True. Two large studies support such a link. (NIH-American Association of Retired Persons Diet and Health Study of 293,888 men and the Multiethnic Cohort Study of 82,483 men.)

○ **True/False: An MRI of the axial skeleton can show bone metastases earlier than bone scans in patients with hormone refractory prostate cancer.**

True (Lecouvet, 2007).

○ **What common drugs have shown activity in reducing biochemical recurrences in high-risk prostate cancer patients receiving high-dose definitive radiation therapy and how? (Hint: it's not an antiandrogen.)**

Statins, presumably through a reduction in antiapoptotic pathways or increased cancer cell sensitivity to radiation. 10-year survival is also increased slightly.

○ **True/False: Diabetic patients have a higher risk of poorly differentiated prostate cancer than nondiabetics.**

True.

○ **A single core from a 12-specimen TRUS-guided prostate biopsy shows Gleason 6 prostate cancer. How often will patients ultimately demonstrate higher Gleason scores, bilaterality, or multifocal disease?**

Slightly less than 50% will develop higher Gleason scores, more than 50% will become bilateral, and up to 100% eventually become multifocal.

○ **According to the Baltimore Longitudinal Study of Aging and the National Comprehensive Cancer Network Clinical Practice Guidelines, for men with a total PSA <4 and a benign rectal examination, what PSA velocity should be used as a threshold for a prostate biopsy?**

A PSA velocity of more than 0.35 ng/mL/year has been recommended.

○ **What percentage of cancers detected in patients with a PSA <2.5 are thought to be clinically significant based on pathological features?**

More than 70%.

○ **What secondary malignancies following definitive external beam radiation therapy for prostate cancer have the greatest potential impact on survival and how often do they occur?**

The most dangerous secondary malignancies are bladder, colorectal, and skin (melanoma). The risk is roughly double the risk of nonradiated controls.

○ **The National Comprehensive Cancer Network currently recommends a baseline PSA level starting at what age?**

At 40 years.

○ **What is the most important risk factor for prostate cancer: a positive family history of prostate cancer, race, or baseline PSA level?**

Baseline PSA level is the strongest predictor of prostate cancer risk.

○ **What is the current 10-year cure rate in radiation therapy patients who undergo salvage cryotherapy and what is their disease-specific survival?**

The 10-year cure rate is approximately one-third and disease-specific survival is 80%.

○   **What membranous urethral length after radical prostatectomy appears to be a good predictor of postoperative continence?**

>11 mm.

○   **Is PSA significantly influenced by circulating testosterone levels?**

No significant influence is noted in PSA levels across a wide range of testosterone readings.

○   **According to the American Cancer Society, what is the estimated number of new cases of prostate cancer and the number of prostate cancer deaths expected in 2008 in the United States?**

More than 186,000 new prostate cancer cases and 28,000 deaths in the United States are predicted.

CHAPTER 45

Radiation Therapy for Prostate Cancer

Gregory J. Kubicek, MD and
Ashraf Youssef, MD, MBA

○ **List the most important clinical prognostic factors predicting disease-free survival for prostate cancer?**

T stage, biopsy Gleason score, pretreatment PSA.

○ **Describe the most important clinical prognostic factors predicting disease-free survival for prostate cancer?**

T stage, biopsy Gleason score, and pretreatment PSA have been the most extensively studied 3 factors. They provide reproducible outcomes among prostate cancer patients treated with radiation therapy alone. Several investigators (D'Amico) have used a combination of these factors to stratify disease-free survival according to low, intermediate, and high-risk groups. Such a strategy is helpful in providing prognostic information for patients and in stratifying patients for prospective trials.

○ **What other clinical prognostic factors can help predict prostate cancer survival?**

PSA doubling time, percent of biopsy cores positive for disease, patient age, comorbidities, and obesity. Race is an unclear prognostic factor with some studies showing a worse clinical outcome for African Americans.

○ **Which of these factors is the single, strongest predictor of death from prostate cancer?**

The Gleason score is the clinical prognostic factor that has consistently been shown to best predict death from prostate cancer. While pretreatment PSA has been shown to correlate with biochemical recurrence, no investigation has yet been able to demonstrate that pretreatment PSA reliably predicts prostate cancer death rate.

○ **How would this affect treatment recommendations for radiation therapy?**

In recommending radiation therapy for prostate cancer, more weight should be given to the Gleason score over any other factor. Dose escalation studies have shown more benefit for high-risk and high-grade cancers than for low- or intermediate-risk groups. Also, several prospective randomized trials have shown that patients with high Gleason score tumors have a survival benefit from the use of long duration adjuvant hormonal therapy.

○   **A 65-year-old male has Gleason 6 prostate cancer involving 2 of 12 cores, PSA 7.5. What is the ideal treatment for this patient?**

The patient has multiple options including active surveillance. There are no data to support one form of treatment (surgery, external beam radiation, and brachytherapy) over another one for this patient. Treatment decisions should be based on patient preference, quality of life, performance status, comorbidities, etc, with an understanding of differences in logistics for the different treatments and side effect profile.

○   **What are the different forms of treatment for nonmetastatic prostate cancer?**

Accepted options for prostate cancer exist including active surveillance, surgery (radical prostatectomy), and several forms of radiation (see the next question). Several other forms of treatment include cryotherapy and high intensity focused ultrasound (HIFU), these treatments are not considered standard at this time and are not recognized by NCCN.

○   **What are the different forms of radiation in the treatment of prostate cancer?**

Accepted forms of radiation include external beam radiation (most commonly intensity modulated radiation therapy [IMRT]) and brachytherapy (low dose and high dose rate). Other types of radiation include proton beam therapy and stereotactic radiosurgery (ie, cyberKnife). These treatments are not considered standard at this time.

○   **What is the difference between 3D and IMRT?**

These are 2 types of radiation used for external beam radiation. The difference is in how the radiation energy is delivered. With IMRT multiple small radiation beams (called beamlets) are used from different angles with different radiation intensities. In effect, IMRT allows the radiation to bend and curve around normal structures.

○   **Is there an advantage of IMRT over 3D?**

Yes, IMRT has been shown to reduce side effects and toxicity when compared to 3D. Because it is more conformal it also allows for radiation doses to be more safely increased. 3D conformal techniques allow a dose 75 to 76 Gy, and IMRT doses can be in excess of 80 Gy with essentially equivalent side effects.

○   **What is IGRT?**

IGRT stands for image guided radiation therapy. IGRT uses various techniques in order to ensure that patient set-up and positioning are correct and that the radiation is being delivered with a high degree of precision. IGRT can take several forms, including daily imaging using cone beam CT scan (CBCT), rectal ultrasound, or placement of fiducial markers into the prostate. IGRT is considered a standard treatment option when using external beam radiation.

○   **What are the typical side effects of external beam radiation?**

During radiation side effects are fairly minimal, the majority of patients can continue to work full time during the entire course of treatment. After radiation long-term side effects can include toxicity to bowel and bladder and erectile dysfunction (ED). Bladder toxicity includes urinary urgency and frequency, this will typically resolves after 1 year. Bowel toxicity includes rectal urgency, frequency and pain, fecal incontinence, or hematochezia can occur; unlike bladder toxicity, bowel toxicity may not resolve. The incidence of grade 2 or great toxicity is less than 10%.

○ **What is the incidence of potency after external beam radiation therapy for prostate cancer?**

Depending on patient age, comorbid conditions, and the use of other medications, potent patients undergoing external beam radiation therapy for prostate cancer have a 50% to 75% chance of remaining potent after treatment.

○ **What is the mechanism by which radiation therapy causes ED?**

Radiation therapy causes ED primarily through arteriogenic and vascular means as opposed to radical prostatectomy, which affects the nerves.

○ **What is the difference between external beam radiation therapy and brachytherapy?**

External beam radiation consists of 8 weeks of daily (M to F) treatment. Brachytherapy (low dose rate) consists of a single procedure in which multiple radioactive seeds are inserted into the prostate. The 2 can be done together but not simultaneously.

○ **What is the cyberKnife?**

CyberKnife is the trademark name of a linear accelerator that can be used to deliver stereotactic body radiotherapy (SBRT), also known as stereotactic radiosurgery (SRS). Because of the high degree of precision in tracking and immobilization, the degree of accuracy with this treatment technique is within millimeters. This allows for very high doses of radiation to be delivered in a short number of treatments (typically 5).

○ **How is radiosurgery delivered?**

Radiosurgery consists of 5 fractions of radiation (as opposed to 8 weeks of conventional external beam) delivered over 2 weeks.

○ **What is proton therapy and how is this different than conventional external beam radiation?**

Conventional external beam uses photons to deliver the radiation as opposed to proton beam, which uses the much heavier proton. The theoretical advantage is that protons will deposit all of their energy at a very specific point and that the dose to nearby tissue is minimal. There are only a small handful of proton centers, but this list is growing. At this time, there is no clinical evidence that protons are any better than photons.

○ **If the above patient is interested in brachytherapy, what other information needs to be looked at?**

Prostate brachytherapy is indicated for patients with low-risk disease ($G < 7$, PSA, 10), but there are also some treatment factors for predicting which patients will do well with brachytherapy implants including prostate size and AUA score. Patients should have a prostate ultrasound to measure the size of the prostate. It has been found that patients with prostates larger than 50 cm^3 tend to have poorer quality outcomes and more toxicity. Also, patients with significant obstructive symptoms (as measured by AUA score >15) tend to have significant toxicity from prostatic swelling.

○ **Which patients with clinically localized disease are most suitable for prostate seed implantation alone?**

The patient most suited for an implant alone has a tumor with a clinical stage T1-T2a, biopsy Gleason score <7, prostate size <50 cm^3, AUA symptom score <15, and PSA <10 ng/mL. Such patients would be considered optimal for any therapy. Interestingly, a prostate that is too small may not provide enough room for an optimal number of seed implants.

○ **What is the difference between high and low dose rate brachytherapy?**

Low dose rate (LDR) and high dose rate (HDR) differ in the half-lives and dose rates of the isotopes they use. HDR dose rates are greater than 12 Gy per hour while LDR dose rates are less than 2 Gy per hour. LDR brachytherapy consists of permanently inserted radioactive seeds. HDR brachytherapy consists of temporarily placed needles into the prostate, the radioactive isotope is inserted into the prostate via these needles and then extracted a few minutes later, and the needles are removed. At this time, LDR can be used as monotherapy or as a boost in combination with external beam therapy. HDR can be used as a boost with external beam. The half-life of a typical LDR isotope (iodine-125) is 59.6 days while the half-life of a typical isotope used in HDR (cobalt 60) is 5.2 years.

○ **For LDR brachytherapy what happens to the radioactive seeds?**

In LDR brachytherapy for prostate cancer, the radioactive seeds (usually iodine-125 although some institutions use palladium-103) are permanently left in the prostate. The half-lives of the LDR brachytherapy sources are much shorter than that for HDR (59 days for iodine-125 and 17 days for palladium-103) which means that after 298 days for an iodine-125 implant (85 days for palladium-103), the radioactive seeds have 3% of their initial radiation dose.

○ **Is there any advantage to combination therapy using external beam and brachytherapy?**

Unclear. A short course external beam (5 weeks) can be used in combination with a brachytherapy boost (using either low dose or high dose brachytherapy). The theory behind this is that it allows for an overall higher dose of radiation than is possible to be delivered with external beam alone. Ongoing studies are addressing whether this technique has any advantage over external beam or brachytherapy alone. Prospective data suggest that this approach may increase toxicity, but have equivalent outcomes.

○ **What is the incidence of ED after prostate seed implantation (brachytherapy)?**

The incidence is approximately 20% to 25%.

○ **What is the best way to determine the actual dosing given after brachytherapy and which dosage parameter is the most useful?**

A CT scan can be used to calculate the actual dose given by the actual seed placement. The most useful number is the D90, which is the dosage given to 90% of the prostate. Optimal cancer survival results are generally found when the D90 is 140 Gy or more. This dosage can only be achieved with radioactive seed implants either alone or in combination with external beam therapy.

○ **What is the maximal safe calculated dose to the urethra?**

The urethral dose should be <150% of the maximal dosage.

○ **Which form of radiation treatment may lead to a higher incidence of urinary incontinence?**

Prostate seed implantation. The incidence can be as high as 50% if the patient had a prior TURP although such patients infrequently get seed implants due to technical difficulties. External beam radiation therapy causes urinary incontinence in less than 5% of the patients. However, if a TURP is done shortly after external beam radiation therapy, the incontinence rate can be quite high. At least 6 months and preferably a year should elapse between any definitive radiation therapy and a TURP.

○ **In a 70-year-old male with Gleason 7, PSA 12, if the patient elects to have external beam radiation, what else should be considered?**

This patient has intermediate-risk prostate cancer, and should also have a short course (6 months) of hormone therapy. While data from a previous study (D'Amico) had shown overall survival advantage with 6 months of hormonal treatment in a population mostly consisting of intermediate-risk patients, further confirmatory data are now available that have also shown an advantage to 6 months of hormonal therapy in intermediate-risk patients treated with external beam radiation.

○ **A 50-year-old has a PSA of 15.0 ng/mL, Gleason 8, and clinical stage T1cNxM0 prostate cancer. How does the PSA influence your treatment decision?**

This patient has high-risk prostate cancer. Whether the patient has monotherapy with standard dose (78-80 Gy) radiation therapy or surgery, his chances of freedom of biochemical failure at 5 years are under 25%. This most likely translates into a 15-year overall survival of 50%. Due to the high-risk category, most oncologists would recommend combined modality therapy with long duration (>2 years) hormonal therapy and radiation therapy. Other therapies that can be considered include radical prostatectomy with adjuvant radiation for pathological high-risk features (extracapsular extension, seminal vesicle invasion, and positive margins).

○ **At what point after beginning hormone therapy should radiation therapy be started?**

There is no clear answer at this point. While most will arbitrarily wait 2 to 3 months, others believe that it is best to wait until the PSA nadir is reached. Monthly PSA checks can be used to determine when the PSA nadir has been attained. Depending on initial PSA levels and other factors, this may take 3 to 12 months but averages about 6 months.

○ **A 61-year-old man undergoes hormonal downsizing (3 months) and has a radical prostatectomy. Pathologically, he is found to have extensive capsular penetration and positive surgical margins. His surgical Gleason score cannot be classified by his pathologist. His postoperative PSA at 10 days is 0.4 ng/mL. What are your recommendations?**

No trials with preoperative hormonal therapy have shown a clinical benefit and thus the hormones that the patient has received are not likely to have any effect on clinical outcome or future treatment recommendations. This patient will likely benefit from salvage external beam radiation to the prostatic bed based on his risk factors including positive margins and capsular extension. The PSA should also be repeated since the biological half-life after a radical prostatectomy is probably no less than 2.2 days. In actuality, his PSA was less than 0.2 ng/mL on repeat measurement a week later.

○ **Same patient as in the previous question and tumor characteristics, but the PSA is undetectable. What are your recommendations?**

The recommendations for this patient are still external beam radiation, but in this case it would be termed "adjuvant" rather than "salvage" since there is no evidence of disease at the time of treatment (using PSA as a disease surrogate). Because of the high preoperative PSA value and the presence of capsular penetration and surgical margin positivity, his risk of biochemical failure at 5 years is greater than 50%. There have been 3 randomized prospective trials randomizing patients with postradical prostatectomy risk factors (extracapsular extension, positive margins, and seminal vesicle invasion) to observation versus external beam radiation. These trials have shown a benefit in biochemical-free survival in the radiation arm.

○ **What radiation dose range is effective adjuvant postoperative radiation therapy and why?**

Radiation doses from 60 to 66.6 Gy in 1.8 to 2 Gy fractions appear safe and effective. Randomized trials all used 60 to 64 Gy to the prostatic bed. Retrospective evidence shows that a radiation dose >64.8 Gy appears to be more effective than lower doses.

○ **What are the clinical benefits from adjuvant radiation therapy?**

All of the randomized adjuvant trials have shown that adjuvant postprostatectomy radiation therapy reduced the risk of biochemical failure and local progression, long-term follow-up of the SWOG study has shown an overall survival advantage.

○ **Would an isolated local recurrence after a radical prostatectomy require higher radiation doses for biochemical control?**

Larger tumor volumes require more radiation dose than smaller tumors for the same probability of local control. Several authors have reported on radiation dose response for patients with rising PSA after radical prostatectomy and have found that doses higher than 64 Gy are necessary.

○ **What are the important predictors of response to salvage radiation therapy for patients with a rising PSA after a radical prostatectomy?**

A nomogram by Stephenson has shown that preradiation PSA >2.0, Gleason score >8, negative surgical margins, and PSA doubling time <10 months were adverse prognostic factors for biochemical relapse at 6 years. Positive margins as a favorable prognostic factor may appear nonintuitive but is related to the presence of local disease that is thus potentially amenable to cure from radiotherapy.

○ **Which factor is perhaps the strongest predictor?**

The magnitude of the PSA elevation prior to radiation is the strongest predictor of a positive response to salvage radiation therapy. Several reports have shown that initiating radiotherapy at a lower postradical prostatectomy PSA level is more beneficial. However, there is no universal agreed upon definition of what a PSA should be to initiate treatment. Most institutions would push for treatment at a PSA of 0.2.

○ **What would combined modality treatment provide over monotherapy for an isolated biochemical failure after a radical prostatectomy?**

There has been no completed prospective trial of combined modality therapy for patients with an isolated biochemical failure after a radical prostatectomy. Decisions regarding management thus depend on clinical judgment. Since approximately half of patients fail after salvage radiation therapy, either insufficient radiation therapy is delivered or subclinical distant metastases are already present. If there is still androgen-sensitive prostate cancer clones, there may be a benefit to use hormonal therapy to both potentiate radiation therapy locally and reduce disseminated disease.

○ **A 70-year-old man has a T1cNxM0 Gleason 8 prostate cancer in 5% of one of 6 cores. His prebiopsy PSA level was 0.9 ng/mL and prostate gland size was 30 cm³. Would you expect this patient to have a large tumor burden?**

The patient has findings suggestive of having low-volume prostate cancer. A single core biopsy containing 5% or less cancer correlates with low volume of disease and a low risk of capsular penetration.

○ **What is his risk of having lymph nodal metastases?**

He has less than 15% risk of having lymph nodal involvement. Since the risk is relatively low, evaluation of the pelvic lymph nodes with either ProstaScint or pelvic lymph node dissection probably would not provide useful information for guiding therapy.

○ **What are the radiation fields used?**

Two prospective randomized trials (RTOG 94-13 and GETUG 01) have addressed the question of radiation to the prostate only or to the whole pelvis followed by a boost to the prostate. Both trials failed to find any improvement with the whole pelvis field, although RTOG 94-13 did note an unexpected benefit to the combination of whole pelvis radiation and adjuvant hormone use that warrants further study. However, at this time this is controversial about when to treat prostate alone versus prostate and pelvis.

○ **A 55-year-old man is diagnosed with T3bN1M0 Gleason 8 prostate cancer, PSA of 29 ng/mL. What is his prognosis with radiation therapy alone?**

Although there appears to be a wide range of estimates made in the literature, nomograms (for example, from Memorial Sloan-Kettering) predict that this patient has approximately a 50% chance of having disease progression at 5 years.

○ **What is his prognosis with combined hormonal therapy and radiation therapy?**

Several retrospective and prospective studies purport 70% to 80% expected survival at 5 years.

○ **For locally advanced prostate cancer is there any advantage to radiation over hormones alone?**

Yes. Several studies have shown a survival advantage when radiation is combined with hormonal therapy for patients with locally advanced disease.

○ **What is the role of radiation in metastatic prostate cancer?**

External beam radiation can be used to resolve pain from metastatic disease to bone, a single fraction of 8 Gy is the ideal dose and fractionation in this palliative setting.

Surgical Therapy for Prostate Cancer

George P. Hemstreet III, MD, PhD and Sudhir Isharwal, MD

○ **What are the newest treatments of prostate cancer?**

- Proton beam therapy
- High frequency ultrasound (HFU)

○ **What are the 3 major goals of surgery in the order of importance?**

- Cancer control
- Preservation of urinary incontinence
- Preservation of sexual function

○ **Describe the arterial blood supply to the prostate and surrounding nearby structures.**

The prostate receives its primary blood supply from the inferior vesicle artery, which is the third major branch of the internal iliac artery. It provides small branches to the seminal vesicle and base of the bladder as well as the prostate. The inferior vesical artery terminates into the prostatic artery, which is typically only 1 cm long before it divides into its 2 primary branches: the urethral and capsular vessel groups.

○ **What is the blood supply for the corpora cavernosa?**

It is derived from the internal pudendal arteries, which can arise from the obturator inferior vesicle or superior vesicle arteries.

○ **Why are these aberrant branches important?**

They are important because they travel along the lower part of the bladder and anteriolateral surface of the prostate and are frequently divided during radical prostatectomy.

○ **What new therapies are on the horizon for improving the function of the striated urethral sphincter, which have the potential for treating incontinence following radical prostatectomy?**

- Stem cell therapy
- Adjustable transobturator male system (ATOMS)

○ **What nerve innervates the striated sphincter and levator ani muscles?**

The pudendal nerve provides the major nerve supply to the striated sphincter and levator ani muscle groups.

○ **How does one decide when to excise the neurovascular bundle?**

Consider if there is a palpable apical lesion, if preoperatively the Gleason score is higher than 6, if the average percentage of poor biopsy core on the side involved greater than 20%, or the percentage of cores with tumor on that side is greater than 33%, or there is an abnormal finding on digital rectal examination on that side.

○ **What is the best way to control the vascular branches to the neurovascular bundle?**

It is recommended that small hemoclips be placed parallel to the bundle and that thermal energy (cautery, laser) of any form should never be used on the neurovascular bundle or its branches.

○ **What are the criteria for salvage radical prostatectomy with the goal of successfully eradicating locally recurrent cancer following definitive radiotherapy?**

The procedure is reserved for patients in excellent health with a life expectancy of more than 15 years, and patients must have no evidence of metastatic disease. Patients should have unequivocally clinically localized prostate cancer at the time of initial therapy and current prostate biopsies should be negative. There must also be no clinical findings to support metastatic disease.

○ **What percentage of patients are incontinent following salvage prostatectomy and remain tumor-free after 5 years?**

Approximately 50% to 60%.

○ **What is the main surgical morbidity associated with radical retropubic prostatectomy and what specific measures help to prevent this complication?**

- Thrombophlebitis with pulmonary embolism.
- Prevention is best accomplished by careful positioning of the patient on the operating table, avoidance of venous compression, use of intermittent compression devices with early ambulation, and anticoagulant prophylaxis.

○ **What difference does it make if the seminal vesicles are not totally excised during a radical perineal prostatectomy and what may be one benefit of not removing the seminal vesicles?**

- There can be as much as a 40% higher frequency of PSA recurrence if the seminal vesicles are not removed at the time of surgery.
- One benefit is a possible decrease in urinary incontinence because of lack of damage to the pelvic nerves.

○ **What is the current attitude toward the anatomical preservation of the bladder neck during radical prostatectomy?**

Randomized trials suggest that there is a small but questionable clinical significance in the early return of urinary control with little or no difference in long-term urinary control. Bladder neck contracture and positive margins in some studies suggest the need to weigh the risks versus benefits of bladder neck preservation.

○ **Why is it likely that there will be a decrease in the number of patients undergoing radical perineal prostatectomy?**

The recent US Preventive Services Task Force report strongly suggests active surveillance for individuals with low-risk prostate cancer. This is the group of patients who are candidates for radical perineal prostatectomy because of the infrequency of seminal vesicle invasion, local extension, and nodal involvement.

○ **How effective is orchiectomy?**

Orchiectomy results in a reduction of circulating androgens by approximately 97%. Castrate levels of testosterone are achieved within 24 hours of orchiectomy. The hormonal deprivation results in remission of the hormone-dependent prostate tumor growth. Depending upon the Gleason grade of the cancer, the duration of the remission varies, and biochemical failure/hormone-independent tumor growth will eventually occur.

○ **How do the results of brachytherapy compare with surgical therapy?**

In one report comparing brachytherapy and radial retropubic prostatectomy in patients matched for similar pretreatment clinical pathological characteristics, the results showed a mean 7-year disease-free survival rate of 84% for surgical extirpation versus 79% for the iodine brachytherapy series. Although there was a proportionately higher probability of nonprogression for brachytherapy, this was not statistically significant. In most studies, brachytherapy has compared favorably to radical prostatectomy in biopsy-confirmed patients post-treatment.

○ **How are the lymph nodes assessed for metastatic disease?**

Although CT scan may be used to evaluate for lymphadenopathy, one cannot differentiate pathologic from nonpathologic nodes if they are <1.5 cm in size. Thus, computed tomography is both nonspecific and nonsensitive. To absolutely rule out metastatic disease of the lymph nodes, a lymphadenectomy is required.

○ **What are the options for pelvic lymphadenectomy?**

If the patient is undergoing radical retropubic prostatectomy, a lymphadenectomy may be performed simultaneously and the lymph nodes can be sent for frozen section analysis to rule out micrometastases. Alternatively, a laparoscopic pelvic lymph node dissection or a minilap lymph node dissection may be performed.

○ **How is a laparoscopic lymph node dissection performed?**

Laparoscopic lymph node dissection can be performed transperitoneally or through a preperitoneal approach. The pelvic lymph nodes are removed, and the tissue is sent for analysis.

○ **What are the boundaries for lymph node dissection?**

The distal limit of the dissection is the node of Cloquet located in the femoral canal. The proximal limit of the dissection is the bifurcation of the iliac vessels. The superior limit of the dissection is the external iliac artery, the lateral limit is the pelvic sidewall, and the inferior limit is the obturator vessels. Thus, all the lymph nodes are dissected off of the external iliac vein, the pelvic sidewall laterally, and the obturator nerve and vessels.

○ **Why is laparoscopic pelvic lymph node dissection so infrequently performed now when it was so popular in the early 1990s?**

The surgery was originally intended for patients with a high likelihood of lymphatic metastatic disease where a radical surgery or definitive radiation therapy could be avoided if positive lymph nodes were identified preoperatively. Typical patients would have elevated PSA levels (at least 10 or more) and Gleason sums of 7 or higher. Better understanding of PSA and the use of nomograms like the Partin tables have largely made the laparoscopic pelvic lymph node dissection unnecessary.

○ **What are the complications of pelvic lymph node dissection?**

The most common complication is lymphocele formation. Lymphocele formation can be minimized by clipping or tying feeding lymphatics as coagulation of lymphatics can result in postoperative lymphatic leakage. Damage to the external iliac vein, obturator vessels, and obturator nerve can also occur during pelvic lymphadenectomy.

○ **What are the different methods of radical prostatectomy?**

- Radical retropubic.
- Laparoscopic.
- Perineal.

○ **How is the patient prepared for radical prostatectomy?**

The patient should have adequate cardiac and pulmonary function. If there are any risk factors of cardiopulmonary disease, the patient should be optimized prior to surgery. Screening tests for coagulopathy are mandatory. Preoperative determination should be made of the patient's hemoglobin, hematocrit, and electrolytes. Although the risk of rectal injury is low, patients should undergo bowel prep prior to surgery.

○ **Should the patient donate autologous blood?**

This depends on the surgeon's experience. If the surgeon historically loses more than 500 mL of blood during a radical prostatectomy, it is reasonable to offer the patient the option of donating autologous blood. The blood is commonly donated within the month before surgery. This bears substantial cost, but decreases the risk of a transfusion reaction or a transfusion-associated morbidity.

○ **Are antiembolism precautions necessary for radical prostatectomy/pelvic lymph node dissection?**

Many of the risk factors for deep vein thrombosis (DVT) and pelvic thrombosis are present: general anesthesia, blood loss, pelvic surgery, and possibly a hypercoagulable state. Lower extremity sequential compression devices and antiembolism stockings are commonly employed to help minimize pooling of blood in the deep veins of the legs. This should be used with medical anticoagulation such as subcutaneous heparin or Lovenox. However, risk of bleeding should be considered when starting pharmacological DVT prophylaxis.

○ **What is the positioning for the radical retropubic prostatectomy?**

The radical retropubic prostatectomy is performed through a midline infraumbilical incision extending from the umbilicus to the pubic symphysis. The patient is placed supine or in a low lithotomy position with the kidney rest or a rolled towel just above the sacrum with the table slightly hyperextended. During the procedure, reverse Trendelenburg may be helpful in visualizing the apex of the prostate.

○ **Describe the approach to the prostate in a retropubic prostatectomy.**

The radical retropubic prostatectomy is an extraperitoneal procedure. The rectus muscles are split in the midline and the space of Retzius is developed. The bladder is freed from the posterior surface of the pubic symphysis and cleared from the lateral pelvic sidewall. At this time, if so indicated, a bilateral lymph node dissection is performed. After the lymph node dissection is complete and the pathological results obtained, incisions are made in the endopelvic fascia, lateral to the apex of the prostate to gain exposure to the apex of the prostate. If the apex of the prostate is not easily visualized, the puboprostatic ligaments are divided.

○ **Are the puboprostatic ligaments vascular structures?**

No. These are fibrous bands that connect the prostate to the underside of the pubic symphysis. They may be incised without causing excessive bleeding.

○ **What is the structure that is most likely to cause significant bleeding?**

Santorini plexus, which is a continuation of the dorsal vein of the penis. This is the structure found in the midline that drains between the puboprostatic ligaments and forms the dorsal venous complex, which is anterior to the urethra at the apex of the prostate gland.

○ **How is bleeding prevented from the dorsal venous complex?**

A variety of techniques for controlling the dorsal venous complex have been described. In the radical retropubic prostatectomy and laparoscopic prostatectomy, the dorsal venous complex must be transected in order to visualize the apex of the prostate. Bunching sutures paced deeply into the dorsal surface of the prostate from the level of the bladder neck and continuing distally to the apex of the gland are helpful in controlling back bleeding. A right-angle clamp is passed between the dorsal vein complex and the anterior surface of the urethra and the dorsal vein complex is tented up and ligated.

○ **What if these measures do not control bleeding from the dorsal venous complex?**

Direct visualization suture ligation of the transected veins under the pubic symphysis is the best means of stopping the bleeding. Rarely, temporary compression of and possibly suture ligation of the deep dorsal vein of the penis below the level of the pubic symphysis may be helpful in gaining control of bleeding from the dorsal venous complex. Suture ligation will require dissection of the veins at the base of the penis at the dorsal vein.

○ **Aside from the dorsal vein complex, what other important structures are located at the level of the apex of the prostate?**

The external sphincter is located distal to the apex of the prostate. Injury to this muscle can cause permanent urinary incontinence. The neurovascular bundles that supply the erectile function run laterally along the apex of the prostate from 3- and 9-o'clock positions at the level of the external urinary sphincter and 5- and 7-o'clock positions at the base of the gland. If both neurovascular bundles are transected, impotence results.

○ **What is the major blood supply to the prostate?**

The main blood supply to the prostate is from the inferior vesical artery, which is a branch of the hypogastric artery. This penetrates the substance of the prostate at the prostatovesical junction at 8- and 4-o'clock positions posteriorly.

○ **Describe the technique for avoiding injury to the external sphincter and the neurovascular bundles.**

The anterior urethra is incised under direct vision. The Foley catheter is delivered through the urethrotomy and transected while maintaining the fluid in the balloon. The posterior urethra is carefully dissected off of the rectum and is divided. The rectourethralis muscle is divided at apex of the gland in the midline and then the midportion of the dorsal surface of the prostate or Denonvilliers fascia can be freed in the midline from the rectal surface. Dissection is then carried out along the posterolateral prostate sharply freeing it off of the neurovascular bundles. When vascular branches are identified, they are controlled with fine ligatures or clips. Cautery should be avoided to prevent injury to the neurovascular bundles. As the base of the prostate is reached, the main prostatic pedicle is encountered. The prostatic pedicle at this point should be secured with ligatures or clips. The prostate is then carefully dissected at the level of the prostatovesical junction, starting anteriorly and progressing posteriorly.

○ **What structures are important to preserve at the base of the prostate?**

The bladder neck, trigone, and ureteral orifices.

○ **What can one do to prevent damage to the ureteral orifices?**

Bladder neck preservation is the safest way to preserve the ureteral orifices. Indigo carmine or methylene blue may be administered intravenously to identify the ureteral orifices. If there is any question subsequently whether the ureteral orifices have been violated, placement of ureteral stents prior to the urethrovesical anastomosis should be entertained.

○ **After freeing up the apex of the prostate, the prostatic pedicles and the prostatovesical junction, what structures remain to be dissected free to allow the prostate to be removed?**

The seminal vesicles and ductus differentia. The ductus differentia are identified in the midline and transected. These are then used to delineate the medial side of the seminal vesicles. The seminal vesicles are dissected free from the surrounding tissue and the apical artery identified, controlled, and divided.

○ **What is the blood supply to the seminal vesicle?**

The artery to the seminal vesicle is a division of the hypogastric artery. It penetrates the seminal vesicle at its superior end. These need to be secured before removing the seminal vesicle.

○ **How is continuity of the urinary tract restored?**

The urethrovesical anastomosis is performed in 2 steps:

1. The bladder neck is reconstructed so that the opening is approximately 1.2 to 1.5 cm. Typically, this is accomplished by closing the bladder neck in a tennis racquet manner anteriorly and/or posteriorly, with care taken to avoid damage to the ureteral orifices. The mucosa is everted using 4-0 absorbable suture to "stomatize" the bladder neck.

2. Sutures are then placed in the urethral stump; once 4 to 6 sutures are placed in the urethra, they are sewn through the bladder neck. After all sutures have been placed, a Foley catheter is passed per urethra and directed into the bladder. The sutures are then tied down individually with gentle traction on the Foley catheter to bring the bladder down to the urethra.

○ **What sort of drains are necessary for this surgery?**

The 2 potential areas of drainage from radical retropubic prostatectomy are urinary drainage from the urethrovesical anastomosis and lymphatic drainage if a lymphadenectomy was performed. Drains (suction or nonsuction) are placed in the left and right side of the pelvis. The incision is then closed in the midline.

○ **How is laparoscopic prostatectomy different from retropubic prostatectomy?**

It is a transperitoneal approach, the dissection is antegrade (starts from the bladder neck and proceeds toward the apex), and the urethrovesical anastomosis is done with a continuous running suture. It avoids the larger low midline incision instead using 5 or 6 small incisions for the laparoscopic trocars.

○ **What are the advantages of laparoscopic prostatectomy versus radical retropubic prostatectomy?**

- Shorter hospital stay—usually patients spend only one night in the hospital, that is, 2 days less than retropubic prostatectomy.
- Less blood loss.
- Faster recovery and quicker return to normal activities.
- Shorter catheter time postop. Generally, the Foley catheter can be removed on postop day 7.

○ **Is there any difference in positive margin, impotence, or incontinence rates between laparoscopic and retropubic prostatectomy?**

None has been described in any current mature series.

○ **What is a *da vinci* or *robotic* prostatectomy?**

It is a laparoscopic prostatectomy using the *da vinci* surgical system, which is a surgical tool that uses robotic technology to translate hand movements into precise movements of microinstruments within the operative site. It allows freedom of movement and accuracy that is not possible with traditional open surgery or unassisted laparoscopic surgery deep in the pelvis.

○ **What are the complications unique to laparoscopic prostatectomy?**

Only those involved with the laparoscopic approach: bowel injury from trocar placement, diaphragmatic irritation from CO_2, and respiratory (ventilatory) difficulty from Trendelenburg and peritoneal insufflation.

○ **What is the optimal positioning for a perineal prostatectomy?**

The patient is placed in the extreme dorsal lithotomy position with a rolled towel or sheet under the sacrum so that the perineum is parallel to the floor. Allen stirrups are used to stabilize the patient's legs.

○ **What incision is used for perineal prostatectomy?**

The incision is made in a convex curvilinear fashion between the ischial tuberosities, anterior to the anus. Prior to the incision, a curved Lowsley tractor is placed per urethra into the bladder.

○ **What are the "pearly gates"?**

The "pearly gates" are also known as Denonvilliers' fascia. When seen, this indicates that the base of the prostate is in view. The rectum is then dissected off of the posterior surface of the prostate by dividing Denonvilliers' fascia using sharp and blunt dissection.

○ **Can the neurovascular bundles be seen and/or preserved in the perineal prostatectomy?**

Yes. Care must be taken to preserve the neurovascular bundles during dissection of the posterolateral portion of the prostate.

○ **How is the prostatovesical junction delineated?**

The prostatovesical junction can be delineated by rotating the wings of the Lowsley tractor in a circumferential manner. Once the junction is well defined, the detrusorotomy is made in the anterior midline at the level of the prostatovesical junction. The wings of the Lowsley tractor can be delivered through this detrusorotomy and dissection is carried circumferentially around the bladder neck using the Lowsley tractor for retraction.

○ **How is the blood supply to the prostate controlled?**

As large vessels are encountered, they may be suture ligated or clipped prior to dividing the apex. The prostate may be rotated anteriorly and the posterior pedicles at the base of the prostate can be visualized and suture ligated before apical dissection.

○ **Describe the technique for seminal vesicle dissections.**

The seminal vesicle dissection is somewhat more problematic with a perineal prostatectomy than a retropubic prostatectomy. Again, the vasa deferentia and ductus deferens are identified in the midline and clipped. Although the dissection down to the apex of the seminal vesicle may sometimes be awkward, with patience the artery to the seminal vesicle may be ligated at the tip of the seminal vesicle and the prostate gland removed.

○ **How is the urethrovesical anastomosis performed in a radical perineal prostatectomy?**

One of the advantages of the perineal prostatectomy compared with the retropubic prostatectomy is that urethrovesical anastomosis is often easier to perform. The bladder neck is tailored to 1.2 to 1.5 cm in diameter, using a tennis racquet approach to avoid damage to the ureteral orifice. Interrupted sutures are used to reanastomose the bladder neck to the urethra, starting in the anterior midline and extending laterally. However, once three-quarters of the anastomosis has been performed, a Foley catheter is placed per urethra and directed into the bladder and the remainder of the anastomosis is completed.

○ **How is a perineal prostatectomy drained?**

A separate perineal stab incision is made and a Penrose drain is placed at the level of the urethrovesical anastomosis. The wound is closed in layers with absorbable sutures.

○ **How long does the patient typically stay in the hospital?**

Patients stay in the hospital until they are tolerating a diet, drainage has tapered off sufficiently, and they are hemodynamically stable. Patients are discharged with their Foley catheter.

○ **How long does the Foley catheter remain?**

The Foley catheter remains in place for 1 to 2 weeks, and then it is removed in the office.

○ **Do any confirmatory tests need to be performed before the Foley catheter is removed?**

Traditionally, a gravity cystogram was performed before removal of the catheter. Due to refinement in technique, this is not uniformly done. If there is any question of urinary leak, a cystogram should be performed prior to removal of the Foley catheter.

○ **If there is excessive drainage from the wound or drainage sites, how can one tell the origin of the fluid?**

The fluid should be sent for creatinine determination. If the creatinine is equivalent to the serum creatinine, a urine leak is ruled out. The drains should be managed conservatively and left in place until the fluid accumulation has subsided. If the drainage persists without evidence of improvement, a lymphatic source is more likely. The patient should be placed on broad-spectrum oral antibiotics and the drains gradually advanced and removed. The lymphatic leak should subside with time, but a lymphocele may accumulate and require internal drainage.

If the fluid has a markedly elevated creatinine, a urine leak is confirmed. Similarly, the patient should be placed on broad-spectrum oral antibiotics and the drains should be taken off of suction and advanced gradually until they are removed. The Foley catheter should be maintained. With adequate drainage, urinary leakage should subside.

○ **What are the intraoperative complications from radical prostatectomy?**

- Hemorrhage
- Bowel injury
- Ureteral injury

○ **How is hemorrhage handled?**

The source must be identified. Generally, this is from the dorsal vein complex or from the prostatic pedicle. The most important step in controlling hemorrhage is to first make sure that the patient remains hemodynamically stable. Communication with anesthesia is of major importance. Initially, pressure may be placed on the bleeding area so that anesthesia can maintain or reestablish hemodynamic stability. Dorsal vein complex bleeding was previously described. If the prostatic pedicles are bleeding, then they must be suture ligated. Mass ligatures or widespread electrocautery should not be used because it may damage the surrounding structures. If the urine is grossly bloody in the postoperative period, gentle traction on the Foley catheter can be utilized for short periods of time.

○ **How do rectal injuries occur, what is their frequency, and how are they managed?**

The incidence of rectal injury for patients undergoing a radical perineal prostatectomy is 10%. Injury usually occurs during takedown of the rectum and rectourethralis musculature. If an enterotomy occurs, it is safe to continue with the dissection of the posterior surface of the prostate unless there is fecal soilage. If feces contaminate the wound, the area should be thoroughly irrigated and the operation ended after formation of a diverting colostomy.

The prostatectomy may be continued in the absence of fecal soilage. The rectum should be closed in 2 layers. Some urologists favor the input of a general surgeon. Assuming that the patient has had preoperative bowel prep, a primary repair should be safe. In addition, a manual dilation or defunctionalization of the anal sphincter should be performed following closure of the incision, and the patient should be kept on a low residue diet for 1 to 2 weeks postoperatively.

Rectal injuries are rare during radical retropubic prostatectomy with an incidence of 5% to 7%. Generally, this occurs during apical dissection in the midline. Following closure of the injury, the anus should be manually dilated and the patient kept on a low residue diet.

○ **What if the patient has fecal drainage from his wound or his drain postoperatively?**

Provided the patient is clinically stable and fit for anesthesia, a diverting colostomy is indicated. The only way to heal a rectal fistula is by complete diversion.

○   **How is ureteral injury handled?**

Ureteral injury is best handled by ureteral reimplantation in the standard fashion.

○   **What are the postoperative complications of radical prostatectomy?**

As with any major pelvic surgery for cancer, DVT of the lower extremity and femoral veins is always a possibility. thromboembolic deterrent (TED) hose and sequential compression devices can be useful intraoperatively. If DVT is clinically suspected, a Doppler ultrasound of the lower extremities and pelvic veins should be ordered immediately.

○   **What are the complications of a DVT?**

The catastrophic complication of DVTs is a pulmonary embolus, which is life threatening. Pulmonary embolus causes circulatory collapse and should be suspected when a patient has shortness of breath, tachypnea, tachycardia, and unexplained fever. A confirmatory study is a spiral chest CT. Pulmonary embolism is an emergent situation that should be treated initially with anticoagulation and urgent cardiac or general surgery consultation.

○   **What if the Foley catheter is removed accidentally or falls out prematurely?**

If the catheter falls out, a coude catheter may be gently passed. If it does not pass easily on the first gentle attempt, the patient should be taken to the cystoscopy suite and under direct visualization a guide wire is placed in the bladder and a council-tipped catheter can be placed into the bladder. This prevents any disruption of the vesicourethral anastomosis.

○   **What if the patient does not void after removal of the Foley catheter?**

If the patient does not void or is uncomfortable, a catheter can be gently passed per urethra. If this does not pass easily, a suprapubic tube can be placed into the patient's bladder, and trials of voiding can be carried out at a later date. Edema at the site of the urethrovesical anastomosis is usually the etiology of failure to void in this situation.

○   **What if the patient develops urinary retention 3 months after surgery?**

A bladder neck contracture is the likely etiology. The urethra may be gradually dilated with filiforms and followers. Alternatively, a direct vision internal urethrotomy may be performed, but this must be done carefully to avoid injury to the sphincter.

○   **What is the major complication risk of a direct vision internal urethrotomy for bladder neck contracture after radical prostatectomy?**

Urinary incontinence. The urethrovesical anastomosis is very close to the external urinary sphincter and when incising an anastomotic stricture, the sphincter may be damaged leading to urinary incontinence.

○   **What if the stricture occurs 3 years after surgery?**

Cystoscopy should be performed to evaluate the stricture. It should be handled with care to avoid incontinence. The surgeon should also be cognizant that this may represent a local recurrence of disease and a PSA should be checked to evaluate this possibility and a biopsy of the stricture may be considered.

○ **What is the incidence of urinary incontinence following radical prostatectomy?**

Depending on the study, continence rates have been reported between 100% and 45% with most studies describing full continence in 85% to 90% of the patients treated with radical prostatectomy. It takes a while to establish continence, and surgeons feel that some stress incontinence between the catheter removal and 6 months postsurgery is not worrisome or negatively prognostic in terms of the patient's overall continence rate postoperatively.

○ **How is incontinence managed?**

For the first year postoperatively, anticholinergics or α-agonists can be used to try to minimize the incontinence. Pelvic physical therapy and kegel exercises should be done in early postoperative period. If the incontinence persists, management with an artificial urinary sphincter, a suburethral sling (InVance, AMS), or a trial of submucosal collagen injections at the bladder neck may be indicated.

○ **What is the incidence of impotence following nerve sparing radical prostatectomy?**

Impotence rates for preoperatively potent patients are between 25% and 40%.

○ **Who is the optimal candidate for prostate cryotherapy?**

Patients with localized high-grade prostate cancer, or with recurrent cancer after radiation therapy.

○ **How well does cryotherapy work as a salvage modality?**

Undetectable PSA levels are formed in approximately 65% of patients at 3 years post-therapy.

○ **What is the principle of cryotherapy for prostate cancer?**

Rapid freezing and thawing causes cancer cell death by crystal formation and cell disruption.

○ **What are the theoretical advantages of cryotherapy?**

It is effective even in high Gleason score cancers. It can be used after radiation therapy. If unsuccessful, it can be repeated. It is relatively noninvasive with few complications.

○ **What are the disadvantages of cryotherapy?**

Almost 100% incidence of ED. There is still the possibility of less common complications like incontinence or urethrorectal fistula.

○ **What elements are used for cooling and thawing?**

Liquid Argon is used for cooling and helium for heating/thawing.

○ **What other improvements have made prostate cryotherapy a viable option?**

Temperature probes placed strategically at the apex and rectal wall can automatically stop the freezing at a preset temperature. A urethral warming catheter prevents urethral sloughing. Helium heating elements allow more precise control of the freeze zone.

○ **After radiation therapy, if a reoccurrence is biopsied, how does the recurrent prostate cancer compare to the original cancer?**

There is frequently an increase in the Gleason score.

○ **Is obesity an independent predictor of biochemical failure after radical prostatectomy?**

Yes. Obese patients were found to have a higher rate of biochemical failure after their radical prostatectomy surgery than normal weight patients. Obesity has also been associated with higher-grade tumors and a higher risk of positive surgical margins.

○ **True/False: Following definitive therapy, a PSA doubling time of 1 year or less is associated with a high risk of dying from prostate cancer.**

True. If the PSA doubling time is over 1 year, they are unlikely to die from prostate cancer within the next 10 years.

○ **True/False: Men older than age 70 are more likely to have an upgraded Gleason score on final pathological examination after radical prostatectomy than men younger than 70.**

True. A large study of 4000 men who had all received radical prostatectomy found a substantially higher incidence of Gleason score upgrading in the older age cohort.

○ **Is bladder neck invasion an independent predictor of PSA recurrence after radical prostatectomy?**

While some of the data is conflicting, the more recent studies suggest that bladder neck invasion by prostate cancer is associated with a higher preoperative PSA level, a higher incidence of extraprostatic extension in areas other than the bladder neck, a larger overall tumor volume, and a higher incidence of positive surgical margins and a higher rate of PSA recurrence.

CHAPTER 47

Treatment of Locally Advanced or Recurrent Prostate Cancer

Himanshu Aggarwal, MD, MSc and
Badar M. Mian, MD, FACS

○ **What is the definition of locally advanced prostate cancer?**

Clinically detectable locally advanced prostate cancer includes cases with clear evidence or a high likelihood of cancer extension beyond the prostate capsule into the periprostatic tissue (T3a), involvement of the seminal vesicles (T3b), or involvement of adjacent organs (T4). Patients with locally advanced disease also are at higher risk of regional (lymph node) or distant (bone) metastases. For patients treated with radical prostatectomy, histological evidence of extraprostatic extension and surgical margin status are used to define locally advanced disease.

○ **How is locally advanced prostate cancer diagnosed?**

Historically, the identification of patients with locally advanced prostate cancer has been based on clinical examination (digital rectal examination, DRE) and/or CT scan demonstrating clinical stage T3 or T4. Clinical surrogates have been used to identify patients who are "likely" to harbor locally advanced disease including PSA >20 ng/mL and/or Gleason score ≥8. The term "high-risk cancer" may encompass those with evidence of or a high likelihood of locally advanced disease.

○ **How do you estimate the likelihood of having a locally advanced disease?**

Clinical examination (DRE) alone can be quite subjective and imaging such as ultrasound or CT scans lack the resolution to provide sufficient accuracy in predicting locally advanced disease, especially when its microscopic. Due to its improved resolution MRI for staging has been expanding especially since 2T and 3T scanners with surface coils (as opposed to endorectal coils) have become more readily available. Several risk assessment tools have been developed over the last 10 years to predict the likelihood of locally advanced disease. The tools (tables, nomograms, neural networks, etc) incorporate several clinical variables, such as clinical stage, PSA, biopsy Gleason score, and biopsy cores with cancers, to predict locally advanced or high-risk cancer. Most of these tools, that are now available online, tend to provide a more accurate risk-assessment than any individual parameter alone.

○ **What is the incidence of locally advanced prostate cancer and how has it changed over the last 2 decades?**

The incidence of clinical stage T3-4 has decreased from 11.8% to 3.5% over the last 15 to 20 years. This reduction is thought to be largely due to the use of the PSA test for early detection of prostate cancer.

491

○   **What is the incidence of pathological T3 disease in patients who are initially treated with radical prostatectomy for clinically localized prostate cancer?**

The incidence of pathological extraprostatic disease has decreased from nearly 40% (1983-1991) to 31% (1992-2003). In a recent surgical series (2008), the incidence of T3a was 13.8% and T3b was 5.7%. This may in part be due to the use of careful selection criteria and risk stratification before surgery. Further, the extent of extraprostatic cancer in the contemporary (PSA) era is often focal and microscopic as opposed to large multifocal areas of extraprostatic disease noted in the earlier series.

○   **What is the extent of clinical staging error for locally advanced prostate cancer?**

Clinical over staging occurs in up to 7% to 20% of patients who are subsequently found to have organ-confined prostate cancer. Under staging has been reported in 20% to 35% of patients who are found to have T3-4 lesions or microscopic nodal metastases, depending upon the criteria used to select surgical candidates.

○   **Does PSA level reliably predict pathological stage?**

Up to 70% of patients with locally advanced prostate cancer may have a serum PSA level of >10 ng/mL, but serum PSA level alone cannot reliably predict pathological stage.

○   **What are the pitfalls of seminal vesicle biopsies to assess local tumor extent in patients suspected of harboring locally advanced prostate cancer?**

A significant number of *false-negative* biopsy results can occur due to sampling error in the presence of focal or microscopic seminal vesicle invasion (SVI). Even when biopsies are performed due to clinical suspicions of SVI, only 50% of patients will have positive biopsy results. *False-positive* results can occur because of a drag-through artifact where the needle goes through the base of the prostate. Due to architectural similarities between SV and low-grade cancers or benign glands, the diagnosis can sometimes be challenging, resulting in false-positive SV biopsy. Lipofuscin staining can identify seminal vesicle tissue and help minimize the *false-positive* results.

○   **What percentage of patients with locally advanced prostate cancer will require surgical or medical intervention for disease progression if initially placed on watchful waiting?**

Over 70% will require some form of intervention secondary to local or distant disease progression depending upon the length of follow-up and life expectancy of the patient. Depending upon the extent of disease progression, most patients are treated with hormonal ablation therapy or with radiation therapy plus hormonal ablation therapy. If initially left untreated, up to 50% of patients may need transurethral resection of the prostate (TURP) for obstruction or hematuria or nephrostomy tube placement for ureteral obstruction.

○   **A 67-year-old patient presents with Gleason score 9, clinical stage T2b, N0, M0 prostate cancer. After a lengthy discussion of treatment options, the patient decides to pursue initial observation. What are the disease-specific and metastasis-free survival rates at 10 years for patients with high-grade, clinically localized prostate cancers that are managed with watchful waiting?**

Patients with clinically localized (clinical stage ≤T2) high-grade prostate cancer who are treated conservatively will have a disease-specific survival rate of only 34% at 10 years, and only 26% of these patients will be free of metastasis at 10 years. Patients with high-grade prostate cancers are over 6 times more likely to die of prostate cancer than are patients with low-grade tumors.

○ **What is the survival of patients with locally advanced disease for 5, 10, and 15 years without immediate or early treatment?**

Overall survival is reported from 25% to 92% at 5 years and 14% to 78% at 10 years for patients who harbor cancers of high Gleason grade or stage who are treated only when clinical disease progression is noted. Of all patients with locally advanced prostate cancer, 15-year mortality rates of 6%, 17%, and 56% are noted for well-differentiated, moderately differentiated and poorly differentiated tumors, respectively.

○ **What is the incidence of SVI when performing radical retropubic prostatectomy in patients with clinical T3a disease?**

Approximately 5% to 15% of patients will have SVI after radical prostatectomy.

○ **What are the long-term results following radical prostatectomy for clinical T3 disease without adjuvant therapy?**

Cancer-specific survival rates are 85% to 92% and 79% to 82% at 5 and 10 years, respectively, regardless of adjuvant therapy. However, without any adjuvant treatment, biochemical (PSA) relapse is noted in about 50% of men by 5 years.

○ **What is the PSA relapse-free survival patients undergoing radical prostatectomy for clinically localized disease that are noted to have pathological T3 disease?**

The 5-year PSA relapse-free survival is 76% for PT3a, 37% for PT3b, and 18% for node positive men after radical prostatectomy for clinically localized disease.

○ **What is the role of adjuvant radiation therapy in pathological T3 disease?**

It has been shown in 2 RCT (EORTC 22911 and SWOG 8794) that adjuvant RT leads to improved biochemical-free survival, from 50% to 88% at 5 years. This appears to be an improvement (30%-50%) compared with the results of surgery alone in high-risk patients. In EORTC 22911, immediate RT was associated with improved biochemical relapse-free survival (74% vs 53% without RT, $P < 0.001$) at 5 years. Similarly, SWOG 8794, with 10.6 years median follow-up, supported immediate RT with a nearly 50% reduction in biochemical recurrence (BCR; 35% vs 64% without RT, $P < 0.001$). In addition, both metastasis-free and overall survival were improved with adjuvant RT (HR, 0.71 and 0.72, respectively).

○ **Which subgroups of pT3 patients may benefit the most with adjuvant RT after radical prostatectomy?**

Men with SVI who achieve a low PSA level (<0.3 ng/mL) after prostatectomy or those positive surgical margins may be a more favorable group in whom adjuvant RT may be considered.

○ **A 60-year-old man presents with palpable extracapsular extension, PSA 15 ng/mL, and Gleason score 7 prostate cancer. He inquires about the use of androgen suppression therapy for few months prior to radical prostatectomy. Is there any evidence that neoadjuvant hormonal therapy results in downstaging of clinical stage T3 prostate cancer?**

There have been many studies of neoadjuvant hormonal therapy in patients with clinical stage T3 disease. These studies showed a drop in PSA level in more than 90% of cases, with a 30% to 50% decrease in prostate volume after neoadjuvant hormonal therapy. However, only about 21% of these patients had organ-confined disease, which is not substantially different from the frequency of organ-confined disease noted in patients undergoing surgery without neoadjuvant hormonal therapy for stage T3 disease. Thus, there is no clear evidence to support the use of neoadjuvant hormonal therapy for downstaging of T3 prostate cancer.

○   **The use of neoadjuvant hormonal therapy prior to radical prostatectomy has been shown to reduce the risk of positive surgical margins in which patients?**

In clinically localized (T2) cancers, there was decrease in the rate of positive surgical margins. For locally advanced tumors (specifically cT3), current data, both retrospective and prospective, do not support a significant benefit of neoadjuvant androgen ablation before surgery.

○   **Is there any proven reduction in the rate of biochemical failure for patients treated with 3 months of neoadjuvant hormonal therapy prior to radical prostatectomy?**

There is no overall benefit of short-term neoadjuvant therapy as measured by BCR (34%-38%), regardless of the clinical stage or any reduction in the positive margin rate. The use of long-term (neoadjuvant and adjuvant) androgen suppression with radical prostatectomy has not been studied systematically.

○   **What is the role of adjuvant androgen deprivation therapy (ADT) in locally advanced prostate cancer after radical prostatectomy?**

In a randomized controlled trial (ECOG 7887) men found to have lymph node metastases during radical prostatectomy (cT1-T2) were randomized to immediate (adjuvant) or delayed (salvage) ADT. At a median follow-up of 11.9 years, men receiving adjuvant ADT had improved overall, cancer-specific, and progression-free survival.

○   **What is the biochemical disease-free survival rate for patients with high-risk prostate cancer who undergo external beam radiation therapy (EBRT) alone?**

Overall survival after RT alone for stage III cancer is approximately 60% to 70% at 5 years and less than 50% at 10 years. In high-risk patients, defined by individual parameters alone or in combination, the 5-year progression-free survival rates after RT are typically less than 50%. Because the results of EBRT alone for locally advanced prostate cancer have been disappointing, there has been a dramatic shift toward treating patients with combined androgen ablation and radiation therapy.

○   **Is there convincing evidence to indicate that the combined use of androgen ablation therapy along with radiation therapy is superior to radiation therapy alone?**

Based on several randomized control trials, a limited period of hormonal ablation (4-6 months) appears to be appropriate for those men with intermediate-risk cancers. More prolonged hormonal ablation (up to 3 years) is beneficial for those with high-risk disease characteristics, including locally advanced cancers or very high pretreatment serum PSA values.

○   **What is the effect of combined ADT and radiation therapy on survival for patients with locally advanced prostate cancer?**

Typically, ADT is started before XRT and is continued during and after the XRT for a total of 28 to 36 months. In a recent RCT combined ADT and RT improved overall survival in patients with locally advanced prostate cancer compared to RT alone at 7 years (74% vs 66%). In a different RCT of locally advanced cancers, XRT plus long-term ADT for 28 months was compared to the group receiving short-term ADT for only 4 months. The disease-free, disease-specific, local progression-free, and metastases free survival were improved, but overall survival was similar. Another landmark RCT (by EORTC) comparing ADT for 6 months versus 3 years plus XRT reported that both the clinical disease-free (40% vs 74%) and overall survival (62% vs 78%) were improved with longer ADT.

○ **What effect does local failure have on quality of life after EBRT?**

A significant decrease in quality of life is noted secondary to pelvic pain, hematuria, bladder outlet obstruction, and ureteral obstruction requiring nephrostomy tube placement. There is a significantly higher incidence of metastatic progression with bone pain and pathological progression.

○ **A patient with recurrent prostate cancer after radiation therapy does not want to undergo salvage radical prostatectomy but does desire further local therapy. Other than salvage radical prostatectomy, what salvage therapies are available?**

Salvage cryotherapy and salvage brachytherapy have been used to salvage local cancer recurrences. Approximately 50% of patients undergoing salvage cryotherapy will have a durable biochemical response. The 5-year biochemical disease-free survival rate following salvage brachytherapy is only 34%, which appears lower than the biochemical disease-free survival rates reported for salvage prostatectomy or cryotherapy. One of the most important predictors of successful salvage procedure is the extent of cancer volume in the prostate and preprocedure PSA level.

○ **What percentage of patients with local disease progression following EBRT may require surgical intervention for symptom control?**

Local recurrence rates after EBRT for cT3 range from 24% to 74%. It is reported that 36% of patients required TURP because of urinary obstruction after RT without hormonal ablation therapy. Other morbidities included hydronephrosis (20%) and incontinence (13%). Due to the technological advances in radiation therapy and more frequent use of hormonal ablation, these complications have become less frequent in contemporary series of patients.

○ **What is the percentage of patients who will become incontinent if they have a TURP after EBRT?**

Some degree of incontinence may be noted in approximately 30% of such patients. The incidence is higher if the TURP is performed less than 1 year after the radiation therapy.

○ **What are the results of cryotherapy for patients with clinical stage T3 prostate cancer?**

For men with high-risk features, those with PSA $\geq$10 ng/mL or Gleason score $\geq$8, 6-year biochemical disease-free rates of 35% can be achieved. Reported recurrences are more common in cancers located at the apex and the seminal vesicles in contrast to those cancers located in the mid gland and base.

○ **What are the most common complications following cryotherapy?**

As with other treatments for prostate cancer, the most common complication is erectile dysfunction. Other complications include tissue sloughing, perineal ecchymosis, incontinence, strictures, and pelvic or urethral or rectal pain. Rectal fistulas are rare with modern equipment and intraoperative temperature monitoring. Incontinence is more common in patients undergoing salvage cryotherapy who previously had received radiation therapy. Hydronephrosis may be noted in those with extensive damage to the trigone or bladder neck area.

○ **What is the definition of BCR after radical prostatectomy?**

The most commonly accepted threshold is PSA >0.2 ng/mL. The AUA guidelines recommend using a threshold of $\geq$0.2 ng/mL, with a second confirmatory level of >0.2 ng/mL, to define surgical failure. Some authors have recognized that low levels such as 0.01 to 0.07 ng/mL noted with the super-sensitive PSA assays can also represent failure especially if there has been a continuous upward trend even at these extremely low values.

○ **What is the definition of BCR after RT?**

ASTRO Phoenix Criteria recommend that biochemical failure be defined as a PSA rise of 2 ng/mL above the post-treatment nadir, whether or not the patient received hormonal therapy in conjunction with radiation therapy.

○ **What is the role of imaging studies in diagnosis of local versus distant recurrence in patients with rising PSA level?**

Current methods of detecting disease, whether in the prostatectomy bed, an irradiated gland, or metastatic sites such as bone or lymph nodes, are of very limited value. Moreover, the finding of local disease on an imaging study does not exclude systemic progression. Traditionally, bone scan and CT scan are the 2 most commonly used imaging modalities for staging. Usually, it takes a PSA above 20 ng/mL before bone scintigraphy will demonstrate metastatic disease. However, based on recent CAPSURE data, a PSA ≥5 ng/mL and a PSA doubling time (PSADT) (<10 months) predicted positive imaging results including both bone scan and CT with a high concordance index in a multivariate model.

○ **What is the role of MRI in the diagnosis of local recurrence in BCR?**

The role of MRI is not well defined in the diagnosis of local recurrence. In a small prospective study of men who had undergone a prostatectomy, endorectal MRI detected locally recurrent disease in all 31 men with clinical evidence of locally recurrent disease, as confirmed by biopsy. Endorectal MRI may be able to identify sites of disease that would otherwise not be sampled by routine blind biopsies of the prostate bed and therefore may be useful for identifying areas suggestive of locally recurrent disease or for guiding biopsies.

○ **What is the value of the ProstaScint scan?**

It is approved for the evaluation of soft tissue metastases in high-risk patients and for patients with rising PSA levels after definitive therapy. Fusing the ProstaScint scan with CT and particularly MRI increases its usefulness. It may be useful in locally advanced cancers to detect extraprostatic disease, or when clinical parameters suggest a high likelihood of advanced disease despite negative conventional imaging. However, there is very high rate of false-positive and false-negative results.

○ **A patient with clinical stage T3 prostate cancer undergoes EBRT and is noted to have a rising PSA level. The patient elects to undergo observation only with serial PSA tests. What is the time interval from the rise in the PSA level to the development of clinically detectable prostate cancer?**

A rising PSA level after initial radiation therapy precedes clinically detectable disease (ie, on DRE or radiographic metastasis) relapse by 3 to 5 years on average. In the absence of salvage therapy (eg, androgen suppression), up to 3 quarters of men will have clinical evidence of recurrent disease within 5 years after PSA elevation is detected.

○ **A 55-year-old man with Gleason score 7, clinical stage T2a prostate cancer elects to receive initial EBRT. His pretreatment PSA value was 7.5 ng/mL and it declines to a nadir level of 1.2 ng/mL. It then rises to 3.5 ng/mL. The patient is now 60 years old. What staging studies should be performed to assess the feasibility of salvage radical prostatectomy?**

Restaging for patients with rising PSA levels after radiation therapy should include a bone scan and a CT scan or an MRI of the abdomen and pelvis to rule out metastatic disease. The role of a ProstaScint scan is not entirely clear as it is of limited value, in general. Although it is well established that bone scans rarely detect metastasis in a treatment-naive patient with a PSA value below 20 ng/mL, this has not been established for patients with rising PSA levels after previous definitive local therapy. For patients who are candidates for salvage radical prostatectomy, prostate biopsies and a cystoscopic examination are helpful to define the volume of recurrent disease and to rule out bladder neck involvement.

○ **For the patient described above, what is the role for prostate biopsies and what is the likelihood that prostate biopsies will be positive in this clinical setting?**

A biopsy is indicated only in those patients who are considering further aggressive local therapy, namely salvage prostatectomy or cryotherapy. Performing a prostate biopsy under transrectal ultrasound (TRUS) guidance is important, as 50% to 80% of patients with a rising PSA after initial radiation therapy are reported to have positive biopsies, depending upon the PSA level at the time of biopsy. Gleason scores usually are increased compared to the original untreated tumor; however, this may be due in part to the therapy-related tissue architectural changes.

○ **The above-described patient elects to undergo a salvage radical prostatectomy. What are his chances of having an undetectable serum PSA 5 years later?**

The 5-year biochemical disease-free survival rate is 60% to 70% for patients undergoing salvage prostatectomy with a presalvage PSA <5 ng/mL compared with 25% to 40% for patients with a presalvage PSA >10 ng/mL.

○ **In salvage prostatectomy series performed in the PSA era, what are the rates of capsular penetration, positive margins, and seminal vesicle involvement?**

Many patients with recurrent prostate cancer after radiation therapy have larger cancers with more advanced pathological stage than what is anticipated from the preoperative clinical staging. Adverse pathologic features are commonly present. Series that include patients diagnosed in the PSA era have shown a 26% to 43% rate of capsular penetration, a 32% to 36% rate of positive surgical margins, and a 28% to 49% rate of seminal vesicle involvement. The biochemical outcome after salvage prostatectomy appears superior to the biochemical outcome after salvage cryotherapy or brachytherapy. Salvage radical prostatectomy may cure approximately 50% of well-selected patients (early treatment, low PSA, lower volume disease).

○ **A patient undergoes salvage radical prostatectomy following radiation therapy. The final pathologic evaluation shows Gleason score 9 prostate cancer with extracapsular extension and a positive surgical margin. The seminal vesicles and lymph nodes are negative. Is a positive surgical margin in a patient undergoing salvage radical prostatectomy biologically significant?**

A positive surgical margin in a previously irradiated patient is biologically more significant than those patients with positive surgical margin after primary radical prostatectomy. Salvage prostatectomy patients with positive margins have a worse cancer-specific survival rate. In previously irradiated patients, there are no other curative treatments to fall back on should the surgery fail to remove all the cancer. Thus, complete excision is paramount in this situation.

○ **What is the risk of urinary incontinence following salvage radical prostatectomy?**

Some recent series have reported lower rates and less severe incontinence. But in general, incontinence after salvage prostatectomy remains high at almost 50%, despite improvements in the operative technique.

○ **What is the role of robotic computer-assisted surgery in salvage prostatectomy?**

Several reports of small series of patients undergoing a robotic salvage prostatectomy have been published. Although there are no direct comparisons, the perioperative complication rates are similar to those noted with open salvage radical prostatectomy. Thus, in the properly selected patients, the robotic approach seems quite feasible and as safe as open surgery if it's performed by experienced surgeons.

○ **What are the biochemical disease-free survival rates and complications of nonsurgical salvage local therapies?**

The main complications of salvage cryotherapy are urinary incontinence, obstructive symptoms, impotence, and perineal pain. The incidence of serious gastrointestinal or genitourinary complications following salvage brachytherapy is about 37%. Obstructive symptoms are common, and up to 14% of patients undergo a transurethral resection for relief of obstructive symptoms following salvage brachytherapy, with an increased risk of post-TURP incontinence. Four percent of patients develop significant rectal ulceration, and there are reports of patients undergoing colostomy for rectal bleeding.

○ **Pathological features are extremely important in establishing risk for local versus distant recurrence after radical prostatectomy. For patients with a rising PSA level after radical prostatectomy, which pathological features of the radical prostatectomy specimen support the presence of distant metastases?**

Patients with radical prostatectomy specimen Gleason score of ≥8, SVI, or positive pelvic lymph nodes are at higher risk for distant metastasis. Patients with a specimen Gleason score ≤7, positive surgical margins, no SVI, and negative pelvic lymph nodes may be at higher risk for local recurrence rather than distant metastases.

○ **Does the presence of negative surgical margins in a radical prostatectomy specimen preclude the development of a local recurrence?**

Of patients with an elevated PSA level and negative bone scan following radical prostatectomy, the chances of a biopsy-proven local recurrence have been reported to be 10% to 30%. This rate depends entirely upon the degree and velocity of PSA rise (ie, PSA kinetics). Therefore, patients should not be excluded from salvage radiation therapy only on the basis of negative surgical margins. At present, patients are often treated early and the PSA is not allowed to rise to any sufficiently high levels. Thus, a biopsy of the prostatic fossa is often not helpful and is usually not required prior to pelvic XRT.

○ **What are the PSA kinetics of local versus distant disease recurrence following radical prostatectomy?**

Short interval from surgery to detectable PSA is often indicative of distant metastasis. The development of a detectable PSA ≤1 year following radical prostatectomy and a PSA doubling time ≤6 months have all been associated with significant risk for distant metastasis. By comparison, patients who develop a detectable PSA >1 year following radical prostatectomy, or have a PSA doubling time >12 months are more likely to harbor local recurrence. It should be noted that there can be a significant overlap in these PSA kinetics which define local versus distant disease.

○ **A 70-year-old man develops rising PSA levels after radical prostatectomy. This patient elects to undergo observation. What is the median actuarial time from postsurgical PSA elevation to the development of clinically evident metastasis?**

In numerous studies, PSADT has been shown to be the dominant factor used to assess the risk of developing metastasis-free survival. Median time to metastatic disease is 10 years for all comers. Those with <3-month PSA doubling time developed metastatic disease at a median of 1 year, whereas those with a 15-month or more doubling time may not develop metastases for up to 10 years after biochemical relapse.

○ **A 60-year-old patient has a rising PSA value of 1.2 ng/mL 4 years after radical prostatectomy. The patient is concerned about the possibility of metastasis, and staging studies including a bone scan and CT scan are ordered. What is the likelihood that a bone scan, ProstaScint nuclear scan, or CT scan will be positive in this patient?**

Although bone scans and CT scans of the pelvis are often recommended for patients with a rising PSA value after surgery, results of these studies are initially negative in the vast majority of patients, particularly in those with lower PSA values (<10 ng/mL). There have been anecdotal cases of patients who had positive bone scans with an undetectable PSA levels, although this is extremely rare. The literature supports the low likelihood of a positive bone scan (<5%) in this setting until the PSA rises to over 20 ng/mL. Furthermore, CT scans of the pelvis are often inaccurate for assessing microscopic lymph node metastasis. A ProstaScint scan may be helpful in select situations, but its use is not widely recommended due to the associated false-negative rates and some false-positive results.

○ **What proportion of patients with a detectable PSA level after radical prostatectomy will experience a decrease in their PSA level following salvage radiation therapy?**

Approximately 35% to 75% of patients with rising PSA who receive postoperative radiation therapy to the prostatic bed experience a decrease in their serum PSA. This fact objectively demonstrates that at least some cancer cells persisted in the local field after radical prostatectomy. This depends upon whether the PSA ever declined to undetectable level or if it began to rise at some interval from the surgery. As mentioned above, PSA kinetics (timing and rate of rise) are extremely important in determining the usefulness of salvage XRT for presumed local recurrence.

○ **Five years after radical prostatectomy, a patient has a PSA value of 0.4 ng/mL. What is his likelihood of having a durable biochemical response to salvage radiation? What would his chance of having a durable biochemical response be if his PSA value was 3.5 ng/mL?**

The preradiation PSA value has a profound effect on the outcome following salvage radiation therapy. It is clear that the lower the preradiation PSA value, the greater the likelihood of achieving a durable biochemical response. If the preradiation PSA is <2 ng/mL, then 83% of such patients can be expected to demonstrate biochemical control compared with only 33% of patients with a PSA >2 ng/mL. Patients with a PSA of 0.5 ng/mL or lower have nearly double the likelihood of remaining disease free compared to those treated at higher PSA levels >1 ng/mL.

○ **What clinical parameters have demonstrated prognostic value for patients undergoing salvage radiation therapy?**

Patients with Gleason score of 8 to 10, preradiotherapy PSA level greater than 2.0 ng/mL, negative surgical margins, PSADT (doubling time) of 10 months or less, and SVI have been associated with lower rate of response following salvage radiation.

○ **What are the complications of salvage radiation therapy to the pelvis for a rising PSA level following radical prostatectomy? If a patient has normal continence, is he likely to develop incontinence?**

In general, salvage radiation therapy is extremely well tolerated with few serious side effects. The most common side effects are related to radiation-induced cystitis and proctitis, which is often mild, and may cause irritative voiding symptoms and diarrhea. The irritative voiding symptoms and diarrhea typically resolve within 3 months of therapy. A worsening of incontinence has been noted in approximately 4% to 8% of patients undergoing salvage radiation therapy. In general, however, most patients who have good urinary control following radical prostatectomy continue to maintain urinary control after salvage radiation therapy. The salvage radiation therapy also has an adverse effect on the erectile function in men who may have regained their potency following surgery.

○   **What is the optimal time of ADT for biochemical relapse after radical prostatectomy?**

There is no strong or level I evidence regarding the optimal PSA value at which to initiate treatment. In a large study of 1350 patients initiating "early" hormonal therapy did not appear to impact time to metastatic disease in the entire study group. However, time to metastatic disease was delayed in patients with Gleason score 8 to 10 cancers and those with PSADT of 12 months or less if ADT was initiated at a PSA level of 5 ng/mL. The decision to initiate ADT for presumed micrometastatic disease must take into consideration not only the PSA level, but also PSA velocity, Gleason score, pathologic stage, patient's comorbidities, side effects of androgen deficiency, effect on patient's quality of life, and patient's wishes.

○   **Can intermittent hormones be used for androgen deprivation in BCR?**

In a study on men with a rising PSA >3 ng/mL who biochemically relapsed after radiation therapy were randomized to either intermittent hormones or continuous androgen deprivation. At median follow-up of 6.9 years the 2 had no difference in overall survival. Time to castration resistance was improved in the intermittent hormonal therapy arm, and while more deaths from prostate cancer were seen in the intermittent therapy arm, there were fewer unrelated deaths in the intermittent arm as well.

CHAPTER 48

Testicular and Paratesticular Tumors

John D. Seigne, MB, FACS and Johann P. Ingimarsson, MD

○ The following are the number of new cancer cases for several urinary cancers in men in the United States in 2011. Match the number of cases to the tumor type.

Number of Cases	Tumor Type
1570	**Bladder**
8590	**Penis**
37,120	**Prostate**
52,020	**Renal**
240,890	**Testis**

Number of Cases	Tumor Type
52,020	Bladder
1570	Penis
240,890	Prostate
37,120	Renal
8590	Testis

○ **The reported incidence of testicular cancer varies greatly between countries. Within the United States, what, if any, is the effect of race on testicular cancer incidence?**

The incidence of testicular cancer in the United States in non-Hispanic whites is 5 times higher than the incidence in African-Americans, 4 times higher than the incidence in Asians, and 78% higher than in Hispanics.

○ **What are the most common genetic alterations found in testis cancer?**

An isochromosome of the short arm of chromosome 12, i (12p), is a relatively frequent finding in germ cell tumors. Tumors not containing i (12p) generally have additional genetic material located on the short arm of chromosome 12. Isochromosome 12p is found in up to 80% of germ cell tumors. Interestingly, neither gain nor amplification of 12p material is commonly seen in intratubular germ cell neoplasia (although many other germ cell genomic changes are already present) suggesting that gain of genetic material from 12p is associated with the progression from intratubular germ cell neoplasia to invasive disease.

○ **A 2-year-old child undergoes a right orchiopexy for a high inguinal undescended testicle. What is his risk of developing testis cancer in that testicle at some point in the future?**

Patients with cryptorchidism have a 2.7 to 8 times increased risk of developing testicular cancer. The lifetime probability of developing testis cancer is therefore between 0.6% and 1.6%.

○ **A 2-year-old child with a high inguinal undescended testicle has an orchiopexy. To what degree will the orchiopexy affect his future risk of developing testis cancer and what effect, if any, does puberty have on this risk?**

There is controversy about the degree to which orchiopexy decreases the risk of testis cancer. Orchiopexy certainly allows for easier examination of the affected testicle and potentially earlier detection. A large population-based study showed children who had an orchiopexy prior to age 13 had an increased relative risk of testis cancer of 2.2, whereas those who had an orchiopexy after age 13 had an increased relative risk of 5.4 when compared to the general population.

○ **A 2-year-old child undergoes a right orchiopexy for a high inguinal undescended testicle. He is at increased risk of developing testis cancer in the right testicle. Is he at greater risk than the general population of developing a tumor in his normal descended left testicle?**

Although it has been previously thought that the normal descended testicle contralateral to an undescended testicle has an increased risk of developing cancer, this is now being challenged. Although a case–control study from the Danish Cancer Registry found an increased risk (HR of 3.6), other studies have not consistently confirmed these findings. Combined data from numerous large case series now suggest that the incidence may in fact be similar to that of the general population.

○ **What is/are the peak age group(s) for the development of Leydig cell tumor and how do these tumors present?**

Leydig cell tumors have a bimodal distribution, with an initial peak in the prepubertal age group, 4 to 10 and then a second peak between the ages of 30 and 60. They present most often with gynecomastia, precocious puberty, or breast tenderness.

○ **β-hCG is a tumor marker that is commonly measured in patients with testis cancer. What cells produce β-hCG? What percentage of patients will demonstrate an elevated β-hCG with pure seminoma and nonseminomatous germ cell tumor (NSGCT)?**

β-hCG is produced by syncytiotrophoblastic cells. β-hCG is elevated in approximately 15% of patients with pure seminoma and 40% to 60% of those with a NSGCT.

○ **Alpha-fetoprotein (AFP) is a tumor marker that is commonly measured in patients with testis cancer. What percentages of patients with pure seminoma have an elevated AFP and what percentage of patients with NSGCT have elevated AFP levels?**

AFP is not elevated in patients with pure seminoma. AFP is elevated in 50% to 70% of patients with NSGCT.

○ **A 25-year-old has a right orchiectomy for a NSGCT. Prior to orchiectomy, his AFP was 124 and his β-hCG was 88. What is the half-life of AFP and β-hCG? Assuming that he has no metastatic disease, when should his AFP and β-hCG return to normal?**

The metabolic half-life of AFP is 5 to 7 days. Thus, using conservative estimates, the AFP should be normal (<9) in about 4 weeks. The serum half-life of β-hCG is 24 to 36 hours. Thus, using conservative estimates, the β-hCG should be normal (<2) in about 9 days.

○ **A family practitioner refers a 3-month-old boy to you for evaluation of a left testis mass. He was concerned about a testis tumor and sent tumor markers. AFP was 57 and β-hCG was <2. On examination, the infant has a swollen left testis that is twice the size of the right testis. The epididymis cannot readily be distinguished from the testis. What is the next step in the evaluation and how likely is this child to have testicular cancer?**

The next step in evaluation is a testicular ultrasound. The child is very unlikely to have testis cancer. The physical examination is much more suggestive of epididymitis or a missed torsion. Testicular cancer is unusual in infants. The most common testicular cancer would be a yolk sac tumor where the peak incidence is 2 years of age. AFP is produced by the fetus and is measurable at very high levels from the 12th week of gestation. The level gradually falls thereafter and reaches normal levels by the end of the first year of life.

○ **A 22-year-old college student was playing a vigorous game of touch football. He does not specifically remember being hit in the genital area but following the game he has an aching pain in his right testicle. He performs a testicular self-examination and feels a testicular mass. Your examination confirms that the right testicle is larger than the left with some thickening at the lower pole. How should the testicle be evaluated?**

Scrotal ultrasound should be the next step in the evaluation. Many testis tumors are noticed after only minor trauma, but in this case, the diagnosis is uncertain. Therefore, the initial evaluation should be the inexpensive, noninvasive, and sensitive screening study of a scrotal ultrasound.

○ **A 24-year-old has a testicular ultrasound for evaluation of a dragging sensation in his right testicle. He is referred to see you as the ultrasound showed "bilateral microlithiasis." The patient has no other complaints or problems. His discomfort is improving and has been attributed to a sports injury. His physical examination is normal with no testicular masses. The ultrasound is a good-quality study and shows approximately 15 to 20 small (<2 mm) microcalcifications distributed throughout the body of both testes. What is the risk of testicular cancer and what should be the next step in his evaluation? What is the recommended follow-up?**

Instruct the patient to perform regular testis self-examination and seek prompt evaluation if he notices a mass. Large studies of army recruits have demonstrated that testicular microlithiasis is not associated with a substantially increased risk of subsequent testis cancer development. Thus, no further evaluation is necessary, short of teaching the patient to perform testicular self-examination.

○   **A 62-year-old man has gradual painless swelling of his left testicle. Physical examination is noticeable for diffuse enlargement and firmness of the left testicle. The right testis is normal. The remainder of his physical examination is normal. A left radical orchiectomy is performed. A low-power photomicrograph is shown below (Fig. 1). What is the diagnosis?**

Figure 1.

Lymphoma. It is the most common testicular tumor in men older than 60 years. The photomicrograph shows tubules surrounded by monotonous blue staining cells, an appearance that is characteristic for testicular infiltration by lymphoma.

○   **What is the rationale for performing an inguinal approach to orchiectomy as part of the treatment of testicular cancer when a scrotal approach is appropriate when performing an orchiectomy as part of the treatment for prostate cancer?**

When operating on testicular cancer, a trans-scrotal approach is contraindicated as it may alter the lymphatic drainage of the testis, increasing the risk of local recurrence and pelvic or inguinal lymph node metastasis. There are no such concerns in prostate cancer as in that scenario the procedure is being done solely for the removal of the androgen producing components of the testes.

○ **A 59-year-old man noticed a mass at the upper pole of the right testicle. He is otherwise healthy and asymptomatic. β-hCG is 110 (normal <2). AFP is 256 (normal <9). His ultrasound is shown below (Fig. 2). He undergoes a right radical orchiectomy. What is the most likely diagnosis?**

Figure 2.

RT TRV MID_

15fps   6cm

Mixed germ cell tumor. A seminoma would be a more common tumor in this age group. However, the presence of an elevated AFP excludes this diagnosis. The presence of elevated tumor markers essentially rules out a lymphoma and a Leydig cell tumor.

○ **A 35-year-old man has a right testis biopsy as part of an evaluation for infertility and is found to have testicular intraepithelial neoplasia (TIN) (or intratubular germ cell neoplasia). Prior to the testis biopsy, he had a small right testis but no masses were palpable. A right testis U/S showed a decrease in testicular volume with normal echo texture throughout. As a child, he had a left undescended testicle that was removed at age 8. He is otherwise healthy. His physical examination is normal. He is azoospermic. His FSH is elevated at 3 times normal. Serum testosterone is normal. What are the treatment options and what is his best option to both minimize his risk of developing testis cancer and maintain as much physiological function as possible?**

The best option to minimize testis cancer risk and preserve as much physiological function as possible is low-dose radiation to the testicle (16-20 Gy). The patient is almost certainly infertile given his elevated FSH and azoospermia. Therefore, preservation of endocrine function and eradication of TIN are the primary goals of therapy; 16 to 20 Gy of irradiation has been shown to effectively achieve this goal in European studies. Chemotherapy can also eradicate TIN. However, the optimal schedule is not known and it is less reliable than radiation. Observation is an option, but the patient is quite likely to develop a germ cell tumor at a future date. Radical orchiectomy will cure the cancer but not preserve his endocrine function.

○ **A 32-year-old man undergoes a right orchiectomy for a stage I NSGCT and enters a surveillance protocol. At the end of 1 year, he is asymptomatic, all radiologic and laboratory studies are negative. He asks you what his chances are of developing a tumor in the opposite testicle.**

Approximately 2% to 4% of patients develop a contralateral germ cell tumor which is a 20- to 40-fold increased risk compared to the general population. For this reason, it is important to teach patients with testicular tumors to perform regular contralateral testicular self-examination.

○ **A 28-year-old man who, 2 years previously, had a left orchiectomy following a traumatic testis injury presents with a 2-cm right lower pole testicular mass. Tumor markers are negative. An ultrasound demonstrates a solid mass located on the anterior surface of the lower pole of the right testis. The remainder of the testis is normal. The patient is recently married and is interested in having children in the future. What are the management options?**

There are 3 management options:

1. Radical orchiectomy, which is associated with significant permanent endocrine abnormalities and sterility but assures local control.

2. Partial orchiectomy followed by low-dose radiation (16-20 Gy), which is associated with sterility but preserves endocrine function and is associated with a low incidence of local recurrence.

3. Partial orchiectomy alone, which preserves endocrine function and may preserve fertility but is associated with a higher risk of local failure. As this patient has a favorably located tumor, partial orchiectomy with negative margins preceded by sperm banking would be a good therapeutic choice, if the patient desires to father a child. He should subsequently be advised to have delayed low-dose radiation after he completes his family.

○ **A 22-year-old man has a right orchiectomy for a pT2 mixed germ cell tumor. Prior to orchiectomy, his β-hCG was 256, AFP was 58, and lactic dehydrogenase (LDH) was normal. He is asymptomatic and his physical examination is unremarkable. All of the following are imaging options; chest x-ray, CT of chest and abdomen, PET/CT fusion imaging of chest and abdomen. Which is the most appropriate choice?**

CT of the chest and abdomen: The most common sites of disease in a patient with a newly diagnosed NSGCT are the retroperitoneal lymph nodes and the lungs. These areas should be routinely imaged. In the past, investigators have argued that a chest x-ray is sufficient for lung imaging in the absence of disease in the retroperitoneum. However, a chest CT has a much higher sensitivity than a chest x-ray and is almost certainly a better choice. A PET CT fusion study is much more expensive and in a prospective study has not been shown to provide reliable additional information in patients with NSGCT.

○ **A 19-year-old man has a right orchiectomy for a pT2 NSGCT. His tumor markers, which were previously elevated, have returned to normal as predicted by their half-lives. His CT scan of the chest and abdomen are normal. He has seen a medical oncologist, who, after reviewing the pathology report, told him that if he had an retroperitoneal lymph node dissection (RPLND) the chances that microscopic disease would be found in his lymph nodes were approximately 40% to 60%. What additional information in the pathology report allowed the medical oncologist to draw this conclusion?**

The presence of vascular invasion and the percentage of embryonal cancer. The combination of vascular invasion and a high percentage (>40%) of embryonal cancer in the primary tumor is associated with an elevated risk of finding disease in the retroperitoneum at RPLND.

○ **A 22-year-old single student has a newly diagnosed International Germ Cell Cancer Consensus (IGCCC) low risk metastatic testis cancer. He has seen a medical oncologist and is fit for and understands the risks of chemotherapy. However, prior to initiating chemotherapy, he should consider what additional precautionary procedure?**

Sperm banking. Treatment of testis cancer has the potential to lead to azoospermia. Therefore, all patients should be encouraged to consider sperm banking prior to initiating therapy. Between 40% and 60% of patients with testicular cancer are hypofertile at diagnosis with sperm counts returning to normal in 75% of patients following orchiectomy. With newer reproductive technologies, fertility is likely to be possible for more than 80% of patients. Sperm banking is a sensible precaution as the sperm can be discarded after 2 to 3 years if the patient remains disease-free and the sperm count reverts to normal.

○ **A 30-year-old man presents with a left testicular mass. He undergoes a left orchiectomy. Pathology shows a 4-cm embryonal cancer invading the tunica albuginea. Vascular invasion is noted. Metastatic workup consists of an abdominal MRI scan (Fig. 3). Chest CT scan shows 5 0.5 cm to 2 cm lung nodules. LDH is 3 times normal. β-hCG is 3000. AFP is 1500. What stage is the patient according to the 7th edition (2010) of the Manual of American Joint Commission on Cancer TNM staging system?**

Figure 3.

MRI shows a 9-cm intra-aortocaval nodal mass. The patient has a T2N3S2M1a, stage IIIB tumor.

○ **A 35-year-old man is diagnosed with a T1N0M0S1 pure seminoma. His β-hCG was 56 at diagnosis and 14 days later is <2. His CT scan of the chest, abdomen, and pelvis are normal. What is his risk of recurrence if he has no further treatment? How does this risk change if he elects to receive 20 to 25 Gy of radiation therapy to the standard retroperitoneal field?**

The risk of recurrence for a patient with a stage I seminoma on surveillance is approximately 15%. In large studies, the risk of recurrence with adjuvant radiation for stage I seminoma is 1% to 3%.

○ **The same patient as in the previous question is considering either adjuvant radiation or a single dose of carboplatin as adjuvant therapy for his stage I seminoma. Should he choose radiation, what is the recommended field of radiation and why?**

He should be treated with a para-aortic field, alone, rather than a "dog leg" field that had been recommended in the past. A large randomized trial comparing para-aortic radiation to para-aortic and ipsilateral iliac lymph node irradiation found no difference in relapse free survival (96% at 5 years). Acute toxicities were less common and sperm counts higher in the para-aortic only group.

○ **The same patient as in the previous question continues to consider either adjuvant radiation or a single dose of carboplatin as adjuvant therapy for his stage I seminoma. What are the advantages, if any, of single dose of carboplatin when compared to radiation therapy?**

A large, randomized study demonstrated equivalence of 20 Gy of retroperitoneal irradiation to a single dose of carboplatin with regards to cancer control. Subjects in the carboplatin arm had less of a decrease in their quality of life scores and had a decrease in the frequency of secondary contralateral testis tumors.

○ **A 28-year-old man is diagnosed with an anaplastic seminoma after a left radical orchiectomy. Tumor markers are normal. A CT scan of the chest is normal. A CT scan of the abdomen demonstrated a 2-cm left para-aortic lymph node just below the left renal vein. The patient is asymptomatic and otherwise healthy. What is the recommended treatment? How would this be different if the patient had a pure seminoma as compared to an anaplastic seminoma?**

The recommended treatment is 30 to 36 Gy of retroperitoneal radiation to a retroperitoneal and ipsilateral iliac field. There is no evidence that anaplastic seminomas should be treated differently to standard seminomas stage for stage. There is some evidence that seminomas with an anaplastic histology present at a more advanced stage. Standard therapy for a low-volume stage II seminoma is retroperitoneal irradiation.

○ **A 63-year-old man is diagnosed with a spermatocytic seminoma after a left radical orchiectomy. Tumor markers are normal. His CT scan of the chest, abdomen, and pelvis are normal. What is the recommended treatment? How would this be different if the patient had a pure seminoma as compared to a spermatocytic seminoma?**

The risk of metastatic disease associated with spermatocytic seminoma is extremely low. Thus, surveillance is the recommended course of action. If the patient had a pure seminoma, the risk of recurrence is approximately 15%, thus a discussion of adjuvant radiation or single dose of carboplatin is appropriate.

○ A 44-year-old man has a right orchiectomy for a 4-cm testis tumor. A representative high power micrograph is shown below (Fig. 4). Preoperative tumor markers were notable for a β-hCG of 200. AFP is normal and LDH is 1.3 times normal. A CT scan of the chest is normal. A CT scan of the abdomen and pelvis shows a large 7-cm mass surrounding the aorta and inferior vena cava, just below the renal vessels. The patient is otherwise healthy and asymptomatic. One week after his orchiectomy, his β-hCG is 108. What is the diagnosis, tumor stage, and recommended therapy?

Figure 4.

The slides show a pure seminoma, thus the patient has bulky stage II seminoma (T1N3M0S1). In the past, treatment would have consisted of retroperitoneal irradiation (35-40 Gy). Now, most centers recommend chemotherapy (3 cycles bleomycin, etopides, cisplatin (BEP) or 4 cycles etopides cisplatin (EP)). Results with retroperitoneal irradiation are variable with recurrence-free survival rates ranging between 45% and 100%. Most patients who fail radiation are salvaged with subsequent chemotherapy. Initial chemotherapy in patients with bulky (>5 cm) disease avoids the necessity for dual treatment in 20% to 50% of patients.

○ A 28-year-old man is found to have a mediastinal mass on CT obtained for shortness of breath. His CT scan of the abdomen and pelvis are normal. Biopsy of the mass shows NSGCT with a predominant yolk sac component. AFP is 1600, but β-hCG is normal. Bilateral testicles are normal on examination. How does the location of the tumor affect treatment and prognosis?

Extra-gonadal NSGCTs are less sensitive to chemotherapy and have a poor prognosis than those that arise from the testicle. The 5-year overall survival of patients with mediastinal NSGCT is only about 45%. In contrast to NSGCT, mediastinal seminomas carry a similar prognosis to testicular seminomas.

○ **A 38-year-old man has a right orchiectomy for a 5-cm pure seminoma. Preoperative tumor markers were notable for a β-hCG of 200. AFP is normal and LDH is 1.5 times normal. A CT scan of the chest shows 3 separate 1-cm lung nodules. A CT scan of the abdomen and pelvis shows a large 9.8-cm mass surrounding the aorta and inferior vena cava just below the renal vessels. The patient is otherwise healthy and asymptomatic. He completes 3 cycles of BEP chemotherapy. Restaging CT scans show resolution of the lung nodules. The mass in the abdomen has shrunk to 3.4 cm in maximum diameter 2 weeks after completing chemotherapy. Tumor markers are normal. What additional testing should be performed and how will this be used in decision making regarding further therapy?**

There is considerable controversy about the best management of a residual mass after chemotherapy for a pure seminoma with some groups suggesting resection of residual masses >3 cm in size and others recommending observation or irradiation. A PET/CT scan can help assess the risk that the mass contains residual active germ cell tumor. Recent reports indicate that a PET scan has 80% sensitivity and 100% specificity for the detection of viable germ cell tumor in a retroperitoneal mass following chemotherapy for pure seminoma.

In general, surgery should be confined to resecting residual masses. A bilateral retroperitoneal lymph node dissection is not recommended after the chemotherapy for seminoma because of the increased risk of complications due to the extensive fibrosis and desmoplastic reaction.

○ **A 37-year-old patient has an orchiectomy for a 6-cm pure seminoma. He refuses additional therapy and is lost to follow up. Two years later, he is admitted to the hospital with extensive metastatic seminoma with bone and liver metastases. AFP is <6, β-hCG is normal, and LDH is 13 times normal. Liver biopsy confirms metastatic seminoma. What is his IGCCC risk level? What is the recommended therapy and what is the patient's likelihood of cure?**

The patient has intermediate risk disease by the IGCCC. Although the patient has what would be considered to be high-risk disease if he had a NSGCT, no seminoma is considered high risk. The recommended therapy for intermediate risk disease is 4 cycles of BEP, which is likely to achieve about an 80% cure rate.

○ **A 19-year-old man has a right orchiectomy for a mixed NSGCT (40% embryonal, 20% teratoma, 30% seminoma, and 10% yolk sac). Vascular invasion is noted on pathology. Prior to orchiectomy, β-hCG was 4 and AFP was 52. His CT scan of the chest, abdomen, and pelvis show no evidence of disease. He decides to proceed with a nerve sparing RPLND. He comes for his preoperative visit 3 weeks after his orchiectomy and 1 week prior to surgery. He feels well and his examination is completely normal. His β-hCG is <2 and his AFP is 40. On the morning of surgery his AFP is 56. How should you proceed?**

Cancel the surgery and proceed with 3 cycles of bleomycin, etoposide, and cis-platinum chemotherapy or 4 cycles of etoposide and cis-platinum. Patients with clinical stage I NSGCT who have persistently elevated markers prior to RPLND have a higher incidence of microscopic metastatic disease outside the retroperitoneum; therefore, primary chemotherapy is the preferred alternative.

○ **A 27-year-old has a left orchiectomy for a mixed NSGCT (10% embryonal, 50% teratoma, 20% seminoma, and 20% yolk sac). Vascular invasion is not noted on pathology (T1N0M0). AFP was 200 and β-hCG was 60 prior to orchiectomy. Both tumor markers are now normal. The patient is otherwise healthy. What is the likelihood of finding retroperitoneal disease if he has an RPLND?**

Approximately 15%. The patient has a low percentage of embryonal cancer and no vascular invasion, thus is at lower risk of retroperitoneal disease and a candidate for surveillance.

○   **A 27-year-old has a left orchiectomy for a mixed NSGCT (10% embryonal, 50% teratoma, 20% seminoma, and 20% yolk sac). Vascular invasion is not noted on pathology (T1N0M0). AFP was 200 and β-hCG was 60 prior to orchiectomy. Both tumor markers are now normal. The patient is otherwise healthy. He elects surveillance. If he has a normal physical examination, tumor markers, and CT scan of the chest abdomen and pelvis at 1 year, what is his likelihood of having a recurrence now?**

The patient has low-risk NSGCT with only a 15% chance of relapse in total. Of those that do relapse on surveillance 85% will relapse within the first year. Thus, with no evidence of relapse at 12 months, his risk of relapse in the future is <3%.

○   **A 36-year-old homeless alcoholic undergoes a left orchiectomy for a pathological stage T1 NSGCT (20% embryonal, 40% seminoma, and 40% yolk sac). Tumor markers prior to orchiectomy were β-hCG 30 and AFP 45. An abdominal CT scan and chest x-ray show no evidence of disease. He is lost to follow up. Five-years later he returns to your office and wants follow-up. He has recently married and is currently working. He has no complaints and physical examination is normal. Tumor markers are notable for an AFP of 20 (normal <9). β-hCG is normal. Chest X-ray and abdominal CT scans are normal. What is the cause of his AFP elevation and what further management is necessary?**

Elevated AFP can be seen in patients with hepatocellular, pancreatic, gastric, and lung carcinomas as well as benign conditions such as cirrhosis and hepatitis. This patient had a low-risk tumor at diagnosis (T1, low percentage of embryonal cell) and has negative evaluation 5-years after diagnosis. He is unlikely to have recurrent testicular cancer and should be evaluated for liver disease due to his history of alcohol abuse.

○   **A 25-year-old male receives 4 cycles of chemotherapy for a stage III NSGCT. At diagnosis, both β-hCG and AFP were markedly elevated. He is now 1 month after completing chemotherapy and his β-hCG has been stable for 2 months but slightly elevated at 4 (normal <2). He has no complaints. Physical examination is notable only for an absent right testicle and a small soft left testicle. An extensive radiologic evaluation demonstrates a complete response. What is the next step in this patient's management?**

Low-level β-hCG elevations following treatment of germ cell tumors have been divided into 3 categories: (1) false-positive (phantom β-hCG), (2) quiescent germ cell tumor, and (3) unexplained increase in β-hCG. In general, false-positive assays can be diagnosed by demonstrating that β-hCG cannot be measured by (a) a different assay or (b) cannot be measured simultaneously in the urine. Differentiating between quiescent germ cell tumors and an unexplained increase can be more difficult. The diagnosis often only becomes clear by either resolution of the elevation (unexplained increase) or successive increases (quiescent germ cell tumor).

○ **A 29-year-old has a left orchiectomy for a mixed germ cell tumor (70% embryonal, 30% yolk sac). Tumor markers are negative. Laboratory tests and chest x-ray are normal. A CT scan of the abdomen and pelvis is shown below (Fig. 5). What is the likelihood that the patient will be found to have metastatic germ cell tumor at the time of RPLND?**

Figure 5.

The CT scan shows a 1.5-cm node in the primary landing site of the left testicle. The likelihood that this contains tumor is approximately 75%.

○ **A 27-year-old man undergoes a left orchiectomy. Pathology shows a T1 NSGCT (50% teratoma, 40% embryonal cell carcinoma, and 10% seminoma. Vascular invasion is noted). Within the teratomatous component, foci of dedifferentiation to squamous cell carcinoma are noted. Metastatic evaluation including chest x-ray, abdominal CT scan, and tumor markers are all normal. How does the presence of the squamous cell carcinoma effect the management of this patient?**

The presence of dedifferentiation into another malignant tumor type within a teratoma is found in approximately 2% of patients. If the patient has stage I disease the current recommendation is to treat these patients as you would a patient with a standard NSGCT. Thus, the recommendation would be for the patient to undergo nerve-sparing RPLND, given the vascular invasion. In the presence of metastatic disease, most patients do not respond to primary cisplatin-based chemotherapy. In these cases, the treatment needs to be tailored to the stage and histologic subtype of the tumor.

○ **A 28-year-old man with an embryonal carcinoma of the left testicle, normal tumor markers, and negative metastatic evaluation undergoes a modified template RPLND. What are the chances that he will have normal antegrade ejaculation? If the surgeon prospectively preserves the sympathetic nerves at the time of the template RPLND, how much will that improve the rate of antegrade ejaculation?**

A template RPLND will result in approximately 90% of patients ejaculating normally. If prospective nerve sparing is performed, this will increase up to approximately 98%.

○ **RPLND can be performed in either an open or laparoscopic fashion. What is the major criticism that open surgeons have of a laparoscopic RPLND?**

Although many criticisms have been leveled at laparoscopic surgery, the main concern is that the completeness of the laparoscopic dissection is less than that of an open procedure, thus the recurrence rates in the retroperitoneum may turn out to be higher. Open surgeons claim that the low recurrence rates reported in laparoscopic RPLND series are a reflection of the increased use of chemotherapy for patients found to have pN1 disease. The validity of these claims is uncertain and this is an area of continuing controversy.

○ **A 25-year-old man is undergoing an RPLND for a clinical stage I testis cancer. On abdominal exploration, you note he has a 4 cm healthy appendix. Should an appendectomy be performed at the time of RPLND?**

An incidental appendectomy performed at the time of RPLND increases the risk of an infectious complication from 2% to approximately 10%. Therefore, incidental appendectomy at the time of RPLND is not recommended.

○ **You are planning a left modified nerve-sparing template RPLND for a T2N0M0 NSGCT in a 24-year-old, newly married man who desires 4 children. What are your boundaries of the dissection?**

The boundaries of dissection are superiorly the renal artery and vein, inferiorly the bifurcation of the common iliac artery, laterally the ureter, and medially the medial boarder of the aorta to the level of the inferior mesenteric artery. Below the inferior mesenteric artery, the boundaries are the lateral aspect of the aorta and the common iliac artery. Additional inter aortocaval nodes should be removed below the right renal artery. More recently some surgeons have argued that all template dissections should be replaced by bilateral nerve-sparing dissections, as some mapping studies have demonstrated positive nodes outside the traditional templates and a properly performed nerve-sparing procedure results in comparable rates of preservation of ejaculation.

○ **A 25-year-old man with an embryonal carcinoma of the right testicle, normal tumor markers, and negative metastatic evaluation undergoes a modified right nerve sparing templated RPLND. What are the boundaries of dissection?**

The boundaries of dissection are superiorly the right renal artery and vein, inferiorly the bifurcation of the common iliac artery, laterally the ureter, and medially the midpoint of the aorta to the level of the inferior mesenteric artery. Below the inferior mesenteric artery, the boundaries are the lateral aspect of the aorta and the common iliac artery. As noted above some surgeons have argued that all template dissections should be replaced by bilateral nerve-sparing dissections.

○ **What are the anatomical/physiological types of the nerves that control emission and ejaculation that are preserved at the time of a nerve-sparing RPLND?**

Postganglionic sympathetic fibers originating from the T12 through L4 vertebral levels.

○ **A 23-year-old man with a stage I NSGCT undergoes an RPLND for a final pT1N0M0 NSGCT. Twenty-six nodes are resected and all are negative. What is his risk of relapse? If a relapse were to occur, what anatomical site would be the most likely?**

His risk of relapse within 2 years is between 5% and 10% and the likely site of relapse is the lungs. Approximately 75% of these patients relapsed in the lungs and approximately 15% of patients developed a marker-only recurrence. A properly performed negative RPLND makes patient follow-up substantially easier as it makes relapse in the retroperitoneum unlikely. Thus, follow-up can be focused with tumor markers and chest x-rays.

○ **A 25-year-old man with an embryonal carcinoma of the left testicle, normal tumor markers, and negative metastatic evaluation undergoes a modified left template nerve-sparing RPLND. At the time of RPLND, gross nodal disease is unexpectedly discovered in the interaortocaval area. What is the appropriate course of action?**

The surgeon should abandon the plan to perform a modified left template operation and proceed with a full bilateral node dissection (nerve sparing if possible).

○ **After the case your colleague suggests that you should not have attempted a modified template procedure to begin with and should as a routine do full bilateral nerve-sparing node dissection in all but selected RPLND cases. What would be the main argument for such a statement?**

Lower risk of disease recurrence. Although a nonrandomized prospective trial did not show a recurrence difference between unilateral and bilateral RPLND, a retrospective mapping of lymph nodes in 500 men after bilateral RPLND showed that 3% to 23% of patients had positive nodes in the extra template regions.

○ **One or 2 cycles of BEP chemotherapy is an option for adjuvant therapy in a patient with a stage I NSGCT with high-risk features in the primary tumor. What are the primary advantages of adjuvant BEP as compared to RPLND?**

The primary advantage of chemotherapy, especially for high-risk patients (>40% embryonal cancer and vascular invasion), is the avoidance of surgery and the decreased risk of systemic relapse.

○ **A 32-year-old man is referred to you after undergoing a trans-scrotal exploration followed by an inguinal orchiectomy for an unsuspected NSGCT. After orchiectomy, his tumor markers remain persistently elevated and he receives 3 cycles of BEP chemotherapy. Clinical, laboratory, and radiological examination show no evidence of disease 1 month after completion of his chemotherapy. He is referred to you for a hemiscrotectomy. What is your recommendation?**

Reports indicate that scrotal violation at the time of orchiectomy demonstrated no evidence of local recurrence in those patients who had received subsequent chemotherapy. Therefore, no surgery is indicated and the patient should be observed.

○ **A 24-year-old man has a right orchiectomy for a T1 NSGCT (40% embryonal, 40% teratoma, and 20% yolk sac). Tumor markers prior to orchiectomy were AFP 78 and a β-hCG of <2. Following orchiectomy, his tumor markers return to normal. A CT scan of the chest is normal. A CT of the abdomen demonstrates a single 1.3-cm lymph node in the intra-aortocaval area at the level of the inferior mesenteric artery. He undergoes an RPLND. He has 3/18 lymph nodes that demonstrate <1 cm of embryonal cancer. What is the likelihood of a relapse following adjuvant therapy? What is the recommended adjuvant therapy and what are the chances of a relapse without it? What is the overall difference in survival for such patients treated with immediate adjuvant therapy versus surveillance and definitive therapy if relapse occurs?**

In several series, RPLND has been shown to cure 85% to 90% of patients with low-volume N1 testis cancer. However, in a large randomized trial, about 48% of patients with N1-3 disease relapsed following RPLND. Two cycles of adjuvant BEP chemotherapy prevented relapse in 98% of pN1-3 patients. Both an initial observation (followed by chemotherapy on relapse) and an immediate adjuvant approach cured a similar proportion (>97%) of patients.

○   **A 28-year-old, newly married patient is diagnosed with a low-risk metastatic NSGCT. He has fathered a child in a previous relationship. His wife wants to know what are his chances of future fertility and how long will it take his sperm count to recover from chemotherapy. She also wants to know if future children will be at increased risk of developing congenital abnormalities.**

Combination chemotherapy for testis cancer is toxic to both spermatogenesis and Leydig cell function. Almost all patients become azoospermic during chemotherapy. The toxicity is usually reversible with approximately 50% of patients having normal sperm counts at 2 years. Approximately 25% of patients have persistent azoospermia. The couple should be advised to delay conception for at least 6 months after completing chemotherapy as there is a risk of congenital malformations during this period. Children conceived after 6 months of patients been treated for testis cancer do not appear to be at increased risk of congenital malformations.

○   **A patient with intermediate risk NSGCT is about to start BEP chemotherapy. He requests that you inform him of the major long-term risks of this treatment.**

There are 6 major long-term risks:

1. Infertility—Combination chemotherapy for testis cancer is toxic to spermatogenesis. Almost all patients become azoospermic during chemotherapy. The toxicity is usually reversible with approximately 50% of patients having normal counts at 2 years. Approximately 25% of patients have persistent azoospermia.

2. Nephrotoxicity—70% to 80% patients have a reversible decline in renal function after cisplatin chemotherapy. However, for those with irreversible decline, this is subclinical.

3. Raynaud phenomenon, which occurs in 20% to 50% of patients following cisplatin and bleomycin chemotherapy.

4. Neurotoxicity—Clinically relevant peripheral neuropathy occurs in 10% to 40% of patients. Injury to the 8th cranial nerve from cisplatin causes tinnitus in up to 30% of patients. However, major hearing loss is rare.

5. Pulmonary toxicity—Bleomycin-induced pulmonary fibrosis occurs when the dose exceeds 450 to 500 units (4 cycles of standard BEP contains 360 units of bleomycin). Bleomycin pulmonary toxicity is fatal in 1% to 2% of patients and clinically significant fibrosis occurs in an additional 2% to 3%.

6. Cardiovascular toxicity—Cis-platinum-based chemotherapy is associated with a relatively small risk of short-term cardiovascular toxicity (MI, thromboembolic disease). However, more concerning is the apparent long-term increased risk of hypertension, hyperlipidemia, and the metabolic syndrome with a consequent increased risk of early cardiovascular morbidity and mortality in patients receiving a total dose of greater than 400 mg/m^2 of cis-platinum.

○   **A 29-year-old man has a left orchiectomy for a T2 NSGCT. His AFP prior to orchiectomy is 3517, β-hCG is 286, and LDH is 3.5 times normal. The chest CT shows multiple lung metastases. His abdominal CT scan shows a 6-cm mass surrounding the aorta. He has moderate back pain but is otherwise asymptomatic and healthy. What is his IGCCC risk class? What is recommended therapy? What is his chance of being disease-free in 5 years?**

Intermediate risk. The IGCCC risk category is useful to stage patients with metastatic testis cancer. The patient has an IGCCC intermediate risk category based on his AFP being between 1000 and 10,000 and LDH that is between 1.5 and 10 times normal and no extrapulmonary metastatic disease. The patient should receive 4 cycles of BEP chemotherapy. Progression-free survival at 5 years is about 80%.

○ **A 29-year-old man has a left orchiectomy for a T2 NSGCT. His AFP prior to orchiectomy is 3517, β-hCG is 286, LDH is 3.5 times normal. The chest CT shows multiple lung metastases. His abdominal CT scan shows a 6-cm mass surrounding the aorta. He receives 4 cycles of BEP chemotherapy. Tumor markers are normal and repeat CT scans show a residual 2-cm left lung nodule and a 4-cm intra-aortocaval residual mass. What is the next step in management?**

The next step in management is resection of the residual retroperitoneal mass and bilateral RPLND followed by lung resection. In general, following chemotherapy for metastatic NSGCT, all significant residual masses should be surgically removed. The general recommendation is to resect the retroperitoneal mass prior to proceeding to resection of the lung masses. The reason is that the residual retroperitoneal tissue is more likely to represent viable germ cell cancer. In patients with a NSGCT, it is recommended that a bilateral RPLND be performed in the postchemotherapy setting rather than a modified dissection, as lymphatic channel obstruction by the tumor can result in changes of the lymphatic drainage pattern thus resulting in microscopic residual disease outside the primary lymphatic drainage area of the effected testicle.

○ **In the same patient as above, the retroperitoneal mass is resected followed by a bilateral RPLND and wedge resection of the lung mass. Pathology reveals necrosis and benign teratoma. What is the next step in management and what is the patient's risk of recurrence at 5 years?**

The next best step in management is follow-up with tumor markers and a chest x-ray every 2 to 3 months with an abdomen/pelvis CT scan in 6 months. The final pathology does not show active germ cell tumor; therefore, additional therapy is not necessary. The patient's risk of recurrence at 5 years is <10%.

○ **Resection of residual masses after chemotherapy for seminoma is controversial. However, resection of residual masses after chemotherapy for a NSGCT is not. What is the reason for this controversy?**

The reasons for controversy are 2-fold and related. First, surgery after chemotherapy for seminoma is more difficult and with increased risk due to an extensive fibrotic reaction. Secondly, surgery is less likely to be beneficial to the patient with seminoma as just scar/necrotic tissue is identified in approximately 70% to 80% of patients; therefore, these patients will not benefit from the surgery. In patients with NSGCT, approximately 60% to 70% benefit as benign teratoma or active germ cell tumor is identified and removed.

○ **A 22-year-old man is scheduled for a post-chemotherapy retroperitoneal node dissection. On reviewing the records, it is apparent that he has received a total of 550 units of bleomycin over the course of his chemotherapy. He reports that he noticed a dry cough during the last cycle of chemotherapy, but currently has no respiratory symptoms. What perioperative testing and precautions may aid in the management of this patient?**

A series of 5 deaths after bleomycin chemotherapy in the 1970s drew attention to the problem of postoperative pulmonary problems. The causes of bleomycin pulmonary toxicity are not entirely clear, but an increased incidence occurs once the cumulative dose is greater than 400 to 450 units. Preoperative pulmonary function tests (CO diffusion and forced vital capacity) may be useful in identifying patients at higher risk. Careful management (restriction) of perioperative fluids and transfusions as well as minimizing the operative time are important interventions that may decrease the risk of this complication. More recent studies have questioned the need to maintain low levels of inspired (28%) oxygen during the perioperative period.

○ **A 30-year-old with a clinical stage I NSGCT is considering having an RPLND and asks that aside from ejaculatory problems, what are the most common short- and long-term complications of the procedure. What would you tell him?**

In a report from the Testicular Inter Group Study, 3.4% of patients undergoing RPLND had a prolonged ileus for greater than 7 days, 3.3% developed pneumonia, and 2% a UTI. Long-term complications included a 2.3% incidence of small bowel obstruction for an overall significant complication rate of 13.8%. Rarer complications included ureteral injury, intraoperative hemorrhage, enterotomy, unplanned nephrectomy, thromboembolism, chylous fistula, lymphocele, and pancreatitis.

○ **In patients with NSGCT, 3 things are commonly found in residual masses following chemotherapy: in approximately 10% active germ cell tumor, in about 50% benign teratoma, and in about 40% necrosis. What possible complications can result from failing to resect residual masses that just contain benign teratoma following chemotherapy for testis cancer?**

Benign teratoma can undergo secondary malignant degeneration within one of its elements leading to a carcinoma or sarcoma that, in general, is poorly responsive to chemotherapy. Benign teratomas grow slowly in size and eventually cause symptoms because of a local mass effect. These are the 2 primary rationales for resection of benign teratoma.

○ **An 18-year-old has a T2N3M0 S1 NSGCT. He undergoes a right orchiectomy followed by 3 cycles of BEP. Tumor markers are now normal and a 10-cm retroperitoneal mass has decreased in size to 5.8 cm. He undergoes resection of the mass. Final pathology shows necrosis and benign teratoma with several nodes containing multiple small foci of embryonal cancer. All margins are negative. What is the risk that this patient will have a recurrence of testis cancer following his surgery and what is the next step in his management?**

The patient should receive 2 further cycles of chemotherapy. Due to bleomycin accumulated risk and incomplete response in the primary tumor, guidelines now recommend cisplatin base combinations without bleomycin.

○ **A patient has an RPLND for a NSGCT. At RPLND he is found to have 4/12 nodes containing 1 cm of tumor each. Two cycles of BEP chemotherapy are recommended to the patient. He is reluctant to undergo the treatment as he has heard that chemotherapy can give you cancer. What information can you give him to support or refute this assertion?**

Large databases have suggested that patients treated for testicular cancer incur a near 2-fold risk of secondary malignancies, compared to controls. Etoposide treatment is associated with an increased risk of developing a secondary leukemia. However, the rate is less than 0.5% and would probably not occur unless additional cycles of etoposide-based chemotherapy are required.

○ A 35-year-old man presents with back pain. Physical examination is notable for a palpable abdominal mass. External genitalia are notable for bilaterally small testes, but no palpable testis mass. Testis U/S is normal. A CT scan shows a 12-cm left para-aortic mass (Fig. 6). β-hCG is 55 and AFP is 187. A CT biopsy of the retroperitoneal mass is consistent with a germ cell tumor, embryonal type. He attempts sperm banking but insufficient sperm are identified on semen analysis. He receives 3 cycles of BEP. Tumor markers normalize and his mass shrinks to 6 cm (Fig. 7). Testis U/S continues to be normal. If he has a left orchiectomy, what is the chance evidence of a prior germ cell tumor will be found in his testicle on pathological assessment?

Figure 6.

Figure 7.

It is unclear if the patient has a primary germ cell tumor of the retroperitoneum or a testis cancer that arose in the testicles and has since undergone regression at the primary site. In small series, in which there is a clinical suspicion that the tumor arose in one particular testicle based on the pattern of the retroperitoneal nodal disease and no primary can be seen on testis U/S, a simultaneous orchiectomy identifies germ cell tumor or prior evidence of germ cell tumor in >70% of the resected testicles.

○ **A 26-year-old man has a right orchiectomy for a NSGCT. Metastatic workup reveals a 10-cm interaortocaval mass and multiple 1-cm pulmonary nodules. β-hCG is 25,000, AFP is 2000, and LDH is 6 times normal. He receives 4 cycles of BEP with shrinkage of pulmonary metastases and the retroperitoneal mass. However, the β-hCG, which had been falling at the appropriate rate, is now noted to be increasing significantly. How should this patient be treated and what is his chance of a complete response?**

The patient is showing signs of progression upon completion of chemotherapy. The optimum treatment would be carboplatin and etoposide, either in high-doses, or in combination with vinblastine or paclitaxel. Such regimens have reported long-term survival rates of up to 70%.

○ **A 37-year-old male comes for routine follow-up 7 years following treatment of a stage IB NSGCT. His treatment consisted of an orchiectomy and BEP. The patient is asymptomatic. Lab results are notable for an AFP of 376 and β-hCG of <2. A CT of the abdomen is shown (Fig. 8). Chest CT is normal. How should this recurrence be managed?**

Figure 8.

The patient has a late recurrence (ie, greater than 2 years following primary treatment) of testis cancer. The pathology of late recurrence is most commonly a yolk sack tumor that is resistant to chemotherapy. The primary therapy of late recurrence is, if feasible surgical resection.

○ **Sertoli cell tumor of the testis in prepubertal boys is associated with what genetic disorder?**

Peutz–Jeghers syndrome.

○ **A 50-year-old man with a 3-year history of gynecomastia discovers a left testicular mass. A radical orchiectomy is performed. On bisecting the testicle, a 2-cm homogeneous brown tumor is seen in the upper pole. Pathology shows closely packed uniform cells with eosinophilic cytoplasm and Reinke crystals. What is the diagnosis and malignant potential of this tumor?**

The patient has a Leydig cell tumor. Approximately 10% of Leydig cell tumors are malignant. The malignant potential of these tumors is difficult to predict based on histology. However, in the absence of a histological suspicion of malignancy (no hemorrhage, uniform cells, few mitoses), observation is the preferred form of management.

○ **A 30-year-old man is referred to you by his family physician for a 1.5-cm epididymal mass. The patient has no complaints and did not notice anything unusual himself. Physical examination reveals a 1.5-cm mass in the epididymis that does not transilluminate. Ultrasound confirms a 1.5-cm homogeneous, solid, intraepididymal mass. What are the differential diagnoses and which is most likely?**

The most likely diagnosis is an adenomatoid tumor since it is the most common solid epididymal tumor. The differential diagnoses are para-testicular sarcoma, cystadenoma, atypical spermatocele, or epididymal cyst. The mass is probably growing very slowly as the patient has not noticed a change. Therefore, it is likely a benign process and transscrotal excision is appropriate. If there is any suspicion of malignancy, an inguinal exploration is indicated.

○ **A 40-year-old man notices a mass in his right groin that has doubled in size in the last 2 months. He otherwise feels well. A radical orchiectomy is performed. Final pathology demonstrates a rhabdomyosarcoma. What are the major determinants of prognosis in patients with sarcomas?**

The main prognostic determinants of sarcomas are tumor grade, tumor size (greater or less than 5 cm), depth of invasion, surgical margin status, and the presence of metastases. Complete surgical resection with wide margins holds the best prospect for cure.

○ **What are epidermoid cysts of the testicle?**

Testicular epidermoid cysts are round, hard, well-circumscribed, and encapsulated intratesticular masses. They account for about 1% of all testicular tumors. They have a claylike, yellow center on cut section and are thought to be a monolayer form of teratoma. They are generally considered to be benign, although they may be associated with germ cell elements. Treatment is usually by radical orchiectomy because of the germ cell elements that may be present. However, local excision is possible and appropriate in select cases.

○ **How is teratoma in children different from teratoma in adults?**

In the pediatric age group, teratoma is almost always benign.

○ **What are the most common mesenchymal tumors of the testis?**

Fibromas, angiomas, leiomyomas, and neurofibromas. They are important mainly because they need to be distinguished from germ cell tumors.

○ **Gonadoblastoma is a mixed germ cell, sex cord, and stromal cell tumor. It is predominantly found in which patient population?**

Gonadoblastomas occur almost exclusively in patients with dysgenic gonads and intersex syndromes.

○ **In a patient diagnosed with gonadoblastoma, some authors have suggested bilateral orchiectomy. What is the basis for that suggestion?**

Generally gonadoblastomas should be treated as germ cell tumors as about 50% are found to have dysgerminoma and another 8% of nonseminomatous tumors. As up to one-third of patients are found to have bilateral tumors, bilateral orchiectomy has been advised.

Penile Cancer

Michael B. Williams, MD, MS
and John W. Davis, MD

○ **True/False: Bowenoid papulosis of the penis is a premalignant condition with the natural history of progression to invasive disease.**

False. Bowenoid papulosis has the histologic criteria of carcinoma in situ, but usually has a benign course. Malignant transformation occurs only in 2.6%.

○ **What causes Bowenoid papulosis?**

It is caused by human papilloma virus, most often type 16.

○ **What is the best palliative treatment for a patient with acquired immunodeficiency syndrome (AIDS) and Kaposi sarcoma (KS) of the glans penis causing obstruction?**

Radiation therapy.

○ **Which forms of KS are associated with AIDS?**

Classic KS, immunosuppressive treatment-related KS, African KS, and epidemic KS.

○ **True/False: Verrucous carcinoma is a well-differentiated variant of squamous cell carcinoma (SCC) with similar metastatic potential.**

False. Verrucous carcinoma of the penis invades locally and can cause local tissue destruction; metastasis does not occur unless invasive SCC coexists.

○ **True/False: Both verrucous carcinoma and condyloma acuminatum typically remain superficial lesions.**

False. Verrucous carcinoma can invade locally causing unrestrained local growth.

○ **Which of the following local treatments is not recommended for verrucous carcinoma and which is the standard recommended therapy: partial or total penectomy, Mohs surgery, radiation therapy, topical podophyllin, 5-fluorouracil, or Nd:YAG laser?**

Radiation therapy has been associated with malignant degeneration and is ineffective. Partial or total penectomy is standard therapy.

○ **What differentiates condyloma acuminata from Buschke–Lowenstein tumors?**

Condyloma never invades adjacent normal tissues and always remains superficial. Buschke–Lowenstein tumors displace and invade adjacent tissues destroying them. Additionally, despite the local invasion, Buschke–Lowenstein tumors do not metastasize.

○ **What other terms are used for penile carcinoma in situ?**

Penile carcinoma in situ is also known as erythroplasia of Queyrat when it involves the glans penis or prepuce, and Bowen disease if it involves the penile shaft.

○ **A 55-year-old uncircumcised male presents with a 0.5-cm reddish, well-defined, barely raised plaque on the glans. The biopsy diagnosis is erythroplasia of Queyrat (CIS). What is the chance of progression to invasive disease and how is the lesion best managed?**

The relative risks of progression to an invasive lesion and development of metastases is 10% and 2%, respectively. Superficial premalignant lesions may be treated with local excision, topical 5-fluorouracil, or laser therapy. Sexual partners should be counseled and examined for CIS.

○ **For the lesion described in the previous question, what is the clinical differential diagnosis?**

Chronic circumscribed balanitis, inflammatory process, drug eruption, psoriasis, and lichen planus, among others.

○ **True/False: The diagnosis of erythroplasia of Queyrat requires a biopsy.**

True.

○ **What is the importance in differentiating Bowenoid papulosis from Bowen disease in the clinical setting?**

Bowenoid papulosis is a dysplastic lesion of the epithelium involving the penile shaft in younger men. The histopathologic appearance may be similar to other forms of CIS. The lesions are light brown to gray papules that may coalesce to form plaques. These lesions generally have an indolent course, respond well to excision or podophyllin, may spontaneously regress, and do not usually progress to invasive cancer. Bowenoid papulosis is similar to multifocal vulvovaginal dysplasia in young women.

○ **How does the incidence of SCC of the penis differ in the United States and Europe versus African and South American countries?**

In the United States and Europe, SCC of the penis accounts for only 0.4% to 0.6% of all male malignancies. In some African and South American countries, SCC accounts for up to 10% of all diagnosed malignancies in men.

○ **In the United States, what is the ethnic population with the highest age-adjusted incidence of penile cancer per million?**

Hispanics are the highest at nearly 7 patients per million. This is followed by blacks, whites, American Indians, and Asian Pacific islanders.

○ **What is the breakdown of likely tumor subtype between younger patients (~50) and older patients (~70)?**

Younger patients have basaloid and warty carcinomas whereas older patients have verrucous and pseudohyperplastic carcinomas.

○ **Which age range has the highest incidence of penile cancer?**

If broken down by age, males older than 85 years of age have the highest incidence.

○ **Over the past 3 decades, is the incidence of penile carcinoma in the United States increasing, decreasing, or remaining constant?**

Based on SEER data, penile carcinoma rates are decreasing.

○ **Describe the relationship between penile cancer and circumcision.**

Chronic exposure to smegma in the prepubertal period is thought to contribute to the development of penile cancer. Phimosis may accentuate this effect, as it is a finding in up to 50% of cases of penile cancer. Neonatal circumcision virtually eliminates the risk of penile cancer, whereas adolescent or adult circumcision has no protective effect.

○ **True/False: In populations that practice good hygiene but are uncircumcised, the incidence of penile carcinoma is similar to that of circumcised populations.**

True.

○ **Name the risk factors for penile carcinoma.**

Sexually transmitted human papilloma virus (HPV), phimosis (smegma accumulation), lack of childhood circumcision, and smoking have been associated.

○ **What is human papilloma virus (HPV)? Approximately how many HPV subtypes are known and which are well known to be benign versus malignant?**

HPV is a double-stranded, supercoiled DNA virus with more than 65 subtypes identified. "Low risk" strands HPV-6 and HPV-11 are associated with benign condylomata of the anogenital area. "High-risk" types such as HPV-16, -18, -31, -33, -35, and -39 are associated with premalignant lesions of the cervix and penis.

○ **HPV has been identified in what percentage of penile cancers?**

HPV has been demonstrated in 50% of penile SCC cases.

○ **True/False: Penile carcinoma secondary to HPV infection causes p53 and retinoblastoma (Rb) dysregulation.**

True. Cells that are infected with high-risk HPV (ie, 16, 18, 31, 33, 35, and 39) continue to make viral genes known as E6 and E7. These genes have products that act to disrupt apoptotic pathways and proliferation pathways via Rb and p53 tumor suppressors.

○ **How are penile cancer and cervical cancer related?**

Both cancers have HPV as a potential etiology. In some studies, female sexual partners of men with SCC of the penis have a 3-fold increased risk of invasive cervical carcinoma. However, there are key differences as cervical carcinoma is much more common and affects younger women whereas penile cancer is rare and affects older men.

○   **Describe the lymphatic spread of penile cancer.**

Lymphatics from the glans and shaft drain to the superficial inguinal, deep inguinal, and pelvic lymph nodes. Drainage is bilateral, and crossover may occur.

○   **What is the natural history of untreated penile cancer?**

Untreated penile cancer progresses to death in the majority of patients within 2 years. Local and regional nodal enlargement and complications predominate over distant metastases to lung, liver, bone, or brain. Death may occur by erosion into the femoral vessels with subsequent hemorrhage. Spontaneous remission has not been reported.

○   **List the sites of the primary tumor in penile cancer in order of frequency.**

Glans (48%), prepuce (21%), glans and prepuce (9%), coronal sulcus (6%), and shaft (<2%).

○   **What types of invasive penile carcinomas are associated with lichen sclerosus?**

Verrucous, papillary, and pseudohyperplastic carcinomas.

○   **What precautions should be taken to prevent dissemination of tumor during biopsy of a penile lesion?**

None. Tumor dissemination due to a biopsy has not been reported.

○   **True/False: The most important factors in determining prognosis in penile cancer are stage and presence of lymph node metastasis.**

True. Of the 2, the presence or absence of nodal metastases is the strongest predictive factor for survival. Additionally, the histologic characteristics of the primary tumor provide further valuable prognostic information.

○   **How does the appearance of well-differentiated (grade 1) SCC differ from poorly differentiated (grade 3)?**

Grade 1 SCC shows downward finger-like projections of atypical squamous cells from the papillomatous epidermis. Keratin pearls are present, and there is limited cellular atypia and mitotic figures. Grade 3 SCC shows little to no keratin pearls and marked cellular nuclear pleomorphism, mitoses, necrosis, and deep invasion.

○   **Compare the 5-year survival for the following groups of patients with SCC of the penis: all patients, negative nodes, positive inguinal nodes, and positive pelvic nodes.**

All patients = 50%, negative lymph nodes = 66%, positive inguinal nodes = 27%, positive pelvic lymph nodes = rare.

○   **What are the most important pathological predictors of nodal spread, and thus, cancer-specific mortality?**

Perineural invasion, lymphovascular invasion, and histologic grade.

○ **What radiologic studies have proven useful in staging penile cancer?**

Lymphangiography has been replaced by CT and MRI due to their technical ease and ability to image the hypogastric and presacral nodes. Ultrasound and MRI can stage the depth of invasion of the primary lesion. Ultrasound and CT scan image the inguinal nodal regions, where physical examination is hindered by obesity or prior surgery. However, do not forget that lymph nodes can undergo reactive changes yielding higher false-positive rates with these modalities.

○ **What is the utility for PET in the assessment of patients with penile cancer?**

Several small studies have demonstrated that F^{18}-FDG uptake is found in lymph nodes with metastatic deposits of SCCs.

○ **Describe the utilization of lymphotropic nanoparticle-enhanced MRI with Ferumoxtran-10 in the evaluation of lymph nodes.**

This new method of MRI utilizes iron particle injection with subsequent imaging 24 hours later. The goal is to limit the number of individuals that undergo lymph node dissection that do not require such a treatment.

In lymph nodes that are metastatic, an area of hypointensity will be seen, whereas normal lymph nodes take up the iron particle. One case series demonstrated a negative predictive value of 100% with high sensitivities. Further research is ongoing and appears promising.

○ **Assessment of the primary tumor is important in deciding whether to perform inguinal lymph node dissections. List the TNM staging system for penile cancer (UICC, 7th edition, 2010).**

- *Primary tumor:*

  Tx = Primary tumor not assessed.

  T0 = No evidence of primary tumor.

  Tis = Carcinoma in situ.

  Ta = Noninvasive verrucous carcinoma.

  T1a = Tumor invades subepithelial connective tissue without lymphovascular invasion (LVI) and not poorly differentiated.

  T1b = Tumor invades subepithelial connective tissue with LVI or is poorly differentiated.

  T2 = Tumor invades corpus spongiosum or cavernosum.

  T3 = Tumor invades urethra or prostate.

  T4 = Tumor invades other adjacent structures.

- *Lymph nodes:*

  Nx = Regional nodes cannot be assessed by palpation or imaging.

  N0 = No palpable or visibly enlarged inguinal lymph nodes.

  pN0 = No regional lymph node metastasis.

  N1 = Palpable and mobile and unilateral inguinal lymph node.

  pN1 = Metastasis in a single inguinal lymph node.

  N2 = Palpable and mobile multiple or bilateral inguinal lymph nodes.

  pN2 = Metastasis in multiple or bilateral inguinal lymph nodes.

  N3 = Palpable fixed inguinal nodal mass or pelvic lymphadenopathy unilateral or bilateral.

  pN3 = Extranodal extension of lymph node metastasis or pelvic lymph node unilateral or bilateral.

- *Distant metastases:*

  MX = Distant metastasis not assessed.

  M0 = No distant metastases.

  M1 = Distant metastases (lymph node metastasis outside the true pelvis, visceral or bone sites).

  Here invasive = destructive; broad pushing borders causing penetration is ok.

○ **What is the Staging based off of the above TNM in the UICC 7th edition. What is the Jackson staging system and why should it not be utilized currently?**

- Stage 0 = Tis-Ta N0M0.
- Stage I = T1aN0M0.
- Stage II = T1b-3N0M0.
- Stage IIIa = T1-3N1M0.
- Stage IIIb = T1-3N2M0
- Stage IV = T4anyNM0 or AnyTN3M0 or AnyTAnyNM1.

The Jackson system has the disadvantage of conveying less information about the tumor and makes interpretation of studies using different staging systems difficult.

○ **What is the gold standard treatment for the primary tumor in penile cancer?**

The gold standard is resection of the primary tumor with a 2-cm margin to ensure complete resection of microscopic finger-like projections of tumor that may extend from the grossly evident tumor. This goal can be accomplished with a partial penectomy if the residual stump is serviceable for upright voiding and/or sexual function. Otherwise, total penectomy is indicated.

○ **What surgical margin is required when performing tumor excision for localized penile cancer?**

Historically, teaching has emphasized a 2-cm margin at the time of excision. However, this has recently come into question with new studies demonstrating a more conservative approach to radical disfiguring surgery. Although a definitive margin has not yet been established, it appears a 1-cm margin with close oncologic follow-up can be implemented safely in localized penile cancer (ie, Tis, Ta, and T1) with low grades (1-2). Local recurrence rates have been found to be between 0% and 8%.

○ **When is circumcision appropriate treatment for penile cancer and what are the risks/benefits?**

Circumcision is less disfiguring than partial penectomy and may be appropriate for small lesions of the prepuce. However recurrence rates are as high as 50%. Close patient follow-up and low threshold for biopsy and additional surgery is necessary for this approach to the primary tumor.

○ **When should topical agents be utilized for the treatment of penile cancer? What agents are used, how long is the treatment period and what is the most common side effect?**

In patients not able to undergo primary surgery, topical therapies are indicated in the treatment of CIS found on penile shaft skin or on the glans penis.

The most commonly used agents are 5-flurouracil and 5% imiquimod cream on either daily or every other day regimens for up to 6 weeks. The primary side effect is skin irritation and this leads to poor compliance.

○ **What is the best management for a primary tumor located on the proximal penile shaft?**

In rare circumstances when the tumor invades only the epidermis, excision of skin only is appropriate. In cases of a deeply invasive tumor of the shaft where a 2-cm margin is not possible, or if the residual stump would not allow upright voiding, then total penectomy with perineal urethrostomy is the best management.

○ **A 70-year-old male underwent a partial penectomy 1 year ago for a T1 N0M0 grade I SCC of the glans penis. He presents with increasing lower urinary tract symptoms. What operative complications apply to this scenario?**

Stricture of the neomeatus is a common complication of partial penectomy and can be avoided by widely spatulating the urethra, performing a tension-free anastomosis, and adequate vascularization of the urethral stump. Strictures are initially managed by dilation or meatotomy. Recurrent local disease must be ruled out.

○ **What are the risks and benefits of Mohs micrographic surgery (MMS) for penile cancer?**

MMS for small, distal lesions in the hands of an experienced Mohs surgeon can provide cure rates equivalent to partial penectomy with a decrease in the amount of tissue that is sacrificed. MMS is less successful for larger (>3 cm) lesions because large resections can create defects in the glans that are difficult to reconstruct. Excessive resections can create significant glans defects and meatal stenosis that is difficult to reconstruct.

○ **What are the risks and benefits of radiation therapy for penile cancer?**

Many patients undergoing radiation therapy (external beam or brachytherapy) refused surgery. Organ preservation is accomplished with cancer control rates for minimally invasive T1-2 lesions that are comparable to conventional surgery. Radiation therapy for larger lesions is less successful and carries higher morbidity. Potential complications include urethral fistula, stricture, penile necrosis requiring penectomy, lengthy treatment schedule, and difficulty distinguishing postirradiation scar from tumor recurrence.

○ **What are the indications for lasers in penile cancer?**

Both CO_2 and Nd:YAG lasers are effective in treating CIS. Select patients with low-stage invasive SCC can be treated as long as they are followed carefully for local recurrence.

○ **What is the major drawback to laser surgery for small SCCs of the penis?**

No histologic specimen to assess stage and grade.

○ **A 40-year-old healthy man presents with a large fungating lesion of the glans penis with erosion into the penile shaft and extensive fungating bilateral inguinal lymphadenopathy. The patient delayed seeing a doctor for a considerable amount of time but now requests maximal therapy. Describe the treatment options.**

In such extreme cases, the anatomy will dictate treatment possibilities. Fixed lymph nodes may require neoadjuvant chemotherapy followed by treatment of the primary lesion and lymphadenectomy (LND). Aggressive approaches for these extreme cases include total emasculation, scrotectomy, resection of the lower abdominal wall and pubic symphysis, and hemipelvectomy.

○ **What is the most common reconstructive option for a patient following partial or total penectomy?**

Free flap reconstruction of the penis with a ulnar forearm flap is the procedure of choice at many centers. Subsequently, a prosthesis can be placed for erectile function.

○ **What is the efficacy of inguinal LND in terms of cure and palliation?**

Inguinal LND is curative in approximately 80% of cases and palliates possible complications of inguinal disease such as ulceration, infection, and vascular compromise.

○ **At the time of diagnosis of an invasive penile cancer, a patient has palpable inguinal lymph nodes. Following 4 to 6 weeks of oral antibiotics therapy, the lymphadenopathy persists. What is the likelihood that the lymph nodes are pathologic?**

Initially: 50%; after 4 to 6 weeks of antibiotics: 70% to 85%.

○ **What are the disadvantages of routine inguinal LND?**

Early complications include phlebitis, pulmonary embolism, wound infection, and flap necrosis. Long-term complications include severe lymphedema from the scrotum to the lower extremities.

○ **Define the terms "early" or "immediate" inguinal LND, and "delayed" LND as they relate to the management of cancer of the penis.**

Early/immediate LND is carried out following 4 to 6 weeks of antibiotic therapy even though the inguinal nodes are not palpably abnormal. Delayed LND is performed when an abnormal inguinal node examination demonstrates lymphadenopathy sometime after penectomy is performed.

○ **True/False: Penectomy and lymphadenectomy should be performed concurrently to maximize staging information.**

False. Mortality from sepsis can occur when a combined procedure is performed. Additionally, the histology of the nodes is often difficult to assess in the presence of severe inflammation. However, this dogma has been challenged in the recent literature. Although, not done concurrently, pathologic staging via penectomy is followed by fine needle aspiration (FNA) of clinical lymphadenopathy. If this is found to be consistent with carcinoma, then proceeding to LND is appropriate following a short course of appropriate antibiotic therapy (ie, not waiting for the full 6 week course of antibiotics to be completed).

○ **What 3 risk factors are the highest predictors of inguinal lymph node metastases?**

Grade III, lymphovascular invasion, $T \geq 2$.

○ **What is the incidence of subclinical metastasis (negative groin examinations) and what factors increase the likelihood of metastatic nodal disease?**

The reported incidence of subclinical metastasis ranges from 2% to 25% in most reports. Primary tumor stage (tumor invading the basement membrane of the penile skin) and higher tumor grade increase the likelihood of nodal disease.

○ **What is the major drawback to the sentinel node concept of penile cancer metastasis?**

Some series have shown metastatic spread to the inguinal nodes without involvement of the sentinel node. Hence sentinel node biopsy alone can miss the diagnosis of inguinal metastasis.

○ **What is the key advantage of prophylactic groin dissections of clinically negative nodes versus delayed dissection if they become palpable?**

Recent studies have pooled results and indicate a potential survival advantage for patients with positive inguinal nodes who underwent prophylactic versus delayed groin dissection. The survival benefit of prophylactic LND, if the nodes are positive, must be weighed against the risk of morbidity in the 75% of patients who will have negative dissections.

○ **What are the key elements of the modified inguinal lymph node dissection?**

Shorter skin incision, skin flaps elevated deep to Scarpa fascia, narrower field of dissection—exclude dissection lateral to the femoral artery and caudal to the fossa ovalis, preservation of the saphenous vein, and elimination of sartorius muscle transposition (unless subsequent deep nodes dissected).

○ **When and why is sartorius muscle transposition performed?**

When standard inguinal LND is performed, the deep nodes and fascia lata over the femoral vessels are resected. In the event of erosion from wound infection or major flap necrosis, a sartorius muscle transposition protects the femoral vessels.

○ **What are the boundaries of the femoral (Scarpa) triangle?**

Base—inguinal ligament; laterally—sartorius muscle, medially—adductor longus muscle; floor—(lateral to medial) the iliacus, psoas major, pectineus, and adductor brevis muscles; roof—fascia lata with small opening (fossa ovalis) through which the greater saphenous vein enters the underlying femoral vein.

○ **What 3 small branches of the femoral artery and vein are usually encountered in inguinal lymph node dissection?**

Circumflex iliac, superficial epigastric, and superficial external pudendal.

○ **A 60-year-old male presents with unilateral inguinal lymphadenopathy. What surgical groin dissection should be performed and why?**

Patients with unilateral groin adenopathy should undergo bilateral inguinal lymph node dissection. This is due to the known crossover of lymphatics at the base of the penis with a reported 60% rate of bilateral disease.

○ **Name the 6 subtypes of SCC of the penis. Which are the most aggressive?**

They are as follows: usual type, papillary, basaloid, warty, verrucous, and sarcomatoid. The basaloid and sarcomatoid variants are the most aggressive with the verrucous being the least. Additionally, the basaloid variant has a strong association with HPV expression (approximately 80%).

○ **A 65-year-old male with SCC of the penis s/p penectomy has bulky eroded groin metastases that would necessitate excision of a large portion of overlying skin. What are treatment approaches?**

Palliative or neoadjuvant chemotherapy/radiation therapy may be given for inoperable nodes. Lymph node dissection is preferred and with the assistance of a reconstructive surgeon to rotate a myocutaneous skin flap such as the tensor fascia lata, gracilis, or rectus abdominis flap, the large defect can be covered.

○ **A 60-year-old male presents with a biopsy-proven SCC of the glans penis and is found to have T1 grade I SCC at partial penectomy. Clinical examination reveals palpable lymphadenopathy on the right and a negative left groin. Describe the management of the lymph nodes.**

Following treatment of the primary tumor, 4 to 6 weeks of oral antibiotics should be administered. If the unilateral lymphadenopathy resolves, then the patient can be carefully followed for recurrence. If the unilateral adenopathy does not resolve, then bilateral superficial inguinal LND should be performed as anatomic crossover of penile lymphatics is well established. If either superficial dissection is positive for malignancy, then a deep inguinal dissection is performed. If any deep dissection is positive, then complete ilioinguinal/pelvic lymph node dissections may be indicated.

○ **How does pelvic LND for penile cancer differ from prostate and bladder cancer?**

Pelvic LND for penile cancer should extend more distally removing all lymph nodes tissue between the deep inguinal node group and the iliac group.

○ **A patient with clinically negative inguinal nodes undergoes resection of a TI grade III penile tumor. During follow-up, he develops unilateral inguinal adenopathy. What is the appropriate management?**

In this setting, unilateral dissection of the palpable lymph nodes is appropriate. The elapsed time has increased the likelihood that the clinically negative side is free of metastasis.

○ **Describe the optimal strategy for surveillance of low stage SCC of the penis and clinically negative inguinal nodes.**

Most inguinal metastases occur within 2 to 3 years of the diagnosis of the primary tumor. Patients must be closely examined during these 2 to 3 years at 2- to 3-month intervals, as well as taught self-examination. Follow-up should continue indefinitely.

○ **A 60-year-old male undergoes partial penectomy for a T2 grade II glanular SCC (corporeal tissue invasion); inguinal nodes are nonpalpable. Appropriate management of the lymph nodes includes:**

T2-3, N0M0 patients have a higher incidence of metastases and should undergo 6 weeks of oral antibiotics followed by bilateral inguinal lymph node dissection even if the nodes remain negative. The extent of dissection varies, but it is common to start with a superficial dissection and only perform a deep dissection if positive nodes are encountered; "skip" metastases are rare.

○ **What role does chemotherapy have in penile cancer?**

Historically, multiagent regimens have yielded partial responses of short duration in most patients (approximately 65%) with advanced disease. Complete responses unfortunately were uncommon (approximately 10%-15%). Various regimens have been utilized to include methotrexate, bleomycin, cisplatin, vinblastine, and ifosfamide. All clinical trials utilize multimodal consolidative approaches with regard to chemotherapy plus either surgery or radiotherapy due to shortened overall responses.

Recently, Pagliaro et al. published a neoadjuvant strategy regimen in patients with advanced disease but not metastatic. The chemotherapy regimen was cisplatin, ifosfamide, and paclitaxel. 50% of patients had a response to chemotherapy and of those that had a response and underwent surgery, 30% were alive at 34-months. This represents a substantial improvement in previous regimens and should be employed in patients with N2 or N3 disease that are not metastatic.

○ **What percentage of patients with metastatic penile cancer exhibit hypercalcemia and what is the mechanism?**

Approximately 20%. The cause is unknown, but systemic release of paraneoplastic hormonal substances is suspected.

○ **How does the incidence of SCC compare with other types of penile cancer?**

SCC accounts for more than 95% of penile cancers. The remaining cancers are rare and include sarcomas, melanomas, basal cell carcinomas, and metastases.

○ **How does malignant melanoma of the penis differ from SCC?**

Malignant melanoma of the penis is rare with <100 cases reported. The glans and prepuce are most common sites. The Breslow thickness scale provides important prognostic information. Most cases of penile melanoma present at an advanced stage with early metastases and poor survival. Hematogenous metastases are more common than lymphatic spread.

○ **How does sarcoma of the penis differ from SCC?**

Sarcomas of the penis are usually locally invasive, low grade, and respond well to local excision. Local recurrence is characteristic, but metastases are rare.

○ **Where do penile metastatic lesions usually originate?**

While rare, metastases to the penis may come from the bladder, prostate, and rectum. The primary disease is usually very advanced when the penis is involved and survival is <1 year.

○ **What is the most common presenting sign of involvement of the penis with metastatic tumor?**

Priapism.

○ **For advanced penile cancer, which chemotherapy agents have shown the most activity?**

Bleomycin, cisplatin, and methotrexate have demonstrated the most activity. Although, recently, the neoadjuvant strategy of cisplatin, ifosfamide, and paclitaxel (TIP) has demonstrated a 50% response rate with 30% being alive at 34 months.

○ **What percentage of patients who ultimately develop SCC of the penis had a preexisting premalignant penile lesion?**

Approximately 30% to 40%.

○ **What is a cutaneous horn and how should it be treated?**

It's a hyperkeratotic growth on the penis that is usually related to a preexisting lesion such as a wart, scratch, or laceration. Due to its malignant potential (up to 30% can have an underlying malignancy associated), local excision is recommended as well as close surveillance postoperatively.

Pediatric Oncology

Miriam Harel, MD and
Fernando A. Ferrer, MD, FAAP, FACS

○ **What is the most common renal tumor of infancy, and which renal tumor is most common during childhood?**

Congenital mesoblastic nephroma is the most common tumor in infants, while Wilms is the most common tumor in children. After the age of 10, renal tumors in children are just as likely to represent a Wilms tumor or a pediatric renal cell carcinoma.

○ **What is the most common extracranial solid tumor of childhood?**

Neuroblastoma is the most common extracranial solid tumor in children. It accounts for 6% to 10% of all childhood malignancies.

○ **The Wilms tumor suppressor gene, WT-1, is located on which chromosome?**

The Wilms tumor suppressor gene (WT-1) is located on the distal portion of the short arm of chromosome 11 in the 11p13 location. A second putative Wilms tumor gene has been found at 11p15 (WT-2). Abnormalities at this location are associated with overgrowth syndrome and Beckwith–Weidemann syndrome.

○ **What congenital anomalies are associated with Wilms tumor, and what chromosomal abnormalities are associated with these anomalies?**

Congenital anomalies are seen in approximately 15% of patients with Wilms tumor. These include the following:
- *WT-1:*
  Aniridia.
  WAGR syndrome (**W**ilms, **A**niridia, **G**enitourinary anomalies, and **R**etardation)—tumor risk 30%.
- *Hemihypertrophy:*
  Denys–Drash syndrome (Wilms, pseudohermaphroditism, glomerulopathy, retardation)—tumor risk 90%.
- *WT-2:*
  Beckwith–Wiedemann syndrome (macroglossia, gigantism, and organomegaly)—tumor risk 5%.
- *Xq26:*
  Simpson–Golabi–Behmel syndrome (organomegaly, renal dysplasia, polydactyly, cardiac defects)—tumor risk 7.5%.

○ **What is the significance of loss of heterozygosity (LOH) at sites 16q and 1p in Wilms tumor?**

LOH at 16q (seen in 20% of all tumors) and 1p (seen in 10% of all tumors) have been identified as biomarkers of worse outcome. When occurring together, they represent an indication for more aggressive therapy.

○ **The histologic picture of Wilms tumor is described as "triphasic." What are these 3 components?**

The classic microscopic appearance of Wilms tumor includes blastemal, epithelial, and stromal components.

○ **What is the significance of nephrogenic rests?**

More than one third of kidneys resected for Wilms tumor contain precursor lesions, known as nephrogenic rests. Nephrogenic rests can be separated into 2 distinct categories: perilobar nephrogenic rests and intralobar nephrogenic rests. These 2 types of rests are distinguished by their location within the renal lobe. Perilobar nephrogenic rests are found only in the lobar periphery, which is elaborated late in embryogenesis, while intralobar nephrogenic rests are found anywhere within the lobe, as well as the renal sinus and the wall of the pelvicalyceal system.

○ **What is the significance of multiple nephrogenic rests within a single kidney?**

Multiple rests in one kidney usually implies that nephrogenic rests are present in the other kidney.

○ **What is the significance of nephrogenic rests in Wilms tumor patients who are less than 12 months old?**

Children less than 12 months of age who are diagnosed with Wilms tumor and also have rests, particularly perilobar nephrogenic rests, have a markedly increased risk of developing contralateral disease and require frequent and regular surveillance for several years. Surveillance is also recommended for those diagnosed after 12 months of age who have nephrogenic rests.

○ **What are the current recommendations regarding screening for Wilms tumor?**

Screening with serial renal ultrasonography has been recommended in children at high risk for development of Wilms tumor, including those with WAGR syndrome, hemihypertrophy, Denys–Drash syndrome, or Beckwith–Wiedemann syndrome. Review of most studies suggests that 3 to 4 months is the appropriate screening interval. Tumors detected by screening will generally be lower stage. Screening of the contralateral kidney following nephrectomy for unilateral Wilms tumor is also recommended. CT or MRI should be performed if ultrasonography demonstrates a suspicious lesion.

○ **How should regional lymph nodes be addressed during surgery for Wilms tumor?**

Selective sampling of lymph nodes is an essential component of local tumor staging and is required by children's oncology group (COG) guidelines. Formal retroperitoneal lymph node dissection (RPLND) is not recommended. Extensive lymph node dissection, particularly above the renal hilum, can result in chylous ascites.

○ **A patient with Wilms tumor undergoes nephrectomy. The tumor penetrates the surface of the capsule. At the time of nephrectomy, there is tumor spillage, which is confined to the flank. Lymph nodes are negative. Contralateral kidney is negative. Chest x-ray is negative. What stage is this tumor?**

This is a stage III Wilms tumor. The staging system is as follows:

Stage I: Tumor limited to kidney, completely resected. The renal capsule is intact. The tumor was not ruptured or biopsied prior to removal. The vessels of the renal sinus are not involved. There is no evidence of tumor at or beyond the margins of resection.

Note: For a tumor to qualify for certain therapeutic protocols as stage I, regional lymph nodes must be examined microscopically.

Stage II: The tumor is completely resected, and there is no evidence of tumor at or beyond the margins of resection. The tumor extends beyond the kidney, as is evidenced by any one of the following criteria:

* There is regional extension of the tumor (ie, penetration of the renal capsule, or extensive invasion of the soft tissue of the renal sinus, as discussed below).
* Blood vessels within the nephrectomy specimen outside the renal parenchyma, including those of the renal sinus, contain tumor.

Note: Tumor spillage confined to the flank, including biopsy of the tumor, is no longer included in stage II and is now included in stage III.

Stage III: Residual nonhematogenous tumor present following surgery and confined to abdomen. Any one of the following may occur:

* Lymph nodes within the abdomen or pelvis are involved by tumor. (Lymph node involvement in the thorax or other extra-abdominal sites is a criterion for stage IV.)
* The tumor has penetrated through the peritoneal surface.
* Tumor implants are found on the peritoneal surface.
* Gross or microscopic tumor remains postoperatively (eg, tumor cells are found at the margin of surgical resection on microscopic examination).
* The tumor is not completely resectable because of local infiltration into vital structures.
* Tumor spillage occurring either before or during surgery.
* The tumor was biopsied (whether tru-cut, open, or fine needle aspiration) before removal.
* Tumor is removed in greater than one piece (eg, tumor cells are found in a separately excised adrenal gland; a tumor thrombus within the renal vein is removed separately from the nephrectomy specimen).

Stage IV: Hematogenous metastases (lung, liver, bone, brain, etc), or lymph node metastases outside the abdomino-pelvic region are present. (The presence of tumor within the adrenal gland is not interpreted as metastasis, and staging depends on all other staging parameters present.)

Stage V: Bilateral renal involvement by tumor is present at diagnosis. An attempt should be made to stage each side according to the above criteria on the basis of the extent of disease.

○ **What hematologic abnormality has been associated with patients with Wilms tumor?**

Acquired von Willebrand disease has been found in 8% of newly diagnosed Wilms tumor patients.

○ **What is the most important factor in the prognosis of patients with Wilms tumor?**

The most important aspect of Wilms tumor is the histology. Unfavorable histology (anaplasia) at any stage is associated with a worse prognosis. Anaplasia is seen in approximately 10% of all Wilms tumors. Anaplasia is defined by the presence of gigantic polyploid nuclei within the tumor sample. It is rare in the first 2 years of life, but the incidence increases to 13% in children older than 5 years old. Anaplasia is further divided into focal and diffuse forms, with diffuse anaplasia carrying a worse prognosis than focal. Anaplasia is believed to be a marker of chemoresistance.

○ **When should partial nephrectomy be considered for Wilms tumor?**

Partial nephrectomy for Wilms tumor should be considered in patients with a solitary kidney, bilateral tumors, and in those with congenital anomalies predisposing them to Wilms tumor development.

○ **How often do synchronous bilateral Wilms tumors occur, and what is the management approach?**

Synchronous bilateral Wilms tumors occur in 5% to 7% of children with Wilms tumor. Children with bilateral tumors should not undergo initial radical nephrectomy. These children should receive preoperative chemotherapy with the goal of tumor shrinkage and renal-sparing surgery. Biopsy is not needed if the radiographic picture is consistent with Wilms tumor. Tumor response is assessed after 6 weeks with CT or MRI to determine the reduction in tumor volume and feasibility of partial resection. Tumors not responding to therapy require bilateral open biopsy to determine histology. Open biopsies are recommended, because they are more accurate than percutaneous needle biopsies when assessing for anaplasia. Failure to achieve a reduction in volume is likely due to tumor differentiation. All patients should undergo definitive surgery by 12 weeks.

○ **What is the current survival in Wilms tumor?**

Data from NWTS IV indicate that for patients with favorable histology and unilateral tumors stages I to IV, 10-year overall survival ranged from 96% to 81%, respectively. For patients with anaplastic tumors stages II and III, survival was 49%, and stage IV patients with anaplasia had a survival rate of 18% at 10 years.

○ **Which patients with Wilms tumor are classified as very low risk, and how does their management differ?**

Children less than 2 years of age with Stage I favorable histology Wilms tumors <550 g are classified as very low risk. They have an excellent prognosis when treated with nephrectomy alone without adjuvant chemotherapy.

○ **An 18-month-old male presents with malaise, weight loss, and diffuse pain. An abdominal mass is palpable. What is the most likely diagnosis?**

Neuroblastoma. At the time of presentation of neuroblastoma, approximately 70% of patients have disseminated disease versus less than 10% to 15% with Wilms. Patients with Wilms tumor generally appear in good health, in contrast to patients with neuroblastoma in whom the tumor may be widespread at presentation, and systemic symptoms are often present.

○ **Congenital neuroblastoma can mimic what other tumor?**

Congenital neuroblastoma may present in a similar fashion as pheochromocytoma, with symptoms produced by secretion of catecholamines (hypertension, tachycardia).

○ **When does the peak incidence of neuroblastoma occur?**

The peak incidence of neuroblastoma is seen in the first year of life. Median age at diagnosis is 19 months. The incidence decreases progressively with age, with 36% occurring in infants, 89% in children younger than 5 years, and 98% diagnosed by 10 years of age.

○ **Neuroblastoma is a malignant neuroendocrine tumor. There is a spectrum ranging from neuroblastoma to other benign tumors. What are these other tumors, and what are their characteristics?**

Ganglioneuroma is the benign counterpart to neuroblastoma. It does not metastasize, but it can envelop adjacent structures and even extend into intervertebral foramina. Histologically, it contains mature ganglion cells in a collagen-rich background. Ganglioneuromas are most often diagnosed in older children and are usually located in the posterior mediastinum and retroperitoneum, with only a small number arising in the adrenal glands.

Ganglioneuroblastoma is intermediate between neuroblastoma and ganglioneuroma. There is a histologic spectrum between these; the outcome for ganglioneuroblastoma is varied.

○ **What is the most common site of occurrence of neuroblastomas?**

Seventy-five percent originate in the abdomen (retroperitoneum). Fifty percent arise in the adrenal, and 25% occur in the paravertebral ganglia.

○ **Is age a significant determinant of outcome in neuroblastoma?**

Yes, age less than 1 year is an indicator of better outcome when compared to older children, likely due to more favorable biology in tumors occurring at a younger age. Other predictive factors include site of origin, with better survival noted for nonadrenal primary tumors. Stage of disease is also an important predictor, as stage I and II patients have excellent survival rates.

○ **When is a bone marrow aspirate and/or biopsy indicated in the evaluation of patients with confirmed or suspected neuroblastoma?**

All patients with neuroblastoma should undergo bone marrow aspirate and/or biopsy. As many as 70% of bone marrow aspirates have been reported to be positive in patients with neuroblastoma.

○ **What molecular markers have been shown to carry prognostic significance in patients with neuroblastoma?**

- N-*myc* amplification is associated with a poor prognosis and is found in about 30% to 40% of patients with advanced disease.
- Hyperdiploid tumors (those that contain more than the normal amount of DNA material found in somatic cells) have demonstrated a favorable outcome.

○ **What are the characteristics of stage IV-S neuroblastoma?**

Stage IV-S describes patients who would otherwise be classified with stage I (tumor confined to the organ of origin) or stage II (tumor extending in continuity beyond the organ of origin, but not crossing the midline; ipsilateral regional nodes may be involved but contralateral nodes must be negative) but who have remote spread of tumor confined to one or more of the following: liver, skin, or bone marrow (without evidence of bony involvement). This stage is restricted to children with less than 10% bone marrow involvement and to patients younger than 1 year. This stage accounts for 7% to 10% of all cases of neuroblastoma. This group typically has an excellent prognosis, with survival rate in excess of 80%. Many of these tumors undergo spontaneous regression.

○ **What diagnostic tests can be useful for making the diagnosis of neuroblastoma, and what specific CT findings would help distinguish neuroblastoma from Wilms tumor?**

- Urinary metabolites of catecholamines. Vanillylmandelic acid (VMA) and homovanillic acid (HVA) are found to be elevated in 90% to 95% of patients.
- Anemia is associated with diffuse bone marrow involvement.
- The finding of intratumoral calcifications, vascular encasement, or both on preoperative computed tomography may help distinguish neuroblastoma from Wilms tumor.
- In addition to standard radiologic imaging tests, metaiodobenzylguanidine (MIBG) scintigraphy can be useful in identifying primary and metastatic lesions.

○ **What is the age distribution among patients with rhabdomyosarcoma?**

A bimodal age distribution exists, whereby peaks in incidence of rhabdomyosarcoma occur in children between the ages of 0 and 2 and then again later in adolescence.

○ **What are the histologic types of rhabdomyosarcoma, and which is most common in childhood?**

The types of rhabdomyosarcoma are embryonal, alveolar, and undifferentiated. Mixed rhabdomyosarcomas also occur, and in about 10% to 20% of cases, the tumor is so undifferentiated that it does not fit into the standard classification.

Embryonal rhabdomyosarcoma is the most common type seen in childhood, accounting for two thirds of genitourinary (GU) rhabdomyosarcomas, and 50% to 70% of all rhabdomyosarcomas in children.

Sarcoma botryoides is a descriptive term for an exophytic embryonal tumor that looks grossly like a cluster of grapes. It tends to arise in hollow organs (bladder, vagina).

Another histologic variant of the embryonal type is the "spindle cell sarcoma." It often arises in a paratesticular location and is associated with an especially favorable outcome.

The second most common form is alveolar, comprising 15% to 20% of cases. Alveolar rhabdomyosarcoma (ARMS) occurs more commonly in the trunk and extremities than in genitourinary sites. ARMS is associated with translocations t(2; 13) and t(1; 13). Translocation fusion positive tumors comprise 80% of ARMS and are more aggressive. Fusion-negative ARMS may have a clinical course similar to embryonal rhabdomyosarcoma.

The third category consists of undifferentiated tumors that also fare poorly.

○ **What are the most common GU sites?**

Prostate, bladder, paratesticular appendages, followed by the vagina and uterus.

○ **If a patient has a post-treatment biopsy indicating mature rhabdomyoblasts, should the patient have exonerative surgery to remove these elements?**

No, current evidence suggests that rhabdomyoblasts alone on biopsy after treatment does not require aggressive surgical treatment. Observation alone is needed.

○ **Besides histologic type, what are some adverse prognostic factors in patients with rhabdomyosarcoma?**

Tumors arising in the prostate, children younger than 1 year, and tumors in adults and older children generally have a poorer prognosis.

○ **A 4-year-old male has a rhabdomyosarcoma of the bladder. At the time of surgery, the tumor appears grossly removed. However, pathological analysis reveals positive margins. Lymph nodes are negative. According to the International Rhabdomyosarcoma Study (IRS) staging system, what stage disease is this?**

This patient is in group IIA. The staging system is as follows:

Intergroup Rhabdomyosarcoma Study Group Clinical Grouping Classification

Group I	Localized disease completely resected
	Confined to the organ of origin
	Contiguous involvement
Group II	
IIA	Total gross resection with evidence of regional spread
	Microscopic residual
IIB	Positive nodes but no microscopic residual
IIC	Positive nodes but microscopic residual in nodes or margins
Group III	Incomplete resection with gross residual disease
	After biopsy only
	After gross or major resection of the primary (>50%)
Group IV	Distant metastasis at diagnosis (lung, liver, bone, bone marrow, brain, and nonregional nodes)
	Positive cytology in cerebrospinal, pleural, or peritoneal fluid or implants on pleural or peritoneal surfaces are regarded as stage IV

○ **What is the primary mode of therapy for patients with stage T2a rhabdomyosarcoma of the bladder?**

Multiagent chemotherapy is the primary mode of treatment for patients with rhabdomyosarcoma. The combination of agents is often determined based on randomized trials but often includes one or more of the following: vincristine, actinomycin D, ifosfamide, etoposide, and/or cyclophosphamide. Radiation therapy may be added, and patients who do not have complete response to these treatments undergo surgical excision. The current trend, however, is toward organ preservation.

○ **A 4-year-old boy is undergoing salvage cystoprostatectomy for rhabdomyosarcoma after failing chemotherapy and XRT. What is the best urinary diversion?**

Transverse colon conduit has the lowest complication rate in this scenario. Once the patient has completed additional chemotherapy and no recurrence of malignancy has occurred for a minimum of 2 years, conversion to a continent urinary diversion can be considered.

○ **What surgical approach is required for paratesticular rhabdomyosarcoma?**

Radical inguinal orchiectomy is recommended for initial treatment of paratesticular rhabdomyosarcoma. If the tumor is removed through a prior transscrotal procedure, the risk of local recurrence and nonregional lymph node spread is increased. If cord elements remain after a transscrotal procedure, an inguinal exploration with removal of the remaining spermatic cord and a partial hemiscrotectomy, including the prior scrotal incision, is performed.

○ **What is the role of RPLND in the management of paratesticular rhabdomyosarcoma?**

Extension to retroperitoneal lymph nodes occurs in up to 20% of patients with paratesticular rhabdomyosarcoma. An imaging evaluation is performed at diagnosis to detect or exclude metastasis. CT is most frequently used to evaluate the retroperitoneum to identify nodal metastases. When enlarged nodes are found on CT, 65% to 94% are confirmed as positive by pathology. The converse is not always true, with studies showing a 14% false-negative rate of CT. The current COG protocols recommend that children 10 years of age and older should undergo ipsilateral RPLND as part of their routine staging prior to chemotherapy. Patients with positive lymph nodes require intensified chemotherapy as well as nodal irradiation.

○ **What is the most common testicular tumor in a prepubertal boy?**

A reporting bias was often present in earlier studies that suggested that yolk sac tumors were the most common tumors in prepubertal males. More recent studies demonstrate that teratoma is the most common testicular tumor in this group. However, yolk sac tumor is the most common malignant testicular tumor in prepubertal males.

○ **What are the histologic hallmarks of yolk sac tumors?**

The characteristic histologic finding in yolk sac tumors is Schiller–Duval bodies. Eosinophilic cytoplasmic inclusions are common, and specialized staining techniques demonstrate the presence of α-fetoprotein (AFP).

○ **What is the recommended treatment for testicular yolk sac tumor?**

The initial treatment for yolk sac tumor is radical inguinal orchiectomy. This treatment is curative in most children. The most common site of distant metastases is the lung, and metastasis to the retroperitoneal lymph nodes occurs in 4% to 6% of children. More than 90% of prepubertal children present with stage I disease. Routine RPLND and/or adjuvant chemotherapy are not indicated.

○ **A 1-month-old boy undergoes left radical orchiectomy for a yolk sac tumor. Chest and abdominal CT scans are normal. Preoperative AFP is 2600 ng/dL, and postoperative levels at 1 and 2 months are 330 and 90 ng/dL (normal <10 ng/dL). What is the next step?**

Repeat AFP in 1 month. AFP is elevated (>10 ng/mL) in 92% of cases of yolk sac tumor. All AFP-positive tumors are considered to contain yolk sac elements. AFP has a half-life of approximately 5 days, and degradation curves are followed after orchiectomy to assess for residual or recurrent disease. It is important to note that AFP levels may be elevated in infant boys and do not always represent the presence of a malignant tumor or persistent disease after orchiectomy for yolk sac tumor. Normal adult reference laboratory values for AFP cannot be used in young children, because AFP synthesis continues after birth. Normal adult levels (<10 mg/mL) are not reached until 8 months of age. However, it should be noted that in children less than 1 year of age, the median AFP is still significantly greater in patients with yolk sac tumor. Furthermore, in children older than 6 months, teratoma patients never had AFP levels greater than 100 ng/mL.

○ **What is the histologic hallmark of a testicular teratoma?**

Teratomas contain elements derived from more than one of the 3 germ tissues: ectoderm, endoderm, and mesoderm.

○ **A 14-month-old male presents with a testicular mass. Tumor markers are negative. Radical orchiectomy is performed, and the pathology reveals a teratoma. What is the next step in management of this patient?**

Observation. Teratomas in prepubertal boys are consistently benign. Either orchiectomy or enucleation of the tumor with preservation of the remaining testicular tissue is curative. An older, postpubertal patient with teratocarcinoma, however, is managed the same as an adult with a nonseminomatous germ cell tumor.

○ **What testicular tumor must be ruled out in boys who present with precocious puberty?**

Leydig cell tumors can produce high levels of testosterone resulting in increased somatic growth, deepening of the voice, phallic growth, and secondary sexual characteristics. Serum levels of testosterone and gonadotropins must be checked, along with testicular ultrasonography. These tumors are generally benign, and testis-sparing surgery with enucleation of the mass is recommended.

○ **What disease can mimic a Leydig cell tumor?**

Congenital adrenal hyperplasia (non-salt-wasting) can present similarly to a Leydig cell tumor. This is particularly true if a hypertrophic adrenal rest is present in the scrotum. These patients will exhibit elevated 17-ketosteroids as well as testosterone; gonadotropin levels will be low. Treatment with corticosteroids usually results in prompt resolution of the scrotal mass (adrenal rest).

○ **When should partial orchiectomy be considered for a prepubertal testicular mass?**

The majority of prepubertal testicular masses are benign, and a testis-sparing approach should always be considered in the absence of evidence of malignancy. The following algorithm can be useful for surgical approach:

If the physical examination and/or testicular sonogram suggest malignancy in conjunction with an abnormal age-specific serum AFP, a radical orchiectomy should be planned.

If the physical examination and testicular sonogram suggest a benign tumor and the age-specific AFP is normal, testis-sparing surgery should be planned. The tumor is excised, and intraoperative frozen section is performed. If the frozen section is concerning for malignancy, a radical orchiectomy is performed. Otherwise, proceed with testis-sparing surgery.

○ **What condition or conditions are associated with the development of gonadoblastoma?**

Gonadoblastoma is a tumor that contains both germ cells and germinal stromal cells (although often the germ cells predominate and the tumor resembles a seminoma). This tumor develops almost exclusively in patients with abnormal gonads. The karyotype of these children contains either a Y chromosome or a translocation, which includes a portion of the Y chromosome, most commonly 46XY or 45XO/46XY. All of these children have genital/sexual abnormalities. Eighty percent are phenotypic females with intra-abdominal testes (or streak gonads); 20% occur in patients with predominantly male phenotype, often with ambiguity. Children with mixed gonadal dysgenesis have a 25% risk of tumor formation, and the incidence increases with age. All streak gonads in patients with gonadal dysgenesis should be removed.

○ **True/False: Younger patient age at the time of diagnosis of a sacrococcygeal teratoma is associated with worse prognosis.**

False. The prognosis for malignant sacrococcygeal teratomas is much worse than that for benign lesions. Malignancy is seen in 7% of girls and 10% of boys diagnosed at less than 2 months of age. In contrast, malignancy is seen in 48% of girls and 67% of boys diagnosed after 2 months of age.

○ **What structure must be excised along with a sacrococcygeal teratoma?**

Resection of the coccyx is an extremely important part of the surgical management of sacrococcygeal teratoma. Failure to resect the coccyx has been associated with a recurrence rate of up to 35%.

○ **What is the primary mode of treatment for a sacrococcygeal teratoma?**

Surgical excision is the mainstay of treatment in patients with sacrococcygeal teratoma. Patients with benign tumors must be followed with imaging to detect any recurrence. Patients with malignant tumors have a poor long-term prognosis despite the multiagent chemotherapy that is required following surgical resection.

Radiology: CT/Ultrasound/MRI

CHAPTER 51

Gopi Kiran Reddy Sirineni, MBBS, MD and Brian J. Hamm, MD

○ **What is the best imaging modality for diagnosing a non-urethral abnormality of the penis?**

Ultrasound is still considered first line when evaluating for abnormal masses, abscesses, or penile hematomas. However, the superior soft tissue contrast and spatial resolution of MRI make it very valuable when ultrasound findings are equivocal. Penile malignancies, periurethral abscesses, hematomas, venous thrombosis, or penile fractures can all be diagnoses with a high degree of accuracy with MRI. T1-weighted contrast-enhanced images below depict a traumatic intracavernosal hematoma (left) with active bleeding (right).

○   **What renal abnormalities are demonstrated below after a blunt abdominal trauma?**

CT images above depict a lacerated right kidney (white arrow) with associated vascular injuries. There is a renal vein psuedoaneursym (black arrow) with an intimal flap extending into the IVC (black dashed arrow) and a renal artery dissection (white dashed arrow).

About 10% of significant blunt abdominal traumatic injuries demonstrate renal injury. Most such cases only manifest with minor lacerations or hematomas but occasionally, the vascular pedicle or any other part of the renal artery and vein can be damaged. Complete transaction of the vascular pedicle is known to occur, but oftentimes vascular injuries such as pseudoaneurysms or dissections can be present. Pseudoaneurysms are collections of blood contained by surrounding tissue and in communication with the vessel. They result from traumatic tears in the vessel wall. They appear as rounded outpouchings from the vessel and fill with IV contrast as the vessel does. Traumatic dissections result when the intimal layer of the vessel wall tears. Blood then "dissects" through the media, separating the intima from the rest of the wall and forming an intraluminal intimal flap. Vascular injuries often must be treated with endovascular catheter embolization, usually of the main renal artery.

○   **What is a Page kidney?**

Occasionally in the setting of trauma, a subcapsular fluid collection can develop around the kidney. These collections are usually hematomas, but can also be urinomas from a damaged collecting system or seromas. The kidney capsule prevents release of the fluid into the retroperitoneum, which causes a buildup of pressure on the kidney itself. If this pressure becomes great enough, blood flow to the kidney is restricted, activating the renin–angiotensin system and causing reactive hypertension. This is referred to as a "Page kidney." On imaging, an encapsulated fluid collected will be seen surrounding and compressing the kidney.

○   **What are the imaging findings below and what diagnosis do they represent?**

Retroperitoneal fibrosis is an idiopathic disorder characterized by desmoplastic bands of fibrous tissue formation in the lumbar retroperitoneum. A mantle of soft tissue encases the aorta, inferior vena cava, and the ureters. CT is the imaging modality of choice for this disorder and will easily demonstrate a fibrous plaque, which can extend from the crus of the diaphragm to the iliac vessels. There is often medial displacement of the ureters with proximal ureteral dilation and often hydronephrosis. Contrast enhancement of the fibrous tissue can be seen if it has recently formed with an active inflammatory response. The axial CT image above demonstrates retroperitoneal fibrosis encasing the aorta and the medial portions of the renal arteries and veins (white arrows). Note that the density of the plaque is similar to muscle.

○   **What are the CT findings demonstrated below?**

The pictures demonstrate an extraperitoneal bladder rupture. Traumatic bladder ruptures are often first diagnosed with the initial CT trauma survey scan. Bladder rupture is best seen on delayed CT images, after contrast has been allowed to accumulate in the bladder and potentially extravasate, revealing the location of the rupture. Bladder rupture is divided into 2 types: intraperitoneal and extraperitoneal. Extraperitoneal rupture occurs more frequently and is usually secondary to fragments of bone from pelvic fractures tearing the bladder wall. Contrast will be seen in the paravesical and presacral spaces and can even track along the retroperitoneum superiorly. Occasionally, such ruptures can dissect into the subcutaneous tissues of the anterior pelvic wall or into the thigh or scrotum. Intraperitoneal ruptures are usually secondary to blunt force against a distended bladder. In these cases, contrast will be seen extravasating into the paracolic gutters, pouch of Douglas, or around the small bowel loops. Intraperitoneal ruptures require surgical repair. The above CT scan depicts an extraperitoneal bladder rupture with contrast extravasating into the subcutaneous anterior tissues from an associated pelvic fracture. Diastatic, displaced pubic symphysis is visible on the left image.

○ **What do the CT findings below represent?**

Prostatic abscess. Occasionally, abscess formation may be a complication of prostatitis. These abscesses appear as unilocular or multilocular rim-enhancing fluid collections usually within the peripheral portion of the gland. The abscess may spread through the prostate capsule and into the periprostate tissue. The CT image below depicts a unilocular rim-enhancing abscess within the prostate. Incidentally, the patient also has fat-filled inguinal hernias.

○ **What is the role of renal CT and MR angiography?**

CT and MR renal angiography are used to diagnose renal artery stenosis (RAS), the most common cause of secondary hypertension. Etiologies include atherosclerosis and fibromuscular dysplasia. Atherosclerotic lesions typically occur at the ostium or within the proximal 2 cm of the renal artery. They present as a focal/segmental stenosis. It typically affects men older than 50 years.

Fibromuscular dysplasia is the second most common cause of RAS and the most common cause in children and young adults. It is bilateral in two-thirds of cases and affects the mid-to-distal renal artery. The renal artery classically has a "string of beads" pattern with stenosis involving a long segment in fibromuscular dysplasia.

CT angiography is also useful in the evaluation of living renal donors prior to surgery to define the anatomy. MR angiography has traditionally also been used to evaluate the vena cava for renal masses, where a suspicion of vena caval thrombus exists.

The above scan is a normal CT angiogram showing arterial and venous anatomy of the left kidney. The appearance of the vena cava is dark due to incomplete mixing with the contrast. The aorta is still bright white indicating an arterial phase picture.

○ **What are the ultrasound findings in renal artery stenosis?**

Direct signs of RAS include increased peak systolic velocity and poststenotic turbulent flow (spectral broadening). Indirect signs or distal manifestations of RAS include a dampened systolic waveform (tardus et parvus waveform) and decreased renal resistive index.

○ **What is the renal resistive index and how is it used?**

The renal resistive index is calculated from Doppler ultrasound studies of the renal vasculature. It is defined as the peak systolic velocity minus the end-diastolic velocity divided by the peak systolic velocity. Resistive index can be elevated in acute obstruction, acute tubular necrosis (ATN), allograft rejection, and cyclosporin toxicity. Resistive index may be decreased in renal artery stenosis due to decreased peak systolic flow.

○ **How does a nuclear medicine study evaluate for renovascular hypertension (RVH)?**

Technetium 99m-DTPA and MAG3 are radionuclide agents cleared by the kidneys. Patients with RVH may show a unilateral reduction in flow, while function is preserved. This study may be performed in conjunction with an ACE inhibitor, such as captopril. The ACE inhibitor blocks efferent arterial vasoconstriction, resulting in a decrease in the glomerular filtration rate (GFR) and effective renal plasma flow (ERPF). The study is considered suggestive of RAS if one of the kidneys GFR drops by 30% after captopril is administered.

○ **What is the role of a renal captopril study in suspected RVH?**

The renal captopril study is a good screening test for those suspected of renal artery stenosis. However, patients with positive studies should undergo additional imaging, such as magnetic resonance angiography or renal angiography.

○ **Which urinary tract stones are radiolucent on CT?**

Indinavir stones can only be seen by secondary findings and usually require an intravenous pyelogram (IVP). Matrix stones are soft tissue attenuation density. Uric acid and cystine stones range from 100 to 300 Hounsfield units (HU), while calcium stones are typically 400 to 600 HU.

Before the widespread use of CT, it was assumed that most calcium stones are visible on plain films. In reality, plain KUB radiography misses many calculi due to their small size and overlying abdominal or bony structures.

○ **What is the advantage of assessing hematuria with CT urogram versus an IVP?**

CT urogram (contrast study) affords improved detection of calculi, better bladder visualization, and demonstrates vascular pathology. Renal masses will be evident on the intermediate contrasted phase where both cortex and medulla are opacified (nephrographic phase). Advances in CT technology have enabled fast acquisition of thin slices that allows improved visualization of the urothelial surfaces.

○ **In the region of the renal medulla, multiple, bilateral calcifications are present. What are the top 3 diagnoses?**

1. Renal tubular acidosis.
2. Medullary sponge kidney.
3. Hyperparathyroidism.

Highly echogenic medullary pyramids suggesting calcification (see below scans).

○ **What are the ultrasound characteristics of renal stones?**

Calculi are seen as crescent-shaped echogenic foci with posterior acoustic shadowing. Posterior shadowing distinguishes small stones from other echogenic structures in the central sinus. Ureteral stones are frequently not seen because of the overlying bowel gas.

Color Doppler is used to visualize ureteric jets of urine into the bladder that excludes high-grade ureteric obstruction. Twinkling artifact or rapid color change posterior to a stone is a useful ancillary finding to confirm a urinary tract stone.

○ **What are the secondary signs of acute obstruction from ureteral calculi on the CT scan?**

Typical findings are renal enlargement, striated cortex, perinephric stranding, and ureteral dilation with hydronephrosis (right image), and a tissue rim sign (left image) around the ureter where the stone is located.

○   **What are the CT characteristics of xanthogranulomatous pyelonephritis (XGP)?**

XGP is a chronic kidney infection resulting in lipid-laden macrophages creating multiple focal low attenuation masses. There is contrast enhancement of the parenchyma surrounding the collections. Cortical involvement is often diffuse, but can be focal. The kidney is usually nonfunctioning or poorly functioning. The process can extend beyond the renal capsule. Renal cutaneous and renal enteric fistulas are a potential complication. Staghorn calculi are associated with XGP. Staghorn calculi fill the collecting system, forming a cast of the pelvis and calyces. Most are composed of struvite and associated with chronic renal infection. XGP can mimic renal cell carcinoma (RCC), transitional cell carcinoma (TCC), lymphoma, metastases, abscess, and pyonephrosis. Treatment always involves antibiotics, which is usually followed by nephrectomy.

Contrast-enhanced CT images below demonstrate XGP in the right kidney with a staghorn calculus.

○   **An adult patient presents with hematuria, hypertension, and an elevated serum creatinine. An ultrasound shows multiple, bilateral large cysts. A representative CT scan is shown as well as a typical renal ultrasound. What is the diagnosis and recommended treatment?**

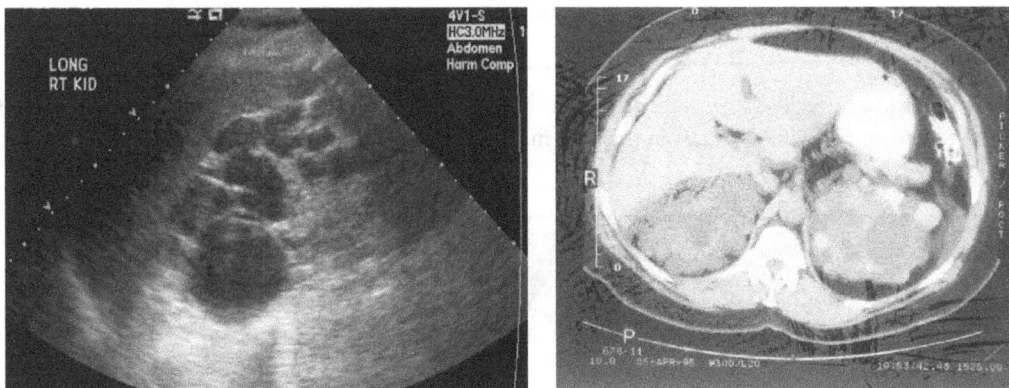

Autosomal dominant polycystic kidney disease (ADPCKD) is the diagnosis. The ultrasound/CT findings are pathognomonic with bilaterally large kidneys containing multiple cysts. The mean age at diagnosis is 43 years. ADPCKD is associated with cysts in the liver and pancreas and saccular berry aneurysms of the cerebral arteries. Renal insufficiency gradually develops. Treatment is a renal transplant.

○ **What other entities present with renal parenchymal cysts?**

Acquired cystic disease from long-term dialysis, multiple simple cysts, von Hippel–Lindau disease, tuberous sclerosis, and medullary cystic disease all cause renal cysts.

○ **What are the characteristics of a simple cyst on renal ultrasound?**

A simple cyst appears as a round or oval anechoic structure, with an imperceptible wall and smooth margins. There is increased through transmission and no internal echoes.

○ **How can one characterize a simple renal cyst on CT?**

Simple cysts are round, low attenuation structures without complexity of the wall. Hounsfield units are less than 20.

○ **What are the typical CT and US findings of renal lymphoma?**

CT demonstrates a homogeneous mass with minimal contrast enhancement. On ultrasound, lymphoma is hypoechoic and may show posterior acoustic enhancement. Diffuse infiltration is characterized by renal enlargement. Primary renal lymphoma is rare. It is most often secondary to hematogenous spread from extra renal lymphoma.

○ **How are renal cystic lesions characterized on CT?**

The Bosniak classification:

- Class I—Benign cysts (well-defined, round, homogeneous, lucent (<HU 20), avascular, thin-walled).
- Class II—Minimally complicated cysts; benign (well-marginated, mildly irregular, calcified, septated, avascular, hyperdense, usually <3 cm).
- Class IIF—Possibly benign (hyperdense, thick or nodular calcifications in wall or septa, vaguely enhanced, may be >3 cm) (see figure below).
- Class III—Indeterminate.
- Class IV—Malignant lesions with large cystic or necrotic components (irregular wall thickening or an enhancing mass).

The CT scan shows right renal cyst with dense calcification centrally and multiple septations (Bosniak IIF-III). This proved to be a cystic RCC. Contrast in this case makes identification of calcification difficult to prove conclusively.

○ **What is the characteristic appearance of RCC on imaging?**

It most often presents as a solid, expansile, hyperenhancing renal lesion: 10% have calcifications and 20% are at least partially cystic. There is often tumor extension into the renal vein and IVC. Lymphatic metastases present as retroperitoneal adenopathy. However, necrotic tumors can illicit reactive hyperplasia in regional nodes.

Patients with acquired cystic renal disease (long-term dialysis), tuberous sclerosis, and von Hippel–Lindau syndrome are predisposed to RCC.

○ **What is the pattern most often seen on CT of distant metastasis in RCC?**

Metastases to the lungs can be solitary or demonstrate a miliary pattern. Bone metastases are lytic, aggressive, and can be solitary or multiple. Hepatic metastases are usually hypervascular.

○ **What is the best imaging test to evaluate for vascular invasion of RCC?**

Both multiphasic contrast-enhanced CT and MRI yield 90% to 95% accuracy in identifying renal vein thrombus. Multislice CT adds the capability of coronal and sagittal reconstructions, which are desirable for surgical planning.

The CT scan (below) showing vena caval thrombus and RCC and another typical CT appearance of a renal cell cancer.

○ **An echogenic, 2-cm renal mass is found on ultrasound. What imaging study should be performed next?**

If fat is found in the mass on CT, the diagnosis of an angiomyolipoma is confirmed. Fat is hypodense on CT and the Hounsfield units should measure less than zero. Angiomyolipomas are benign lesions consisting of fat, smooth muscle, and blood vessels. If they reach a large size they may hemorrhage, therefore, they may be resected.

Ultrasound (below) showing a subtle upper pole hyperechoic angiomyolipoma and a CT scan (below) from a patient with tuberous sclerosis showing multiple bilateral angiomyolipomas.

○ **What renal transplant complications may occur immediately postoperatively and what are their characteristics?**

- Acute tubular necrosis (ATN)—Transient renal enlargement and increased renal resistive index.
- Acute rejection—Similar to ATN but does not resolve.
- Renal artery stenosis—Tardus et parvus waveform distal to stenosis, peak systolic velocity >250 cm/s.
- Renal vein thrombosis—Reversal of diastolic flow on Doppler ultrasound.
- Urine leak—Anechoic collection (urinoma) without septations.

○ **ATN is suspected in a renal transplant patient. What findings would you expect on the nuclear medicine renal scan?**

The classic findings of ATN are blood flow is preserved; however, poor concentration and excretion is present resulting in an increasingly dense nephrogram. Rejection and dehydration can have a similar appearance.

○ **How can one tell the difference on nuclear renal scans between ATN and rejection?**

Subsequent renal scans show improvement in flow and function in the setting of ATN, whereas flow and function continue to decrease with rejection. Serial examinations to differentiate ATN from rejection should be performed with ultrasound, monitoring resistive indices.

○ **What factors are evaluated on a renal transplant ultrasound?**

The kidney is identified, measured, and the flow in the kidney is examined. The flow is evaluated with color and power Doppler imaging. The main renal artery and vein blood flows are evaluated. The resistive index should typically not exceed 0.80. Remember, the resistive index is the peak systolic velocity (PSV) minus the end-diastolic velocity (EDV) divided by the peak systolic velocity or (PSV – EDV)/PSV.

○ **Fluid collections may accumulate around the transplanted kidney. Name the differential for the fluid collections immediately postop, 3 months, and 6 months from surgery.**

- Urinoma—1 to 2 weeks post-transplant.
- Hematoma—1 to 3 weeks post-transplant.
- Lymphocele—A few weeks to several months post-transplant.
- Abscess—4 to 5 weeks post-transplant.

○ **What ultrasound findings are suggestive of obstruction of the transplanted kidney?**

Either increasing dilatation of the renal collecting system on subsequent ultrasounds or significant dilatation of the collecting system may represent obstruction (ureteral stenosis or a blood clot). However, mild dilatation is often seen in normal transplants.

○ **What is the normal appearance of the adrenal glands on CT/MRI?**

Each limb of the adrenal gland has straight or slightly convex borders, may measure up to 4 cm in length, and should measure less than 10 mm in thickness. T1 signal on MRI is homogeneous and slightly less intense than that of a normal liver and renal cortex.

○ **Which imaging study is best to differentiate adrenal masses from upper pole renal masses?**

Historically, multiplanar MRI (coronal, sagittal) has made this modality the best choice in evaluating a renal versus adrenal mass. Newer multislice CT scanners can easily reconstruct axial sequences into coronal and sagittal planes. Subtle fat planes between the renal mass and adrenal gland may be distinguished on a coronal or other planar imaging sequence.

○ **What is the CT imaging characteristic of an adrenal adenoma?**

Adrenal adenomas are typically 3 cm or less and appear as focal low densities with a smooth round margin. Hounsfield units that are less than 10 on noncontrast CT is 95% specific for adrenal adenoma. Adenomas, unlike metastases, demonstrate rapid washout of intravenous contrast. Thus, indeterminate lesions can be evaluated with contrast CT scans. A lesion that demonstrates 60% or greater washout of contrast on the 15 minutes delayed scan compared with the portal venous phase scan will be an adenoma 98% of the time.

○ **What is the MRI characteristic of an adrenal adenoma?**

Chemical shift imaging with in and out of phase sequences is 95% to 100% specific for a diagnosis of adrenal adenoma. False negatives may be encountered in lipid poor adenomas.

○ **What are the CT and MRI characteristic of an adrenal hemorrhage?**

CT demonstrates a round mass with increased attenuation (50-90 HU). The mass does not enhance and will decrease in size over a 6-month period of time.

MRI characteristically demonstrates a ring pattern of high T1 low T2 signal peripherally caused by methemoglobin and hemosiderin.

○ **What are the clinical entities associated with adrenal hemorrhage?**

Adrenal hemorrhage is associated with trauma, anticoagulation, septicemia, burns, recent surgery, and metastatic melanoma. It is more common in the right adrenal gland.

○ **Describe the imaging characteristics of an adrenal pheochromocytoma on CT and MRI.**

Pheochromocytomas are usually greater than 2 cm at presentation. They are indistinguishable from metastases. Larger tumors will have areas of central necrosis. Correlation with blood tests is required to establish the diagnosis. The use of intravenous contrast in patients with pheochromocytoma is controversial in the setting of a history of hypertensive episodes or if the patient has not had adequate adrenergic blockade.

MRI may not be as useful as previously thought secondary to cost, time, and increased artifacts. Furthermore, the classic description of "light bulb" appearance on T2 sequences is seen in less than half of adrenal pheochromocytomas. Other tumors with cystic components will also have a high T2 signal.

A whole body iodine-131–labeled metaiodobenzylguanidine (MIBG) is used when looking for an extra-adrenal tumor. The scan below is an MRI of adrenal pheochromocytoma showing a bright signal on T2-weighted imaging. Note compression of the underlying kidney.

○ **If a single kidney were seen in the abdomen on ultrasound, what differential would one consider?**

- Congenital absence of a kidney.
- Renal hypoplasia or atrophy.
- An ectopic location, such as the pelvis.
- Prior resection.
- Nonfunctioning kidney (trauma or obstruction).

○ **What are the imaging findings in renal trauma?**

Intrarenal hematoma presents as an area of decreased enhancement on nephrographic (parenchymal) phase of contrast CT. Infarct has a similar appearance but is classically a peripheral wedge-shaped defect. Subcapsular hematomas are elliptical or round and have 40 to 70 HU. Lacerations are linear low attenuation areas that can extend into the collecting system and result in contrast extravasation of urine. Delayed phase images should be performed to evaluate collecting system injury when lacerations are present. Extensive areas of devascularization are common in higher-grade lesions.

The CT scan (below) demonstrating a classic right-sided "rim sign," where the external kidney cortex is perfused by cortical perforators. This is a classic sign of an intimal disruption and significant renovascular trauma.

○ **What are the imaging characteristics of a horseshoe kidney?**

The lower poles of the kidneys fuse, creating a single band of tissue crossing the midline. The orientation of the kidneys is altered with the lower poles directed more medial and the collecting systems directed anterior. This condition is associated with an increased incidence of ureteropelvic junction (UPJ) obstruction, recurrent urinary infections, Wilms tumor in children, and is more predisposed to injury in trauma.

○ **What are the characteristics of adrenal myelolipoma on CT?**

Adrenal myelolipoma is a rare benign lesion containing myeloid, fat, and hematopoietic tissue. Size is usually 2 to 10 cm. They demonstrate heterogeneous attenuation and are very rarely bilateral. Large tumors can hemorrhage. Fat content creates increased echogenicity on ultrasound and negative Hounsfield units on CT. It can mimic retroperitoneal lipoma or liposarcoma. They are T1 hyperintense on MRI. Signal drops out on fat suppression sequences.

The scan (below) shows classic right adrenal myelolipoma with fat density.

○ **What are the most common causes of adrenal hemorrhage in pediatric and adult patients?**

In neonates, the most common cause of adrenal hemorrhage is birth trauma, hypoxia, or septicemia. Most cases are bilateral. In neonates, ultrasound is the imaging study of choice. In adults, trauma, anticoagulation, and infection are the most common causes of hemorrhage. Typically, unilateral hemorrhage involving the right adrenal gland occurs in adults. CT is performed in adult patients being evaluating for adrenal hemorrhage.

○ **What are the imaging characteristics of adrenal hemorrhage on ultrasound?**

Ultrasound initially images acute hemorrhage as hyperechoic. Over time, the blood becomes more hypoechoic and smaller.

○ **What are the CT findings of pyelonephritis?**

Imaging studies, including CT, is normal in 75% of cases. However, a contrast-enhanced CT study may show wedge-shaped areas of decreased density (striated nephrogram) or renal enlargement. CT can rule out potential complications of pyelonephritis, such as abscess, hydronephrosis, stones, or scarring. Differential diagnosis for a striated nephrogram includes contusion, infarct, and radiation.

○ **What are the ultrasound and CT findings in emphysematous pyelonephritis?**

Ultrasound demonstrates echogenic foci in the renal sinus and parenchyma with dirty posterior shadowing. Ring down artifacts from trapped air bubbles can be seen. Perinephric gas may obscure visualization of the kidney.

CT demonstrates gas radiating from the medulla to the parenchyma. There is often a crescentic subcapsular gas collection. Gas can extend into the ipsilateral and contralateral anterior pararenal space.

The scan (below) depicts bilateral emphysematous pyelonephritis showing gas in the parenchyma.

○ **What are the imaging findings of medullary sponge kidney?**

CT urogram and IVP: Retained contrast in dilated tubules in renal pyramids. Medullary nephrocalcinosis and urolithiasis may be present. These patients have an increased incidence of urinary tract infections and nephrolithiasis due to renal leak type hypercalciuria and hypocitraturia.

○ **What are the imaging findings of papillary necrosis?**

- Ultrasound shows echogenic foci in renal papillae progressing to cystic cavities in the pyramids.
- CT urogram/IVP demonstrates contrast-filled clefts in the renal parenchyma, sloughed papillae (renal pelvis filling defect), and ring-shaped medullary calcifications.
- Papillary necrosis is associated with analgesic abuse. Diabetic and sickle cell patients are also susceptible.

○ **Unilateral hydronephrosis and hydroureter is identified on an ultrasound. The patient has no history of compromised renal function. Which imaging study should be ordered next?**

A CT urogram with contrast is best to evaluate for the cause of obstruction, such as an obstructing bladder stone or a bladder cancer obstructing the UVJ. If there is a reasonable suspicion for nephrolithiasis, a single phase CT without contrast may be sufficient for diagnosis and save the patient considerable radiation exposure. If there is compromised renal function, consider an MR urogram.

Causes of obstruction include ureteral stricture, sloughed papilla, prior stone, prior infection, pelvic neoplasm, retroperitoneal fibrosis, ureterocele, or prior instrumentation.

○ **What are the ultrasound and CT imaging findings of a ureterocele?**

A ureterocele is a cystic dilatation of the distal ureter with prolapse into the bladder. Orthotopic ureteroceles insert normally at the trigone. Ectopic ureteroceles insert below the trigone and are associated with duplicated collecting systems in 80% of the time.

CT demonstrates an intravesicular mass at the UVJ. CT urogram findings can be similar to the IVP. Orthotopic ureteroceles present as a dilated distal ureter projecting into the bladder. Ectopic variety is often best demonstrated by ancillary findings of duplication.

On ultrasound, an orthotopic ureterocele presents as a round, thin walled sac, continuous with the distal ureter. Size fluctuates with ureteral peristalsis. A full bladder can occasionally cause a ureterocele to invert, giving the appearance of a bladder diverticulum.

Ultrasound (below) showing ureterocele in the base of the bladder.

○ **What are the imaging findings of a collecting system duplication?**

CT demonstrates a duplex kidney. Absence of a renal sinus at the junction of upper and lower pole creates "faceless kidney" appearance. There are 2 ureters. The upper pole is most often obstructed. It can insert medial and caudal to the insertion of the lower pole ureter (Meyer–Weigert rule) or ectopically.

Ultrasound shows 2 renal sinus echo complexes and intervening renal parenchyma as well as upper pole hydronephrosis.

○ **In a duplicated collecting system, hydronephrosis of the upper pole moiety is due to what entity?**

The upper pole ureter inserts ectopically. An ectopic ureter inserting into the bladder (not at the trigone) is usually stenotic at its orifice and may end in an ectopic ureterocele. Extravesicular insertion in males is most common at the prostatic urethra. In females, insertion is most commonly at the urethra or vestibule. Males, unlike females, do not experience incontinence because the ectopic orifice is always above the external sphincter.

○ **What is the preferred imaging modality for suspected urolithiasis?**

The noncontrast CT of the abdomen and pelvis is now the preferred imaging study. A plain x-ray of the abdomen (KUB) is recommended when the CT scan is positive for stones. The KUB is useful to establish the radiopacity or radiolucency of the stone as well as to characterize its shape and surgical orientation. It also provides a simple and inexpensive way to track the progress of the stone.

○ **What is the role of the CT urogram in the evaluation of the patient with microhematuria?**

CT urogram of the abdomen and pelvis is gaining favor over the IVP. The study consists of a noncontrasted scan to look for urolithiasis. If stones are present, the study may be terminated to spare the patient unnecessary radiation exposure. After administration of contrast, the nephrographic phase (maximum cortical enhancement) and excretory phase images are performed. A series of excretory scans are often performed to ensure complete visualization of contrast throughout the renal collecting systems, ureters, and bladder. The nephrographic phase is most sensitive for evaluation of cortical lesions.

The bladder should be carefully evaluated with contrast opacifying the majority of the structure. If contrast is especially dense, bone windows help "see through" the contrast in the bladder so no masses are missed.

CT urogram (below) showing TCC of the right renal pelvis seen as multiple filling defects in the collecting system.

○ **How is TCC distinguished from a blood clot on ultrasound?**

TCC will have color flow on ultrasound and is immobile. Blood clots are immobile and will move as patient changes the position. TCC can involve any part of the urothelium but is most common in the bladder. Lesions can be low-grade papillary or high-grade nonpapillary (nodular or flat). Echogenic polypoid tumor can mimic fungus ball or bladder stone.

○ **What are the CT/MRI characteristics of TCC?**

TCC is a hypovascular, infiltrative tumor. In the renal pelvis, it can present as urothelial thickening or as a polypoid or sessile mass. There may be invasion of the renal cortex and sinus fat. Look for thin rims of contrast filling caliceal spaces around the periphery of the tumor. In the ureter, it presents as circumferential or eccentric wall thickening. Hydronephrosis is often present.

Bladder TCC may enhance and protrude into the bladder lumen. MRI is the study of choice to assess invasion of the bladder wall and adjacent organs. Lesions are hyperintense on T2 sequences compared with normal bladder wall and perivesical tissues. Bladder TCC mildly enhances with gadolinium.

○ **How is TCC distinguished from tuberculosis on CT urogram?**

Strictures are the earliest finding and can result in an amputated infundibulum and irregular caliceal contour. Papillary necrosis results in irregular cavities. Calcifications are common.

○ **What imaging modality is best for evaluation of prostatic cysts? Can you name any of the types of cysts?**

Transrectal ultrasound and MRI with endorectal coil are the best studies for evaluating prostatic cysts.

Utricle and Mullerian cysts are derived from the paramesonephric duct. Utricle cyst will fill on retrograde urethrogram via connection with the posterior urethra. A Mullerian cyst can be larger extending cephalad to the prostate and does not communicate with the urethra.

Cysts associated with benign prostatic hypertrophy and ejaculatory duct cysts are usually paramedian in location. Congenital and retention cyst are usually more lateral.

○ **What neoplasm is associated with a urachal remnant? What are the imaging features?**

Urachal remnants result from persistence of the embryonic connection between the bladder dome and allantoic duct. This can result in a patent urachus, urachal cyst, urachal sinus, or urachal diverticulum. CT demonstrates a midline cystic lesion above the bladder dome. It may have rim calcifications. Urachal carcinoma (adenocarcinoma is most common) presents as a mass in this region and often invades the bladder dome.

The scan (below) shows urachal adenocarcinoma presenting as a mass in the dome of the bladder and space of Retzius.

○ **Which zone of the prostate is the site of benign prostatic hypertrophy?**

The transitional zone is the site of origin (greater than 95%) of benign prostatic hypertrophy.

○ **What is the percentage of prostate cancer arising from each zone?**

- Peripheral zone 70%.
- Central zone 10%.
- Transitional zone 20%.

○ **Which imaging modality is used to evaluate acute scrotal pain?**

Ultrasound.

○ **What are the ultrasound findings of testicular torsion?**

Early torsion (less than 4 hours) may be normal on gray scale images. However, color imaging shows an absence of flow to the affected testis. By 24 hours, the testicle may be hyper- or hypovascular on color images and enlarged with a heterogeneous echotexture on gray scale imaging.

○ **What are the ultrasound findings in epididymitis?**

The epididymis is enlarged and hypervascular. If the testis is involved, increased blood flow will be present. A reactive hydrocele and skin thickening may also be present.

○ **What is the importance of differentiating an extra/intratesticular mass?**

The majority of intratesticular masses are malignant. Most extratesticular masses are benign.

Primary and metastatic malignancies can involve the testicles. The vast majority of testicular neoplasms are primary. The most common germ cell tumors include seminoma, embryonal carcinoma, choriocarcinoma, and teratocarcinomas. Common primaries that may metastasize to the testicles are lymphoma (the most common in patients older than 60), prostate, leukemia, and kidney.

Testicular ultrasound (below) showing an intraparenchymal neoplasm suspicious for a germ cell tumor.

○ **Ultrasound appearance of an epidermoid cyst.**

Layers of keratin and desquamated squamous cells create an "onion skin" appearance.

Other nonmalignant mass-like testicular lesions seen on ultrasound include the following:

- Hematoma—Hypoechoic and avascular.
- Segmental infarct—Focal hypoechoic, avascular area; painful. No palpable abnormality.
- Focal orchitis—Increased vascularity, reactive hydrocele/epididymitis, and scrotal wall thickening.

○ **What is the ultrasound appearance of Fournier gangrene?**

Gas in the scrotum and perineum is echogenic with dirty posterior shadowing. Ring down artifact can also be seen. There is thickening of the scrotum.

○ **An infant's renal ultrasound shows the right kidney to have multiple cysts of varying sizes, which do not communicate. A right renal pelvis is not identified. What is the diagnosis?**

(A) Dysplastic right kidney in newborn infant

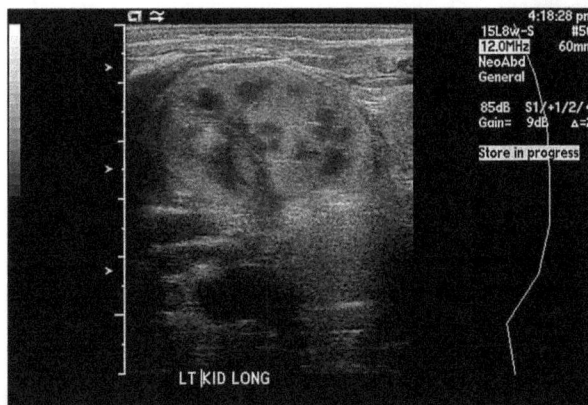

(B) Normal left kidney in the same infant

Multicystic dysplastic kidney (MCDK) is the result of atresia of the renal pelvis. If the disorder is bilateral, it is incompatible with life. MCDK is associated with contralateral renal abnormalities, most commonly UPJ obstruction and vesicoureteral reflux.

It is one of the most common causes of abdominal mass in an infant.

○ **Prenatal ultrasound demonstrates oligohydramnios and large echogenic kidneys. What is the diagnosis?**

Autosomal recessive polycystic kidney disease. Microcystic dilatation of the renal tubules causes an echogenic appearance without visible cysts (macrocysts).

○ **What is nephroblastomatosis and what is its significance?**

Nephroblastomatosis presents in young patients with multiple renal masses and renal enlargement. Nephroblastomatosis are persistent embryonal remnants (metanephric blastoma) in the kidney. Although not malignant itself, nephroblastomatosis is considered a precursor to Wilms tumor. The involved kidney is enlarged with a lobulated contour. Lesions are hypovascular, with little to no enhancement on contrast CT.

○ **What is mesoblastic nephroma and what is its significance?**

It is the most common neonatal renal neoplasm. It is a hamartoma of the kidney. Most are nonfunctioning. It can mimic Wilms tumor. Most are diagnosed pathologically.

○ **What is the typical age range for diagnosing Wilms tumor?**

Wilms tumor is diagnosed between the first and fifth years of life. They are uncommon in the first year of life.

○ **Describe the typical imaging findings of a Wilms tumor.**

Wilms tumor commonly presents as a large (mean 12 cm) mass arising from the renal cortex, displacing and distorting the pelvocaliceal system, with less contrast enhancement than the surrounding parenchyma. There is frequent invasion of the renal vein and IVC. They are poorly enhancing and heterogeneous on CT and usually have well-defined margins.

A large left-sided Wilms' tumor (2) on CT (see below) with a vena caval thrombus (3).

○ **What is the sequence of imaging tests for hydronephrosis found on prenatal ultrasound?**

- Postnatal ultrasound performed 4 to 7 days after birth to avoid false-negatives from physiologic postnatal dehydration.
- Voiding cysto-urethrogram (VCUG) should be ordered in severe cases to evaluate for vesicoureteral reflux and posterior urethral valves.
- If obstruction is suspected, nuclear medicine renogram with diuretics will evaluate the degree of obstruction and differential renal function.

○ **What is the normal appearance of infant kidneys on ultrasound?**

They can have an undulating contour. Renal pyramids are hypoechoic compared with the cortex. This finding can be mistaken for hydronephrosis.

The scan (below) is the ultrasound appearance of a normal infant kidney showing fetal lobulation and hypoechoic renal pyramids. This is due to impaired concentrating ability of these kidneys with a relatively dilute medullary interstitium.

○   A 74-year-old man is admitted to the hospital for treatment of a foot infection. He has noted increasing abdominal distension over the last 3 months, but no pain. He thinks he is just been gaining weight. His voiding is unchanged from his usual habit of small amounts and moderate frequency. Urology is consulted because of hydronephrosis and kidney stones. What is the correct diagnosis?

The images show significant hydronephrosis, renal calculi, a large bladder stone, and an enormous cystic structure extending from the pelvis to the kidneys and beyond. This cystic structure extended beyond the kidneys to the diaphragm. This is his bladder, which has become decompensated and stretched out to an enormous degree. He was catheterized for 9350 cc of urine and developed postobstructive diuresis that lasted another 24 hours. His PSA was 54 and he was diagnosed with prostate cancer as the underlying cause of his prostatic obstruction. He was treated with a suprapubic tube and intensity-modulated radiation therapy (IMRT) for his localized prostate cancer.

Urothelial Carcinoma of the Bladder

Kevin R. Rice, MD and
Michael O. Koch, MD

EPIDEMIOLOGY OF BLADDER CANCER

○ **How many cases of bladder cancer are diagnosed each year in the United States? How many patients die of bladder cancer each year?**

According to current estimates, there will be approximately 73,510 new cases of bladder cancer diagnosed in the United States in 2012. There will be an estimated 14,880 deaths from bladder cancer (Siegel et al., 2012).

○ **What are the top 4 causes of cancer death in the United States? How many cases of bladder cancer are diagnosed each year in the United States? How many patients die of bladder cancer each year?**

Lung cancer is first, followed by breast/prostate, colorectal and then bladder cancer is fourth. (Pancreatic cancer is fifth.) So 2 of the top 4 cancer killers in men are urological cancers.

○ **What are the main carcinogens linked to bladder cancer formation?**

Aromatic amines including benzidine, β-naphthylamine, arsenic, benzopyrene, and 4-aminobiphenyl.

○ **Name some established risk factors for development of urothelial carcinoma.**

- Cigarette smoking
- Occupational exposure to arylamines
  - Textile dying
  - Rubber workers
  - Hairdressers

○ **Approximately what percentage of urothelial carcinomas can be attributed to cigarette smoking?**

While it is impossible to know the exact number, at most, 50% of bladder cancers can be attributed to cigarette smoking.

○ **Which gender is more likely to develop bladder cancer?**

Men have 3 to 4 times a greater risk of developing bladder cancer than women (Siegel et al., 2012).

○ **Which racial group demonstrates the highest incidence of bladder cancer?**

Non-Hispanic whites demonstrate twice the incidence of bladder cancer seen in African American men or Hispanic men and nearly 3 times the incidence seen in Asian men. A similar pattern is seen in women (Yuan and Nelson, 2011).

○ **At what age is bladder cancer typically diagnosed?**

It is most commonly diagnosed in the 8th decade of life with a median age of diagnosis of 70 in both men and women (Parkin, 2008; Siegel et al., 2012).

DIAGNOSIS OF BLADDER CANCER

○ **What percentage of patients with cystoscopically detectable bladder cancer will have gross or microscopic hematuria?**

85% (Varkarakis et al., 1974).

○ **What percentage of patients with gross hematuria are found to have a bladder tumor on evaluation?**

12% will have a bladder tumor (Khadra et al., 2000).

○ **What percentage of patients without gross hematuria, but hematuria detected on urine dipstick tests are found to have bladder cancer? How about patients without gross hematuria, but microscopic hematuria confirmed on laboratory microscopic examination?**

1.3% (0.4%-6.5%) of patients without gross hematuria, but a positive dipstick will be found to have bladder cancer (Golin and Howard, 1980; Messing and Vaillancourt, 1990; Mohr et al., 1986). 4.1% of patients with true microscopic hematuria confirmed in the laboratory will be found to have bladder cancer (Mishriki et al., 2008).

○ **What percentage of patients with carcinoma *in situ* (CIS) report irritative voiding symptoms?**

The Mayo Clinic reported that 80% of patients with CIS presented with irritative voiding symptoms (Zincke et al., 1985).

URINE CYTOLOGY

○ **What is the sensitivity of a positive voided urine cytology?**

- For high-grade disease: sensitivity—70% to 85%.
- For low-grade disease: sensitivity—30% to 40% (Lotan and Roehrborn, 2003).

○ **What are the sensitivity and specificity of urine cytology for CIS?**

Approximately 90% sensitivity and specificity (Sylvester et al., 2005).

FLUORESCENT IN SITU HYBRIDIZATION (FISH)—UROVYSION

○ **What does the UroVysion urine FISH assay test for?**

It is a locus-specific probe to the 9p21 band on chromosome 9 and the aneuploidy for chromosomes 3, 7, and 17.

○ **What are the sensitivity and specificity of the UroVysion (FISH) test for detecting bladder cancer?**

Sensitivity—72% and Specificity—83% (Hajdinjak, 2008). Recent studies have reported that the sensitivity and specificity may be somewhat lower than this, particularly in lower stage tumors (Moonen et al., 2007; Gudjonsson et al., 2008).

○ **What percentage of patients with a positive UroVysion FISH test, but negative cystoscopy and cytology will have bladder cancer?**

65% (Yoder et al., 2007).

STAGING AND GRADING OF BLADDER CANCER

○ **What percentage of bladder tumors are urothelial in origin?**

The histology of approximately 90% of malignant bladder tumors is urothelial carcinoma. This is was previously referred to as transitional cell carcinoma, but the new terminology also includes other epithelial cell types (Lopez-Beltran, 2008).

○ **How is bladder cancer staged clinically?**

Exam under anesthesia (rectal exam and bimanual exam), endoscopic biopsy (transurethral resection of bladder tumor [TURBT] or cystoscopic biopsy), and cytology. Upper tracts should be evaluated with delayed contrast images (eg, intravenous pyelogram, CT urogram, MR urogram) or retrograde pyelogram at time of cystoscopy. Patients with evidence of invasive disease should have chest x-ray to evaluate for pulmonary metastases, and cross-sectional imaging of the abdomen and pelvis to evaluate local extent of disease as well as for the presence of nodal/visceral metastases, comprehensive metabolic panel, and a complete blood count.

○ **Go through 2007 AJCC Staging for bladder cancer:**

- *T stage:*

    Tx—Primary tumor cannot be assessed.
    T0—No primary tumor.
    Ta—Noninvasive papillary carcinoma.
    Tis—Carcinoma in situ.
    T1—Tumor invasion of subepithelial connective tissue (lamina propria).
    T2a—Tumor invasion of superficial muscularis propria (inner half).
    T2b—Tumor invasion of deep muscularis propria (outer half).
    T3a—Microscopic invasion perivesical tissue.
    T3b—Macroscopic invasion of perivesical tissue.
    T4a—Invasion of prostatic stroma, uterus, and vagina.
    T4b—Invasion of pelvic and/or abdominal wall.

- *N stage:*

    Nx—Lymph nodes cannot be assessed.
    N0—No lymph node metastases.
    N1—Single regional lymph node metastasis distal to bifurcation of common iliac arteries.
    N2—Multiple regional lymph node metastasis distal to bifurcation of common iliac arteries.
    N3—Lymph node metastases proximal to the bifurcation of the common iliac arteries, but still within the true pelvis.

- *M stage:*

    M0—No distant visceral or nonregional lymphatic metastases.
    M1—Distant visceral or nonregional lymphatic metastases.

○ **When should a bone scan be considered?**

When patients have symptoms concerning for skeletal metastases (bone pain, neurologic symptoms), when other staging imaging demonstrates lesions suspicious for metastatic disease, or when alkaline phosphatase is elevated.

○ **What is the typical cystoscopic appearance of low-grade bladder tumors?**

Papillary and pedunculated.

○ **How do papillary bladder cancers differ in cystoscopic appearance from benign inflammation?**

Papillary tumors will each have a tiny but separate blood supply and blood vessel while inflammatory growths may have generalized erythema, but will lack the extra vascularity.

○ **What is the typical cystoscopic appearance of high-grade bladder tumors?**

Flat and velvety (CIS), sessile, and/or nodular. They often tend to lose the papillary appearance and appear more solid. Sometimes tumor necrosis is evident.

○ **Which patients should have repeat resections after TURBT? When should this be performed?**

Any patients with bladder cancer, but no muscularis propria in the specimen should undergo re-resection, as their staging is incomplete. Patients with high-grade T1 disease, regardless of whether or not muscularis propria is seen in the specimen, should also undergo re-resection, as initial staging underestimates disease invasion in 30% to 40% of these patients (Dutta et al., 2001; Herr, 1999). Re-resections should be performed 2 to 6 weeks after the initial resection.

○ **What percentage of patients will have residual tumor at re-resection for the above indications?**

Herr reported a 76% incidence of residual tumor at re-resection (Herr, 1999).

○ **How can cautery artifact be minimized?**

Use of cutting rather than cauterizing current, finer diameter cutting loops, and lower cutting currents.

○ **What phenomenon can account for a T1 tumor being falsely read as a T2 tumor?**

Invasion of the muscularis mucosa in the lamina propria rather than the muscularis propria.

○ **Which patients with clinical T1 bladder cancer are at the highest risk for progression?**

Those with prior treatment with Bacillus Calmette–Guérin (BCG) and persistent T1 disease on restaging TURBT, history of multiple T1 recurrences, multifocal T1 disease, extensive concomitant CIS, and vascular invasion. These patients should be considered for immediate cystectomy rather than intravesical treatment (Dalbagni, 2011; Herr et al., 1989, 2007; Lambert et al., 2007).

○ **How many tiers does the current preferred World Health Organization (WHO)/International Society of Urologic Pathology (ISUP) urothelial carcinoma grading system have?**

Two (low or high grade). The previous grading system was 3-tiered (low, intermediate, and high grade) (Epstein, 1998).

○ **What percentage of papillary urothelial neoplasms of low malignant potential (PUNLMP) will recur and how many will progress to invasive disease?**

27% to 47% will recur and 0% to 4% will progress to muscle-invasive disease.

○ **What percentage of patients with low-grade noninvasive (Ta)urothelial carcinoma will recur and how many will progress to invasive disease?**

48% to 71% will recur. 5% will progress to invasive disease.

○ **What percentage of patients with high-grade papillary noninvasive (Ta)urothelial carcinoma will recur and how many will progress to invasive disease? How many will die from disease?**

Approximately 60% to 70% recur and 24% to 40% progress to muscle-invasive disease. Approximately 22% will go on to die of their disease (Lightfoot et al., 2011; Herr, 2000).

○ **Is CIS premalignant or malignant?**

Malignant. CIS is noninvasive high-grade urothelial carcinoma confined to the epithelium.

○ **What factors are associated with recurrence and progression in patients with non-muscle-invasive urothelial carcinoma?**

Multiplicity, prior recurrences, tumor size, concomitant CIS, female gender, tumor grade, and T-stage (Fernandez-Gomez et al., 2008; Sylvester et al., 2006).

○ **What is the most important factor predicting progression of non-muscle-invasive tumors?**

Grade.

○ **What level of bladder tumor invasion does hydronephrosis at staging suggest?**

This is a marker for invasion at least into the muscularis propria of the bladder. However, hydronephrosis can also be associated with more advanced disease and might be due to intraluminal ureteral disease.

○ **What percentage of patients with CIS will recur after intravesical BCG or chemotherapy and how many will progress to invasive disease? Will die of disease?**

Since CIS is extremely difficult (if not impossible) to completely eradicate with TURBT alone, recurrence rates can really only be assessed after treatment with intravesical therapies. In one review of 12 intravesical therapy trials, van der Meijden et al. (2005) found that at a median follow-up of 3.75 years, patients treated with BCG exhibited a 51% recurrence-free survival rate while those managed with intravesical chemotherapy demonstrated a 27% recurrence free survival rate. Forty to eighty percent of patients with CIS will progress to invasive disease (Hudson and Herr, 1995; Lamm et al., 1998; Solsona et al., 1990). Anywhere from 10% to 40% of patients initially diagnosed with CIS will ultimately succumb to bladder cancer (Gofrit et al., 2009; Jakse et al., 2001; Utz et al., 1970).

○ **A patient has completed a 6-week induction course of BCG therapy and is found to have raised velvety patches on cystoscopy as well as positive high-grade cytology. Random bladder biopsies reveal persistent CIS. What management options should you present to this patient?**

Re-induction BCG, maintenance BCG, intravesical chemotherapy (valrubicin), and radical cystectomy. It is possible that this patient will achieve a complete response (CR) with further BCG.

○   **In the above case, what is the expected CR rate to a second 6-week induction course of BCG?**

Up to 50% of those receiving a second 6-week induction course of BCG will achieve a CR (van der Meijden et al., 2005).

○   **What is the most important predictor of progression in CIS and what is the recommended treatment for those who fail to achieve a CR with BCG therapy?**

Patients who fail to achieve a CR by 6 months should undergo radical cystectomy, as 6-month response to BCG has been shown to be the single most important predictor of progression in CIS patients (Herr et al., 1989).

○   **What percentage of patients undergoing radical cystectomy for clinical CIS only will demonstrate upstaging on final pathologic analysis?**

In a study of 243 patients who underwent radical cystectomy for clinical CIS only, 87 patients (36%) demonstrated pathologic upstaging. Additionally, 14 (5.9%) patients demonstrated regional lymph node involvement. The 5-year recurrence-free and cancer-specific survival for the entire study group were 74% and 85%, respectively (Tilki et al., 2010).

○   **How often should patients with high-grade non-muscle-invasive bladder cancer (HG Ta, HG Ta, CIS) undergo upper tract imaging?**

Annually (Babjuk et al., 2008).

○   **What percentage of patients present with non-muscle-invasive bladder cancer?**

70% to 75% (Heney et al., 1983).

○   **How does one differentiate *clinical* T3a versus T3b bladder cancer?**

Clinical T3a refers to an extravesical mass that is palpable on examination under anesthesia, but is no longer palpable after transurethral resection. Clinical T3b disease is still palpable on examination after transurethral resection.

○   **What percentage of clinical stage T1 tumors are upstaged at radical cystectomy? Of clinical T2 tumors?**

Dutta et al., (2001) reported 40% upstaging to T2 or greater in patients with clinical stage T1 or less undergoing cystectomy. In a separate study, Chang et al. (2001) reported 27% of T1 tumors and 49% of T2 tumors were upstaged at cystectomy.

○   **Which pattern of prostatic invasion portends a worse prognosis: (A) direct invasion from the bladder into the prostatic stroma or (B) invasion of prostate from a noncontiguous urothelial carcinoma arising in the prostatic urethra?**

(A) A bladder tumor with direct invasion of the prostatic stroma is associated with 7% 5-year cancer-specific survival compared to a 46% 5-year cancer-specific survival for patients with urothelial carcinoma arising from the urothelium of the prostatic urethra and invading the prostatic stroma (Pagano et al., 1996).

○   **Which lymph nodes are considered regional lymph nodes in the staging of bladder cancer?**

Those that lie within the true pelvis distal to the bifurcation of the common iliac arteries.

○ **What is the distinction between N1 and N2 disease in bladder cancer?**

N1—a single positive lymph node in the true pelvis; N2—multiple lymph nodes in the true pelvis.

○ **What classifies a patient as having N3 disease?**

Positive nodes in the common iliac chain.

○ **What staging designation are patients with positive retroperitoneal lymph nodes given?**

M1.

○ **What percentage of patients with bladder cancer will develop upper tract urothelial tumors?**

A recent study from the Surveillance, Epidemiology, and End Results (SEER) database reported that 0.8% of bladder cancer patients will develop upper tract tumors (Wright et al., 2009). Patients at the highest risk for upper tract disease after bladder cancer are those with high grade, muscle-invasive, multifocal, and/or intravesical therapy refractory tumors. Thus, these patients may require more vigorous upper tract surveillance.

TREATMENT OF NONINVASIVE BLADDER CANCER

○ **What maneuvers should one take to minimize the chance for an obturator reflex when performing TURBT?**

Minimize bladder distension during resection and have the anesthesiologists establish neuromuscular blockade prior to resecting lateral bladder wall tumors. Continuous flow irrigating systems can decrease the level of bladder distension.

○ **Which type(s) of resecting energy can be used to minimize the chance of bladder perforation?**

Bipolar transurethral resection (TUR) has been reported to result in 1.7% of bladder perforation and holmium laser resection has been associated with a 0.9% incidence of perforation (Pu et al., 2008; Zhu et al., 2008).

○ **What maneuvers can be used to assist in reaching anterior wall bladder tumors with the resectoscope?**

Minimize filling of the bladder and external manual compression of the suprapubic area by the surgeon or (preferably) the assistant. Use of video imaging is also very helpful by optimizing surgeon comfort. The use of Trendelenburg positioning is also useful.

○ **How should tumors overlying the ureteral orifice be managed?**

Smaller tumors can be removed with the cold-cup biopsy forceps. However, postbiopsy fulguration should be avoided. Larger tumors should be resected with pure cutting current as this should produce minimal scarring. Complete resection/staging should not be compromised just to preserve the ureteral orifice.

○ **What are some signs of bladder perforation?**

Visible fat or peritoneal contents at the resection bed, difficult bladder filling, abdominal distension.

○ **How does one confirm a suspected bladder perforation during TURBT?**

Intraoperative cystogram.

○ **How should one manage a bladder perforation during TURBT?**

First, immediately stop the TURBT. If the perforation is extraperitoneal (as most will be), Foley catheter drainage followed by a cystogram in 1 to 2 weeks is all that should be required. The traditional management of intraperitoneal rupture has been open surgical repair of the cystotomy. However, smaller injuries with minimal extravasation of contrast can be safely managed in the same manner as extraperitoneal ruptures.

○ **What type of laser is best suited for ablation of bladder tumors? How large of a tumor can this laser effectively ablate?**

The neodymium:yttrium–aluminum–garnet (Nd:YAG) laser. This laser can ablate tumors up to 2.5 cm in greatest dimension (Jones and Larchian, 2011).

○ **What type of patient would be suitable for office ablation/fulguration of a bladder tumor?**

Small <5 mm tumor(s) with a previous tissue diagnosis of low-grade cancer with negative cytology (these findings make high-grade recurrence/progression unlikely). This option is most appropriate for older patients with multiple medical comorbidities that pose a significant surgical/anesthetic risk.

INTRAVESICAL TREATMENT OF BLADDER CANCER

○ **Name 2 intravesical immunotherapy agents.**

BCG and Interferon.

○ **Name 6 intravesical chemotherapeutic agents**

Thiotepa, mitomycin C, valrubicin, epirubicin, doxorubicin, and gemcitabine.

○ **How long should one wait before administering BCG after TURBT?**

At least 2 to 3 weeks to allow healing of the resection site and prevent systemic infection.

○ **What percentage of patients with CIS will experience a CR to intravesical BCG? To intravesical chemotherapy?**

In a meta-analysis of over 600 patients with CIS, 68% of patients receiving BCG achieved a CR while only 49% of those receiving intravesical chemotherapy achieved CR. Of these responders, 68% and 47% demonstrated a durable response to intravesical BCG and intravesical chemotherapy, respectively, at a median follow-up of 3.75 years (Sylvester et al., 2005).

○ **What should be done when a patient suffers a traumatic catheterization immediately prior to intravesical BCG instillation?**

The treatment should be postponed at least 1 week due to risk for BCG sepsis.

○ **How long should BCG stay in the bladder during a single treatment?**

2 hours.

○ **What is the main side effect of intravesical thiotepa?**

Myelosuppression from systemic absorption. Patients should undergo CBC testing prior to each instillation and treatment should be delayed for low blood cell counts (particularly thrombocytopenia and leukopenia are most common).

○ **What is the proposed mechanism by which perioperative intravesical chemotherapy has its effect?**

Perioperative chemotherapy prevents implantation of tumor cells liberated by the surgical manipulation of a bladder tumor.

○ **Which intravesical agents are safe to administer in the perioperative period?**

Chemotherapeutic agents such as mitomycin C, epirubicin, valrubicin, and gemcitabine. BCG can never be safely administered in the perioperative period due to high risk of sepsis and death.

○ **When is it *unsafe* to administer perioperative chemotherapy?**

Suspected or confirmed bladder perforation is a contraindication.

○ **What effect does a single perioperative intravesical chemotherapy treatment have on bladder cancer recurrence?**

The recurrence rate is decreased by 12% (48.4% decreased to 36.7%) (Sylvester et al., 2004).

○ **What measures can be taken to optimize the efficacy of mitomycin in delaying bladder cancer recurrence?**

Patients should be dehydrated receiving no fluids (IV or PO) for 8 hours prior to dosing. Urine should be alkalinized with 1.3 g of sodium bicarbonate taken orally the evening prior, the morning of, and 30 minutes prior to therapy. The bladder should be completely drained (confirmed with ultrasound) prior to instillation of a concentrated dose—40 mg mitomycin C in 20 mL sterile water (Au et al., 2001).

○ **Valrubicin has FDA approval for management of what type of patient? What is the complete response rate?**

Patients with BCG-refractory CIS who are medically unfit or refuse to undergo radical cystectomy. The reported complete response rate in a study of 90 patients with BCG-refractory CIS was 21% (19/90). Seven of these complete responses were durable at a median follow-up of 30 months (Steinberg et al., 2000).

○ **What are the options for treatment in a patient with BCG-refractory CIS?**

Repeat induction course of BCG, BCG and interferon combination therapy, valrubicin, and radical cystectomy.

○ **What is the most common reported side effect of intravesical BCG therapy?**

Lower urinary tract symptoms have been reported to occur in 25.7% to 97.5% of patients receiving BCG (Losa et al., 2000; van der Meijden et al., 2003).

TREATMENT OF HIGH-RISK NON-MUSCLE-INVASIVE BLADDER CANCER

○ **Explain the difference between BCG-refractory, BCG-resistant, and BCG-recurrent disease.**

BCG-refractory bladder cancer refers to disease that is either nonimproving or worsening after BCG therapy. BCG-resistant refers to persistent or recurrent disease to a lesser degree that resolves with further BCG therapy. BCG-recurrent refers to disease recurrence after initial resolution with BCG (Herr and Dalbagni, 2003; Jones and Larchian, 2011).

○ **You are seeing a patient for his 3-month follow-up after completing and induction course of BCG for CIS. His cystoscopy reveals no evidence of recurrent disease. However, his cytology is positive for high-grade urothelial malignancy. How should this patient be managed?**

While it is tempting to rebiopsy this patient to evaluate for recurrence of his CIS, it is reasonable to observe him and follow-up after 3 more months. In a study by Herr and Dalbagni (2003), the response rate in patients with history of high-grade bladder cancer treated with BCG increased from 57% at 3 months to 80% at 6 months without any further intervention (Herr and Dalbagni, 2003).

○ **You perform TURBT on a patient with no history of urothelial malignancies. The pathology reveals a high-grade Ta cancer. There is muscularis propria in the specimen, which is uninvolved. You appropriately administer a single postoperative dose of intravesical mitomycin C. What is your next step in management?**

This patient should receive at least a 6-week induction course of BCG and, preferably, maintenance BCG. Multiple single-institution studies and meta-analyses have demonstrated decreased rates of both recurrence and progression in high-risk non-muscle-invasive tumors given BCG compared to those managed with TURBT and surveillance cystoscopy alone. Notably, decreased rates of progression have only been consistently appreciated in patients receiving maintenance BCG in addition to induction (Bohle and Bock, 2004; Han and Pan, 2006; Sylvester et al., 2002).

○ **What percentage of patients with CIS of the bladder are found to have upper tract CIS? How common is prostatic urethral CIS in patients with CIS of the bladder?**

In 1 study, 34 of 148 patients (24.6%) with CIS in the bladder were found to have occult upper tract CIS (Solsona et al., 1997). Similarly, patients with CIS of the bladder have a 7-fold increased risk of prostatic urethral involvement regardless of stage (Witjes, 2004).

○ **You are managing a patient who initially presented with microscopic hematuria. He has a normal CT urogram and unremarkable clinic cystoscopy. However, his voided urine cytology is read as positive for high-grade urothelial carcinoma. How should you manage this patient?**

Cystoscopy under anesthesia with random bladder biopsies, prostatic urethral biopsy, and selective ureteral cytologies. This patient very likely has CIS. The above evaluation is aimed at localizing the CIS so that appropriate treatment can be administered.

○ **What percentage of bladder CIS diagnoses are likely missed by white light cystoscopy (WLC) alone? What newer technologies have been developed to improve cystoscopic sensitivity for detection of CIS?**

As many as 53% of CIS diagnoses may be missed by WLC (Zaak et al., 2002). Photodynamic diagnosis (PDD) and narrow band imaging (NBI) are new technologies aimed at increasing cystoscopic sensitivity for detecting CIS. Both have demonstrated increased sensitivity in detecting CIS, but more research is necessary before they are reasonably incorporated into routine surveillance for bladder tumors/CIS (Herr, 2010; Jocham et al., 2008).

○ **What are some indications for radical cystectomy in patients with clinical T1 bladder cancer?**

Persistent high-grade T1 disease at re-resection, size >3 cm, presence of micropapillary histology, and lymphovascular invasion (Herr et al., 2007; Lerner and Sternberg, 2011).

TREATMENT OF INVASIVE BLADDER CANCER

○ **What percentage of patients with muscle-invasive bladder cancer have no history of noninvasive bladder cancer?**

80% (Kaye and Lange, 1982; Vaidya et al., 2001).

○ **What is the 2-year cancer-specific survival of untreated muscle-invasive bladder cancer?**

15% (Prout and Marshall, 1956).

○ **What structures are removed when a radical cystectomy is performed in men? In women?**

In men it can also be referred to as radical cystoprostatectomy and includes en bloc removal of the urinary bladder, urachus, prostate, seminal vesicles, and perivesical fat. In women, it can also be referred to as anterior pelvic exenteration and refers to removal of the bladder, uterus, fallopian tubes, cervix, ovaries, anterior vaginal wall, and perivesical fat. Recent modifications of these techniques have led to the development of prostate-, vagina-, and ovary-sparing techniques.

○ **What is the perioperative mortality of radical cystectomy?**

2% to 3% (Hollenbeck et al., 2007; Isbarn et al., 2009; Quek et al., 2006).

○ **Several studies have demonstrated that delaying radical cystectomy more than _____ weeks is associated with worsened survival outcomes.**

12 weeks (Gore et al., 2009; Kulkarni et al., 2009; Lee et al., 2006; Sanchez-Ortiz et al., 2003).

○ **What is the 10-year disease-free survival for patients found to have organ-confined (≤pT2) disease at radical cystectomy?**

82% (Stein et al., 2001).

○ **What is the 10-year disease-free survival for T3 disease found at radical cystectomy?**

48% (Quek et al., 2004).

○ **What is the 10-year recurrence-free survival for T4 disease found at radical cystectomy?**

45% (Stein et al., 2001).

○ **What percentage of patients with organ-confined disease at cystectomy will experience a pelvic recurrence?**

6% (Stein et al., 2001).

○ **What percentage of patients with grossly positive nodes found at surgery are cured by cystectomy with lymph node dissection alone?**

Investigators at Memorial Sloan Kettering Cancer Center (MSKCC) report a 24% durable cure in these patients (Herr and Donat, 2001; Stein et al., 2001).

○ **What is the overall complication rate associated with cystectomy?**

Complications rates reported for cystectomy vary widely. This is likely due to a multitude of factors to include variations in surgeon volume, reporting systems, complication grading systems, and patient populations. However, Konety and Allareddy (2007) reported a 28.4% incidence of inpatient complications occurring in 6577 patients undergoing radical cystectomy from 1998 to 2002 in the inpatient sample. The mortality rate in this study was 2.6%.

○ **A patient is found to have high-grade muscle-invasive urothelial carcinoma on TURBT. Staging reveals a single 1.6-cm hypogastric lymph node. Percutaneous biopsy confirms this node to be positive for urothelial carcinoma. How should this patient be managed?**

This patient should receive systemic chemotherapy followed by consolidative radical cystectomy. The biggest threat to cure for this patient is extravesical and micrometastatic disease, which cannot be addressed with surgical extirpation alone. Thus, chemotherapy should be delivered first to eradicate micrometastatic disease. Following chemotherapy, local control can be achieved with radical cystectomy.

○ **You are performing a radical cystectomy on a patient who had no clinical evidence of extravesical disease on preoperative staging. Unfortunately, the patient has palpably pathologic pelvic lymph nodes. In what situation should cystectomy with extended pelvic lymph node dissection be aborted?**

Unresectable lymph node metastases, extensive periureteral tumor, a bladder which is fixed to pelvic sidewall, and/or tumor invasion of the rectosigmoid colon (Lerner and Sternberg, 2011).

○ **What is the risk of developing urethral recurrence of urothelial carcinoma in patients with prostatic stromal involvement at radical cystectomy?**

30% (Hardeman and Soloway, 1990).

○ **What potentially curative options are available to the patient with muscle-invasive disease who refuses or is medically unfit for radical cystectomy? What associated pathologic finding on TURBT would suggest that a patient is unlikely to benefit from such interventions?**

Radical TURBT, partial cystectomy, chemotherapy/radiation therapy. In general, patients with CIS are not candidates for bladder-sparing approaches to muscle-invasive bladder cancer (Herr, 2001; Holzbeierlein et al., 2004; Shipley et al., 1998; Solsona et al., 1998).

SYSTEMIC CHEMOTHERAPY FOR METASTATIC BLADDER CANCER

○ **List 2 chemotherapeutic regimens considered standard first-line therapy for patients with metastatic bladder cancer.**

Methotrexate, vinblastine, doxorubicin (Adriamycin), cisplatin—MVAC and gemcitabine, cisplatin—GC. A prospective randomized trial comparing the newer regimen (GC) to the standard regimen (MVAC) revealed the GC exhibited similar response rates and overall survival to MVAC while demonstrating better safety and tolerability (von der Maase et al., 2000).

○ **How are these regimens altered in patients with renal insufficiency? Does this have any effect on outcomes?**

Carboplatin may be substituted for cisplatin. Carboplatin is associated with inferior oncologic outcomes compared to cisplatin (De Santis et al., 2012).

○ **What is the median survival time for patients diagnosed with metastatic bladder cancer?**

1 year (Saxman et al., 1997).

○ **List some prechemotherapy characteristics associated with poorer response of metastatic bladder cancer to systemic chemotherapy.**

Karnofsky performance score <80, visceral metastases, elevated alkaline phosphatase levels, and anorexia (Bajorin et al., 1999; Roychowdhury et al., 2003).

○ **Which patients with locally advanced, primarily unresectable, or metastatic bladder cancer appear to be the best candidates for postchemotherapy consolidative cystectomy?**

Patients presenting with locally advanced disease and/or pelvic lymphadenopathy that demonstrates clinical response (decrease in size of measurable disease) have the greatest chance at durable cure from primary systemic chemotherapy followed by consolidative cystectomy. In a series reported by MSKCC, patients found to have a pathologic CR at consolidative surgery demonstrated a 41% 5-year overall survival. Those patients who were able to undergo complete resection of residual viable cancer demonstrated a 33% 5-year overall survival. Patients classified as nonresponders to chemotherapy or those with persistent viable lymphatic metastases did not appear to benefit from consolidative postchemotherapy surgery (Dodd et al., 1999; Donat et al., 1996).

○ **What percentage of patients with advanced/metastatic bladder cancer who demonstrate a major response (complete or partial) to systemic chemotherapy and forego consolidative surgery will die of bladder cancer?**

92% of patients who demonstrate a major response to systemic chemotherapy will go on to die of their disease if they do not undergo consolidative surgery (Dodd et al., 1999; Donat et al., 1996).

NEOADJUVANT AND ADJUVANT CHEMOTHERAPY FOR BLADDER CANCER

○ **What is meant by the term neoadjuvant chemotherapy in the treatment of bladder cancer?**

This refers to chemotherapy given to patients without macroscopic evidence of metastases on staging prior to cystectomy (clinical T2-4N0M0). The aim of neoadjuvant chemotherapy is to treat micrometastatic disease prior to resection of the primary tumor. This term does not refer to chemotherapy given to patients with clinical evidence of metastases.

○ **What are the theoretical advantages to administering chemotherapy in the neoadjuvant setting rather than in the adjuvant setting or waiting for clinical evidence of metastases/recurrence?**

Early administration of chemotherapy prior to gross evidence of metastases allows it to have its effect when the metastatic tumor burden is minimal. Patients are more likely to have better performance status/better able to tolerate chemotherapy prior to undergoing surgery and/or developing macroscopic metastases. There may be better drug delivery to the tumor if the vascular supply is intact. Finally, locally advanced tumors may be downstaged by neoadjuvant chemotherapy, allowing for easier complete resection.

○ **What are the theoretical *disadvantages* to neoadjuvant chemotherapy?**

A significant number of patients will receive chemotherapy without any true survival benefit (those who have chemoinsensitive tumors as well as those who have no micrometastatic disease to begin with). In patients who don't respond to chemotherapy, their definitive local therapy is delayed. Patients who suffer significant toxicity from neoadjuvant chemotherapy may be rendered unfit for cystectomy.

○ **What are the advantages to postcystectomy adjuvant chemotherapy in bladder cancer patients?**

Pathologic examination of the cystectomy and lymphadenectomy specimens allows for the most accurate determination of patients at the highest risk for metastases and/or recurrence. Definitive local therapy (cystectomy) is not delayed, which is particularly advantageous in patients with chemo-refractory tumors.

○ **What are the *disadvantages* of post-cystectomy adjuvant chemotherapy?**

Waiting for the patient to recover from surgery may allow micro-metastatic disease to progress beyond the point of curative disease. Some patients may become so deconditioned by surgery that they are unable to receive the full dose or a sufficient number of courses of chemotherapy. Postoperative scarring may compromise delivery of chemotherapy to the potential sites of residual disease.

○ **What is the absolute 5-year survival advantage associated with neoadjuvant chemotherapy followed by radical cystectomy versus cystectomy alone for patients without evidence of metastatic disease on clinical staging?**

5% (Advanced Bladder Cancer Meta-analysis Collaboration, 2003; Griffiths et al., 2011; Grossman et al., 2003; Winquist et al., 2004).

○ **What percentage of patients with muscle-invasive disease are found to have no residual tumor at cystectomy after having received neoadjuvant cisplatin-based chemotherapy? What percentage who receive no preoperative chemotherapy are found to have no residual tumor?**

Approximately 32% to 38% of patients having received neoadjuvant chemotherapy are found to have no residual tumor at cystectomy (pT0). By contrast just 12% to 15% of patients who proceed directly to cystectomy after being diagnosed with muscle invasive disease on TURBT demonstrate no evidence of residual tumor. This finding strongly correlates with improved survival outcomes with this group of patients demonstrating 85% 5-year survival (Grossman et al., 2003; International Collaboration of Trialists, 1999).

○ **Which group of patients derives greater survival benefit from neoadjuvant chemotherapy: those with locally advanced (clinical T3-4) bladder cancer or those with clinical T2 disease?**

In the Southwest Oncology Group (SWOG) 8710, Intergroup-0080 study patients with locally advanced disease who received neoadjuvant MVAC demonstrated a 20% improvement in 5-year survival compared to those who did not receive neoadjuvant chemotherapy. By contrast, those with clinical stage T2 bladder cancer who received neoadjuvant chemotherapy demonstrated a 5% increase in 5-year survival compared to those who did not receive neoadjuvant chemotherapy (Grossman et al., 2003).

○ **How does the presence of variant histologies mixed at TURBT affect the decision to administer neoadjuvant chemotherapy versus proceeding directly to radical cystectomy?**

The answer to this question depends on the type of variant histology encountered. The interplay of most variant histologies and chemotherapy has not been examined as most are rare and/or very recently described in the literature. Investigators at MD Anderson Cancer Center reported worsened survival outcomes in patients with micropapillary urothelial carcinoma receiving neoadjuvant chemotherapy compared to those who proceeded directly to cystectomy (Kamat et al., 2007). Thus, the micropapillary variant appears chemoresistant and administering chemotherapy may just provide a localized tumor more time to metastasize. Conversely, a secondary analysis of the SWOG 8710 trail of neoadjuvant MVAC suggested that compared to patients with pure urothelial carcinoma, patients with urothelial carcinoma mixed with glandular or squamous cell components enjoyed a greater survival benefit from neoadjuvant chemotherapy (Scosyrev and Messing, 2011).

○ **Summarize the evidence for use of post-cystectomy adjuvant chemotherapy in high-risk patients.**

There is a paucity of prospective randomized trials evaluating the efficacy of adjuvant chemotherapy after cystectomy revealing high-risk bladder cancer (generally, pT3-4 and/or N+ disease). Available trials are compromised by major methodological flaws to include patients not receiving allocated treatments, early trial stoppage, and control arm patients not receiving salvage chemotherapy for disease recurrence. A meta-analysis including 491 patients from 6 prospective trials reported a 9% absolute risk reduction of death from cancer at 3 years. However, the author acknowledged that these data were not sufficient to base clinical recommendations on due to the problems listed above (Advanced Bladder Cancer (ABC) Meta-analysis Collaboration, 2005).

LYMPHADENECTOMY IN THE TREATMENT OF BLADDER CANCER

○ **What is the 5-year cancer-specific survival for patients found to have regional lymphatic metastases at radical cystectomy?**

Approximately 30% (Mills et al., 2001; Stein et al., 2003; Vieweg et al., 1999).

○ **What percentage of patients undergoing cystectomy for clinically organ-confined disease are found to have positive lymph nodes at cystectomy?**

Approximately 25% to 30% (Morgan et al., 2012).

○ **What is the pattern of lymphatic spread from a primary bladder cancer?**

Three successive levels of lymphatic metastases have been described. Level I nodes include the external iliac, hypogastric, obturator, and deep obturator lymph nodes. Level II includes the common iliac, presacral, and presciatic lymph nodes. Level III includes paraaortic, interaortocaval, and paracaval lymph nodes. To put these levels in the perspective of TNM staging, N1 and N2 lesions refer to level I lymphatic metastases, N3 refers to level II nodes, and level III nodal metastases are classified as M1. Lymph node metastases are more common in the lower levels and skip lesions to higher levels are rare. Interestingly, tumor laterality does not correlate reliably with laterality of lymphatic spread (Leissner et al., 2004; Morgan et al., 2012).

○ **What is meant by standard pelvic lymph node dissection, extended pelvic lymph node dissection, and superextended lymph node dissection?**

While a uniform consensus on the meanings of these terms has not been established, in general, a standard pelvic lymph node dissection includes removal of level 1 nodes. An extended pelvic lymph node dissection refers to removal of level I and II nodes. A super-extended pelvic lymph node dissection includes removal of level I, II, and III nodes.

○ **Does a more aggressive lymph node dissection correlate with improved survival?**

This is a very controversial topic. Several studies have reported improved survival outcomes with higher lymph node counts (Konety et al., 2003; Leissner et al., 2000; May et al., 2011). However, lymph node counts within the same template have been demonstrated to vary widely among different institutions and pathologists (Dorin et al., 2011). Thus, many experts believe that the actual extent and thoroughness of the template are more important than the number of nodes counted by the pathologist. Several investigators have demonstrated improved survival and recurrence outcomes when comparing extended and super-extended templates to standard pelvic lymphadenectomy (Abol-Enein et al., 2011; Dhar et al., 2008). However, in a recent study, no improvement in survival or recurrence outcomes was demonstrated for patients undergoing a super-extended lymph node dissection as compared to an extended lymph node dissection (Zehnder et al., 2011).

○ **When examining only patients with pathologic N0 disease, how can one explain the improved survival demonstrated by patients with higher node counts?**

This is most likely an artifact of improved staging. That is, when a more limited node dissection is performed, despite negative nodes being removed, there may be a greater chance of positive nodes being left behind. Those patients who undergo more extensive dissections and have only negative nodes on pathologic examination are more likely to be truly N0 and, thus, demonstrate improved survival.

○ **What is meant by "lymph node density (LND)?" What lymph node density number has been used as a cutoff to stratify lymph node positive bladder cancer patients into good and poor prognostic groups?**

LND is calculated by dividing the number of positive lymph nodes by the total number of nodes removed and multiplying by 100%. Patients with less than 20% positive lymph nodes have demonstrated improved disease-free and disease-specific survival compared to those with greater than 20% positive lymph nodes. Investigators have reported improved prognostic performance of LND compared to the stand N classification of the 1997 TNM staging system (Herr, 2003; Stein et al., 2003).

CHAPTER 53

Laparoscopic and Robotic Urologic Surgery

Chad A. LaGrange, MD, FACS and Justin D. Johnson, MD

○ **What are some general benefits of laparoscopic surgery compared to traditional open surgery?**

Postoperative pain control requirements are approximately 4 times less than with traditional open incisions. Hospital stays have been decreased by 50%, and the time to full convalescence has been reported to be markedly less than with open removal. The laparoscopic approach has been shown to have less blood loss, shorter hospital stay, lower analgesic requirement, and shorter convalescence compared to traditional surgery.

○ **What are the absolute contraindications to perform laparoscopy?**

Any contraindication that would preclude surgery by another approach (ie, severe uncompensated cardiopulmonary disease or uncorrected coagulopathy), significant abdominal wall infection, generalized peritonitis, suspected malignant ascites, massive hemoperitoneum or hemoretroperitoneum, and intestinal obstruction unless intention is to treat at the same time.

○ **What is the standard gas used for insufflation during laparoscopy and what properties of this gas make it the gas of choice?**

Carbon dioxide (CO_2) because it is colorless, odorless, nonflammable, and a readily available gas that is rapidly absorbed into the systemic circulation and quickly eliminated by the lungs.

○ **What is the standard insufflation (intrabdominal) pressure (IAP) and why was this particular pressure selected?**

- Fifteen (15) mm Hg is the standard insufflation pressure.
- Studies have shown cardiopulmonary, renal, and splanchnic effects are minimal and still reversible at an insufflation pressure of ≤ 15 mm Hg.

○ **Can insufflation pressures ever be safely increased higher than 15 mm Hg? If so, what are the indications?**

- Brief increases in intra-abdominal pressure, up to 20 mm Hg, are tolerable for most patients.
- Briefly increasing intra-abdominal pressure can be a helpful maneuver to control intraoperative venous oozing. Central venous pressures range from −1 to 5 cm H_2O and the tamponade effect provided by a slightly higher IAP can yield better visualization by providing a clearer operative field in times of bleeding. Once hemostasis has been achieved, intra-abdominal pressure should be returned to 15 mm Hg.

583

○ **What are the cardiovascular effects of increased intra-abdominal pressure from pneumoperitoneum?**

- Increased preload from increased venous return to the heart with initial increased intra-abdominal pressure. This leads to increased cardiac output, increased stroke volume, and increased mean arterial pressure.
- With continued increased intra-abdominal pressure the venous return to the heart decreases, along with increased arterial resistance, that causes a decreased stroke volume with resultant increased heart rate.
- The overall physiologic response is that there is no clinically significant change in cardiac output—assuming normovolemia and intra-abdominal pressure ≤15 mm Hg.

○ **Immediately upon peritoneal insufflation and prior to any operative steps, the anesthesiologist notes severe bradycardia and hypotension. What is the most likely cause and treatment?**

The most likely cause is vagal stimulation due to abrupt peritoneal stretching. Immediate treatment is to desufflate the abdomen. Anesthesia can give atropine-like agents to reverse the bradycardia.

○ **Can pneumoperitoneum cause cardiac arrhythmias?**

- Carbon dioxide can elicit a sympathetic response, thus leading to tachycardia, vasoconstriction (via stimulation of the renin–angiotensin pathway), and potentially a cardiac arrhythmia.
- The above processes are exacerbated by acidosis.

○ **What are the pulmonary effects of pneumoperitoneum?**

- There are mechanical and metabolic effects.
- Mechanical: Increased intra-abdominal pressures have direct influence on the thoracic cavity by impairing diaphragmatic movement, increasing intrathoracic pressures, and decreasing respiratory compliance. This leads to an increase in airway pressures and a decrease in vital capacity.
- Metabolic: CO_2 absorption leads to hypercarbia and acidosis.

○ **What are the risks of laparoscopy on a patient with chronic obstructive pulmonary disease (COPD)?**

Severe hypercarbia, due to baseline impairment of CO_2 elimination in patients with COPD.

○ **How should CO_2 levels be monitored intraoperatively on patients with pulmonary compromise?**

Arterial CO_2 levels should be checked every 1 to 2 hours. Expired CO_2 levels are unreliable in the presence of COPD due to the diffusion barrier. Arterial blood gas sampling should be continued postoperatively due to continued risk of hypercarbia after extubation due to subsequent mobilization of procedurally absorbed CO_2.

○ **If hypercarbia develops intraoperatively, what steps can be performed to correct the problem?**

Lowering insufflation pressures from 15 mm Hg to just 10 to 12 mm Hg may be helpful. If this fails to correct the hypercarbia, then the insufflation gas should be changed to helium or more likely the surgery should be converted to an open procedure.

○ **What are the renal effects of pneumoperitoneum?**

Impaired glomerular filtration rate, creatinine clearance, sodium excretion, and decreased urine output. There is no permanent renal impairment and all of these problems are reversible with desufflation.

○ **What are the potential factors that cause this transient oliguria?**

Decreased renal blood flow due to direct compression of the renal vasculature and inferior vena cava from the increased intra-abdominal pressure and direct renal parenchymal compression.

○ **Should the oliguria during laparoscopic cases be managed initially with increased intravenous fluids?**

Since the oliguria is transient, the patient should not be over-hydrated as this can lead to fluid overload, CHF, and respiratory compromise.

○ **For prolonged laparoscopic cases, how can the oliguria be addressed to maintain adequate urine output?**

Pharmacologic modalities can be used to prevent intraoperative oliguria:

• Furosemide (Lasix) (mg dose = 20 times the patient's creatinine).
• Mannitol (12.5-25 g).
• Dopamine at 2 μg/kg/min.

○ **What are the splanchnic effects of pnuemoperitoneum?**

• Decreased blood flow has been reported in abdominal organs including the liver, pancreas, stomach, spleen, small intestine, and the colon.
• Delayed mesenteric thrombosis has also been reported, but is not a common complication of laparoscopic surgery.

○ **Is pregnancy a contraindication to laparoscopy?**

No, pregnancy is no longer considered a contraindication to laparoscopy.

○ **What are the preferred sites of laparoscopic access for pregnant patients and should any special technique or approach be used?**

Access should be gained by the Hasson technique in the left or right upper quadrant in the subcostal midclavicular line above the uterine fundus.

○ **Are there any changes needed in insufflation pressures for pregnant patients and what levels would be considered potentially dangerous?**

Insufflation pressures should be kept as low as possible but still allow for adequate visualization and operative space. IAPs >20 mm Hg have significant cardiopulmonary risks to mother and fetus.

○ **Is obesity a contraindication to laparoscopic surgery?**

No, obesity is not considered a contraindication to laparoscopy.

○ **Are prior abdominal surgeries and/or intra-abdominal adhesions contraindications to laparoscopy?**

• No, laparoscopy has been shown to be a safe method for lysis of intra-abdominal adhesions with significantly fewer wound complications with faster convalescence and return of bowel function than open lysis of adhesions.
• Primary intra-abdominal access should be gained at an area away from prior incisions, which have the greatest likelihood of underlying adhesions.
• The Hasson technique should be used to gain intra-abdominal access if it is felt that access cannot be gained safely with the Veress needle.

○   **What is the primary disadvantage of smaller diameter lenses?**

Smaller diameter = Less light transmission (darker image). A darker image may be worsened with blood in the operative field as blood absorbs light.

○   **Where should the laparoscopic tower (insufflator, camera box, and light source) be positioned relative to the surgeon?**

- All components should be in the surgeon's line of view.
- This allows the surgeon to have the ability to assess any equipment-related problems.

○   **Where should the monitor(s) with the laparoscopic images be positioned relative to the surgeon?**

- In the surgeon's direct line of vision at a comfortable distance.
- The monitor should be slightly below eye level and at a slight angle toward the surgeon—most ergonomic position and minimizes neck strain.

○   **If additional monitors are available, where should they be positioned?**

Additional monitors should be placed opposite the assistant if the surgeon and assistant are on opposite sides of the table. Extra monitors can also be placed opposite the surgical scrub technician to allow him/her to anticipate the surgeon's needs and assist more efficiently.

○   **What is a Veress needle and how does it work?**

- A Veress needle is a needle that contains a spring-loaded superficial protective sheath.
- The sheath retracts as the needle is advanced through tissue exposing the needle tip.
- Once the needle enters the peritoneal cavity, and the majority of the resistance on the needle is released, the sheath springs forward and covers the needle.
- When the sheath covers the needle tip, it protects the intra-abdominal organs from being injured by the sharp end of the needle.

○   **Describe the correct technique for gaining laparoscopic access when using the Veress needle.**

- Examination of the Veress needle sheath to ensure it retracts.
- Flushing of the Veress needle to ensure it is patent.
- Pass the Veress needle through abdominal wall with gentle constant pressure.
- Irrigate the needle with saline, aspirate to look for blood, allow a drop of saline to drain by gravity through the needle ("drop test").
- Connect the needle to CO_2 insufflation.
- Once the intra-abdominal pressure reaches 15 mm Hg, withdraw the Veress needle.
- Insert the primary trocar followed by the laparoscope and inspect the abdomen for potential organ and/or vascular injury.

○   **What should be the initial opening pressures of the intraperitoneal space?**

<10 mm Hg, usually 5 to 7 mm Hg.

○   **How many clicks should be felt and/or heard when passing the Veress needle through the abdominal wall and what does each click represent?**

Two clicks is optimal representing the abdominal wall fascia and the parietal peritoneum.

○ **What does the "drop test" represent?**

Confirmation that the distal tip of the Veress needle is within a low-pressure space.

○ **Describe how to perform the "drop test" after the Veress needle has been passed through the abdominal wall.**

- Attach a saline-filled syringe to the Veress needle.
- Aspiration of the needle to confirm no blood, cloudy aspirate, etc.
- Irrigation into the Veress needle of 1 to 2 mL of saline.
- Repeat aspiration of the needle again. No fluid should aspirate.
- Gently advance the needle 0.5 cm. No resistance should be felt.
- Remove the syringe from the needle.
- Fluid within the needle should drop rapidly into the abdominal cavity.

○ **When insufflating through the Veress needle, should you use low-flow or high-flow and explain why.**

- High-flow should be used.
- The size of the Veress needle limits flow to 1.5 to 2 L/min, so low-flow is not needed.

○ **If initial insufflation pressures are greater than 10 mm Hg, what is the next step?**

- The Veress needle should be withdrawn slightly (generally means that it's in the mesentery or omentum).
- If the insufflation pressure drops to <10 mm Hg, continue insufflation as this indicates that the needle tip was against an intra-abdominal structure.
- If the pressure remains ≥10 mm Hg, the needle is not properly placed and should be removed and the above algorithm for initial insertion repeated.

○ **Describe the Hasson technique for gaining laparoscopic access.**

- A small skin incision is made at the planned trocar location.
- Dissection to fascia is performed.
- Fascia is opened under direct vision.
- Peritoneum is identified and a 12-mm open peritonotomy is created.
- Trocar is placed through peritonotomy.

○ **How are Hasson trocars different from conventional trocars?**

The Hasson trocar may have points on the trocar for securing fascial sutures or a retention balloon at the tip to prevent dislodgement. It may also have an adjustable foam collar externally to prevent insufflation gas leakage.

○ **What are the indications for the Hasson technique?**

Children, very thin patients, pregnant women, patients with previous abdominal incisions who are likely to have extensive adhesions, and patients with a distorted anatomy where the spine and great vessels are near the desired primary access site.

○ **What is an optical trocar and what is its purpose?**

Optical trocars have a translucent dilating tip and accommodate a camera so that the trocar can be advanced through the abdominal wall layers under direct vision.

○ **Can and should direct optical trocar insertion be performed *without* pneumoperitoneum?**

- Direct insertion of an optical trocar without prior creation of pneumoperitoneum has been reported.
- However, this technique is discouraged because it is associated with a significantly greater risk of access-related complications.

○ **To which trocar should the insufflation tubing be connected?**

Insufflation tubing should be connected on any trocar *except* the camera trocar. This will minimize the cooling effect and will result in less lens fogging.

○ **What is the risk of trocars when placed through the rectus muscles?**

- Placement of trocars through the rectus muscle potentially could damage the epigastric vessels.
- Lateral trocars should be placed at least 6 cm lateral to the midline to prevent epigastric injury.

○ **What are the most common causes of a gas embolism and how is it recognized?**

- A gas embolism is often caused by direct insufflation of a blood vessel with the Veress needle or via prompt absorption of a large volume of CO_2 after large vessel injury at the time of raised intra-abdominal pressure.
- The most common presentation is sudden hypotension, elevated end-tidal CO_2, cyanosis, and a "mill wheel" murmur at the right ventricular area.
- This is the most serious pulmonary complication that can result in rapid cardiovascular collapse and death.

○ **If a gas embolism is suspected, what are the appropriate steps in intervention?**

- To prevent the gas embolus from entering the right ventricular outflow into the pulmonary vasculature:
  ○ Immediately release the pneumoperitoneum.
  ○ Patient should be positioned in the left lateral decubitus (right side up), head-down position. (This forces the air embolus into the apex of the right ventricle.)
  ○ Anesthesia should increase minute ventilation (hyperventilation) with 100% O_2 administration.
  ○ Central venous line placement may be performed in an attempt to aspirate the gas.
  ○ Cardiopulmonary resuscitation, as necessary.

○ **How should the patient be prepared for laparoscopic surgery after anesthesia induced ? (What tubes should be placed?)**

A bladder catheter and a gastric tube are placed for decompression of the bladder and stomach during insufflation, trocar placement, and dissection to prevent injury to a distended bladder or stomach.

○ **During robotic surgery, it is important that anesthesia maintains deep sedation and paralysis. Why?**

The robotic system is "docked" to the patient and immobile. If the patient moves or begins breathing or coughing, inadvertent organ injury can occur due to violent movement of the robotic instruments or movement of the patient with robotic arms fixed in place.

○ **How do you determine which port sites should be formally closed and how should this be done?**

- As a general rule, all midline ports ≥10 mm and all nonmidline ports ≥12 mm should have the fascia closed.
- In thin patients, the fascia is easily seen and a single figure-of-eight suture will suffice. In more obese patients, the Carter-Thomason (Inlet Medical, Eden Prairie, MN) device can be used to place 1 to 2 simple sutures through the fascia under direct vision.

○ **What is the presenting sign of a trocar site hernia?**

A bulge at the trocar site; independent of signs of small bowel obstruction.

○ **Shoulder pain, specifically in the area of the scapula, can be caused from?**
- Diaphragmatic irritation due to residual pneumoperitoneum.
- If associated with a sensory or motor deficit, then it could be related to neuromuscular injury from inappropriate positioning.

○ **What is the most effective way to prevent neuromuscular injuries?**

Proper positioning and padding.

○ **How do most neuromuscular injuries present?**

Paresthesias and weakness in the affected extremity.

○ **What is the general course of neuromuscular injuries?**
- Mild injuries frequently resolve over a few weeks and may benefit from physical therapy.
- Severe injuries may result in permanent neurological dysfunction.

○ **During renal surgery, what can be done during positioning to decrease the risk of a brachial plexus injury?**

Placement of an axillary roll significantly reduces the risk of brachial plexus injuries. The upper arm should not be abducted more than 90° and should not be externally rotated as this can cause the head of the humerus to impinge upon the brachial plexus.

○ **How can peroneal nerve injuries be prevented for patients in the lithotomy position?**
- Proper padding of the lateral surface of the leg.
- Ensuring that the weight of the lower leg rests upon the heel rather than the lateral surface of the leg.

○ **What are the risk factors for rhabdomyolysis during surgery?**
- Prolonged operative time, especially in lithotomy or flank positions.
- Increased body weight (particularly large muscular patients).
- Use of the kidney rest.
- Male gender.

○ **What are the presenting symptoms of rhabdomyolysis?**

Acute muscular pain immediately postoperatively along with "tea-colored" urine—due to the presence of myoglobinuria.

○ **What is the classic presentation of myoglobinuria on urinalysis—dipstick and microscopy?**

Positive urinary dipstick analysis for blood in the absence of red blood cells on microscopy.

○ **What are other possible presenting clinical scenarios with rhabdomyolysis?**
- Compartment syndrome: General, vascular, or orthopedic surgery consultation is warranted for possible fasciotomy.
- Acute renal failure: Treatment includes hydration, diuretics, alkalinization, and potentially dialysis.

○   **What is the risk of major vascular injury during laparoscopic surgery?**

Only 0.05% of all laparoscopic cases.

○   **What is the mortality rate of a major vascular injury during laparoscopic surgery?**

8%. Major vascular injuries account for 81% of all deaths associated with laparoscopy.

○   **At what point during laparoscopic surgeries do most major vascular injuries occur?**

- Approximately 75% occur while obtaining access.
- The remaining 25% occur during dissection.

○   **Does the Hasson (open) laparoscopic access technique eliminate the risk of a major vascular injury?**

No.

○   **If blood is aspirated from the Veress needle during placement or if blood is filling a trocar, what are the next steps in management?**

- The needle or trocar should not be insufflated as this may cause CO_2 embolization.
- The surgeon should resist the temptation to remove the needle or trocar as it can be used to help identify the site of injury once proper laparoscopic access has been successfully gained or the procedure converted to open.

○   **How do major vascular injuries from the Veress needle and trocar differ in management?**

- Vascular injury caused by trocar placement should be treated by an open exploration, which is usually best performed via a midline laparotomy incision.
- Vascular injury from the Veress needle may be able to managed laparoscopically.

○   **Where is the most common site of vessel injury with the blind Veress needle insertion?**

The vessel most prone to injury is the right common iliac artery as it crosses midline at the level of the umbilicus.

○   **What is the incidence of bowel injury in laparoscopic cases?**

0.13% to 0.9%.

○   **What percentage of bowel injuries are due to cautery?**

50%.

○   **Of the bowel injuries, what percentage are recognized intraoperatively?**

33%.

○   **What are the presenting symptoms of a bowel injury secondary to laparoscopic surgery?**

Single trocar-site pain, low-grade fever, abdominal distention, diarrhea, and leukopenia. Generalized peritoneal signs may be *absent*.

○ **If a bowel injury is suspected, what test(s) should be ordered?**

CT of abdomen/pelvis with oral contrast. If it does not demonstrate signs of a bowel injury such as a gross leak or thickening of the bowel, a delayed film obtained 6 hours later increases the probability of identifying a site of bowel perforation.

○ **What is the mortality rate for laparoscopic bowel injuries?**

3.6%.

○ **How should recognized bowel injuries due to a Veress needle be managed?**

Most can be managed with a oversewing if the injury is recognized intraoperatively.

○ **How should a bowel injury due to trocar placement be managed?**

A trocar injury to the bowel requires formal repair. General surgery consultation is recommended and wise.

○ **How should a cautery/thermal bowel injury be managed?**

If the injury is not full thickness, it may be treated with interrupted sutures. These patients should be monitored closely postoperatively because energy-based injuries may result in delayed perforation of the bowels. Full thickness bowel injuries should be treated with resection and formal repair.

○ **Is conversion to an open approach considered a laparoscopic complication?**

No, but failing to recognize the need to convert to an open procedure could lead to a complication!

○ **What should be expected if the initial aspiration of the Veress needle has colored or malodorous fluid?**

An injury to the colon, stomach, or bladder.

○ **How is an injury to the gallbladder managed?**

Most injuries to the gallbladder require cholecystectomy because even a small perforation in the gall bladder may result in a bile leak and peritonitis.

○ **What is the operating room setup for a laparoscopic prostatectomy?**

- The surgeon typically stands on the patient's left side.
- The assistant stands on the patient's right side.
- A single monitor is placed between the patient's legs or at the foot of the bed.

○ **What is the chance of rectal injury with laparoscopic and robotic-assisted laparoscopic prostatectomies?**

- Laparoscopic radical prostatectomy: 0.7%.
- Robot-assisted radical prostatectomy: 2.4%.

○ **If an intraoperative rectal injury is noted *without* gross fecal spillage, what is the recommended management?**

- Area of rectal injury can be closed primarily in 2 layers with interposition of omentum between the rectum and anastomosis, which can usually avoid long-term problems.
- Closed suction drain must be placed near the repair and the patient's antibiotic coverage must be broadened for several days.
- Stool softeners and low-residue diet are given postoperatively.

○ **How do the recommendations change if there is gross fecal contamination noted during laparoscopic surgery?**

Requires open conversion and a diverting colostomy

○ **If a small rectal injury is suspected but not identifiable, how can you potentially identify the site of injury?**

Insufflation of air through a catheter inserted into the rectum with irrigation fluid filling pelvis may exhibit small bubbles at the site of the injury.

○ **During laparoscopic radical prostatectomy what is the open conversion rate?**

<2%.

○ **If the patient develops a postoperative deep venous thrombosis in the lower extremities, what other problem should you be worried about?**

Possible lymphocele, hematoma, or urinoma that could be compressing the external iliac vein.

○ **What are the steps used to gain access when performing an extraperitoneal approach for laparoscopic radical prostatectomy?**

- A 1.5-cm umbilical incision is carried out down through the anterior rectus sheath.
- Blunt finger dissection is performed to create a space anterior to the posterior rectus sheath and the underlying peritoneum.
- A trocar-mounted balloon dilator device is inserted into the preperitoneal space anterior to the posterior rectus sheath.
- Balloon dilator is advanced down to the pubis along the midline.
- Approximately 500 mL of air is inflated to develop the space of Retzius under laparoscopic view.
- The operative steps then proceed just as the transperitoneal approach.

○ **Is there a difference in operative time or perioperative outcomes between transperitoneal and extraperitoneal approaches of laparoscopic radical prostatectomy?**

None significant.

○ **What are the benefits of utilizing an extraperitoneal approach for laparoscopic radical prostatectomy?**

- The peritoneum acts as a natural barrier—minimizing the potential for bowel injury and preventing the bowels from falling into the operative field and obscuring the surgeon's view.
- This can confine any urine leak that may occur from the vesicourethral anastomosis within the extraperitoneal space.

○ **What are the limitations of the extraperitoneal approach for laparoscopic radical prostatectomy?**

- Reduced working space (compared with the entire peritoneal cavity when using transperitoneal access).
- Higher CO_2 absorption compared to transperitoneal insufflation, which may require a higher ventilator minute volume to resolve the hypercarbia and acidosis.

○ **Why do patients with a prior history of laparoscopic inguinal hernia repair, potentially represent difficult laparoscopic radical prostatectomy cases?**

A prior history of laparoscopic extraperitoneal mesh herniorrhaphy obliterates the space of Retzius, which is the working space during radical prostatectomy.

○ **Laparoscopic radical prostatectomies are performed with patients in the Trendelenburg position. What are the risks to the eyes while in this position and how can they be prevented?**

- Corneal abrasion—the anesthesiologist should maintain good eye lubrication and protection.
- Increased intraocular pressure—does not appear to have any apparent clinical long-term consequence.

○ **What other patient safety risks are present from an extreme Trendelenburg position during laparoscopic or robotic prostatectomy?**

- Brachial plexus neuropraxia due to compression on the shoulders without proper padding.
- Patients not properly secured may slide off bed!

○ **During a pelvic lymph node dissection, if a small venotomy or arteriotomy is encountered how is it managed?**

- Most can be closed laparoscopically with a fine polypropylene (Prolene) suture.
- A major vascular injury may require conversion to an open approach.

○ **Does a transperitoneal approach to pelvic lymph node dissection preclude pelvic lymphocele formation?**

No.

○ **How do symptomatic pelvic lymphoceles present?**

Infection, pain, lower extremity swelling, fever, or DVT.

○ **What is the management algorithm for symptomatic pelvic lymphoceles?**

Early percutaneous drainage should be done for any infected or symptomatic lymphoceles, followed by aspiration, sclerosis and eventually more formal management techniques if refractory, such as laparoscopic or open marsupialization into the peritoneal cavity.

○ **What are the indications for laparoscopic adrenalectomy?**

AM, adrenal mass, without radiographic evidence of local invasion.

○ **What are the contraindications to laparoscopic adrenalectomy?**

Known adrenal vein or vena caval involvement. Large tumors, especially large pheochromocytomas or suspected adrenal cancers, may be more safely managed via open adrenalectomy.

○ **What is the most common complication of a laparoscopic adrenalectomy?**

Bleeding (4.7%).

○ **What are the surgeon and assistant locations for laparoscopic renal surgery?**

- For transperitoneal approach renal laparoscopic cases—the ventral aspect of the patient.
- For retroperitoneal approach renal laparoscopic cases—the dorsal aspect of the patient.

○ **Is more carbon dioxide absorbed during transperitoneal or retroperitoneal laparoscopic access?**

Retroperitoneal.

○ **How is the patient positioned when performing transperitoneal renal surgery?**

- 30° to 45° flank position.
- Table break should be at the level of the anterior superior iliac spine and the table is angled at the hip to accentuate the distance between the 12th rib and the iliac crest, thus maximizing the distance to allow for adequate distance between ports.
  - Extreme-flexion of the table should be avoided as it may limit the expansion of the abdominal wall, thus limiting the working space during the procedure.
- The patient's ventral surface should be on the edge of the table to allow the surgeon to drop his/her instruments when gaining access to the most lateral/anterior aspects of the surgical field.
- Patient's dependent leg should be flexed at the knee and hip with the top leg extended and padded.

○ **What are the indications to perform retroperitoneal renal surgery?**

- Same as for open retroperitoneal surgery.
- May be preferred for selected cases of laparoscopic partial nephrectomy for posterior tumors, renal cyst marsupialization, pyeloplasty, biopsy, or in patients with prior peritonitis or history of multiple abdominal surgeries.

○ **What is the positioning of the patient for retroperitoneal renal surgery?**

- Full-flank position with an axillary roll and arms secured on pillows or armrest.
- Table flexion can help increase the distance between the 12th rib and iliac crest to allow for better trocar placement.

○ **What are the limitations of performing retroperitoneal renal surgery?**

- Limited working space and more subtle anatomic landmarks.
- The smaller working space limits the distance between trocars, potentially leading to awkward hand positioning.

○ **If additional operating space is needed what options does the surgeon have?**

The retroperitoneal access can be expanded to a transperitoneal approach through opening the peritoneum under direct vision.

○ **A small hole is made in the peritoneum during a retroperitoneoscopic nephrectomy. This leads to collapse of the retroperitoneal space and poor visualization. What can the surgeon do to re-expand the retroperitoneal space?**

An 18-gauge angiocath can be placed through the abdominal wall into the peritoneal cavity to vent the trapped gas out of the peritoneal cavity and equalize retroperitoneal and intraperitoneal insufflation pressures.

○ **What are the advantages of hand-assisted laparoscopic renal surgeries?**

- Offers a link between open surgery and laparoscopy.
- Allows for concurrent tactile feedback.
- Can simplify surgical dissection in patients with significant scarring around the kidney.
- Can be used in the event of bleeding by extending a trocar site and placing a hand port.

○ **What is the incidence of hernia at the hand-port site and when do they most commonly present?**

4%. Hernias usually present 3 months or more postoperatively.

○ **What are the indications for laparoscopic renal or ureteral stone extraction?**

- Indications for laparoscopic stone extraction may vary, but primarily include patients with renal stones who are undergoing simultaneous laparoscopic pyeloplasty. Patients should always undergo a complete nephroscopy to ensure stone clearance.
- Other patients who may benefit include those with unusual anatomy (pelvic kidney), stones resistant to fragmentation, and failed extracorporeal shock wave lithotripsy (ESWL), ureteroscopy, or percutaneous procedures.

○ **During laparoscopic (including robot-assisted) partial nephrectomy, what are the options to assist in tumor localization?**

Laparoscopic ultrasonography and Fluorescence imaging (Firefly™) with the da Vinci Si Surgical System.

○ **When the collecting system has been entered during partial nephrectomy there is a risk of urine leakage postoperatively. When do most urine leaks present?**

About 1 week postoperatively. That's why some surgeons recommend keeping postoperative drains for 7 to 10 days.

○ **How do you confirm a urine leak after partial nephrectomy?**

- Check drainage fluid for creatinine, which would be significantly higher in urine than serum creatinine.
- Check drainage fluid color for blue after administration of intravenous indigo carmine.

○ **If a urine leak is suspected and the patient does not have a drain, what is the next step?**

- Intravenous or retrograde pyelogram.
- Imaging will also rule out ureteral obstruction (ie, blood clot).

○ **What is the treatment for renal leaks/fistulas after laparoscopic/robotic partial nephrectomy?**

- Ureteral stent or less commonly a percutaneous nephrostomy tube to allow upper tract drainage.
- Foley catheter to allow the collecting system to remain at low pressure.
- Retroperitoneal closed system drain if the patient is symptomatic or drainage is infected.

○ **A patient continues to have high urine output from the perinephric drain after the above measures have been performed. What is the next step?**

After initial drainage and management, gradually retract drain away from the area of leakage to prevent suction of urine through the defect. Output usually decreases over several days.

○ **With conservative management, what is the usual outcome of urinary fistulas?**

Most urine leaks resolve within 1 month and rarely require reoperation.

○ **Postoperative (delayed) bleeding can occur after a partial nephrectomy. How is it managed?**

- Initial management is conservative; including thorough clinical monitoring, being placed on bed rest, and frequent checks of blood counts.
- More serious bleeding, indicated by the requirement of less than two units of transfused blood, is an indication for angioembolization to be attempted.
- If a life-threatening hemorrhage is suspected, then complete angioinfarction of the kidney or reoperative exploration may be required.

LAPAROSCOPY IN CHILDREN

○ **How does gaining laparoscopic access differ in children versus adults?**

- Children have a shorter distance between the anterior abdominal wall and the great vessels and the organs.
- Making a small paraumbilical incision first allows the insufflating needle to be passed by direct observation.
- If the Veress needle is used, it requires less pressure because the child's fascia is less resistant.

○ **Why is it particularly important to place an orogastric tube and a urinary catheter prior to gaining laparoscopic access in children?**

- The urinary bladder is intra-abdominal.
- Children have increased tendency to swallow air, thus their stomachs are pushed more inferior.
- Both the urinary bladder and the stomach are at increased risk of injury during gaining laparoscopic access unless they are decompressed.

Urological Grab Bag Challenge

Stephen W. Leslie, MD, FACS

○ **What is the most common cause of urinary retention in pregnancy and at what gestational age is it most likely to occur?**

An impacted retroverted uterus is the most common cause of urinary retention in pregnancy. Most of these cases will present at approximately 16-week gestational age.

○ **The bladder may become palpable if it holds what minimum amount of urine?**

Usually, the bladder is palpable if it contains at least 200 mL of urine. It can be percussed if it is holding at least 150 mL of urine.

○ **True/False: Acute urinary retention can raise PSA levels.**

True, so do not bother checking the PSA level in situations of acute urinary retention.

○ **What is the clinical significance of "atypical small acinar proliferation" on a prostate biopsy and how often is it found?**

It represents approximately 2% of cases and has a 60% chance of developing into prostate cancer.

○ **What percentage of low-risk prostate cancer patients with focal or localized disease who undergo saturation prostatic biopsies are ultimately found to have significantly higher Gleason scores or previously undetected contralateral cancer?**

Nineteen percent would have their Gleason scores upgraded and approximately 30% will have contralateral disease.

○ **True/False: The bladder should always be emptied rapidly and completely, without clamping the Foley catheter, in cases of acute urinary retention even when the volume is well over 1000 mL.**

True. There is no benefit and possibly some harm if the catheter is clamped.

○ **α-Adrenergic blockers are often started immediately after placing a catheter for acute urinary retention. What is the recommended optimal duration of α-blocker therapy before removing the catheter for a voiding trial after an episode of acute retention?**

Three days appears to be the reasonable minimum time period to wait for the α-blocker therapy to be effective before catheter removal in most cases of acute retention.

○ **Is mumps orchitis more common in prepubertal or postpubertal boys and what percentage of boys with mumps will get mumps orchitis?**

Mumps orchitis is rare in prepubertal boys. Approximately 30% (20%-40%) of boys with mumps will get mumps orchitis.

○ **What cardiac drug at what dosage can cause a chemical epididymitis, what portion of the epididymis is involved most often and how should it be treated?**

Amiodarone at dosages more than 200 mg/day can cause a chemical epididymitis in 3% to 11% of patients on the medication. This type of chemical epididymitis typically involves the head of the epididymis. Treatment is discontinuation of the drug.

○ **Pyuria is present in roughly what percentage of patients with acute epididymitis?**

Only approximately 25%.

○ **What exactly is the function of fructose in the semen and what is the significance of its absence?**

Fructose nourishes the sperm. Absence of fructose in the semen suggests the absence of the seminal vesicles.

○ **What 3 medical diseases or disorders can cause calcification of the vas deferens?**

Tuberculosis, diabetes, and gonorrhea.

○ **Which kidney is affected most often with angiomyolipomas and with what other disease is it closely associated?**

The right kidney is affected 80% of the time. Approximately 20% of renal angiomyolipomas are associated with tuberous sclerosis and 80% of patients with tuberous sclerosis have angiomyolipomas.

○ **What percentage of patients with renal tuberculosis present with hematuria?**

Approximately 30%.

○ **What is the normal volume of the renal pelvis?**

The normal value is 5 to 8 cm^3.

○ **What are the most common benign and malignant tumors of the spermatic cord?**

The most common benign tumors are adenomatoid tumors and lipomas. Malignancies are uncommon in the spermatic cord, but the most frequent malignant tumor is a liposarcoma.

○ **Painful ejaculation is caused by what problems?**

Ejaculatory duct obstruction, prostatitis, BPH, and chronic pelvic pain syndrome.

○ **Are adult men with cystic fibrosis sterile and, if so, why?**

Adult cystic fibrosis men are sterile because of the absence of the vas deferens.

○ **A patient getting a TURP under spinal anesthetic develops epigastric and/or chest pain radiating to the left shoulder. What has probably happened?**

While a cardiac event is possible, it is far more likely that there has been an intraperitoneal bladder rupture.

○ **What is Dietl crisis?**

Recurrent renal colic pain caused by intermittent kinking or twisting of the ureter, associated with nephroptosis.

○ **Fanconi syndrome is sometimes associated with what other disorder sometimes in kidney stone disease?**

Cystinuria.

○ **How does vaginal atresia differ from vaginal agenesis?**

Vaginal atresia involves only the distal vagina. The Mullerian structures are not affected. The uterus, cervix, and proximal vagina are all normal and intact.

Vaginal agenesis is the absence of a proximal vagina in a normal 46 XX female with normal hormones. A hymenal fringe and a small distal vaginal pouch are usually present.

○ **What is Mayer–Rokitansky–Kuster-Hauser (MRKH) syndrome?**

Another name for vaginal agenesis.

○ **What urological problems are most commonly associated with vaginal agenesis?**

Unilateral renal agenesis or ectopia of one or both kidneys occurs in 74% of patients.

○ **What are Fordyce spots and how are they treated?**

Fordyce spots are the small, 1- to 3-mm painless fleshy bumps commonly found on the shaft of the penis. They are a form of ectopic sebaceous gland and are not considered pathologic so no treatment is necessary or recommended. A CO_2 laser can be used to remove them for cosmetic reasons if desired.

○ **True/False: The ascending loop of Henle contains active sodium transport and is impermeable to water.**

True.

○ **What are Tyson glands?**

These are identical to Fordyce spots, except that they are located on the glans.

○ **Gadolinium can cause what potentially serious complication when used in patients with renal failure?**

Nephrogenic systemic fibrosis.

○ **What is NAION, what causes it, and how is it treated?**

Non**A**rteric **I**schemic **O**ptic **N**europathy, a type of blindness, has been associated extremely rarely with PDE5 inhibitors. There is no effective treatment.

○ **What is Stauffer syndrome?**

Stauffer syndrome is a paraneoplastic liver disorder associated with renal cell carcinoma.

○ **What are the 4 major effects of angiotensin II?**

Arteriolar vasoconstriction, decreased renal blood flow, sodium retention, and stimulation of aldosterone synthesis.

○ **What is Balkan nephropathy and why is it important urologically?**

Balkan nephropathy is a rare degenerative interstitial nephritis found typically in rural areas of the Balkans. It is urologically significant because of its associated 100- to 200-fold increase in the risk of upper tract transitional cell carcinoma.

○ **What type of renal tumor is associated with staghorn calculi?**

Squamous cell carcinoma.

○ **Describe the mechanism of action of thiazides.**

Thiazide diuretics inhibit NaCl reabsorption from the luminal side of the early segments of the distal convoluted tubule, resulting in a diuresis. This causes a compensatory increase in the proximal tubular reabsorption of calcium and NaCl, which explains the hypocalciuric effect of thiazides and why it is blunted by excess NaCl.

○ **What is the ipsilateral recurrence rate of transitional cell cancer when a segmental ureterectomy is done for distal ureteral disease?**

Approximately 25%.

○ **What is the most common site of ureteral TB?**

At the UVJ.

○ **What is the most common tumor metastatic to the kidneys?**

Lymphoma.

○ **Eighty percent of angiomyolipomas are associated with what other disorder?**

Tuberous sclerosis.

○ **What is the nephrectomy rate in major renal trauma cases that are surgically explored?**

Approximately 18%.

○ **Identify the most common location for iatrogenic injury to the ureter.**

At the pelvic brim, where the ureter crosses the iliac artery and courses posterior to the broad ligament and ovarian vessels in women.

○ **A retrocaval ureter develops due to the persistence of what vein?**

The subcardinal vein.

○ **What percentage of chronic dialysis patients developed renal failure due to polycystic kidney disease?**

Approximately 10%.

○ **Explain the underlying pathophysiology of polycystic kidney disease and how it causes renal cysts expansion and growth.**

Excessive expansion of renal cysts is due to a heightened sensitivity to the proliferative stimulation of epidermal growth factor.

○ **Explain the underlying etiology of hypertension in polycystic kidney disease, and is it renin mediated?**

As the renal cysts enlarge, they stretch the renal tubules, which causes ischemia to the distal portions of the renal parenchyma resulting in renin release and hypertension.

○ **Name at least 4 other disorders besides hypertension and renal failure that are associated with polycystic kidney disease.**

Circle of Willis and Berry aneurysms, subarachnoid bleeds, colonic diverticula, and mitral valve prolapse.

○ **A simple renal cortical cyst will have what kind of T2-weighed image on an MRI?**

Homogenous hyperdense image.

○ **Name 9 separate treatments to help control bleeding in hemorrhagic cystitis.**

1. Continuous bladder irrigation.
2. Intravesical therapy with alum, formalin, or silver nitrate.
3. Systemic therapy with Elmiron and Amicar.
4. Electrocautery.
5. Laser coagulation therapy.
6. Hydrodistension.
7. Hyperbaric oxygen.
8. Urinary diversion.
9. Hypogastric artery embolization.

○   **"Moth-eaten" calices on IVP are typical of what disease and how is it treated?**

Renal tuberculosis. Treatment is with INH, rifampin, and pyrazinamide.

○   **Physiologic hydronephrosis of pregnancy affects which side most often and why?**

The right side is affected approximately 3 times more often than the left. The left ureter is partially protected from compression by the sigmoid colon.

○   **Which antibiotics are preferred during pregnancy for UTIs?**

Penicillins and cephalosporins are preferred. Nitrofurantoin is acceptable but may be more likely to cause gastrointestinal (GI) upset. Sulfa can be used except near term. Avoid quinolones and tetracyclines.

○   **Can aminoglycosides be used during pregnancy?**

Yes, but only when other agents are not suitable in patients with normal renal function.

○   **What is the average number of sperm that ultimately reach the site of fertilization in the fallopian tube?**

Only approximately 300.

○   **When is INH therapy useful in urology?**

INH can be used in TB but is most useful as the primary antibiotic for severe side effects of BCG therapy.

○   **What complication of INH therapy can be prevented with pyridoxine therapy?**

Peripheral neuropathy.

○   **What is the significance of poor endothelial cell functional testing in men with ED?**

Poor endothelial cell function would suggest a higher risk of cardiovascular disease.

○   **After a vasectomy, what percentage of men develop antisperm antibodies?**

Approximately 60%.

○   **What is the most common epididymal tumor?**

A benign adenomatoid tumor.

○   **Incomplete dissolution of Chwalla membrane will cause what?**

A ureterocele.

○   **What is the most common renal tumor in infants?**

Congenital mesoblastic nephroma.

○ **Which is more sensitive in the detection of vesicoureteral reflux: a radionuclide cystogram or a VCUG, and which delivers less radiation to the patient?**

The radionuclide cystogram is more sensitive and more specific than a VCUG in the detection of vesicoureteral reflux. It also delivers considerably less radiation exposure to the patient.

○ **Explain the differences among detrusor overactivity, overactive bladder, detrusor hyperreflexia, and detrusor instability. (Warning: this could be the toughest single question in the whole book!)**

Detrusor overactivity describes the urodynamic observation of involuntary detrusor contractions during bladder filling which may be spontaneous or provoked. It requires urodynamic testing.

Overactive bladder is a symptomatic diagnosis secondary to detrusor overactivity usually defined as urgency with or without incontinence usually associated with frequency and nocturia.

Detrusor hyperreflexia is defined as bladder overactivity or increased bladder contractile activity caused by a disturbance in the nervous control mechanism. It requires identification of a relevant, underlying neurologic disorder. If no neurologic disorder is identified, then the term idiopathic detrusor hyperreflexia should be used.

Detrusor instability has previously been used to describe uninhabitable bladder contractions typically occurring at bladder volumes below capacity. Idiopathic detrusor hyperreflexia describes the same situation although the term idiopathic detrusor overactivity is now preferred.

○ **Angiomyolipomas are associated with what disease?**

Tuberous sclerosis.

○ **Calcification of the vas occurs in association with what 3 disorders?**

Diabetes, TB, and gonorrhea.

○ **The majority of the calcium ultimately excreted in the urine is determined where in the nephron?**

The distal convoluted tubule and proximal collecting tubule. No significant changes in calcium occur anywhere else in the nephron.

○ **Tuberous sclerosis is an inheritable autosomal dominant disorder associated with angiomyolipomas and what other renal problems?**

Cysts and renal cell carcinoma.

○ **What tumors are associated with von Hippel–Lindau disease?**

Renal cell carcinomas, pheochromocytomas, and hemangioblastomas of the central nervous system.

○ **Topamax (topiramate), a drug used for migraine and epilepsy, causes what specific GU problem and how?**

Calcium phosphate nephrolithiasis. It is a carbonic anhydrase inhibitor that causes metabolic acidosis resulting in hypocitraturia and increased urinary alkalinity. This results in calcium phosphate stones. The increase in risk is roughly 2 to 4 times normal.

○ **True/False: Measuring bone mineral density is recommended before long-term, androgen-deprivation therapy?**

True.

○ **Name 3 oral drugs that can be used specifically for prostatic bleeding.**

Dutasteride (Avodart), finasteride (Proscar), and epsilon-aminocaproic acid (Amicar).

○ **What is the treatment for stuttering (intermittent) priapism?**

Intermittent intracorporal self-injection with a diluted α-agonist solution. LHRH therapy can also be used in resistant or persistent cases.

○ **In which gender and racial group is nocturia most common?**

It is most common in non-white females.

○ **True/False: Diuretics increase nocturia by approximately 40%.**

True.

○ **Nocturia is associated with what chronic conditions? (Name 10.)**

Diabetes, cardiac disease, hypertension, sleep disorders such as sleep apnea, overactive bladder, neurogenic bladder, urinary retention, interstitial cystitis, radiation cystitis, renal disease, diabetes insipidus, and depression.

○ **True/False: Evening fluid restriction is a reasonably effective initial treatment for nocturnal polyuria.**

False. It is reasonable but usually ineffective.

○ **Differentiate between nocturnal polyuria and global polyuria.**

Nocturnal polyuria is a relative increase in nocturnal urinary volume but with a normal 24-hour urine total volume. Global polyuria has an abnormally high 24-hour urine volume, usually >40 mg/kg/24 h.

○ **What does a "beehive in the bladder" on cystogram or cystoscopy typically indicate?**

A colovesical fistula.

○ **Colovesical fistulas are typically located in what part of the bladder?**

The dome.

○ **Is there any clinical significance to a colovesical fistula that involves the right side versus the left side of the bladder?**

Lesions on the right side (dome or posterior wall) are most likely due to Crohn disease, while left-sided lesions are typically due to diverticular disease.

○ **An acute left varicocele suggests what underlying pathology?**

Testicular vein occlusion from a renal cell tumor thrombus extending into the left renal vein.

○ **What common urologic anomaly can mimic a sacral metastasis on a bone scan?**

A pelvic horseshoe kidney.

○ **Patients treated with sorafenib for renal cell carcinoma have a significant higher risk of what common medical disorder?**

Hypertension.

○ **Is testicular cancer more common on one side?**

The right side is involved more often.

○ **What is a Quackel shunt and what is it used for?**

It is a cavernosal–spongiosum shunt used for priapism performed through a perineal approach.

○ **What is the preferred intracavernosal injection agent for reversal of low-flow priapism and why?**

Diluted phenylephrine solution is preferred due to its pure α-agonist activity with minimal β effects.

○ **True/False: Cranberry juice and tablets are recommended for both recurrent UTIs and nephrolithiasis patients.**

False. Cranberry juice has a relatively high oxalate content and therefore is not recommended for kidney stone patients. It may be of some use in UTIs.

○ **True/False: A 24-hour urine for metabolic kidney stone risk factors is required in renal transplant patients.**

True.

○ **True/False: Tetracycline lowers testosterone levels by approximately 20% and nitrofurantoin depresses spermatogenesis.**

True.

○ **What is the mortality rate associated with urinary retention?**

12.5% without comorbidities and 28.8% with comorbidities.

○ **Define and differentiate the following terms: microhematuria, dipstick hematuria, dipstick pseudohematuria, and significant microhematuria.**

Microhematuria is the presence of red blood cells in the urine.

Dipstick hematuria means a positive dipstick test for urinary blood with or without any actual RBCs on microscopic examination.

Dipstick pseudohematuria is defined as a positive dipstick test for urinary blood with no RBCs actually present on microscopic examination.

Significant microhematuria, according to the Official AUA Panel Definition, means an average of 3 or more RBCs/HPF in 2 of 3 properly collected urine specimens.

○ **Is the incidence of penile cancer in the world increasing, decreasing, or stable and what is the incidence in the United States?**

Decreasing in the world. Approximately 1200 cases are reported yearly in the United States.

○ **Name 7 risk factors for penile cancer.**

Age (incidence increases significantly after age 60), smoking, poor personal hygiene, phimosis, increased number of sexual partners, balanitis xerotica obliterans (BXO), HPV infection, lichen sclerosis, giant condyloma, bowenoid papulosis, and penile intraepithelial neoplasia.

○ **What is the overall mortality rate from penile cancer?**

The National Cancer Institute's Surveillance, Epidemiology and End Results program found a mortality rate of 22.4%, while the National Cancer Database (2007) reported a 5-year mortality rate of 25%.

○ **True/False: Circumcision offers almost complete protection from penile cancer.**

False. Adult circumcisions offer no significant protection. To be effective as a prophylactic measure, circumcision must be done during the neonatal period. When circumcision is done at puberty, the risk is reduced but if done while the patient is a neonate, penile cancer almost never develops.

○ **What is the difference between erythroplasia of Queyrat and Bowen disease?**

Both are histologically carcinoma in situ intraepithelial neoplasms. Erythroplasia of Queyrat involves the foreskin and glans, while Bowen disease affects the penile shaft and the remainder of the male genitalia and perineum.

○ **Most (95%) of penile cancers are squamous cell cancers. What other primary cell type tumors can occur in the penis?**

Carcinoma in situ (Queyrat, Bowen), adenocarcinoma (from sweat glands), melanoma, basal cell, and sarcomas (from blood vessels, smooth muscle, and connective tissue).

○ **Does circumcision reduce the risk of HIV transmission and, if so, by how much?**

Circumcision reduces HIV transmission by approximately 50% to 60%.

○ **Rate the risk of chemotherapy-induced nausea and vomiting from highest to lowest for the following chemotherapy agents: cisplatin, cyclophosphamide, adriamycin, docetaxel, mitomycin, mitoxantrone, bleomycin, vincristin, and vinblastin.**

They are in correct descending order with cisplatin having the highest risk. The risk is low to minimal from docetaxel on.

○ **What is a Page kidney, what is its most common cause, how is it diagnosed, and how should it be treated?**

A Page kidney is a kidney exposed to external compression of the renal parenchyma resulting in renin-mediated hypertension and renal ischemia. The most common example would be a subcapsular hematoma following a trauma, but it can also be caused by a needle biopsy. Compression by a cyst or tumor is also possible, but less common. Doppler ultrasound typically shows no or diminished diastolic renal blood flow. Treatment is surgical decompression. It was named after Dr Irvine Page (1901-1989) who demonstrated in 1939 that wrapping cellophane tightly around an animal kidney would cause hypertension.

○ **What is the ipsilateral recurrent rate for ureteral cancers treated by segmental or partial ureterectomy?**

The recurrent rate is 45% to 50%.

○ **True/False: Statins are harmful to patients receiving BCG therapy for superficial bladder cancer.**

True. Studies suggest that the use of statins is associated with a 3-fold increased risk of tumor progression and subsequent need for radical cystectomy.

○ **True/False: Epirubicin intravesical chemotherapy has recently been shown to have comparable recurrence rates to BCG therapy for superficial bladder cancer and CIS.**

False. BCG remains superior.

○ **Describe the "trigger and maintenance" theory of hyperoxaluric nephrolithiasis and what causes the "trigger." (For extra credit, who first suggested this theory and when?)**

Vermeulen et al. (1967) first suggested that many calcium oxalate stone formers would have mild or borderline hyperoxaluria with transient spikes in urinary oxalate excretion caused by "dietary indiscretions."

○ **True/False: According to the Stress Incontinence Surgical Treatment Efficacy Trial (SISTEr), overall success from the Burch colposuspension and the pubovaginal sling are roughly comparable.**

False. The sling procedure had significantly better success rates for controlling stress incontinence than the Burch.

○ **Male slings are most useful and effective for men with what severity level of incontinence?**

Male slings are best suited for men with mild-to-moderate incontinence. Artificial urinary sphincters are the preferred treatment for more severe male incontinence.

○ **Does the percentage of smooth muscle and α-adrenergic receptors in the prostate change with age and, if so, how?**

The percentage increases with age.

○   **True/False: A slower ESWL rate of 60 shocks per minute achieves better stone fragmentation and higher stone-free rates than 120 shocks per minute.**

True. An 18% improvement in stone-free rate has been reported with the slower shock wave frequency.

○   **True/False: Osteopenia is more prevalent in infertile, oligospermic men than in normal men.**

True. Low total sperm counts and low FSH levels have been reported to correlate to decreased bone mineral density.

○   **True/False: Coenzyme Q10 (Co Q10) can increase sperm motility in idiopathic asthenozoospermia.**

True.

○   **What infertility treatments, if any, are available to a man with nonmosaic Klinefelter syndrome?**

Microdissection testicular sperm extraction (Micro-TESE) and intracytoplasmic sperm injection (ICSI) have demonstrated success.

○   **Which of the following have been found to be good predictors of sperm detection during microscopic sperm extraction surgery: serum inhibin, spermatogenic cells in semen, Y chromosome microdeletions, testicular size, FSH level, and positive testicular histopathology.**

Only the first 3 listed.

○   **What is the significance of Yq11.23 (interval 6)?**

This is the designated area on the long arm of the Y chromosome considered critical for male fertility.

○   **Which is more common: ED or premature ejaculation?**

ED is more common in the older age group, but overall premature ejaculation is the most common male sexual disorder.

○   **Premature ejaculation is often associated with ED and what other urologic problem?**

Chronic prostatitis is present in more than 55% of men with premature ejaculation.

○   **Daily use of what drug appears to yield the longest ejaculatory delay when used for premature ejaculation?**

Paroxetine (Paxil).

○   **What is the major contraindication for daily SSRI medication?**

The presence or reported history of bipolar depression.

○   **True/False: Oxytocin analogues may be possible future treatments for premature ejaculation.**

False. Oxytocin analogues may prove useful for stimulating ejaculation in patients with delayed ejaculation, while oxytocin inhibitors may play a future role in premature ejaculation treatment.

○ **In postobstructive diuresis, what IV fluid should be used for fluid replacement and how should the rate be calculated?**

The recommended replacement fluid in postobstructive diuresis is half-normal saline. The suggested rate of fluid replacement is 50% of the hourly urinary output up to 1000 mL less than the 24-hour total urine output. Check electrolytes at least every 6 to 8 hours.

○ **How long does postobstructive diuresis typically last?**

24 to 72 hours.

○ **What relationship, if any, has been established between FSH, LH, inhibin, testosterone, free T4, and abnormal semen parameters in infertile men?**

No clear association has been found.

○ **Which vasopressin subtype affects the renal collecting duct cells causing increased free-water reabsorption?**

Type V2. (A type V2 antagonist is now available as conivaptan (Vaprisol) to treat persistent or refractory hyponatremia but only in hospitalized patients with hypervolemia or euvolemia without congestive heart failure.) Type 1a increases platelet aggregation and vasoconstriction, while type 1b increases release of ACTH and B-endorphins.

○ **What is the nocturnal polyuria index and what is normal?**

It is the percentage of the 24-hour urinary volume that is produced during sleep. Normal is 35% or less. A higher percentage would be diagnostic of nocturnal polyuria.

○ **Compared to normal controls, do patients with nocturnal polyuria demonstrate different patterns of water intake or body water distribution?**

No difference in water intake is found, but patients with nocturnal polyuria generally demonstrate increased water volume in the lower extremities compared to controls. This process usually begins at about noon and gradually increases through the afternoon and evening until bedtime. This may explain the observed benefits noted with lower extremity elevation and evening walks in patients with nocturnal polyuria.

○ **Which condition tends to lose urinary and rectal continence earlier and why: Shy–Drager syndrome or amyotrophic lateral sclerosis (ALS)?**

ALS tends to preserve urinary and rectal continence until very advanced stages of the disease. Shy–Drager syndrome patients lose continence early in the course of the disease. The difference is due to preservation/destruction, respectively, of Onuf nucleus in the sacral spinal cord. The nucleus is preserved in ALS but destroyed early in Shy–Drager syndrome.

○ **Which of the following is NOT a treatment for nocturia:**

1. Vasopressin (DDAVP) therapy.
2. Decreased oral fluid intake before bedtime.
3. Elevation of the lower extremities before bedtime.
4. Taking an afternoon nap.
5. Changing the timing of daily furosemide from early morning to midafternoon.
6. Use of anticholinergics or imipramine.
7. Use of sleeping pills/aids.

None of the above. All are possible therapies for nocturia.

○ **What is the recommended number of ejaculations needed to achieve azoospermia after a bilateral vasectomy?**

Approximately 32.

○ **What is cabergoline (Dostinex) and what urologic problem does it address?**

Cabergoline is an ergot-derived dopamine receptor agonist that is used primarily in the United States as a second-line oral agent for hyperprolactinemia when bromocriptine alone is insufficient. It has also been used in Parkinson. There is also some evidence that it may be reasonably effective in the treatment of ED in PDE5 inhibitor failures.

○ **What is the specific medical risk for cabergoline (Dostinex)?**

It has been associated with an increased risk of heart valve disease, although this usually occurs only at the higher dosages.

○ **What is the most common cause of male infertility and what is its frequency in infertile men?**

Varicocele, which is found in approximately 40% of all male infertility cases.

○ **Renal colic from intractable stone disease can be treated with what last resort surgical procedure?**

Renal autotransplantation with a pyelovesicostomy.

○ **Intracorporeal laser lithotripsy of cystine and uric acid stones produces what chemicals?**

Laser treatment of cystine stones produces hydrogen sulfide, while treatment of uric acid stones can make cyanide.

○ **MUSE is contraindicated in what conditions?**

Abnormal penile anatomy, allergy to alprostadil, multiple myeloma, sickle cell anemia or trait, thrombocythemia, and polycythemia.

○ **What is the "poppy seed" test?**

Visual inspection of the urine after oral ingestion of poppy seeds. It is a simple, cost-effective screening test for colovesical fistula.

○ **True/False: Renal cell cancer patients with a positive family history for renal cell carcinoma have a greater risk of dying from that cancer than renal cell cancer patients without a positive family history.**

False. However, those with a positive family history are more likely to develop bilateral disease.

○ **What factors are associated with the degree or severity of the penile deformity/curvature in Peyronie disease?**

Age, lateral location of the plaque, and ED.

○ **BXO has been linked to what other urological disorder?**

Hypogonadism that may play a significant role in the development, progression, and recurrence of BXO. Application of 2% testosterone cream and testosterone-replacement therapy has shown normalization of tissue in BXO cases who are hypogonadal.

○ **Children with nocturnal enuresis have a higher incidence of what other disorders?**

Obesity and sleep apnea.

○ **What percentage of patients with gross hematuria and a totally negative initial urological workup will eventually be diagnosed with a urological cancer?**

Approximately 3.4%.

○ **Which has shown, so far, better rates of suppressing local tumor progression and metastases in renal tumors: cryoablation or radiofrequency ablation?**

Cryoablation appears to be significantly better in reducing tumor progression according to most studies.

○ **Capsular invasion in renal cell cancer has what impact on tumor recurrence and survival? How does it change the staging?**

Capsular invasion does not change the staging, but it tends to indicate more aggressive disease.

○ **Obstructive azoospermia due to ejaculatory duct obstruction should be suspected in azoospermic men with what clinical findings?**

At least one palpable vas, low semen volume, acidic semen pH, and low or absent semen fructose.

○ **What is the expected pregnancy rate after ejaculatory duct resection in men with ejaculatory duct obstruction?**

Only approximately 20% to 30%.

○ **You are called by a patient on a PDE5 inhibitor such as sildenafil (Viagra) about sudden blindness or hearing loss. According to the pharmaceutical's manufacturer, what advice should you give the patient?**

Stop taking the medication. They offer no other advice. However, referral to an appropriate specialist (ENT or ophthalmology) would seem reasonable, as there might be other treatable causes of the patient's problem.

○ **During a long laparoscopic procedure, the patient's blood pressure starts to drop slowly and ventilation is becoming more difficult according to the anesthesiologist. New cardiac arrhythmias have been detected. You have encountered no obvious problems with the surgery and no significant bleeding. What is the diagnosis, pathophysiology, and treatment for this condition?**

Most likely, the patient is developing a tension pneumoperitoneum due to the persistently elevated intra-abdominal pressure. High intraperitoneal pressures over time lead to vena caval compression that decreases the venous return, resulting in hypotension as well as direct pressure on the diaphragm making ventilation more difficult. Higher amounts of carbon dioxide are absorbed into the blood eventually causing acidosis, hypoxia, and arrhythmias. Cardiovascular collapse will ultimately develop if recognized and treated promptly. Treatment involves immediate desufflation, correcting any Trendelenburg position, IV fluids, and hyperventilation with 100% oxygen.

○ **What is the "eggplant sign" and what problem does it indicate?**

This is the typical appearance of the penis immediately after a penile fracture with extensive hematoma formation and extravasation of blood.

○ **What is tumor necrosis factor-α (TNF-α), what does it normally do, and why is it important urologically?**

TNF-α is a cytokine that is involved with homeostasis of the immune system, inflammation, and host defense as well as malignant disease. TNF is secreted by a number of tumor cells including renal cell carcinoma where it appears to act as an autocrine growth factor. The presence of TNF in tumors is associated with cachexia, hormone resistance, and more aggressive disease with a poorer prognosis. TNF-α is one of the targets of renal cell cancer chemotherapy along with vascular endothelial growth factor and mammalian target of rapamycin (mTOR).

○ **True/False: Tumor necrosis factor-α is elevated in prostate cancer patients with advanced or extensive disease.**

True.

○ **What is the most common site of malignant melanoma in the urinary tract?**

The urethra. In men, it is most often in the fossa navicularis.

○ **What is the overall incidence and significance of testicular microcalcifications on testicular ultrasound examinations? How should it be treated and followed?**

Testicular microcalcifications are not rare and occur in approximately 0.6% to 9% of men. There is an increased risk of testicular cancer associated with these microcalcifications. α-Fetoprotein and β-HCG tumor markers along with yearly follow-ups are suggested.

○ **What is the medication and recommended dilution formula for intracorporeal injection therapy of priapism?**

The most commonly used medication is phenylephrine. Typically, the standard ampule is 10 mg/mL, which is too concentrated to use directly. One-half a milliliter of the drug in 9.5 mL of NS provides sufficient dilution to use safely. 0.5 to 1 mL is injected directly into the corpora every 15 minutes until the priapism is resolved, up to a maximum of 3 injections. If this fails, then a shunt will be needed. Vital signs should be checked regularly during this process because of the risk of hypertension when injecting an α-agonist.

○ **What is the modality of choice for evaluating the nodal status of penile cancer patients with impalpable nodes?**

Dynamic sentinel node biopsy.

○ **True/False: α-Blocker therapy reduces the incidence of ureteral colic after ureteroscopy and improves the stone-free rate after both ESWL and ureteroscopy.**

True.

○ **True/False: Shockwave therapy has shown slight benefits when used for Peyronie disease.**

False. No benefit has been demonstrated from shockwave therapy in Peyronie disease.

○ **True/False: Testosterone does not influence PSA levels in older men.**

True. For men older than 50 years, testosterone does not appear to affect PSA levels.

○ **What is the cause of nephrogenic systemic fibrosis?**

Use of gadolinium-contrast in patients with azotemia or renal failure. First recognized in 1997, the typical patient is already on dialysis. It begins with subacute swelling of the distal extremities and progresses to severe skin induration, which can spread to internal organs. Transmetallation from prolonged exposure to gadolinium-contrast media is thought to be the underlying cause.

○ **Can nephrogenic systemic fibrosis occur in patients without significant renal failure?**

Apparently not, since no confirmed cases have been reported without severe azotemia or end-stage renal disease.

○ **True/False: C-reactive protein is an independent prognostic variable for outcomes in renal cell carcinoma and can be used to monitor response to chemotherapy in metastatic disease.**

True.

○ **True/False: Cryoablation of small renal tumors has similar outcomes to radiofrequency ablation.**

False. Cryoablation appears to have better outcomes according to meta-analysis.

○ **When performing a partial nephrectomy, what is the maximum recommended warm ischemia time?**

No more than 36 to 40 minutes are recommended.

○ **What is elastography, how does it work, and what is its urological application?**

Elastrography is thought to be potentially helpful in identifying prostate cancer. It is performed by compressing prostate tissue, then measuring its tissue strain and degree of elasticity. It is thought that areas of increased stiffness would indicate prostate cancer due to the increased cell density present in cancer tissue.

○ **True/False: Penile ultrasonography can be useful in categorizing and following Peyronie disease.**

True. The density of echogenic areas and acoustic shadows can be easily followed.

○ **What are the contraindications for laparoscopic radical nephrectomy?**

Need for nephron-sparing surgery, locally advanced (T4) disease with tumor invasion of surrounding tissues, and significant vena caval tumor thrombus or vena caval wall invasion. Tumor size is a relative contraindication if more than 20 cm in size.

○ **What are the characteristics and differential diagnosis of inflammatory myofibroblastic tumors of the bladder?**

These are rare, benign tumors that typically occur in younger patients. The most common bladder location is the posterior lateral wall. The etiology is thought to be inflammatory, but there is evidence of a neoplastic process as well. The main differential diagnosis is sarcoma where the treatment is more surgically aggressive. The correct diagnosis of inflammatory myofibroblastic tumor of the bladder often requires a final histologic confirmation, so this entity must be considered when dealing with bladder masses of undetermined etiology to avoid overtreatment if benign, and potentially dangerous undertreatment if it is ultimately determined to be a malignant sarcoma.

○ **Micturition syncope is classically caused by what disorder?**

Pheochromocytoma involving the bladder.

Getting to the Top of Google in 5 Steps

Ron Romano and Neil Baum, MD

Whenever the topic of the Internet surfaces, everyone wants to know, how do you reach the Holy Grail of being at the top of the Google search? The truth is that it's not a mystery or a secret, but there is a process. This article is intended to provide you with the "secrets" of how to reach the top of Google.

Let's begin with a question. When was the last time that you went to the second or third page of a Google search? Like most of us, you probably seldom or never get past the first page. That is the mindset of nearly 85% of the population. So if you want to get your site and your practice recognized, you have to be on the first page of the Google search and ideally at the very first position. If you're not on the first page of Google, you are invisible to most potential new patients who are looking specifically for you and your practice. And more importantly, can your urology practice even survive without a steady flow of new patients?

Now that we've explained why you want to be on the first page, let's share with you how it can be done. So, how do you get Google to rank your website, in your local area, so it gets in the top 10 which are shown on the first page? Consider the fact that Google uses over 200 different algorithms to rank websites, and most of these are not published. To make things harder, many of these algorithms are changed on a regular basis to plug loopholes that programmers and website operators discover to trick or game the system. Only the really important ones are more or less permanent and these are the ones that Google will share and tell us what they want the website owners to do!

65.09% OF ALL SEARCHES ARE THROUGH GOOGLE

We live in an information technology world today with nearly everyone of us connected to the information superhighway. Whether you want to find a product or service, book a flight, or just research any topic at all, we Google it. According to all the statistics, approximately 65.09% of all searches are done through Google. Google is still by far the most dominant search engine in the United States followed by Yahoo with 15.89% and Bing at 13.10%.

And if that's not enough for you, according to a recent study by BIA/Kelsey, "nearly all consumers (97 percent) now use online media (whether it is online or on smart phones) when researching products or services (including medical services) in their local area."

Wayne Gretzky, one of the greatest hockey players of all time, was asked about his skills and he said, "I don't skate where the puck is, but where the puck is going to be." That same approach applies to doctors and practices trying to attract new patients. The patients are going to be on the Internet and will be mostly looking at the first page of Google, which is why you try to achieve that coveted top spot! Google has the overwhelming ability to send you an endless and enormous supply of patients if you can get on their first page. Now, here's how to do it.

FIVE STEPS TO GET TO THE TOP OF GOOGLE

Getting to the top of Google is a system and a process. As we mentioned, there are over 200 different algorithms but here are the top 5 tried and tested steps for search engines to find and rank you:

1. Keywords in your website coding
2. Keywords in website copy
3. In-bound Links
4. New keyword related content
5. Social media sites

Keywords are Key!

Just as proper and accurate coding of your diagnoses and procedures are vital to the financial success of your urology practice, using keywords are at the top of the list and probably the most important part of the search engine optimization (SEO) process. Keywords are what your patients enter when searching for your services. This is what the search engine spiders are looking for so they can direct the person who typed in that keyword phrase to the website they perceive as the best source of information to answer the website surfer's inquiry.

For example, if you are a Urologist and your practice was in Houston the website surfer might type in "*Urologist Houston Tx*", or simply "*Urologist Houston.*" Search engines look at these as 2 separate and distinct search terms. For "*Urologist Houston Tx*" Google tells us there are 880 searches per month and for "*Urologist Houston*" there are 3600 searches per month.

Google has an on-line tool that not only tells us how many people are searching a particular keyword every month; they also give you other related keywords that other people are searching for. In that same search above, Google also reports that 480 people are typing in the keyword phrase "*Vasectomy Houston.*" For more information on keywords, you can go to www.instantmarketingsystems.net/tool and get connected to Google's Keyword page.

Keywords in Your Website Coding and in the Website Copy

Unless you have some experience in this area you might consider hiring a professional for the coding. Website coding and placement includes places like Meta tags (*Meta tags* are HTML codes that are inserted into the header on a web page), Anchor text, sitemap, and many more that would be beyond the scope of this introductory article. You can easily incorporate your keywords in the copy of your articles and text.

However, a warning, you don't want to game the system by overwhelming the Google search process by inserting too many keywords as their search system picks this up and recognizes that you are trying to manipulate the search and will not recognize your content or your website. We recommend that the keyword density should be no more than approximately 3% to 5% of the total copy. This means that if you are writing an article on prostate cancer and the article has 300 words, you should not use the term prostate cancer more than 15 times in the body of article.

In-bound Links

Google wants users to have a positive experience so that the website surfer will continue to use Google as their primary search engine. Google wants to make sure that the websites they have ranked highly are considered by other websites to be an authority on the subject being searched.

The measurement Google uses is the number of websites that have links (your website address on their website) to your website. But not just the number of links, it is also the quality of the links. That means, are the websites that provide a link to your website in a related field. *Example:* Google would give a high ranking if you had an *in-bound* link from a medical website such as Mayo Clinic or American Cancer Society. They would penalize you and pull down your rankings if you had an in-bound link from a pest control or a day spay for pets!

This means you want to submit your website address with a description of your keywords that you want to get ranked for, on a regular monthly basis, to on-line medical directories, to medical publications, and to medical blogs. You should also write a minimum of 250 to 400 word keyword-rich articles with your submissions. Press releases with professionally written articles are another strategy to use and can be very powerful for search engine optimization (SEO) purposes.

New "Keyword Related" Content
To position yourself and your website as the knowledgeable expert in your field, add new content that has your keywords in it. Google wants to see an active website, one that has "keyword relevant" updated information. This is best accomplished through a blog. A blog that is attached to your website is easy for anyone to add content. You don't have to be a programmer or know HTML. The key to success is regularity and frequency. Depending on what your competition is doing your can get an immediate bump in your rankings with your blog.

CASE STUDY GETTING TO THE TOP OF GOOGLE IN 2 WEEKS
One of us, NHB, wanted to find out how long it would take to get to the first page of Google for a certain keyword phrase.

June 1, 2012: On June 1, he took a topic "scrotal pain" that wasn't on his radar and typed in the key words in the Google search bar. Now this keyword phrase is not as competitive a phrase as "Urologist," but, nonetheless his name and practice was nowhere to be found on the first page.

June 2, 2012: He wrote a 300-word blog, "*An Ouch In the Pouch-Acute Scrotal Pain and What To Do About It*," on his Word Press Blog.

June 9, 2012: A second blog of approximately 200 words was written. The title was "*When It Really Hurts Down There— Epididymitis*" again with key words "scrotal pain," "testicle," "painful testicle," and "epididymitis" included as tags for the blog.

June 10, 2012: A third blog was written, "*Pain In the Pouch May Be Coming From Somewhere Else.*"

June 14, 2012: A YouTube video was created with the topic of acute pain in the scrotum.

June 15, 2012: A repeat Google search was conducted on June 15, 2012 which showed, just like magic, that a search for "*scrotal pain New Orleans*" demonstrated that his practice was at the very top of the Google search page in the first position! What's the bottom line: You can go from obscurity to visibility in just 2 weeks. Just follow the few steps we have recommended and you can do it too.

Social Media Sites
There is a lot of hype about social media sites such as Facebook, Twitter, and YouTube, etc with good reason. Although they won't produce the number of patients that comes from being on the first page of Google, these sites are very important for 2 very good reasons.

First, Google likes them and Google likes them even more when they link back to your website. That means these in-bound links with keyword relevance from Facebook and Twitter are good for your rankings!

Second, Facebook, twitter, and YouTube are search engines within themselves. There's almost a billion Facebook users, hundreds of millions on twitter and YouTube gets as much traffic as Facebook does. People using these sites search your keywords looking for information.

If you have a social media presence and you regularly add new keyword-related content that is informative, relevant, and fun, over a period of time you will build up followers who will share your information with their friends.

These sites give you a forum to position yourself as the expert in your field and will give your rankings a boost!

MAXIMIZE YOUR GOOGLE RANKINGS WITH A PATIENT CONVERSION WEBSITE

Whether you like it or not, the success of you practice depends on how well you manage search engines and the quality of your website. Google is one piece of the Internet Marketing Puzzle. Once you have invested in mastering the Google rankings either by doing it yourself or getting professional help to get there, now it's up to your website to convert the visitor to a paying patient.

However, if your website does not have any patient conversion processes on it then you will have wasted your time, effort, and money. Success depends on not only getting on the first page of Google so prospective patients will go to your website but also on the conversion quality of your website. To maximize your return on investment (ROI), you need to implement marketing strategies, techniques, and systems such as email capture and automated follow-up in your website.

Bottom Line

All of us have skills and training for diagnosing and treating urologic diseases. In that arena, we are, indeed, experts. However, few of us have the skills necessary to navigate the information superhighway. However, as Mr Gretzky suggests, the Internet is where the patients are going to be and we have to develop skills or hire those who can help us harness this important aspect of medical marketing. See you all at the top of the Google first page!

Just for Fun: Urology Trivia

Stephen W. Leslie, MD, FACS

○ **Who first coined the name "nephrostomy" and was the first to actually do this as a planned surgical procedure? For extra credit, what is this urologist's full name, his nationality, when did this happen, and what is he better known for?**

The first nephrostomy was done by Joaquin Albarran Maria y Dominguez in 1896. He was a prominent French urologist born in Cuba. He is better known for inventing the deflecting cystoscope lever or bridge.

○ **What is Gerota's full name and nationality?**

Dimitrie Gerota was Romanian.

○ **What is another name for Highmore body?**

The hilum of the testis.

○ **What is the Fick principle and what is its urological application?**

Developed by Adolf Eugen Fick. It is the basic principle and formula used to measure blood flow to an organ. Originally used for cardiac output, a modified form of Fick formula is currently used to calculate the creatinine clearance.

○ **What is pilimiction and how does it happen?**

Pilimiction means hair passing in the urine. It is most commonly caused by a pelvic dermoid cyst that breaks through into the bladder.

○ **"Suprasegmental reflex mechanisms becoming integrated with the spinal reflex arc" describes what urological milestone event?**

Toilet training.

○ **Annual amount of money spent on urology-related medical care in the United States is?**

$11 billion.

○ **Harrison Ford came up with the idea for the famous scene in "Raiders of the Lost Ark" where Indiana Jones shoots the big swordsman. What was his inspiration?**

He urgently needed a bathroom break.

○ **The first episode of "Joanie Loves Chachi" was the highest rated American program ever in the history of Korean television. How come?**

Chachi is Korean for "penis."

○ **True/False: Dutch researchers have found a way to measure the resistance of the urethra using sound via a microphone placed behind the scrotum.**

True. Apparently, the sound's frequency varies according to the degree of urethral narrowing.

○ **Birt–Hogg–Dube syndrome, a type of small papular skin lesion on the scalp, forehead, face, and neck, is associated with what 2 urological conditions?**

Multiple or bilateral renal cell carcinomas and renal oncocytomas.

○ **Lo Prado, Chile, a suburb of Santiago, was the first city in the world to do what?**

Give all its senior male residents free Viagra.

○ **What does "cock-throppled" mean?**

That your Adam's apple is larger than normal.

○ **Who first placed the eyes or openings on a catheter on opposite sides instead of just using a terminal opening? (Hint: He was also the first to use a catheter introducer and a stylet.)**

Rhazes, an Arab physician who lived in 850 to 923 AD.

○ **What is the origin of the word penis? (Hint: It is Latin.)**

It is Latin for "tail."

○ **How far would the seminiferous tubules reach if fully stretched out?**

Approximately one-fourth mile.

○ **What is the total lifetime male semen production volume?**

Approximately 18 quarts.

○ **What is the average speed of a sperm and how far can a sperm swim in an hour?**

Approximately 1/8 in/min or approximately 7 in/h.

○ **Who performed the first successful artificial insemination in a human and when?**

Scottish surgeon John Hunter in the 1780s.

○ **Where did the term "missionary position" come from?**

It came from Trobriand Islanders, who were urged by missionaries to adopt the "man on top" position as the only morally acceptable way to have intercourse.

○ **What is a spermologer? (Hint: The editor of this book is one.)**

A person who collects trivia.

○ **What is the most common neoplastic condition affecting males?**

BPH.

○ **Hypospadius is associated with how many other syndromes, anomalies, and congenital malformations?**

49.

○ **What is "Tire Pump syndrome," how does it happen, who gets it, and when?**

It refers to abdominal and shoulder pain after sexual activity, which improves quickly on its own without further treatment. It occurs only in females, usually after hysterectomy. The abdominal and shoulder pain is caused by pneumoperitoneum produced by the sexual intercourse in the presence of a salpingovaginal fistula. It is quite rare, but reported.

○ **Living, laboratory-grown skin for skin grafts has been successfully developed using what original source for the cellular material?**

Neonatal foreskin.

○ **What age group is affected most often by acute urinary retention?**

From 75 to 84 years.

○ **What is the world's largest recorded human urinary bladder volume from retention?**

So far, the largest documented human bladder capacity was 9350 cm^3. The patient never went to the physician and thought his increasing abdominal distension was just gaining weight. He might have gone on for several more months except he got a severe foot infection that required hospitalization. The underlying cause of his retention was found to be prostate cancer. If anyone has found a larger bladder, please inform the editor!

○ **What noted urologist was able to achieve a BA, MA, and an MD degree from the University of Virginia in only 4 years?**

High Hampton Young.

○ **What is "Soot Wart," what causes it, and why did it affect people in England more than in other countries? (For extra credit, who discovered it and when?)**

Soot wart was the original name for squamous cell carcinoma of the scrotum. It was associated with chimney sweeps in England in the 18th century and was the first proven occupational cancer. Soot from the chimneys would easily penetrate their clothes and reach the scrotum, ultimately causing cancer. English chimney sweeps, unlike those in other countries, were notoriously averse to washing and therefore had much higher scrotal cancer rates. First reported by Sir Percival Pott in 1775.

○ **Name 5 predisposing factors to squamous cell carcinoma of the scrotum.**

Compromised immune system, scrotal trauma, UV and x-ray radiation exposure, chemical exposure, and arsenic.

○ **What is the most common malignancy in men in Uganda? (Hint: It is a urological malignancy.)**

Penile cancer.

○ **Phimosis comes from the Greek word for what?**

Muzzling.

○ **The foreskin represents approximately what percentage of the total skin of the penis?**

Approximately 50%.

○ **Buschke-Lowenstein tumor is another name for what urological neoplasm?**

Verrucous carcinoma of the penis.

○ **Name the 2 urologists who have won the Nobel Prize and describe their contributions.**

Dr Charles Huggins was a Canadian-born urologist who discovered that male sex hormones stimulate prostate growth in dogs while estrogens inhibit it. This finding rapidly became the basis for hormonal therapy for the treatment of prostate cancer. Dr Huggins won the Nobel Prize in 1966.

Dr Werner Forssmann was a general surgery resident during the depression in 1929. He passed a ureteral catheter through his antecubital vein into the right atrium. He then ran to the radiology department to take a picture. Up until that time, it was widely believed that passage of a tube into the heart would be instantly fatal. His goal was to find a better way to deliver drugs directly to the heart for cardiac resuscitation. For this momentous discovery, Dr Forssmann was immediately fired from the hospital and general surgery residency program. He eventually became a urologist (no other surgical field would take him). He later received the Nobel Prize in 1956 for his role in the discovery of cardiac catheterization.

○ **Several decades ago, then AUA President Dr Logan Holtgrewe surveyed practicing urologists approximately the minimum number of TURP cases necessary to achieve minimal proficiency. What was the consensus conclusion?**

A minimum of 80 TURP cases.

○ **What is the average total number of TURP procedures currently done by urology residents in a 4-year urology residency training program?**

Approximately 60 and decreasing.

○ **Claudius Galen, the famous Roman physician from 200 AD, died from what urological disorder?**

Hydrocele. His hydrocele was so large that he had to drain it periodically. Eventually, it got infected and he succumbed to sepsis.

○ **What animals have a urogenital diaphragm similar to humans?**

None.

○ **Which medical specialty is the least likely to refer a patient with hematuria to urology or order any imaging studies?**

Ob-Gyn. Their usual treatment is to repeat the urinalysis or send a urine culture.

○ **How did syphilis contribute to modern urography and who was responsible?**

In 1923, a dermatology resident named Earl Osborne was experimenting with intravenous sodium iodide as a possible treatment for syphilis. He discovered that the x-rays he obtained on patients given the sodium iodide showed clearly opacified urinary tracts.

○ **Who first correctly described Gerota fascia? (Hint: It was not Gerota!)**

Emil and Otto Zuckerkandl in 1883. Dimitrie Gerota description of the same entity was not published until 1895.

○ **What famous and momentous urological event occurred on Monday, April 18, 1983 at exactly 7 PM in Las Vegas, NV; who did it, and what medication was involved?**

That was when British neurophysiologist Dr Giles Brindley injected his own penis with phenoxybenzamine and then showed the entire AUA meeting delegates his induced erection!

○ **What is the precise, formal chemical descriptive name for conivaptan hydrochloride (Vaprisol), what is it, and what is it used for?**

[1,1'-biphenyl]-2-carboxamide, N-[4-[(4,5-dihydro-2-methylimidazo[4,5-d][1]benzazepin-6(1H)-yl)carbonyl] phenyl]-monohydrochloride is the chemical formula. It is a type V_2 vasopressin antagonist that is approved for the treatment of hyponatremia. It increases free-water excretion while retaining sodium.

○ **Who was the first Board certified female urologist?**

Dr Elisabeth Pauline Pickett was the first female certified in urology in 1962.

○ **As of 2008, how many Board certified women urologists are there in the United States?**

324, not counting the 237 who are Board eligible and another 229 still in urology residency.

○ **What is the association between snoring and male sexual function?**

Heavy snoring is associated with decreased ejaculatory function and overall sexual satisfaction. There does not appear to be a relationship between snoring and libido or erectile function.

○ **What is the Nutcracker syndrome, how is it diagnosed and what is the treatment?**

It is left renal venous hypertension caused by compression of the left renal vein between the aorta and superior mesenteric artery. This causes left-sided hematuria, left gonadal vein varices, varicoceles in men, and possibly pain. Diagnosis is difficult but may be picked up with CT or MR angiography. Current treatment is with stents as a minimally invasive option, but embolization and vascular repositioning are acceptable alternatives.

○ **What is the most commonly litigated procedure that involves urologists, how many are done annually, and how many does the average urologist do a year?**

Vasectomy is the most commonly litigated procedure routinely performed by urologists. Approximately 527,000 are done yearly in the United States with the average urologist doing approximately 70 annually.

○ **What is infibulation?**

The placement of a ring or stick through the foreskin, presumably to prevent masturbation, sexual activity, and the spread of STDs by the ancient Greeks and Romans. It was done permanently in slaves and entertainers, but was removable for soldiers at age 25.

○ **Was infibulation ever accepted medical practice in the United States?**

It was commonly practiced starting in the 1860s and was not totally abandoned until 1929.

○ **What is an escutcheonectomy and what is its urological application?**

Excision of excessive suprapubic fat. It is one of several procedures to treat adult acquired buried penis. (The other procedures are scrotoplasty, split-thickness skin grafts, Y-V plasty, and panniculectomy.)

○ **Name the Roman god for lust and the god for marriage.**

Priapus for lust and Hymen for marriage.

○ **The early Christian church allowed sex in marriage only on what days?**

Tuesdays and Wednesdays.

○ **According to the Urologic Diseases in America Project by the NIDDK, what are the 5 most expensive urological conditions (in order) that accounted for more than $9 billion in 2007?**

In order, UTIs, kidney stones, prostate cancer, bladder cancer, and BPH.

○ **What are the estimated total yearly expenditures for overactive bladder in the United States?**

Approximately $16.4 billion.

○ **What percentage of patients can accurately and reliably fill out their AUA symptom scores by themselves without help?**

16%.

○ **What is Zoon balanitis, is it dangerous, and how is it treated?**

Also called plasma cell balanitis, Zoon balanitis is a rare, idiopathic, benign penile dermatocytis. It causes a bright red skin in the glans under the foreskin. Microscopically, it shows significant plasma cell infiltration. The lesion does not respond to steroids. Recommended treatment is a circumcision.

○ **Achille Boari first described his successful method for ureteral extension in dogs in 1894. When was the first human trial of this technique and who did it? (Hint: It was not Boari and it was done somewhere in the United States.)**

The first human case was in 1936 by Ockerblad of Yale.

○ **Describe in detail the unique connection between urine and matches.**

German alchemist Hennig Brand was looking for the "philosopher's stone." In 1669, he distilled a small amount of a glowing chemical that burned brilliantly by boiling a large amount of urine. This new chemical was noticed by Robert Boyle who added it to sulfur-tipped wooden splinters to facilitate ignition—the first matches. (Fortunately, early commercial matches used crushed bone treated with acid instead of urine as a source of this chemical.) Today we call Brand's chemical "phosphorus."

○ **Define "Koro" and "Dhat" and where they are most prevalent.**

"Koro" syndrome is the pathologic fear that the penis is shrinking. "Dhat" is a significant decrease in vitality from excessive loss of semen. Koro is found mostly in Southeast Asia while Dhat is typical of India.

○ **What is a Candiru?**

It is the name of the small catfish of the Amazon that reportedly can swim up the human male urethra.

○ **Premature ejaculation, as defined by the International Society for Sexual Medicine, includes what general time limit for ejaculation after vaginal penetration?**

1 minute.

Bibliography

Abol-Enein H, Tilki D, Mosbah A, et al. Does the extent of lymphadenectomy in radical cystectomy for bladder cancer influence disease-free survival? A prospective single-center study. *Eur Urol.* 2011;60:572–577.

Advanced Bladder Cancer (ABC) Meta-analysis Collaboration. Adjuvant chemotherapy in invasive bladder cancer: a systematic review and meta-analysis of individual patient data. *Eur Urol.* 2005;48:189–199; discussion 199–201.

Advanced Bladder Cancer Meta-analysis Collaboration. Neoadjuvant chemotherapy in invasive bladder cancer: a systematic review and meta-analysis. *Lancet.* 2003;361:1927–1934.

Akerlund S, Campanello M, Kaijser B, et al. Bacteriuria in patients with a continent ileal reservoir for urinary diversion does not regularly require antibiotic treatment. *Br J Urol.* 1994;74:177–181.

Aparicio AM, Elkhouiery AB, Quinn DI. The current and future application of adjuvant systemic chemotherapy in patients with bladder cancer following cystectomy. *Urol Clin North Am.* 2005;32:217–230.

Au JL, Badalament RA, Wientjes MG, et al. Methods to improve efficacy of intravesical mitomycin C: results of a randomized phase III trial. *J Natl Cancer Inst.* 2001;93:597–604.

AUA. *Guidelines for the Management of Nonmuscle Invasive Bladder Cancer (Stage Ta, T1, and Tis).* Linthicum, MD: AUA; 2007.

Babjuk M, Oosterlinck W, Sylvester R, et al. EAU guidelines on non-muscle-invasive urothelial carcinoma of the bladder. *Eur Urol.* 2008;54:303–314.

Bajorin DF, Dodd PM, Mazumdar M, et al: Long-term survival in metastatic transitional-cell carcinoma and prognostic factors predicting outcome of therapy. *J Clin Oncol* 1999;17:3173–3181.

Barzon L, Boscaro M. Diagnosis and management of adrenal incidentalomas. *J Urol.* 2000;163:398–407.

Baseman AG, Young RR Jr, Young AK, et al. Conservative management of spontaneous rupture of Kock orthotopic ileal reservoir. *Urology.* 1997;49:629–631.

Bauer SB. Anomalies of the kidney and ureteropelvic junction. In: Walsh PC, Retik AB, Vaughan ED, Wein AJ, eds. *Campbell's Urology.* 7th ed. Philadelphia, PA: W.B. Saunders; 1998.

Bearhs OH, Hanson DR, Hutter RVP, Kenedy BJ. *Manual for Staging of Cancer.* 4th ed. Philadelphia, PA: J.B. Lippincott; 1992:181.

Beilby JA, Keogh EJ. Spinal cord injuries and an ejaculation. *Paraplegia.* 1989;27:152.

Benson MC, Olsson CA. Continent urinary diversion. In: Walsh PC, Retik AB, Vaughan ED, Wein AJ, eds. *Campbell's Urology.* 7th ed. Philadelphia, PA: W.B. Saunders; 1998:3190.

Benson MC, Olsson CA. Continent urinary diversion. *Urol Clin North Am.* 1999;26:125–147.

Bihrle R. The Indiana pouch continent urinary reservoir. *Urol Clin North Am.* 1997;24:773–779.

Bloch MJ, Trost DW, Pickering TG, Sos TA, August P. Prevention of recurrent pulmonary edema in patients with bilateral renovascular disease through renal artery stent replacement. *Am J Hypertens.* 1999;12(1, pt 1):1–7.

Blyth B, Snyder HM. Ureteropelvic junction obstruction in children. In: Krane RJ, Siroky MB, Fitzpatrick JM, eds. *Clinical Urology.* Philadelphia, PA: J.B. Lippincott; 1994.

Bohle A, Bock PR: Intravesical bacille Calmette-Guerin versus mitomycin C in superficial bladder cancer: formal meta-analysis of comparative studies on tumor progression. *Urology.* 2004;63:682–686; discussion 686–687.

Bosl GJ, Motzer RJ. Testicular germ-cell cancer. *N Engl J Med.* 1997;337(4):242–253.

Breneman JC, Donaldson SS, Hays DM. The management of pediatric genitourinary rhabdomyosarcoma. In: Vogelzang NJ, Scardino PT, Shipley WU, Coffey DS, eds. *Comprehensive Textbook of Genitourinary Oncology.* Baltimore, MD: Williams and Wilkins; 1996.

Bricker EM. Bladder substitution after pelvic evisceration. *Surg Clin North Am.* 1950;30:1511–1521.

Brossner C, Bayer G, Madersbacher S, Kuber W, Klinger C, Pycha A. Twelve prostate biopsies detect significant cancer volumes (>0.5 mL). *Br J Urol.* 2000;85(6):705.

Bukowski RM, Klein EA. Management of adrenal neoplasms. In: Vogelzang NJ, Scardino PT, Shipley WU, Coffey DS, eds. *Comprehensive Textbook of Genitourinary Oncology.* Baltimore, MD: Williams and Wilkins; 1996;125–153.

Buvat J, Lemaire A. Endocrine screening in 1022 men with erectile dysfunction: clinical significance and cost-effective strategy. *J Urol.* 1997;158:1764–1767.

Caldamone AA, Woodard JR. Prune belly syndrome. In: Wein AJ, Kavoussi LR, Novick AC, Partin AW, Peters CA, eds. *Campbell-Walsh Urology,* 9th ed. Philadelphia, PA: W.B. Saunders; 2007.

Cameron J, et al. *Current Surgical Therapy.* 8th ed. Philadelphia: Mosby; 2004.

Campbell MF, Wein AJ, Kavoussi LR. In: Wein AJ, Kavoussi LR, Novick AC, Partin AW, Peters CA, eds. *Campbell-Walsh Urology.* 9th ed. Philadelphia, PA: W.B. Saunders; 2007.

Campbell-Walsh Urology. 9th ed. Philadelphia, PA: Saunders-Elsevier Inc.; 2007.

Carroll P, ed. Testis cancer. *Urol Clin North Am.* 1998;23(3).

Carson CC. Management of penile prosthesis infection. *Probl Urol.* 1993;7:368–380.

Cassady JR, Hutter JJ Jr, Whitesell LJ. Neuroblastoma: natural history and current therapeutic approaches. In: Vogelzang NJ, Scardino PT, Shipley WU, Coffey DS, eds. *Comprehensive Textbook of Genitourinary Oncology.* Baltimore, MD: Williams and Wilkins; 1996.

Catalona WJ. Urothelial tumors of the urinary tract. In: Walsh PC, Retik AB, Stamey TA, Vaughan ED Jr, eds. *Campbell's Urology.* Philadelphia, PA: W.B. Saunders; 1992:1094–1158.

CDC Surveillance Reports. Reported Tuberculosis in the United States, www.cdc.gov.

Cendron M, Elder JS, Duckett JW. Perinatal urology. In: Gillenwater JY, Grayhack JT, Howards SS, Duckett JW, eds. *Adult and Pediatric Urology.* Vol III. 3rd ed. St. Louis, MO: Mosby-Year Book, Inc.; 1996:2075–2169.

Cesaro S, Facchin C, Tridello G, et al. A prospective study of BK-virus-associated hemorrhagic cystitis in pediatric patients undergoing allogenic hematopoietic stem cell transplantation. *Bone Marrow Transplant.* 2008;41:363.

Chang BS, Kim HL, Yang XJ, et al. Correlation between biopsy and radical cystectomy in assessing grade and depth of invasion in bladder urothelial carcinoma. *Urology.* 2001;57:1063–1066; discussion 1066–1067.

Chen Z, Lu G, Li X, Li X, Fang Q, Ji H, et al. Better compliance contributes to better nocturnal continence with orthotopic ileal neobladder than ileocolonic neobladder after radical cystectomy for bladder cancer. *Urology.* 2009;73(4):838–843.

Cheville JC. Classification and pathology of testicular germ cell and sex cord-stromal tumors. *Urol Clin North Am.* 1999;26(3):595–609.

Chodak GW, Keller P, Scheonberg HW. Assessment of screening for prostate cancer using digital rectal examination. *J Urol.* 1989;141:1136.

Choong SK, Gleeson M. Conservative management of a spontaneous rupture of a continent cutaneous urinary diversion. *Br J Urol.* 1998;82:592–593.

Clayman RV, McDougal EM, Figenshau RS. Endourology of the upper urinary noncalculous applications. In: Gillenwater JY, Grayhack JT, Howards SH, Duckett JW, eds. *Adult and Pediatric Urology.* 3rd ed. St. Louis, MO: Mosby; 1996.

Cohen MS, Resnik MI. *Reoperative Urology.* Boston: Little, Brown and Company; 1995.

Colding-Jorgensen M, Poulsen AL, Steven K. Mechanical characteristics of tubular and detubularized bowel for bladder substitution: theory, urodynamics and clinical results. *Br J Urol.* 1993;72:586–593.

Connolly JA, Peppas DS, Jeffs RD, Gearhart JP. Prevalence and repair of inguinal hernias in children with bladder exstrophy. *J Urol.* 1995;154(5):1900–1901.

Coplen DE, Snow BW, Duckett JW. Prune Belly syndrome. In: Gillenwater JY, Grayhack JT, Howards SS, Duckett JW, eds. *Adult and Pediatric Urology.* 3rd ed. St. Louis, MO: Mosby; 1996:2297.

Cornu J-N, Neuzillet Y, Hervé J-M, Yonneau L, Botto H, Lebret T. Patterns of local recurrence after radical cystectomy in a contemporary series of patients with muscle-invasive bladder cancer. *World J Urol.* 2012:1–6.

Cruz DN, Huot SJ. Metabolic complications of urinary diversions: an overview. *Am J Med.* 1997;102:477–484.

Dahl DM, McDougal WS. Use of intestinal segments in urinary diversion. In: Wein AJ, Kavoussi LR, Novick AC, Partin AW, Peters CA, eds. *Campbell-Walsh Urology.* 9th ed. Philadelphia, PA: W.B. Saunders; 2007.

Dalbagni G, Reuter VE. Lamina propria: invasive bladder cancer (T1). In: Scardino PT, Linehan WM, Zelefsky MJ, Vogelzang NJ, eds. *Comprehensive Textbook of Genitourinary Oncology.* 4th ed. New York: Wolters Kluwer/Lippincott Williams & Wilkins; 2011:398–404.

Davidson AJ, Hartman DS, eds. *Radiology of the Kidney and Genitourinary Tract.* 3rd ed. Philadelphia, PA: W.B. Saunders; 1999.

Davidsson T, Akerlund S, Forssell-Aronsson E, et al. Absorption of sodium and chloride in continent reservoirs for urine: comparison of ileal and colonic reservoirs. *J Urol.* 1994;151:335–337.

De Santis M, Bellmunt J, Mead G, et al. Randomized phase II/III trial assessing gemcitabine/carboplatin and methotrexate/carboplatin/vinblastine in patients with advanced urothelial cancer who are unfit for cisplatin-based chemotherapy: EORTC study 30986. *J Clin Oncol.* 2012;30:191–199.

deKernion JB, Trapasso JG. Urinary diversion and continent reservoir. In: Gillenwater JY, Grayhack JT, Howards SS, Duckett JW, eds. *Adult and Pediatric Urology.* 3rd ed. St. Louis, MO: Mosby; 1996:1465.

Dhar NB, Klein EA, Reuther AM, et al. Outcome after radical cystectomy with limited or extended pelvic lymph node dissection. *J Urol.* 2008;179:873–878; discussion 878.

Diamond DA, Gosalbez R. Neonatal urologic emergencies. In: Walsh PC, Retik AB, Vaughn ED, Wein AJ, eds. *Campbell's Urology.* Vol II. 7th ed. Philadelphia, PA: W.B. Saunders; 1998:1629–1654.

Diamond M. Pediatric management of ambiguous and traumatized genitalia. *J Urol.* 1999;162(2):1021–1028.

Dodd PM, McCaffrey JA, Herr H, et al. Outcome of postchemotherapy surgery after treatment with methotrexate, vinblastine, doxorubicin, and cisplatin in patients with unresectable or metastatic transitional cell carcinoma. *J Clin Oncol.* 1999;17:2546–2552.

Donat SM, Herr HW. Role of radical cystectomy in patients with advanced bladder cancer. In: Scardino PT, Linehan WM, Zelefsky MJ, Vogelzang NJ, eds. *Comprehensive Textbook of Genitourinary Oncology.* 4th ed. New York, NY: Wolters Kluwer/Lippincott Williams and Wilkins; 2011: 421–428.

Donat SM, Herr HW, Bajorin DF, et al. Methotrexate, vinblastine, doxorubicin and cisplatin chemotherapy and cystectomy for unresectable bladder cancer. *J Urol.* 1996;156:368–371.

Dorin RP, Daneshmand S, Eisenberg MS, et al. Lymph node dissection technique is more important than lymph node count in identifying nodal metastases in radical cystectomy patients: a comparative mapping study. *Eur Urol.* 2011;60:946–952.

Dunnick NR, McCallum RW, Snadler CM. *Textbook of Uroradiology.* 2nd ed. Baltimore, MD: Williams and Wilkins; 1997.

Dutta SC, Smith JA Jr., Shappell SB, et al. Clinical under staging of high risk nonmuscle invasive urothelial carcinoma treated with radical cystectomy. *J Urol.* 2001;166:490–493.

Einhorn LH, Donohue JP. Advanced testicular cancer: update for urologists. *J Urol.* 1998;160(6, pt 1):1964–1969.

Eisenberger CF, Schoenberg M, Fitter D, Marshall FF. Orthotopic ileocolic neobladder reconstruction following radical cystectomy: history, technique and results of the Johns Hopkins experience, 1986–1998. *Urol Clin North Am.* 1999;26:149–156.

El Bahnasawy MS, Osman Y, Gomha MA, et al. Nocturnal enuresis in men with an orthotopic ileal reservoir: urodynamic evaluation. *J Urol.* 2000;164:10–13.

Elder JR, Hladky D, Selzmann AA. Outpatient nephrectomy for non-functioning kidneys. *J Urol.* 1993;154:712–715.

Endogenous Hormones and Prostate Cancer Collaborative Group. *J Natl Cancer Inst.* 2008;100:158.

Epstein JI, Amin MB, Reuter VR, et al. The World Health Organization/International Society of Urological Pathology consensus classification of urothelial (transitional cell) neoplasms of the urinary bladder. Bladder Consensus Conference Committee. *Am J Surg Pathol* 1998;22:1435–1448.

Feldman HA, Goldstein I, Hatzichristou DG, Krane RJ, McKinlay JB. Impotence and its medical and psychosocial correlates. Results of the Massachusetts Male Aging Study. *J Urol.* 1994;151:54–61.

Fernandez-Gomez J, Solsona E, Unda M, et al. Prognostic factors in patients with non-muscle-invasive bladder cancer treated with bacillus Calmette-Guerin: multivariate analysis of data from four randomized CUETO trials. *Eur Urol.* 2008;53:992–1001.

Fitzgerald J, Malone MJ, Gaertner RA, Zinman LN. Stomal construction, complications, and reconstruction. *Urol Clin North Am.* 1997;24:729–733.

Fowler JE, Koshy M, Strub M. Priapism associated with the sickle cell hemoglobinopathies: prevalence, natural history, and sequelae. *J Urol.* 1991;145:65–68.

Furness PD, Cheng EY, Franco I, Firlit CF. The Prune-Belly syndrome: a new and simplified technique of abdominal wall reconstruction. *J Urol.* 1998;160:1195.

Garovic V, Textor SC. Renovascular hypertension: current concepts. *Semin Nephrol.* 2005;25(4):261–271.

Gburek BM, Lieber MM, Blute ML. Comparison of studer ileal neobladder and ileal conduit urinary diversion with respect to perioperative outcome and late complications. *J Urol.* 1998;160:721–723.

Gillenwater JY, GrayhackJT, Howards SS, Duckett JW, eds. *Adult and Pediatric Urology.* 3rd ed. St. Louis, MO: Mosby; 1996: 2061–2758.

Gofrit ON, Pode D, Pizov G, et al. The natural history of bladder carcinoma in situ after initial response to bacillus Calmette-Guerin immunotherapy. *Urol Oncol.* 2009;27:258–262.

Goldfarb DS, Modersitzki F, Asplin JR. A randomized controlled trial of lactic acid bacteria for idopathic hyperoxaluria. *Clin J Am Soc Nephrol.* 2007;2(4):745–749.

Goldstein I, Lue TF, Padma-Nathan H, Rosen RC, Steers WD, Wicker PA. Oral Sildenafil in the treatment of erectile dysfunction. *N Engl J Med.* 1998;338:1397–1404.

Golin AL, Howard RS: Asymptomatic microscopic hematuria. *J Urol.* 1980;124:389–391.

Gonzales ET Jr. Anomalies of the renal pelvis and ureter. In: Kelalis PP, King LR, Belman AB, eds. *Clinical Pediatric Urology.* 3rd ed. Philadelphia, PA: W.B. Saunders; 1992.

Gordon I. Ultrasonography in uronephrology. In: O'Donnell B, Koff SA, eds. *Pediatric Urology.* 3rd ed. Oxford: Butterworth-Heinemann; 1997:41–64.

Gore JL, Lai J, Setodji CM, et al. Mortality increases when radical cystectomy is delayed more than 12 weeks: results from a surveillance, epidemiology, and end results—medicare analysis. *Cancer.* 2009;115:988–996.

Gorelick JI, Goldstein M. Loss of fertility in men with varicocele. *Fertil Steril.* 1993;59:613.

Gow JG. The current management of patients with genitourinary tuberculosis. In: *AUA Update Series.* Lesson 26. Vol. XI. Houston, TX: American Urological Association; 1992.

Granberg CF, Harrison SM, Dajusta D, et al. Genetic basis of Prune Belly syndrome: screening for HNF1β gene. *J Urol.* 2012;187: 272–278.

Graves FT. The anatomy of the intrarenal arteries and its application to segmental resection of the kidney. *Br J Surg.* 1955;2:132.

Gray H. *Grays Anatomy, the Anatomical Basis of Medicine and Surgery.* 38th ed. New York: Churchill Livingstone; 1995.

Gray H, Carter HV, Pick TP, Howden R. *Grays Anatomy.* London: Senate; 2003.

Gray SW, Skandalakis JE. *Embryology for Surgeons.* Philadelphia, PA: W.B. Saunders; 1972.

Greenfield LJ, et al. *Surgery: Scientific Principles and Practice.* 2nd ed. Philadelphia: Lippincott Williams and Wilkins; 1997.

Greskovich FJ, Nyberg LM. The prune belly syndrome: a review of its etiology, defects, treatment and prognosis. *J Urol.* 1988;140:707.

Griffiths G, Hall R, Sylvester R, et al. International phase III trial assessing neoadjuvant cisplatin, methotrexate, and vinblastine chemotherapy for muscle-invasive bladder cancer: long-term results of the BA06 30894 trial. *J Clin Oncol.* 2011;29:2171–2177.

Grossman HB, Natale RB, Tangen CM, et al. Neoadjuvant chemotherapy plus cystectomy compared with cystectomy alone for locally advanced bladder cancer. *N Engl J Med.* 2003;349:859–866.

Gudjonsson S, Isfoss BL, Hansson K, et al. The value of the UroVysion assay for surveillance of non-muscle-invasive bladder cancer. *Eur Urol.* 2008;54:402-408.

Guiney EJ. Emergency room problems. In: O'Donnell B, Koff SA, eds. *Pediatric Urology.* 3rd ed. Oxford: Butterworth-Heinemann; 1997:281–285.

Gulml FA, Felsen D, Vaughan ED. Pathophysiology of urinary tract obstruction. In: Walsh PC, Retik AB, Vaughan ED, Wein AJ, eds. *Campbell's Urology.* 7th ed. Philadelphia, PA: W.B. Saunders; 1998.

Guyton AC. *Textbook of Medical Physiology.* 8th ed. Philadelphia, PA: W.B. Saunders; 1991.

Haas GP, Triest J, Pontes E, Trump DL. Nonsurgical treatment of adrenocortical cancer. In: Raghavan D, Scher HI, Leibel SA, Lange P, eds. *Principles and Practice of Genitourinary Oncology.* Philadelphia, PA: Lippincott-Raven; 1997:1001–1006.

Hajdinjak T. UroVysion FISH test for detecting urothelial cancers: meta-analysis of diagnostic accuracy and comparison with urinary cytology testing. *Urol Oncol.* 2008;26:646–651.

Hall MC, Chang SS, Dalbagni G, et al. Guideline for the management of nonmuscle invasive bladder cancer (stages Ta, T1, and Tis): 2007 update. *J Urol.* 2007;178:2314–2330.

Han RF, Pan JG. Can intravesical bacillus Calmette-Guerin reduce recurrence in patients with superficial bladder cancer? A meta-analysis of randomized trials. *Urology.* 2006;67:1216–1223.

Hanno PM. Diagnosis of interstitial cystitis. *Urol Clin North Am.* 1994;21(1):63.

Hardeman SW, Soloway MS. Urethral recurrence following radical cystectomy. *J Urol.* 1990;144:666–669.

Hassett S, Smith GHH, Holland AJA. Prune belly syndrome. *Pediatric Surg Int.* 2012;28:219–228.

Hautmann RE. The ileal neobladder to the female urethra. *Urol Clin North Am.* 1997;24:827–835.

Hautmann RE, Abol-Enein H, Hafez K, et al. Urinary diversion. *Urology.* 2007;69(1 suppl):17–49.

Hautmann RE, Simon J. Ileal neobladder and local recurrence of bladder cancer: patterns of failure and impact on function in men. *J Urol.* 1999;162:1963–1966.

Hedge GA, Colby HD, Goodman RL. *Clinical Endocrine Physiology.* Philadelphia, PA: W.B. Saunders; 1987.

Hendren WH. Historical perspective of the use of bowel in urology. *Urol Clin North Am.* 1997;24:703–713.

Hendren WH. Urinary undiversion: refunctionalization of the previously diverted urinary tract. In: Walsh PC, Retik AB, Vaughan ED, Wein AJ, eds. *Campbell's Urology.* 7th ed. Philadelphia, PA: W.B. Saunders; 1998:3247.

Heney NM, Ahmed S, Flanagan MJ, et al. Superficial bladder cancer: progression and recurrence. *J Urol.* 1983;130:1083–1086.

Henly DR, Farrow GM, Zincke H. Urachal carcinoma: role of conservative surgery. *Urology.* 1993;42:635–639.

Hensle TW, Bingham JB, Reiley EA, et al. The urologic care and outcome of pregnancy after urinary tract reconstruction. *BJU Int.* 2004;93:588–590.

Herr HW: Narrow-band imaging cystoscopy to evaluate the response to bacille Calmette-Guerin therapy: preliminary results. *BJU Int.* 2010;105:314–316.

Herr HW. Restaging transurethral resection of high risk superficial bladder cancer improves the initial response to bacillus Calmette-Guerin therapy. *J Urol.* 2005;174:2134–2137.

Herr HW. Superiority of ratio based lymph node staging for bladder cancer. *J Urol.* 2003;169:943–945.

Herr HW. The value of a second transurethral resection in evaluating patients with bladder tumors. *J Urol.* 1999;162:74–76.

Herr HW. Transurethral resection of muscle-invasive bladder cancer: 10-year outcome. *J Clin Oncol.* 2001;19:89–93.

Herr HW. Tumor progression and survival of patients with high grade, noninvasive papillary (TaG3) bladder tumors: 15-year outcome. *J Urol.* 2000;163:60–61; discussion 61–62.

Herr HW, Badalament RA, Amato DA, et al. Superficial bladder cancer treated with bacillus Calmette-Guerin: a multivariate analysis of factors affecting tumor progression. *J Urol.* 1989;141:22–29.

Herr HW, Dalbagni G. Defining bacillus Calmette-Guerin refractory superficial bladder tumors. *J Urol.* 2003;169:1706–1708.

Herr HW, Donat SM. Outcome of patients with grossly node positive bladder cancer after pelvic lymph node dissection and radical cystectomy. *J Urol.* 2001;165:62–64; discussion 64.

Herr HW, Donat SM, Dalbagni G. Can restaging transurethral resection of T1 bladder cancer select patients for immediate cystectomy? *J Urol.* 2007;177:75–79; discussion 79.

Hinman F. *Atlas of Urosurgical Anatomy.* Philadelphia, PA: W.B. Saunders; 1993.

Hinman F Jr. *Atlas of Urologic Surgery.* 2nd ed. Philadelphia, PA: W.B. Saunders; 1998.

Hoffman DM, Resnick MI. Return of perineal prostatectomy. *MediGuide Urol.* 1993;6(3).

Hollenbeck BK, Wei Y, Birkmeyer JD. Volume, process of care, and operative mortality for cystectomy for bladder cancer. *Urology.* 2007;69:871–875.

Holzbeierlein JM, Lopez-Corona E, Bochner BH, et al. Partial cystectomy: a contemporary review of the Memorial Sloan-Kettering Cancer Center experience and recommendations for patient selection. *J Urol.* 2004;172:878–881.

Horgan JD, Smith AD. Endopyclotomy and pyeloplasty. In: Krane RJ, Siroky MB, Fitzpatrick JM, eds. *Clinical Urology.* Philadelphia, PA: J.B. Lippincott; 1994.

Hudson MA, Herr HW. Carcinoma in situ of the bladder. *J Urol.* 1995;153:564–572.

Husmann DA, Levy JB, Cain MP, et al. Micropenis: current Concepts and Controversies. In: *AUA Update Series.* Lesson 10, Vol. XVII. Houston, TX: American Urological Association; 1998:74–79.

Iborra I, Casanova JL, Solsona E. Tolerance of external urinary diversion (Bricker) followed for more than 10 years. *Eur Urol.* 2001;39(suppl 5):146–147.

Inman BA, Harel F, Tiguert R, et al. Routine nasogastric tubes are not required following cystectomy with urinary diversion: a comparative analysis of 430 patients. *J Urol.* 2003;170:1888–1891.

International Collaboration of Trialists: Neoadjuvant cisplatin, methotrexate, and vinblastine chemotherapy for muscle-invasive bladder cancer: a randomised controlled trial. International collaboration of trialists. *Lancet* 1999;354:533–540.

Isbarn H, Jeldres C, Zini L, et al. A population based assessment of perioperative mortality after cystectomy for bladder cancer. *J Urol.* 2009;182:70–77.

Jakse G, Hall R, Bono A, et al. Intravesical BCG in patients with carcinoma in situ of the urinary bladder: long-term results of EORTC GU Group phase II protocol 30861. *Eur Urol.* 2001;40:144–150.

Jocham D, Stepp H, Waidelich R. Photodynamic diagnosis in urology: state-of-the-art. *Eur Urol.* 2008;53:1138–1148.

Johnson DE, Hodges GB, Abdul-Karim FW, et al. Urachal carcinoma. *Urology.* 1985;26:218–221.

Jones JS, Larchian, WA. Non-muscle-invasive bladder cancer (Ta, T1, and CIS). In: Wein AJ, Kavoussi LR, Novick AC, Partin AW, Peters C A, eds. *Campbell-Walsh Urology.* 10th ed. Philadelphia, PA: Elsevier Saunders, 2011:2335–2354.

Kabalin JN. In: Walsh PC, Retik AB, Vaughan ED Jr, Wein AJ, eds. *Campbell's Urology.* Vol I. 7th ed. Philadelphia, PA: W.B. Saunders; 1998.

Kaefer M, Retik AB. The Mitrofanoff principle in continent urinary reconstruction. *Urol Clin North Am.* 1997;24:795–811.

Kamat AM, Dinney CP, Gee JR, et al. Micropapillary bladder cancer: a review of the University of Texas M. D. Anderson Cancer Center experience with 100 consecutive patients. *Cancer.* 2007;110:62–67.

Kass EJ. Megaureter. In: Kelalis PP, King LR, Belman AB, eds. *Clinical Pediatric Urology.* 3rd ed. Philadelphia, PA: W.B. Saunders; 1992.

Katz MD, Imperato-McGinley J. Adrenal cancer: endocrinology, diagnosis and clinical staging. In: Raghavan D, Scher HI, Leibel SA, Lange P, eds. *Principles and Practice of Genitourinary Oncology*. Philadelphia, PA: Lippincott-Raven; 1997:981–992.

Kaye KW, Lange PH. Mode of presentation of invasive bladder cancer: reassessment of the problem. *J Urol*. 1982;128:31–33.

Kelalis PP, King LR, Belman AB, eds. *Clinical Pediatric Urology*. Vol. 2. 3rd ed. Philadelphia, PA: W.B. Saunders; 1992.

Khadra MH, Pickard RS, Charlton M, et al. A prospective analysis of 1,930 patients with hematuria to evaluate current diagnostic practice. *J Urol*. 2000;163:524–527.

Khafagy M, Shaheed FA, Moneim TA. Ileocaecal vs ileal neobladder after radical cystectomy in patients with bladder cancer: a comparative study. *BJU Int*. 2006;97(4):799–804.

Kim J-H, et al. Contemporary management of renovascular hypertension. In: *AUA Update Series*. Lesson 14. Houston, TX: American Urological Association;2007:26.

King LR. Vesicoureteral reflux, megaurter and ureteral reimplantation. In: Walsh PC, Retik AB, Vaughan ED Jr, Wein AJ, eds. *Campbell's Urology*. 6th ed. Philadelphia, PA: W.B. Saunders; 2007.

Koch MO, Gurevitch E, Hill DE, et al. Urinary solute transport by intestinal segments: a comparative study of ileum and colon in rats. *J Urol*. 1990;143:1275–1279.

Koch MO, McDougal WS. Chlorpromazine: adjuvant therapy for the metabolic derangements created by urinary diversion through intestinal segments. *J Urol*. 1985;134(1):165–169.

Koch MO, Smith JA. Surgical management of adrenal tumors. In: Raghavan D, Scher HI, Leibel SA, Lange P, eds. *Principles and Practice of Genitourinary Oncology*. Philadelphia, PA: Lippincott-Raven; 1997:993–1000.

Kogan BA. Disorders of the ureter and ureteropelvic junction. In: Tanango EA, McAnich JW, eds. *Smith's General Urology*. 14th ed. Norwalk, CT: Appleton and Lange; 1995.

Kogan S, Hadziselimovic F, Howards SS, Snyder HM, Huff D. Pediatric andrology. In: Gillenwater JY, Grayhack JT, Howards SS, Duckett JW, eds. *Adult and Pediatric Urology*. 3rd ed. St. Louis, MO: Mosby; 1996:2623–2674.

Konety BR, Allareddy V. Influence of post-cystectomy complications on cost and subsequent outcome. *J Urol*. 2007;177:280–287; discussion 287.

Konety BR, Joslyn SA, O'Donnell MA. Extent of pelvic lymphadenectomy and its impact on outcome in patients diagnosed with bladder cancer: analysis of data from the Surveillance, Epidemiology and End Results Program data base. *J Urol*. 2003;169: 946–950.

Koo HP, Bloom DA. Laparoscopy for the nonpalpable testis. *Semin Laparosc Surg*. 1998;5:40–46.

Korman HJ. *Monographs in Urology*. Vol. 17. 1996b:83–95.

Korman HJ, Watson RB, Soloway MS. Bladder cancer: clinical aspects and management, 1996. In: Stamey TS, ed. *Monographs in Urology*. Vol. 17. 1996a:6, 81–110.

Koziol JA. Epidemiology of interstitial cystitis. *Urol Clin North Am*. 1994;21(1):1–7.

Kramer SA. Vesicoureteral reflux. In: Kelalis PP, King LR, Belman AB, eds. *Clinical Pediatric Urology*. 3rd ed. Philadelphia, PA: W.B. Saunders; 1992.

Krane RJ, et al., eds. *Clinical Urology*. Philadelphia, PA: J.B. Lippincott; 1994.

Kristjansson A, Bajc M, Wallin L, et al. Renal function up to 16 years after conduit (refluxing or anti-reflux anastomosis) or continent urinary diversion. 2. Renal scarring and location of bacteriuria. *Br J Urol*. 1995b;76:546–550.

Kristjansson A, Wallin L, Mansson W. Renal function up to 16 years after conduit (refluxing or anti-reflux anastomosis) or continent urinary diversion. 1. Glomerular filtration rate and patency of uretero-intestinal anastomosis. *Br J Urol*. 1995a;76:539–545.

Kulkarni GS, Urbach DR, Austin PC, et al. Longer wait times increase overall mortality in patients with bladder cancer. *J Urol*. 2009;182:1318–1324.

Lambert EH, Pierorazio PM, Olsson CA, et al. The increasing use of intravesical therapies for stage T1 bladder cancer coincides with decreasing survival after cystectomy. *BJU Int*. 2007;100:33–36.

Lamm D, Herr H, Jakse G, et al. Updated concepts and treatment of carcinoma in situ. *Urol Oncol*. 1998; 4:130–138.

Lecouvet FE, Geukens D, Stainier A, et al. Magnetic resonance imaging of the axial skeleton for detecting bone metastases in patients with high-risk prostate cancer: diagnostic and cost-effectiveness and comparison with current detection strategies. *J Clin Oncol*. 2007;25:3281–3287.

Lee CT, Madii R, Daignault S, et al. Cystectomy delay more than 3 months from initial bladder cancer diagnosis results in decreased disease specific and overall survival. *J Urol*. 2006;175:1262–1267; discussion 1267.

Lee PA. Fertility in cryptorchidism: does treatment make a difference? *Endocrinol Metab Clin North Am*. 1993;22:479.

Leissner J, Black P, Fisch M, et al. Colon pouch (Mainz Pouch III) for continent urinary diversion after pelvic irradiation. *Urology*. 2000;56:798–802.

Leissner J, Ghoneim MA, Abol-Enein H, et al. Extended radical lymphadenectomy in patients with urothelial bladder cancer: results of a prospective multicenter study. *J Urol.* 2004;171:139–144.

Leissner J, Hohenfellner R, Thuroff JW, et al. Lymphadenectomy in patients with transitional cell carcinoma of the urinary bladder; significance for staging and prognosis. *BJU Int.* 2000;85:817–823.

Lerner SP, Sternberg CN. Management of metastatic and invasive bladder cancer. In: Wein AJ, Kavoussi LR, Novick AC, Partin AW, Peters CA, eds. *Cambell-Walsh Urology.* 10th ed. Philadelphia, PA: Elsevier Saunders; 2011:2355–2374.

Levy DA, Resnick MI. Laparoscopic pelvic lymphadenectomy and radical perineal prostatectomy: a viable alternative to radical retropubic prostatectomy. *J Urol.* 1994;151:905.

Licht MR, Lewis RW, Wollan PC, Harris CD. Comparison of RigiScan and sleep laboratory nocturnal penile tumescence in the diagnosis of organic impotence. *J Urol.* 1995;154:1740–1743.

Lightfoot AJR, HM, O'Donnell, MA. High-risk non-muscle-invasive bladder cancer: Ta high grade and carcinoma in situ. In: Scardino PT, Linehan WM, Zelefsky MJ, Vogelzang NJ, eds. *Comprehensive Textbook of Genitourinary Oncology.* 4th ed. New York, Wolters Kluwer/Lippincott Williams & Wilkins; 2011:390–397.

Lopez-Beltran A. Bladder cancer: clinical and pathological profile. *Scand J Urol Nephrol Suppl.* 2008:95–109.

Losa A, Hurle R, Lembo A. Low dose bacillus Calmette-Guerin for carcinoma in situ of the bladder: long-term results. *J Urol.* 2000;163:68–71; discussion 71–72.

Lotan Y, Roehrborn CG. Sensitivity and specificity of commonly available bladder tumor markers versus cytology: results of a comprehensive literature review and meta-analyses. *Urology.* 2003;61:109–118; discussion 118.

Madersbacher S, Mohrle K, Burkhard F, et al. Long-term voiding pattern of patients with ileal orthotopic bladder substitutes. *J Urol.* 2002;167:2052–2057.

Malone MJ, Izes JK, Hurley LJ. Carcinogenesis: the fate of intestinal segments used in urinary reconstruction. *Urol Clin North Am.* 1997;24:723–728.

Mansson W, Colleen S, Mardh PA. The microbial flora of the continent cecal urinary reservoir, its stoma and the peristomal skin. *J Urol.* 1986;135:247–250.

Mansson W, Davidsson T, Konyves J, et al. Continent urinary tract reconstruction—the Lund experience. *BJU Int.* 2003;92:271–276.

Manyak MJ, Hinkle GH, Olsen JO, et al. Immunoscintigraphy with indium-111-capromed pendetide: evaluation before definitive therapy in patients with prostate cancer. *Urology.* 1999;54(6):1058.

Matzkin H, Moinuddin SM, Soloway MS. Value of urine cytology versus bladder washing in bladder cancer. *Urology.* 1992;39:201–203.

May M, Herrmann E, Bolenz C, et al. Association between the number of dissected lymph nodes during pelvic lymphadenectomy and cancer-specific survival in patients with lymph node-negative urothelial carcinoma of the bladder undergoing radical cystectomy. *Ann Surg Oncol.* 2011;18:2018–2025.

McDougal WS. Metabolic complications of urinary intestinal diversion. *J Urol.* 1992;147:1199–1208.

McDougal WS. Use of intestinal segments and urinary diversion. In: Walsh PC, Retik AB, Vaughan ED, Wein AJ, eds. *Campbell's Urology.* 7th ed. Philadelphia, PA: W.B. Saunders; 1998:3121.

McDougal WS, Koch MO. Effect of sulfate on calcium and magnesium homeostasis following urinary diversion. *Kidney Int.* 1989;35:105–115.

Messing EM, Vaillancourt A: Hematuria screening for bladder cancer. *J Occup Med.* 1990;32:838–845.

Meyers RP. Practical pelvic anatomy pertinent to radical retropubic prostatectomy. In: *AUA Update Series.* Lesson 4. Vol. XIII. Houston, TX: American Urological Association; 1994.

Mills RD, Studer UE. Metabolic consequences of continent urinary diversion. *J Urol.* 1999;161:1057–1066.

Mills RD, Turner WH, Fleischmann A, et al. Pelvic lymph node metastases from bladder cancer: outcome in 83 patients after radical cystectomy and pelvic lymphadenectomy. *J Urol.* 2001;166:19–23.

Mishriki SF, Nabi G, Cohen NP. Diagnosis of urologic malignancies in patients with asymptomatic dipstick hematuria: prospective study with 13 years' follow-up. *Urology.* 2008;71:13–16.

Mohr DN, Offord KP, Owen RA, et al. Asymptomatic microhematuria and urologic disease. A population-based study. *JAMA.* 1986;256:224–229.

Montorsi F, Brock G, Lee J, et al. Effect of nightly versus on-demand vardenafil on recovery of erectile function in men following bilateral nerve-sparing radical prostatectomy. *Eur Urol.* 2008;54(4):924–931.

Moonen PM, Merkx GF, Peelen P, et al. UroVysion compared with cytology and quantitative cytology in the surveillance of non-muscle-invasive bladder cancer. *Eur Urol.* 2007;51:1275–1280; discussion 1280.

Morgan TM, Kaffenberger SD, Cookson MS. Surgical and chemotherapeutic management of regional lymph nodes in bladder cancer. *J Urol.* 2012;188:1081–1088.

Morris PJ, ed. *Kidney Transplantation: Principles and Practice.* 4th ed. Philadelphia: WB Saunders; 1994.

Muruve NA. E-medicine: radiation cystitis. Feb 7, 2008.

Narayan P, Konety BR. Surgical treatment of female urethral carcinoma. *Urol Clin North Am.* 1992;19(2):373–382.

Nieh PT. The Kock pouch urinary reservoir. *Urol Clin North Am.* 1997;24:755–772.

Nippgen JB, Hakenberg OW, Manseck A, et al. Spontaneous late rupture of orthotopic detubularized ileal neobladders: report of five cases. *Urology.* 2001;58:43–46.

Noh PH, Cooper CS, Winkler AC, et al. Prognostic factors for long-term renal function in boys with prune-belly syndrome. *J Urol.* 1999;162:1399.

Norman DJ, Suki TO, eds. *Primer on Transplantation.* Thorofare, NJ: American Society of Transplant Physicians; 1998.

Novick AC, Howards SS. The adrenals. In: Gillenwater JY, Grayhack JT, Howards SS, Duckett JW, eds. *Adult and Pediatric Urology.* 3rd ed. Chicago: Mosby; 1996:587–616.

Novick AC, Streem SB. Surgery of the kidney. In: Walsh PC, Retik AB, Vaughan ED, Wein AJ, eds. *Campbell s Urology.* 7th ed. Philadelphia, PA: W.B. Saunders; 1998.

Oates RD, Lipshultz LI. Fertility and testicular function in patients after chemotherapy and radiotherapy. *Adv Urol.* 1989;10:52.

O'Donnell B, Koff SA, eds. *Pediatric Urology.* 3rd ed. Oxford: Butterworth Heinemann; 1997.

Pagano F, Bassi P, Ferrante GL, et al. Is stage pT4a (D1) reliable in assessing transitional cell carcinoma involvement of the prostate in patients with a concurrent bladder cancer? A necessary distinction for contiguous or noncontiguous involvement. *J Urol.* 1996;155:244–247.

Pagliaro LC, Williams DL, Daliani D, et al. Neoadjuvant paclitaxel, ifosfamide, and cisplatin chemotherapy for metastatic penile cancer: a phase II study. *J Clin Oncol.* 2010;28(24):3851–3857. doi: 10.1200/JCO.2010.29.5477. Epub 2010 Jul 12. PMID:20625118.

Pandha H, Sorensen KD, Orntoft TF, et al. Urinary engrailed-2 (EN2) levels predict tumor volume in men undergoing radical prostatectomy for prostate cancer. *BJU Int.* 2012;110(6 Pt B):E287–E292.

Parekh DJ, Gilbert WB, Koch MO, et al. Continent urinary reconstruction versus ileal conduit: a contemporary single-institution comparison of perioperative morbidity and mortality. *Urology.* 2000;55:852–855.

Parkin DM. The global burden of urinary bladder cancer. *Scand J Urol Nephrol Suppl.* 2008;218:12–20.

Parsons CL, Parsons JK. Interstitial cystitis. In: Shlomo Raz, ed. *Female Urology.* 2nd ed. Philadelphia, PA: Saunders; 1996.

Partin AW, Yoo J, Carter HB, et al. Letter to the editor. *J Urol.* 1994;152:172.

Partin AW, Yoo J, Carter HB, et al. The use of prostatic specific antigen, clinical stage and Gleason's score to predict pathological stage in men with localized prostate cancer. *J Urol.* 1993;150:110.

Penn I. Renal transplantation in patients with pre-existing malignancies. *Transplant Proc.* 1983;15:1079.

Peters P. "Ball Peen Hammer" appearance of the duplicated collecting system. Personal communication.

Pisansky T, Kahn MJ, Bostwick DG. An enhanced prognostic system for clinically localized carcinoma of the prostate. *Cancer.* 1997;79:2154–2161.

Presti JC, Chang JJ, Bhargava V, Shinohara K. The optimal systematic prostate biopsy scheme should include 8 rather than 6 biopsies: results of a prospective clinical trial. *J Urol.* 2000;163(1):163.

Prout GR, Marshall VF. The prognosis with untreated bladder tumors. *Cancer.* 1956;9:551–558.

Pryor JP, Hendry WF. Ejaculatory duct obstruction in subfertile males: analysis of 87 patients. *Fertil Steril.* 1991;56:725.

Pu XY, Wang HP, Wu YL, et al. Use of bipolar energy for transurethral resection of superficial bladder tumors: long-term results. *J Endourol.* 2008;22:545–549.

Quek ML, Stein JP, Clark PE, et al. Microscopic and gross extravesical extension in pathological staging of bladder cancer. *J Urol.* 2004;171:640–645.

Quek ML, Stein JP, Daneshmand S, et al. A critical analysis of perioperative mortality from radical cystectomy. *J Urol.* 2006;175: 886–889; discussion 889–890.

Racioppi M, D'Addessi A, Fanasca A, et al. Acid–base and electrolyte balance in urinary intestinal orthotopic reservoir: ileocecal neobladder compared with ileal neobladder. *Urology.* 1999;54:629–635.

Ramos CG, Carvalhal GF, Smith DS, Mager DE, Catalona WJ. Retrospective comparison of radical retropubic prostatectomy and 125-iodine brachytherapy for a localized prostate cancer. *J Urol.* 1999;161(4):1212–1215.

Ravi R, Dewan AK, Pandey KK. Transverse colon conduit urinary diversion in patients treated with very high dose pelvic irradiation. *Br J Urol.* 1994;73:51–54.

Redman JF. In: Raghavan D, Scher HI, Leibel SA, Lange P, eds. *Principles and Practice of Genitourinary Oncology.* Philadelphia, PA: Lippincott-Raven; 1997.

Resnik MI, Kursh ED. Extrinsic obstruction of the ureter. In: Walsh PC, Retik AB, Vaughan ED, Wein AJ, eds. *Campbell s Urology.* 7th ed. Philadelphia, PA: W.B. Saunders; 1998.

Retik AB, Peters CA. Ectopic ureter and ureterocele. In: Walsh PC, Retik AB, Vaughan ED Jr, Wein AJ, eds. *Campbell s Urology.* 6th ed. Philadelphia, PA: W.B. Saunders; 1992.

Ritchie JP. Testicular neoplasms. In: Walsh P, Retik A, Vaughan E, Wein A, eds. *Campbell s Urology.* 7th ed. Philidelphia, PA: W.B. Saunders; 1998:2411.

Rob DH, Blascoe JC, Grim PD, et al. Interstitial iodine-125 radiation without adjuvant therapy, the treatment of clinically localized prostate. *Cancer.* 1997;80:442.

Routh JC, Huang L, Retik B, Nelson CP. Contemporary epidemiology and characterization of newborn males with prune belly syndrome. *Urology.* 2010;76:44–48.

Roychowdhury DF, Hayden A, Liepa AM. Health-related quality-of-life parameters as independent prognostic factors in advanced or metastatic bladder cancer. *J Clin Oncol.* 2003;21:673–678.

Sadler TW. *Langmans Medical Embryology.* 6th ed. Baltimore, MD: Williams & Wilkins; 1990:260–296.

Sanchez-Ortiz RF, Huang WC, Mick R, et al. An interval longer than 12 weeks between the diagnosis of muscle invasion and cystectomy is associated with worse outcome in bladder carcinoma. *J Urol.* 2003;169:110–115; discussion 115.

Sarosdy MF. Immunotherapy of superficial bladder carcinoma. In: *AUA Update Series.* Lesson 209. Vol. XIV. Houston, TX: American Urological Association; 1995:234–239.

Saxman SB, Propert KJ, Einhorn LH, et al. Long-term follow-up of a phase III intergroup study of cisplatin alone or in combination with methotrexate, vinblastine, and doxorubicin in patients with metastatic urothelial carcinoma: a cooperative group study. *J Clin Oncol.* 1997;15:2564–2569.

Schaeffer AJ. Infections and Inflammations of the genitourinary tract. In: Walsh PC, Retik AB, Vaughan ED, Wein AJ, eds. *Campbell's Urology.* Philadelphia, PA: W.B. Saunders; 1998.

Schaeffer AJ. Urinary tract infections. In: Gillenwater JY, Grayhack JT, Howards SH, Duckett JW, eds. *Adult and Pediatric Urology.* 3rd ed. Mosby, MO: St. Louis; 1996.

Scosyrev E, Messing EM. Do mixed histological features affect survival benefit from neoadjuvant platinum-based combination chemotherapy in patients with locally advanced bladder cancer? *BJU Int.* 2011;108:700.

Shaaban AA, Abdel-Latif M, Mosbah A, Gad H, Eraky I, Ali-El-Dein B. A randomized study comparing an antireflux system with a direct ureteric anastomosis in patients with orthotopic ileal neobladders. *BJU Int.* 2006;97(5):1057–1062.

Shipley WU, Winter KA, Kaufman DS, et al. Phase III trial of neoadjuvant chemotherapy in patients with invasive bladder cancer treated with selective bladder preservation by combined radiation therapy and chemotherapy: initial results of Radiation Therapy Oncology Group 89-03. *J Clin Oncol.* 1998;16:3576–3583.

Shokeir AA. The diagnosis of upper urinary tract obstruction. European Urology Update Series 1999:3. *Br J Urol.* 1999;83:893.

Siegel R, Naishadham D, Jemal A. Cancer statistics, 2012. *CA Cancer J Clin.* 2012;62:10–29.

Singh G, Wilkinson JM, Thomas DG. Supravesical diversion for incontinence: a long-term follow-up. *Br J Urol.* 1997;79:348–353.

Siroky MB, Edelstein RA, Krane RJ, eds. *Manual of Urology.* 2nd ed. Philadelphia, PA: Lippincott Williams & Wilkins; 1999.

Smith RB, Ehrlich RM, eds. *Complications or Urologic Surgery: Prevention and Management.* 2nd ed. Philadelphia, PA: W.B. Saunders; 1990:386–411.

Snyder HM III, D'Angio GJ, Evans AE, Raney RB. Pediatric oncology. In: Walsh PC, Retik AB, Vaughan ED, Wein AJ, eds. *Campbell's Urology.* 7th ed. Philadelphia, PA: W.B. Saunders; 1998.

Sobin LH, Wittekind CH, eds; International Union Against Cancer. *TNM Classification of Malignant Tumours.* New York: Wiley-Liss; 1997:187–190.

Soloway MS. Expectant treatment of small, recurrent, low-grade, noninvasive tumors of the urinary bladder. *Urol Oncol.* 2006;24:58–61.

Solsona E, Iborra I, Ricos JV, et al. Biological behavior of untreated bladder carcinoma in situ. *Arch Esp Urol.* 1990;43:643–645.

Solsona E, Iborra I, Ricos JV, et al. Upper urinary tract involvement in patients with bladder carcinoma in situ (Tis): its impact on management. *Urology.* 1997;49:347–352.

Solsona E, Iborra I, Ricos JV, et al. Feasibility of transurethral resection for muscle infiltrating carcinoma of the bladder: long-term followup of a prospective study. *J Urol.* 1998;159:95–98; discussion 98–99.

Splinter TA, Scher HI. Adjuvant and neoadjuvant chemotherapy for invasive (T3-T4) bladder cancer. In: Vogelzang NJ, Scardino PT, Shipley WU, Cofffey DS, Miles BJ, eds. *Comprehensive Textbook of Genitourinary Oncology.* Baltimore, MD: Williams and Wilkins; 1996:464–471.

Stamey TA, Yang N, Hay AR, McNeal JE, Freiha FS, Redwine E. Prostate-specific antigen as a serum marker for adenocarcinoma of the prostate. *N Engl J Med.* 1987;317:909.

Stamm WE. Treatment of acute uncomplicated urinary tract infection. In: Bergan T, ed. *Urinary Tract Infections.* Basel, Switzerland: Karger; 1997.

Stampfer DS, McDougal WS, McGovern FJ. Metabolic and nutritional complications. *Urol Clin North Am.* 1997;24:715–722.

Stein BA, Harel F, Tiguert R, et al. Routine nasogastric tubes are not required following cystectomy with urinary diversion: a comparative analysis of 430 patients. *J Urol.* 2003;170:1888–1891.

Stein JP, Cai J, Groshen S, et al. Risk factors for patients with pelvic lymph node metastases following radical cystectomy with en bloc pelvic lymphadenectomy: concept of lymph node density. *J Urol.* 2003;170:35–41.

Stein JP, Cai J, Groshen S, Skinner DG. Risk factors for patients with pelvic lymph node metastases following radical cystectomy with en bloc pelvic lymphadenectomy: concept of lymph node density. *J Urol.* 2003;170:35.

Stein JP, Clark P, Miranda G, Cai J, Groshen S, Skinner DG. Urethral tumor recurrence following cystectomy and urinary diversion: Clinical and pathological characteristics in 768 male patients. *J Urol.* 2005;173:1163–1168.

Stein JP, Lieskovsky G, Cote R, et al. Radical cystectomy in the treatment of invasive bladder cancer: long-term results in 1,054 patients. *J Clin Oncol.* 2001;19:666–675.

Stein R, Fisch M, Beetz R. Urinary diversion in children and young adults using the Mainz Pouch I technique. *Br J Urol.* 1997;79: 354–361.

Steinberg G, Bahnson R, Brosman S, et al. Efficacy and safety of valrubicin for the treatment of Bacillus Calmette-Guerin refractory carcinoma in situ of the bladder. The Valrubicin Study Group. *J Urol.* 2000;163:761–767.

Stenzl A, Burger M, Fradet Y, et al. Hexaminolevulinate guided fluorescence cystoscopy reduces recurrence in patients with nonmuscle invasive bladder cancer. *J Urol.* 2010;184(5):1907–1913. Epub 2010 Sep 17.

Stephens FD. *Congenital Malformations of the Urinary Tract.* New York: Praeger; 1983.

Studer U, Danuser H, Thalmann G, Springer J, Turner W. Antireflux nipples or afferent tubular segments in 70 patients with ileal low pressure bladder substitutes: Long term results of a prospective randomized trial. *J Urol.* 1996;156:1913–1917.

Studer UE, Burkhard FC, Schumacher M, Kessler TM, Thoeny H, Fleischmann A, Thalmann GN. Twenty years experience with an ileal orthotopic low pressure bladder substitute—lessons to be learned. *J Urol.* 2006;176(1):161–166.

Studer UE, Hautmann RE, Hohenfellner M, et al. Indications for continent diversion after cystectomy and factors affecting long-term results. *Urol Oncol.* 1998;4:172–176.

Studer UE, Zingg EJ. Ileal orthotopic bladder substitutes: what we have learned from 12 years experience with 200 patients. *Urol Clin North Am.* 1997;24:781–793.

Sylvester RJ, Oosterlinck W, van der Meijden AP. A single immediate postoperative instillation of chemotherapy decreases the risk of recurrence in patients with stage Ta T1 bladder cancer: a meta-analysis of published results of randomized clinical trials. *J Urol.* 2004;171:2186–2190, quiz 2435.

Sylvester RJ, van der MA, Lamm DL. Intravesical bacillus Calmette-Guerin reduces the risk of progression in patients with superficial bladder cancer: a meta-analysis of the published results of randomized clinical trials. *J Urol.* 2002;168:1964–1970.

Sylvester RJ, van der Meijden A, Witjes JA, et al. High-grade Ta urothelial carcinoma and carcinoma in situ of the bladder. *Urology.* 2005;66:90–107.

Sylvester RJ, van der Meijden AP, Oosterlinck W, et al. Predicting recurrence and progression in individual patients with stage Ta T1 bladder cancer using EORTC risk tables: a combined analysis of 2596 patients from seven EORTC trials. *Eur Urol.* 2006;49: 465–475; discussion 475–477.

Tanagho EA, McAninch JW, eds. *Smith's General Urology.* 14th ed. Norwalk, CT: Appleton & Lange; 1995.

Tchetgen MB, Sanda MG, Montie JE, et al. Collagen injection for the treatment of incontinence after cystectomy and orthotopic neobladder reconstruction in women. *J Urol.* 2000;163:212–214.

Tilki D, Reich O, Svatek RS, et al. Characteristics and outcomes of patients with clinical carcinoma in situ only treated with radical cystectomy: an international study of 243 patients. *J Urol.* 2010;183:1757–1763.

Tolkoff-Rubin NE, Rubin RH. Urinary tract infection in the renal transplant recipient. In: Bergan T, ed. *Urinary Tract Infections.* Basel, Switzerland: Karger; 1997.

Turek PJ, Lipshultz LI. Immunologic infertility. *Urol Clin North Am.* 1994;21:447.

Utz DC, Hanash KA, Farrow GM. The plight of the patient with carcinoma in situ of the bladder. *J Urol.* 1970;103:160–164.

Vaidya A, Soloway MS, Hawke C, et al. De novo muscle invasive bladder cancer: is there a change in trend? *J Urol.* 2001;165:47–50; discussion 50.

Valicenti RK, Gomella LG, Ismail M, et al. Effect of higher radiation dose on biochemical control after radical prostatectomy for PT3N0 prostate cancer. *Int J Rad Oncol Biol Phys.* 1998;42(3):501–506.

van der Meijden AP, Sylvester RJ, Oosterlinck W, et al. Maintenance Bacillus Calmette-Guerin for Ta T1 bladder tumors is not associated with increased toxicity: results from a European Organisation for Research and Treatment of Cancer Genito-Urinary Group Phase III Trial. *Eur Urol.* 2003;44:429–434.

van der Meijden AP, Sylvester RJ, Oosterlinck W, et al. EAU guidelines on the diagnosis and treatment of urothelial carcinoma in situ. *Eur Urol.* 2005;48:363–371.

Varkarakis MJ, Gaeta J, Moore RH, et al. Superficial bladder tumor. Aspects of clinical progression. *Urology.* 1974;4:414–420.

Varol C, Studer UE. Managing patients after an ileal orthotopic bladder substitution. *BJU Int.* 2004;93:266–270.

Vates TS, Steinberg GD. Testicular, sacrococcygeal, and other tumors. In: Vogelzang NJ, Scardino PT, Shipley WU, Coffey DS, eds. *Comprehensive Textbook of Genitourinary Oncology.* Baltimore, MD: Williams and Wilkins; 1996.

Vaughan ED, Blumenfeld JD. The adrenals. In: Walsh PC, Retik AB, Vaughan ED, Wein AJ, eds. Campbell's Urology. 7th ed. Philadelphia, PA: W.B. Saunders; 1998.

Vermeulen CW et al. *J Urol.* 1967;97(7):573–582.

Vieweg J, Gschwend JE, Herr HW, et al. Pelvic lymph node dissection can be curative in patients with node positive bladder cancer. *J Urol.* 1999;161:449–454.

Vogelzang NJ et al., eds. *Comprehensive Textbook of Genitourinary Oncology.* 2nd ed. Philadelphia, PA: Lippincott Williams & Wilkins; 1999.

Vogelzang NJ, Scardino P, Shipley WU, Coffey DS, eds. *Comprehensive Textbook of Genitourinary Oncology.* Baltimore, MD: Williams & Wilkins Press; 1996.

von der Maase H, Hansen SW, Roberts JT, et al. Gemcitabine and cisplatin versus methotrexate, vinblastine, doxorubicin, and cisplatin in advanced or metastatic bladder cancer: results of a large, randomized, multinational, multicenter, phase III study. *J Clin Oncol.* 2000;18(17):3068–3077.

Walsh PC, Retik AB, Vaughn ED Jr, Wein AJ. *Cambell's Urology.* 6th ed. Philadelphia, PA: W.B. Saunders; 1992:1194–1221.

Walsh PC, Retik AB, Vaughan ED Jr, Wein AJ, eds. *Campbell's Urology.* 7th ed. Philadelphia, PA: W.B. Saunders; 1998.

Wein AJ, Broderick GA. Interstitial cystitis: current and future approaches to diagnosis and treatment. *Urol Clin North Am.* 1994;21(1):153.

Weiss RE, Fair WR. Urachal anomalies and urachal carcinoma. In: In: *AUA Update Series.* Lesson 38. Vol. XVII. Houston, TX: American Urological Association; 1998.

Williams JA, Greenwald CA, Rao BK. Wilms' tumor. In: Vogelzang NJ, Scardino PT, Shipley WU, Coffey DS, eds. *Comprehensive Textbook of Genitourinary Oncology.* Baltimore, MD: Williams and Wilkins; 1996.

Williams O, Vereb MJ, Libertino JA. Noncontinent urinary diversion. *Urol Clin North Am.* 1997;24:735–744.

Williamson MR, Smith AY. *Fundamentals of Uroradiology.* Philadelphia, PA: W.B. Saunders; 2000.

Winquist E, Kirchner TS, Segal R, et al. Neoadjuvant chemotherapy for transitional cell carcinoma of the bladder: a systematic review and meta-analysis. *J Urol.* 2004;171:561–569.

Witjes JA. Bladder carcinoma in situ in 2003: state of the art. *Eur Urol.* 2004;45:142–146.

Woodard JR, Smith EA. Prune-Belly syndrome. In: Walsh PC, Retick AB, Vaughan ED, Wein AJ, eds. *Campbell's Urology.* 7th ed. Philadelphia, PA: W.B. Saunders; 1998:1917.

Woodard JR, Zucker I. Current management of the dilated urinary tract in prune belly syndrome. *Urol Clin North Am.* 1990;17:407.

Woods AG, Brandon DH. Prune belly syndrome. *Adv Neonatal Care.* 2007;7(3):132–143.

World Health Organization (WHO) Consensus Conference on Bladder Cancer, 2010.

World Health Organization. A double-blind trial of clomiphene citrate for the treatment of idiopathic male infertility. *Int J Androl.* 1992;15:299.

Wright JL, Hotaling J, Porter MP. Predictors of upper tract urothelial cell carcinoma after primary bladder cancer: a population based analysis. *J Urol.* 2009;181:1035–1039; discussion 1039.

Wu FC, Tajar A, Beynon JM, et al. Identification of late-onset hypogonadism in middle-aged and elderly men. *N Engl J Med.* 2010;363:123–135.

Yeung CK, Sihoe JDY. In: Wein AJ, Kavoussi LR, Novick AC, Partin AW, Peters CA, eds. *Campbell-Walsh Urology.* 9th ed. Philadelphia, PA: W.B. Saunders; 2007:3605–3624.

Yoder BJ, Skacel M, Hedgepeth R, et al. Reflex UroVysion testing of bladder cancer surveillance patients with equivocal or negative urine cytology: a prospective study with focus on the natural history of anticipatory positive findings. *Am J Clin Pathol.* 2007;127(2):295–301.

Yossepowitch O, Dalbagni G, Golijanin D, et al. Orthotopic urinary diversion after cystectomy for bladder cancer: implications for cancer control and patterns of disease recurrence. *J Urol.* 2003 Jan;169(1):177–181.

Young RH. Pathology of carcinomas of the urinary bladder. In: Vogelzang NJ, Scardino PT, Shipley WU, Coffey DS, eds. *Comprehensive Textbook of Genitourinary Oncology.* Philadelphia, PA: Lippincott Williams & Wilkins; 2000.

Yuan JM, Nelson, HH. The epidemiology of bladder cancer. In: Scardino PT, Linehan WM, Zelefsky MJ, Vogelzang NJ, eds. *Comprehensive Textbook of Genitourinary Oncology.* 4th ed. New York: Wolters Kluwer/Lippincott Williams & Wilkins; 2011: 287–294.

Zaak D, Hungerhuber E, Schneede P, et al. Role of 5-aminolevulinic acid in the detection of urothelial premalignant lesions. *Cancer.* 2002;95:1234–1238.

Zehnder P, Studer UE, Skinner EC, et al. Super extended versus extended pelvic lymph node dissection in patients undergoing radical cystectomy for bladder cancer: a comparative study. *J Urol.* 2011;186:1261–1268.

Zhu Y, Jiang X, Zhang J, et al. Safety and efficacy of holmium laser resection for primary nonmuscle-invasive bladder cancer versus transurethral electroresection: single-center experience. *Urology.* 2008;72:608–612.

Zincke H, Utz DC, Farrow GM. Review of Mayo Clinic experience with carcinoma in situ. *Urology.* 1985;26:39–46.

Zuckerman JM, Tisdale B, McCammon K. Advance male sling in irradiated patients with stress urinary incontinence. *Can J Urol.* 2011;18(6):6013–6017.

Zugor V, Schott GF, Labanaris AP. The prune belly syndrome: urological aspects and long-term outcomes of a rare disease. *Pediatr Rep.* 2012;4(2):e20.

INDEX

Page numbers followed by *fig* indicate figures.